PRINCIPLES
OF NEURAL
AGING

少年易老学難成

一寸光陰不可軽

This ancient Chinese proverb attributed to Confucius is a compound of images that tell us about this paradox of aging: 'One becomes rapidly old, but learning is slow; (therefore) never waste a moment.'

The photograph by Chen Anding (entitled 'Blood Relation') reproduced at the opposite page was awarded a 'Grand Prix' at the UNESCO/ACCU World Photo Contest in 1993 for its use of the contrast between the skin of a woman near the end of her time and that of her great-grandchild to hint at a bright family future.

Together, the ancient proverb and the photograph from China convey our feeling about the value of the human efforts to understand aging and the nature of the risk that aging may eventually overwhelm our most precious faculties - those conferred by our brain.

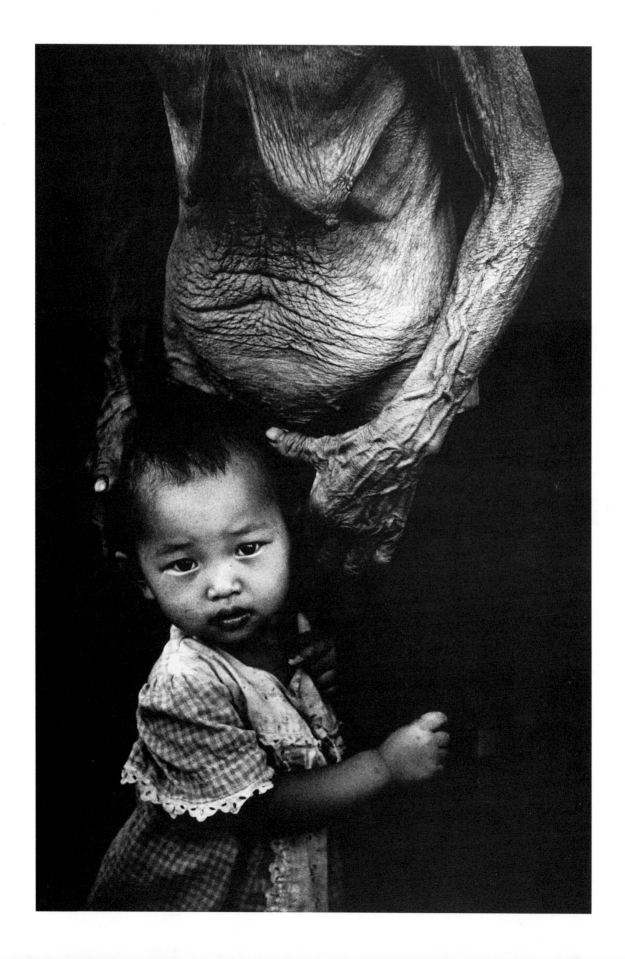

It is a natural tendency of the mind to come to and remain at a complete standstill. This is a principle of Newtonian stature. Prolonged disuse of the brain is also bad for you. Try therefore to think or converse about something other … than your own piteous plight.

Peter Medawar

Medawar, P. *Son of Stroke.* World Medicine, 18 Oct. 1972.

PRINCIPLES OF NEURAL AGING

Edited by

SERGIO U. DANI
AKIRA HORI
GERHARD F. WALTER

Institute for Neuropathology of the
Hannover Medical School, Germany

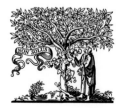

1997

ELSEVIER

Amsterdam • Lausanne • New York • Oxford • Shannon • Singapore • Tokyo

Elsevier Science B.V.
P.O. Box 211, 1000 AE Amsterdam, The Netherlands

© 1997 Elsevier Science B.V.
All rights reserved

ISBN 0 444 82329 8

Cover: A pyramidal neuron in the human parahippocampal gyrus. The soma of this neuron is completely filled with neurofibrillary tangles, stained by colloidal silver impregnation. Prepared and photographed by S.U. Dani. Cover design by Studio Jan de Boer BNO.

We dedicate this book to our families,
and to our contributors from many parts
of the World.

Contents in Brief

Section IV
Neural Aging, From Perception to Behavior

Contents

xiv   Contents

Preface

The ultimate goal of neurogerontology is to understand the principles governing the longevity and loss of maintenance capacity of nervous systems, including that one biological structure we always marvel at, not less for its astonishing complexity, than because it is what makes us humans: our brain.

The ways to accomplish that immense goal are being patiently and resolutively led; they are not straight, nor have they been paved in many tracks, but much ground has definitely been covered, mainly in the basic principles of gerontology. In its early years, gerontology was mainly concerned with descriptive and correlative approaches. Now a major paradigm shift to experimental designs has occurred. Whereas we come to this realization, we also realize that, if progress has been achieved, it is because gerontology is not an independent field, but a synthesis of distinct branches of knowledge. Looking back at the history of modern biology, we come to the conclusion that when disciplines are maintained apart from each other, less progress is attained. It is thus no wonder that an astonishing progress has been achieved with molecular biology, whose interdisciplinary nature is an extremely important element. Then, it is time for researchers in the field of neural aging to become aware of this fact of life: If an ultimate understanding of the longevity and aging of the human brain is to be hoped, it is likely to come through interdisciplinarity.

Relevant for the study of neural aging are a number of distinct disciplines, from the obvious evolutionary biology, genetics, biochemistry, biophysics, embryology, neurology, pathology and toxicology, to the less obvious but not less important paleontology, ecology, and the social sciences, to name some. We tried to capture some of these disciplines here in such an interdisciplinary and synthetic way that could fit, on the one hand, the needs of a critical review and, on the other hand, the aims of an introductory course on the biology of neural aging.

To that aim we found it appropriate to divide this volume into four sections. Section I, *General Theory of Aging*, introduces the problem of aging in general, and aging of the nervous system in particular, in biophysical and biochemical perspectives. Section II, *Ontogeny, Evolution and Neural Aging*, addresses evolutionary and ontogenetical topics to some depth. Section III, *Tissue and Cellular Changes*, presents the issue of neural aging, starting from the early neurogenetic events which are responsible to mold the adult brain, and terminating with a description of histological and metabolic changes in the aging human brain. Finally, Section IV, *Neural Aging, From Perception to Behavior*, discusses, in brief, the importance of some age related changes to our capacity to perceive and interact with the environment. At the end of each chapter there is a list of selected readings followed by the reference list.

We are convinced that, in many as yet partly understood ways, the brain regulates the rates of longevity and aging. Although new relevant data are coming out every week in dozens of specialized journals, a great deal of the knowledge on the aging human brain is still elusive, and the field is open for major contributions. It is therefore possible that some of the considerations put forward in many chapters may sound speculative. However, speculations reflect the stand of our knowledge, and seem to be justified in view of the fact that, with the progressive aging of the world population, there is an absolute need for a better understanding of the causes of longevity and the means to promote it. Therefore, we hope the hypotheses will stimulate research and thus be useful for those who intend to initiate or proceed in the fascinating field of neural aging. We strongly encourage the readers to contribute critiques.

Sergio U. Dani
Akira Hori
Gerhard F. Walter

Acknowledgements

A book by authors of different parts of the world reflects the worldwide determination to understand our common nature, and to improve upon it. We were fortunate to have recruited renowned colleagues from the Americas, Europe, Africa and Asia who friendly and in such a distinguished manner have contributed chapters for this book. It is therefore a great pleasure to express our indebtedness to all of them.

We are grateful to the following friends and colleagues who have made constructive comments or suggestions on matters pertaining to chapters: Mike Cahill, Caleb Finch, Mizuki Hara, Yasuo Ihara, Alfred Nordheim, Manuel Graeber, Michael Rose, and José E. H. Pittella.

We are also indebted to Hannelore Rylands, Marcus Vinicius S. Maciel, Ronaldo Lazzarotti, and Aderivaldo S. Santos, for their help with the preparation of artwork, to Renato U. Dani, for assistance in computer matters, and to Eliane L. Ribeiro, for secretarial assistance.

During the last four years, we benefitted greatly from the support of the following institutions, whose help was instrumental for the execution of this book: CAPES-Fundação Coordenação de Aperfeiçoamento de Pessoal de Nível Superior, Fundação Acangaú, and FAPESP-Fundação de Amparo à Pesquisa do Estado de São Paulo, Brazil; Gesellschaft der Freunde der Medizinischen Hochschule Hannover, and DAAD-Deutscher Akademischer Austauschdienst, Germany; Monbusho-Japanese Ministry for Education, and JSPS-Japan Society for the Promotion of Science. UNESCO-ACCU, in the person of Akiko Narita, helped us with the picture by Chen Anding which opens this volume.

Finally, we are obliged to Nello J. Spiteri, M. Tanke, Cathalijne van Doorne and Ruud de Boer of Elsevier, for their participation in producing this book.

Contributors

Abass Alavi, M.D.
Division of Nuclear Medicine
University of Pennsylvania School of Medicine, USA

Hartmut Becker, M.D.
Department of Neuroradiology, Hannover Medical School,
Germany

Fabio Blandini, M.D.
Neurological Institute C. Mondino, University of Pavia, Italy

Irina N. Bogolepova, M.D.
Institute of Brain Research of the Russian Academy of Sciences,
Moscow, Russia

Jürgen Bohl, M.D.
Institute of Neuropathology of the University of Mainz,
Germany

Ashley I. Bush, M.D., Ph.D.
Laboratory of Genetics and Aging, Massachusetts General
Hospital, Harvard University, USA

Sergio U. Dani, M.D., D.Sc.
Institute for Neuropathology, Hannover Medical School,
Germany, and
Ludwig Institute for Cancer Research, São Paulo, Brazil

Setsuya Fujita, M.D., Ph.D.
Kyoto Pasteur Institute, Japan

Bernd Gallhofer, M.D.
Psychiatry Clinic, University of Gießen, Germany

Joseph L. Graves, Jr., Ph.D.
Department of Life Sciences, Arizona State University West,
Phoenix, USA

John Timothy Greenamyre, M.D., Ph.D.
Department of Neurology, Emory University School of
Medicine, Atlanta, USA

Herbert W. Haug, M.D.
Institute of Anatomy, University of Lübeck, Germany

Jean-Jacques Hauw, M.D.
Laboratory of Neuropathology Ramon Escourolle, University of
Paris, France

Akira Hori, M.D.
Institute for Neuropathology, Hannover Medical School,
Germany

Kenji Ikeda, M.D.
Tokyo Institute of Psychiatry, Japan

Rafael Linden, M.D., D.Sc.
Department of Neurobiology, Carlos Chagas Filho Institute of
Biophysics, Federal University of Rio de Janeiro, Brazil

Alvaro Macieira-Coelho, M.D., D.Sc., D.h.c.
INSERM, Versailles, France

Thierry Maisonobe, M.D.
Laboratory of Neuropathology Ramon Escourolle, University of
Paris, France

Carl R. Merril, PhD.
Laboratory of Biochemical Genetics, NIMH, Bethesda, USA

Andreas Meyer-Lindenberg, M.D.
Psychiatry Clinic, University of Gießen, Germany

Fabiola Müller, Dr. habil. rer. nat.
University of California School of Medicine
Davis, California, USA

Andrew B. Newberg, M.D.
Division of Nuclear Medicine
University of Pennsylvania School of Medicine, USA

Ronan O'Rahilly, M.D., D.Sc., Dr.h.c.
University of California School of Medicine
Davis, California, USA
and Institut d'Anatomie et d'Embryologie Spéciale
Université de Fribourg, Fribourg, Switzerland

José Eymard H. Pittella, M.D.
Department of Pathological Anatomy and Forensic Medicine,
Federal University of Minas Gerais, Brazil

Davide Schiffer, M.D.
Neurological Clinic, University of Turin, Italy

Andrew J. G. Simpson, Ph.D.
Ludwig Institute for Cancer Research, São Paulo, Brazil

Romeu R. de Souza, M.D.
Department of Anatomy, University of São Paulo, Brazil

Rudolph Tanzi, M.D., Ph.D.
Laboratory of Genetics and Aging, Massachusetts General
Hospital, Harvard University, USA

Cristina Tassorelli, M.D.
Neurological Institute C. Mondino, University of Pavia, Italy

Phillip V. Tobias, D.Sc., Ph.D., M.B.B.Ch., FRCP,
OMSG, Sc.D. h.c., D.Sc. h.c.
Palaeo-Anthropology Research Unit, University of
Witwatersrand Medical School, Johannesburg, South Africa

Gerhard F. Walter, M.D., Ph.D.
Institute for Neuropathology, Hannover Medical School,
Germany

Kazuaki Yoshikawa, M.D.
Institute for Protein Research, Osaka University, Japan

Steve Zullo, Ph.D.
Laboratory of Biochemical Genetics, NIMH, Bethesda, USA

PRINCIPLES OF NEURAL AGING

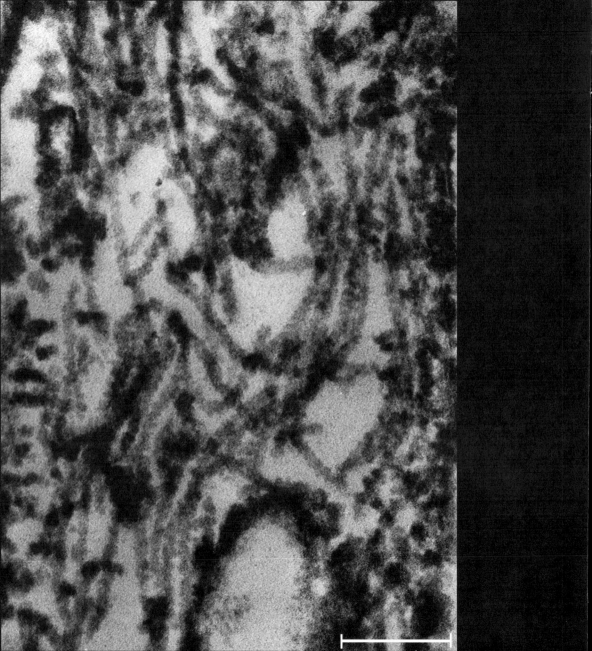

I

General Theories of Aging

Formation of amyloid fibril-like structure within the cells over-expressing a carboxyl-terminal fragment of APP. A complementary DNA (cDNA) encoding carboxyl (C)-terminal 100 amino acid residues of APP was transfected into cultured monkey kidney cells (COS-1). The cells overexpressing the C-terminal sequence of APP were selected by immunostaining with an anti-body against the C-terminus of APP. An ultra-thin section of the cell having the intense inclusion-like deposit was stained with lead citrate and uranyl acetate, and observed under a transmission electron microscope. Note the accumulation of single helical fibers, which resemble Aβ amyloid fibrils. Scale bar: 200 nm. Photomicrograph by K. Yoshikawa.

PART I – General Theories of Aging

Chapter 1:   **Mechanisms of Aging: A Survey**
Chapter 2:   **Biophysical Principles of Aging**
Chapter 3:   **Mutation, Evolution and Aging**
Chapter 4:   **General Theories of Aging:**
                        Unification and Synthesis

Sergio U. Dani

Mechanisms of Aging: A Survey

Aristotle, in his book entitled *De Longitudine et Brevitate Vitae*, originally posed the fundamental problem of Biogerontology as 'it is not clear whether in animals and plants universally it is a single or diverse cause that makes some to be long-lived, others short-lived.' While aging apparently remains as one of the least understood biological phenomena, a number of theories on the mechanisms of biological aging have been proposed in this century based on an ever growing set of mainly correlative data. Although much of the theories have limited value as 'theories of aging', they opened the way to experimental Biogerontology. In the first three chapters of this book, we shall present the main so-called mechanistic theories, as a basis for a better understanding of the pathobiology of neural aging. Chapter 4 is a unification and synthesis of the main theories, in light of the evolutionary theory of aging.

In Search of a Lexicon

As in every branch of science, also in gerontology, or the biology of aging, there is a need for a lexicon. However, the reader should be cautioned that terminology not always describes accurately complex phenomena such as aging. Some terms can be even misleading, specially in fields where important scientific evidence is still lacking. The most accepted definition of aging, which is also the one used throughout this book is that of Comfort (1979). He defined aging as a progressive increase throughout life, or after a given stadium, in the likelihood that a given individual will die, during the next succeding unit of time, from randomly distributed causes. In Comfort's view, this happens as a result of a *progressive loss of physiological functions* that culminates in death.

The progressive loss of physiological functions that occurs with aging has been termed *senescence*. The force acting to prevent or delay the onset of senescence, is sometimes referred to as *longevity*, or less commonly, vitauct (Latin *vita*, life + *auctum*, enhancement). The aged phenotype would then arise as the result of a concerted action of senescence and longevity. A corollary to Comfort's view is that putative age-specific fitness components (longevity) are overwhelmed by the progressive internal physiological deterioration (senescence) to cause the individual to grow older. The balance between senescence and longevity mechanisms may be viewed as the basis of the great variability of aging, giving rise to a classification that takes not only chronological parameters into account, but also the maintenance status of the individual.

Longevity and Life Span

At the outset, a distinction must be made between the two related concepts, *longevity* and *life span*. Life span is simply the life time of an organism, measured in hours, days, months or years. Longevity is the age-related resistance to failure, in other words, the maintenance capacity of an organism, measured by physiologic parameters such

as muscular strength and physical activity, or the incidence of pathologic markers such as cancer, neurodegeneration, etc. Life span is not necessarily a measure of longevity: whereas in the wild, life span usually corresponds to longevity for a great number of organisms, in domestication life span usually surpasses longevity.

However, *maximum life span* (MLS) is usually employed as a measure of longevity in a given taxon, because it is readily measurable in units of time, and also because it serves as a reference value. While MLS, or the maximum age at death observed in a given taxon, is an index which can be easily obtained from records of animals living in captivity, the assessment of longevity, or the age-specific resistance to metabolic failure, is a more complex issue. Data on MLS are useful as an indirect estimate of longevity, but they can tell us only part of the story.

Observing the Phenomenon

The phenomenon of aging can be best observed in organisms presenting a life-history: birth, development, maturation and death, being hardly detected in less specialized organisms, or in organisms placed at lower evolutive steps, such as some coelenterates. Strehler (1977) distinguished three categories of organisms: '(i) those which clearly never have an opportunity to age because they divide and yield two new growing organisms before aging processes can produce change; (ii) those which clearly do age, primarily because they do no replace damaged or lost parts at a rate sufficient to compensate for the assaults of time and environment; and (iii) a class of organisms which fail to show aging as a whole because of a continual replacement regimen, even though there is an attrition of their constituent parts, either, for example, molecules or subcellular organelles in the case of single-celled organisms or even large groups of cells in multicellular organisms'.

The predominant cause of death is species specific, being defined by a composite of environmental factors and genetic background. Causative agents which are internal and external to the individual may participate in determining the rate of aging. A dramatic example is the 'postponement' of aging in laboratory rodents through nutritional restriction (Masoro, 1988). It has been put forward that longer-lived nutrition-restricted rodents were, in fact, healthy controls of laboratory animals that usually receive larger nutritional intake than they would usually have, if living in the wild. Aging is thus characterized for its determinism, provided that each individual is somehow programmed to age, according to well defined stages for his own species (Table 1-1). It is also characteristic of aging that it is a multifactorial process, inasmuch as the original programmation can be influenced in variable degree by the environment which surrounds the individual. In a general multilevel scheme, the hypotheses on the possible mechanisms involved in biological aging can be classified at the population genetic (evolutionary), the or-

TABLE 1–1.   Mean maximum recorded life spans for various metazoan

Phylum	Species (class)	Mean maximum recorded life spans (in years)
Rotifera	*Rotaria macrura*	0.16
Porifera	*Suberites carnosus*	15
Echinodermata	*Marthasterias glacialis*	7+
Coelenterata	*Cereus pedunculatus*	85-90
Mollusca	*Venus mercenaria*	40+
	Megalonaias gigantea	54
Helminthes	*Wuchereria bancrofti*	17
	Taeniorrhynchus saginatus	35+
Annelida	*Sabella pavonia*	10+
Arthropoda	*Periplaneta americana* L.(insecta)	1.1
	Tarantula (arachnida)	11-20
	Stenamma westwoodi (hymenoptera)	16-18
	Homarus americana (crustacea)	50
Chordata	*Poecillia reticulata* (osteictes)	3
	Mus musculus (mammalia)	3.5
	Canis familiaris (mammalia)	12+
	Thraupis sayaca (aves)	25+
	Bos indicus (mammalia)	27+
	Gallus domesticus (aves)	30
	Equus cabalus (mammalia)	25-35
	Rhea americana (aves)	40+
	Megalobatrachus (amphibia)	52+
	Silurus glanis (osteictes)	60+
	Bubo bubo (aves)	68+
	Homo sapiens (mammalia)	118+
	Testudo sumeiri (reptilia)	152+
	Galapagos turtoise (reptilia)	175+

(after several sources; most evidence compiled from Strehler, 1977).

ganismal or physiological, the cellular and the molecular aspects.

Population (Evolutionary) Level

The Gompertz Equation

The survival of well-nourished and protected populations of several mammalian species, including *Homo sapiens*, can be described by an equation formulated by British actuary Benjamin Gompertz in 1825. The Gompertz equation has the property that the logarithmic derivative of the survival (S) increases exponentially with age (t). This is equivalent to the statement for a real population that its age-specific death rate $\mu(t)$ increases exponentially (Figure 1–1).

May Aging be Selected For or Against?

Most current evolutionary biologists do not accept that aging could be selected for or against in natural populations of animals, since death by disease, accidents, and predation occurs long before organisms become senescent. However, there are examples which show that longevity may have significance for evolutionary fitness. There are hospitable environmental conditions allowing individuals to grow old which include absence of decimation by pre-

dators. Conversely, a participation of predators or other agents may be important in establishing an evolutionary pressure on the species' life span. The species-specific environment must be considered in the evaluation of possible selective or non-selective forces impinging on a particular species' life span. For example, there are annual life cycle fishes of the family Cyprinodontidae in regions of Africa marked by seasonality. These fishes are born during the wet season and must attain reproductive maturity just before the dry season, when they mate, lay their eggs and die. The eggs remain desiccated until the next wet season comes, when the cycle reinitiates. The life span of these fishes must have been selected in a way that only the most precocious and consequently short-lived specimens could reproduce before they die in the drought.

There appears to be support for the hypothesis that longevity evolved by selection of positive longevity-assurance systems. While senescence would have evolved as the result of the accumulation of deleterious genes, longevity would have evolved as the result of the accumulation of genetic systems that govern positive enzymatic mechanisms for the protection, regulation and repair of the longevity-assurance systems at all levels of organization (Sacher, 1978). Alternative views have been proposed (Dykhuisen, 1974; Sager, 1991), in which an evolutionary advantage of senescence is to suppress tumorigenesis,

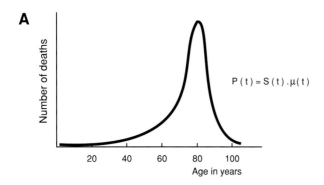

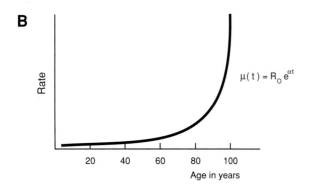

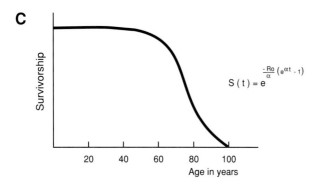

FIGURE   1-1

Three forms of the Gompertz equation to describe mortality in a given human population.

A. P(t) is the number of deaths in a given interval at age t.

B. μ(t) is the age-specific death rate. The parameter R_0, the death rate extrapolated back to birth, is an estimate of initial vulnerability of the population to the causes of senescent death in adults, in other words, it measures the vulnerability of the population before the onset of aging; the parameter α, the rate of increase of the death rate, is a measure of the actuarial aging rate. Note that the the age-specific death rate μ(t) for the population increases exponentially.

C. S(t) is the number of individuals living at age t.

thereby allowing young organisms to survive to reproductive years. This view is however controversial. Rose (1991) envisages that 'aging may be as physiologically diverse as other whole-organism attributes, if not more so, because it is produced by evolutionary forces acting on the full range of genetic variability present in each species'. This evolutionary approach suggests further that there are no ineluctable physiological causes of aging, but a failure of natural selection to 'pay attention' to the problem.

Organismal (Physiological) Level

Wear and Tear: Aging is Submitted to the Second Law of Thermodynamics

Wear and tear must affect all machinery in a world subjected to the Second Law of Thermodynamics. For example, horses and kangoroos die due to starvation after their teeth have worn down. The capacity that some organisms have to repair damage seems not to be a problem to this theory, since all living things, including their repair mechanisms, are susceptible to damage, in varying degree.

Rate-of-Living

It is generally known that animals with small body size have higher metabolic rate per unit of body mass and shorter life spans as compared to large animals. According to the view defended in 1928 by Pearl, the lenght of life depends inversely on the rate of living; in other words, on the metabolic rate. Although metabolic rate per unit of body mass varies greatly from animal to animal across and within species, there is a remarkable constancy of the daily expenditure of energy (Kcal) expressed per metabolic mass, i.e., body weight (g) raised to the 0.75 power, when animals are permitted to eat freely. The ratio is approximately 70, and the relationship is sometimes called *Kleiber's rule* (Figure 1-2). Since some of the experiments supporting this theory have been conducted at extreme temperature ranges required to experimentally accelerate metabolism, it remains elusive whether thermal injury might have not been involved in reducing life span. Moreover, exercise in rats seems to have no effect on life span (Holloszy and Smith, 1987). Reproductive exhaustion, however, seems to play an important part in reducing life span. For example, captive salmons that are castrated live as much as 18 years longer than those that are not (Robertson, 1961), and virgin *Drosophila* females live longer than those that are mated (Maynard Smith, 1958; Partdrige, 1986).

Nutrition Alters the Rate of Organismal Development, Aging and Onset of Diseases

Simple nutrient depletion critically alters the rate of organismal aging. In an extreme situation, some adult insects of the orders Ephemeroptera and Lepidoptera lack or have atrophied mouthparts. Contrarily to juvenile forms, that live in average 2-3 years in aquatic environment, the adult forms of Ephemeroptera live just a couple of hours, or a few days or weeks, in the long-lived species. They apparently don't take solid food, imbibing only water in their short lives, and dying probably due to starvation (Figure 1-3).

On the other hand, if the supply of food during laboratory rearing is restricted in a balanced manner, then life span is prolonged in a wide range of invertebrates, and in some mammalian species (Finch, 1991). Nutritionally balanced diet restriction also reduces and delays many age-related diseases (Weindruch and Walford, 1988, for reviews). Some cases of life span prolongation do not result from prolonged adult life; instead, prolongation of juvenile development may be involved.

Allometrical Relations

Some organisms pose some difficulty to the assessment of aging, or are indeed free from aging, because they do not stop growing, like nonsenescent protozoa, sea anemones and sponges. Multicellular organisms with indefinite growth like giant trees, however, do grow senescent. While some species may not age, these are cases in which the germ- and somatic-cell lineages are not fully distinct.

In 1932, Bidder proposed that a mechanism may exist to stop natural body growth after specific body size has been reached. He called it regulator. In Bidder's view, senescence would be the result of the continued action of the regulator after the growth is stopped. Studying total life spans in a sample of 63 mammal species, Sacher (1959) found that maximum life span is allometrically related to adult brain weight and body weight, in other words, there appears to be a linear relationship of the logarithm of life span to the logarithm of brain weight and of body weight. In most groups of mammals, there appears to be an overall evolutionary trend toward increase in body size and brain size, and decrease of reproductive rate.

Autoimmune Malfunction

The immune system of vertebrates undergoes a process of somatic recombination and mutation as an integral part of the production of antibodies (Baltimore, 1981; Hood, Weissman and Wood, 1982; Tonegawa 1983). The level of autoantibodies tends to increase with age in man, which may play some role in the onset of senescence. However, the lack of etiological relationships between autoantibodies and aging in man and mouse suggests that autoimmune pathology cannot be considered the primary cause of normal vertebrate aging. But this in no way rules out the contributory role of autoimmune pathology in aging. The process of somatic recombination and mutation in cells of the immune system provide additional rationales to explain the aging process of these cells.

Aging May be a Result of Global Feedforward Failure in a Real System that has Too Many Degrees of Freedom

Aging is the result of mechanisms acting at the highest levels of organismal integration, with consequences that are expressed in diverse ways in the wide array of tissues and structures making up complex organisms such as metazoa or metaphyta. Changes in hepatic, kidney, and en-

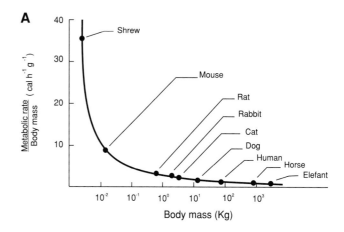

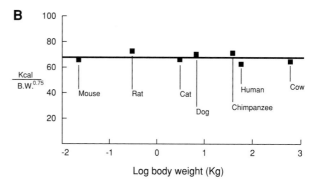

FIGURE 1–2

Body weight and daily energy expenditure of various species of mammals. (Adapted from Kleiber, 1947; compare with life spans listed in Table 1-1).

A. Metabolic rate per gram of body increases exponentially with decreasing body mass. The smaller extant mammals are the shrews, with approximately 4 g body weight. Their metabolic rate per gram is so high, that they have to intake a daily amount of food which almost equals their body mass to remain alive.

B. Daily energy expenditure, when expressed per metabolic body size (body weight$^{0.75}$) is relatively constant over a wide range of body size. This relationship is sometimes called Kleiber's rule.

docrine functions might well interact with age changes in brain mineral metabolism and other functions. Loss of feedforward control may occur throughout aging, that may be not a result of a complete failure to function. Rather, it is a result of the necessary imperfections of any feedforward control system for real systems that have too many degrees of freedom (Rosen, 1978).

Cellular Level

Non-Neoplastic Cells Have Limited Life Spans in Culture

Leonard Hayflick, working in the early 60's first demonstrated that limited life span in culture is a hallmark of di-

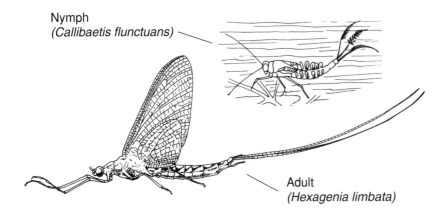

Nymph
(Callibaetis flunctuans)

Adult
(Hexagenia limbata)

FIGURE   1–3
Mayflies (Insecta, Ephemeroptera), adapted from Ross, Ross and Ross, 1982. A juvenile form or nymph (*Callibaetis flunctuans*) and an adult form (*Hexagenia limbata*) from two species are represented. Mayflies, together with chironomids (midges), are the two most important insect groups from the standpoint of fish food in many continental waters.

ploid human fibroblasts. These cells exhibit a limited number of proliferation 'passages' in culture that seems to be proportional to life spans in each of many species of metazoa, and also depends on the histological tissue-type and age. This limited passage number, also referred to as the *Hayflick limit* seems to be also regulated by a range of hormonal factors, such as growth factors and insulin (Philips and Cristofalo, 1983). Cells in the end of their life span become arrested in G_0 phase of the cell cycle, but can be artificially arrested in the G_0/G_1 (for example, by serum starvation: Celis *et al.*, 1990). The crucial parameter in cellular aging is not the chronological time in culture, but the number of cell divisions completed (Smith and Lincoln 1984; Hayflick, 1991). It is generally believed that the late passage senescent cells also have a decreased rate of protein synthesis. It is now clear that the same principle applies for a number of different cell types, in a wide variety of species (Smith and Lincoln, 1984; Dice, 1993). The exception are some stem cell lines and certain cancer cells.

Loss of Maintenance Capacity Accompanies Cell Differentiation

Pearl put forward in 1922 that all the essential tissues of the metazoan body are immortal. He sustained that what brings about death is the differentiation and specialization of function of the mutually dependent aggregate of cells and tissues which constitute the metazoan body, and not any inherent or inevitable mortal process in the individual cells themselves. These assertions must be taken with caution. On the one hand, there is evidence that the pattern of gene expression changes with differentiation. For instance, the total amount of facultative heterochromatin is very different in different cell types: embryonic cells seem to have little, whereas some highly specialized cells have a great deal (Chapter 5). This fact indicates that, as cells develop, progressively more genes can be packaged in a condensed form in which they are no longer accessible to gene activator proteins. In addition, whereas it has been possible to maintain tumorous cells indefinitely in culture media, for the time being, no laboratory has discovered a medium for *in vitro* cell cul-

ture that allows indefinite proliferation of diploid cells having normal histological features. Nonetheless, people working intensively with transformed cell lineages in culture are aware of aging changes that sometimes affect these relatively undifferentiated lineages. It is possible that even such cells undergo a process of natural selection and evolution *in vitro*, in the sense that less differentiated and proliferating mutants prevail over the remainder, say, aged cells. The relationship between aging and evolution will be discussed to more depth in the next chapters.

Molecular Level

Codon-Restriction and Age Specificity of Gene Action

The codon-restriction theory, which might be regarded as a corollary of the differentiation and loss of maintenance capacity approach, has been put forward by Bernard Strehler and his colleagues, in the early 70's. According to this theory, a random loss of various isoaccepting tRNAs (of more than 60 types) will progressively restrict the readability of codons resulting in the inefficiency and inaccuracy of protein synthesis.

In Strehler's view, aging would occur as a result of molecular damage to the coded form of the cell's goal, resulting in mistaken redirection of the cell towards loss of specific function. As every constituent of a differentiated cell has its own repair system, aging of differentiated cells could then be a result of the autonomous deterioration of the macromolecules making up such repair structures. The model presumes that 'different cell types possess restricted codon-decoding properties and that these capacities are precisely those required to translate a restricted group of messages - namely, those 'needed' by a cell at a particular time in its ontogeny' (Strehler, 1977). Thus, changes in the pattern of isoaccepting tRNAs and tRNA synthetases may be linked to development and aging. In the view of Strehler and colleagues, aging is part of a larger developmental sequence. Just as some genes control embryonic development, other genes program aging processes in the organism; and the changes of old age might result from the normal expression of a genetic program that begins at conception and ends in death.

The notion of age specificity of gene action provides some useful physiological details to the hypothesis called *antagonistic pleiotropy* (Greek *pleion*, more + *tropos*, tendency = the tendency of an inherited disposition to influence or affect several parts or functions of the organism) or *abiotropic gene action* (*a*, privation; bios, life; *tropos*, tendency), which proposes that some genes would have a benign or innocuous expression during early life, and then acquire another injurious expression at a later life stage, despite that there is no apparent trend to increasingly common genetic disorders with age. Indeed, while there are quite a number of well-characterized human genetic pathologies that arise congenitally or by early adulthood (hemophilia, phenylketonuria, progeria, Tay-sachs, etc), there are only a few that are known to have late onset, Huntington chorea, idiopathic hemochromatosis (Martin, 1978; Albin, 1988), and some cases of Alzheimer disease (Chapter 28) being examples (Roses, 1993). *Fatal familial insomnia*, once believed to belong to this group of late onset congenital diseases, is now known to be a prion disease (Chapter 7).

There is some evidence that a shift in the pattern of isoaccepting tRNAs occurs during development and aging in some plants, nematodes, insects and rat liver and skeletal muscle, but there is no general pattern that emerges from these studies, and the reported changes vary significantly among different species. More recently Jeffrey Powell, a disciple of Dobzansky, studying *Drosophila* evolutionary molecular genetics has collected evidence that some *Drosophila* genes display a *codon usage bias*, i.e., for a given aminoacid in the protein sequence, some of the possible codons are preferred and some are not used at all. The phenomenon is refined further since codon usage bias may vary inversely with the length of the message, i.e., small genes appear to display more codon usage bias than large genes. Thus, codon restriction and codon usage bias may have important repercussions on aging.

Aged Cells are Less Sensitive to Hormones

Probably because hormones are the best understood substances that effect gene control in multicellular organism, a proposal has been made that aging is endocrinally mediated, i.e., mediated by the active action of hormones. Unfortunately, this hypothesis cannot withstand some experimental testing. Simple administration of gonadal hormones, for instance, cannot be used to restore vertebrate fertility directly (Wise, 1983), probably reflecting exhaustion of the oocytes. On the other hand, a reduced sensitivity to a variety of growth factors and hormones is usually found during aging (Carlin *et al.*, 1983; Harley, Goldstein and Posner, 1981; Plisko and Gilchrest, 1983). Age-dependent reduction in the number of receptors has been reported in some cases, but it has also been admitted that additional age-related dysfunctions occur in some post-receptor signal transduction pathways (McCormick and Campisi, 1991).

Naturally Occurring Xenobiotics and Somatic Mutations Alter Cell Life Spans

Toxins or xenobiotics of either chemical (e.g. free-radicals), or biological (e.g. infectious disease, virus, prions) origin, and also physical agents (e.g. temperature, radiation), might act to damage cells and diminish their life spans, presumably by leading to somatic mutations, and also possibly by changing the patterns of gene expression (Figure 1–4). Free radicals and some reactive oxygen species are continuously produced in the living organism. For instance, hydroxyl radicals are produced in living organisms by radiation-dependent splitting of water. As a result, the organisms have evolved not only antioxidant defense systems, but also repair systems that prevent accumulation of oxidatively damaged molecules. Antioxidant defense capacity of the cell is integrated by enzymes

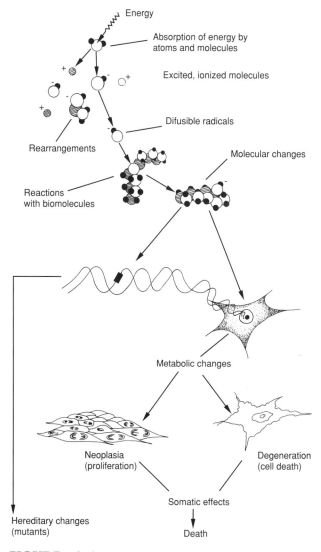

FIGURE 1–4

Free radicals cause molecular changes that, if not repaired, may lead to genetic and metabolic changes characteristic of aging.

such as superoxide dismutase, catalase and glutathione peroxidase, as well as vitamin E and glutathione. Although free radicals, including some reactive oxygen species, are frequently proposed to be involved in the pathology of several tissue injuries in most, if not all, diseases (Halliwell, 1992), it must be considered that free radicals may also have some important role in physiological processes. Therefore it remains to be proved whether the age-related increase in somatic mutations results from an increased level of damaging agents or decreased abilities of senescent cells to repair DNA (Hart and Setlow, 1974; Rattan, 1989; Kirkwood, 1989). For example, damaging effects of oxygen free radicals on nucleic acids, proteins, and lipids may be caused by increased production of oxidatively damaged macromolecules due to an age-related decrease in activity of protective enzymes such as superoxide dismutase and catalase. Support for this hypothesis includes the observations that (i) overexpression of antioxidative enzymes retards the age-related accrual of oxidative damage and extends the maximum life span of transgenic *Drosophila*; (ii) variations in longevity among different species inversely correlate with the rates of mitochondrial generation of the *superoxide anion radical* and *hydrogen peroxide*, and (iii) restriction of caloric intake lowers steady-state levels of oxidative stress and damage, retards age-associated changes, and extends the maximum life span in mammals (reviewed in Sohal and Weindruch, 1996).

Somatic mutations include gene mutations, chromosomal abnormalities, aneuploidies, mitotic recombinations, gene conversions, and gene amplifications, which could play a role in the induction, promotion and progression of aging and a number of diseases. A variety of chromosomal abnormalities (Crowley and Curtis, 1963, Hayflick, 1975, Rattan, 1989, Kirkwood, 1989) and mitochondrial DNA anomalies (Wallace, 1992) are increased in senescent tissues from aged organisms and in cell cultures. Some short-lived mouse strains accumulate chromosomal abnormalities faster than related long-lived strains (Crowley and Curtis, 1963). Human somatic cell cultures, in particular, show great stability of karyotype and proliferative limitation, quite unlike rodent cells (Hayflick, 1977). Hall and colleagues (1984) found that UV-induced DNA repair in primate lymphocytes positively correlates with maximum species life span. Maslansky and Williams (1985) found positive correlations between unscheduled DNA repair and species longevity at low, but not high doses of UV-radiation. An instructive example is the age-related decline in telomerase activity due to expression of a different isozyme or due to its reduced turnover rate with subsequent accumulation of damaging posttranslational modifications in the molecule. This could give rise to shortening of chromosome telomeres (Dice, 1993), with consequences for cellular aging (Harley, Futcher and Greider, 1990). Further aspects of somatic mutations during aging are discussed as follows and in the next chapter.

Changes in DNA During Replication are Rare but Genetic Recombinations Give Rise to Accumulation of Errors with Surprising Frequency

The process of DNA duplication is rather complex but its basic principle is quite simple: the enzyme called DNA helicase controls the unwindling of the double stranded DNA molecule, and DNA polymerase catalyzes the synthesis of new duplicate strands made in a 5' to 3' direction. In the case of the human genome, an exact copy of 6 billion base pairs must be accomplished within 6-12 hours (Ross, 1992). The original single DNA molecule of the genome present in the fertilized zygote at the moment of conception must be copied some 1,015 times during the subsequent course of a human lifetime. One measured error rate in direct copying DNA has been estimated as 0.01 percent or one incorrect base in every 10^4 base pairs. There are systems that maintain the precision of DNA replication such as (i) a proofreading system which checks the tentative match between the template strand and the newly synthesized duplicate strand; (ii) systems that detect chemical modification such as methylation of bases. These systems greatly improve the error rate in DNA replication, so that the final error rate is estimated to be one in 10^8 base pairs (*ibidem*). Other estimates envisage that only about one nucleotide pair in a thousand is randomly changed every 200,000 years (Alberts *et al.*, 1989).

Genetic recombinations, however, cause major rearrangements of the genome with surprising frequency: the genome can expand or contract by duplication or deletion, and its parts can be transposed from one region to another to create new combinations. Although defects in the genome (Gensler and Bernstein, 1981) and in repair systems (Hart and Setlow, 1974) have been reported during aging (particular during aging of mitotic cells), there seems to be no major genome defects which may be responsible for the progressive aging of cells (Rattan, 1989). Instead of random accumulation of DNA errors because of damage and insults that occur with time, most evidence indicates that changes in gene activity during aging, when they occur, are selective for the gene locus and cell type (Reff, 1985). This assertion bears careful consideration as to not oversight the possibility that such changes, when affecting cell cycle regulatory genes may display far-reaching effects.

An alternative scenario is proposed by Strehler (reviewed 1986), according to whom a 30-50 percent age-related loss of rRNA genes occurs in DNA from brain and other tissues. Although the notion that tandemly repeated sequences such as rRNA cistrons or satellite DNAs (highly repetitive simple DNA sequences which are not transcribed *in vivo* and functions presumably to align homologous chromosomes during meiosis and/or to facilitate their recombination) are hypothesized to be at greater risk for excision, this evidence has not yet been rigorously verificated. The exception is the observation that satellite DNAs are largely or entirely eliminated in the somatic cells of a variety of eukaryotes (which are no

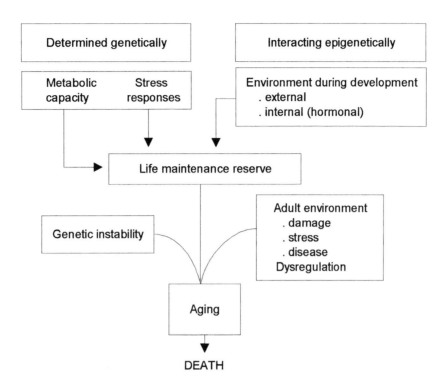

FIGURE   1–5
Determinants of aging and longevity: An overall view. Redrawn
from Jazwinski, S. M., 1996.

longer totipotent) but not in their germ cells (Voet and
Voet, 1990). Some other intriguing putative mechanisms
of age-related change in gene expression seem not to involve the primary sequence, but are thought to be possibly epigenetically attained by differential processing of
hnRNA or by intrachromosomal gene conversions (van
Leeuen *et al.*, 1989) giving rise to abnormal proteins.

*The Translation Error Catastrophe is not Widely
Accepted*

According to the translation error catastrophe advanced
by Orgel in 1963, accumulation of translational errors may
result in senescence, because errors at the level of translation may be subject to positive feedback, leading to an
exponential increase in error levels, an 'error catastrophe',
which results in cellular aging. In support of Orgel's view
is some evidence suggesting that the rates of translation
are usually reduced during aging. Increase in aminoacid
misincorporation in proteins has been reported during cellular aging (Luce and Bunn, 1987), and the aminoglycoside
antibiotic paromycin, which is known to reduce ribosomal
accuracy during translation (Buchanan, Stevens and Sidhu,
1987) induced more errors in translation in cell extracts
prepared from senescent human and rat cells than from
young cells (Luce and Bunn, 1987, 1989; Butzow, McCool
and Eichhorn, 1981). The problem lies in that not only reduced translation but also reduced transcription seem to
be implicated in aging (Nose and Okamoto, 1980; Dice,

1985). For example, ornithine decarboxylase mRNA is reduced only slightly in senescence, but translation of the
mRNA is inefficient, and the protein is rapidly degraded
(Chang and Chen, 1988; Warner and Wang, 1989); the age-
related reduction in thymidine kinase appears to be due to
a combination of reduced transcription, reduced processing
of RNA, and reduced translation (Rittling *et al*, 1986; Stein
et al, 1991; Pang and Chen, 1992).

Rose (1991) presents two lines of evidence against translation error catastrophe: (i) it has not yet been ascertained
whether organisms which can lack aging such as fissile an-
nelids, must have considerably increased translation fidelity compared with closely related organisms that do exhibit aging. It appears that some proteins do undergo some
loss of function with age, but this loss is rarely severe. In
fact, some proteins show no loss of function with age and
in those cases in which the cause of functional deterioration can be ascertained, it seems to be consistently due
to postsynthetic modification (Rothstein, 1983). Whereas
diverse tissues accumulate catalytically inactive enzymes,
the few altered enzymes that have been analyzed in depth
indicate altered conformations, not changes of amino acid
sequence. It has been even possible to recover full enzyme
activity by cycles of denaturation-renaturation (Sharma
and Rothstein, 1980; Rothstein, 1982; Yuh and Gafni,
1987). Moreover, abnormal proteins yielded by defective
translation may be prone to rapid degradation in the cell
(Chapter 7). (ii) It must be borne in mind that all cells that
synthesize proteins are probably selected to minimize error

Gensler, H. L., and Bernstein, H. 1981. DNA damage as the primary cause of aging. Q. Rev. Biol. 56:279-303.

Goldspink, D., Kelly, F. 1984. Protein turnover and growth in the whole body, liver, and kidney of the rat from foetus to senility. Biochem. J. 217:507-516.

Hall, K. Y., Hart, R. W., Benirschke, A. K., and Walford, R. L. 1984. Correlation between ultraviolet-induced DNA repair in primate lymphocytes and fibroblasts and species maximum achievable life span. Mech. Ageing Devel. 24:163-173

Halliwell, B. 1992. Oxygen radicals as key mediators in neurological disease: fact or fiction? Ann. Neurol. 32:S10-15.

Harley, C. B., Goldstein, S., and Posner, B. 1981. Decreased sensitivity of old and progeric human fibroblasts to a preparation of factors with insulin-like activities. J. Clin. Invest. 68:988-994.

Harley, C. B., Futcher, A. B., and Greider, C. W. 1990. Telomeres shorten during ageing of human fibroblasts. Nature 345:458-460.

Hart, R. W., and Setlow, R. B. 1974. Correlation between deoxyribonucleic acid excision repair and lifespan in a number of mammalian species. Proc. Natl. Acad. Sci. USA 71:2169-2173.

Hayflick, L. 1965. The limited in vitro lifetime of human diploid cell strains. Exp. Cell Res. 37:614-636

Hayflick, L. 1975. Current theories of biological aging. Fed. Proc. 34:9-13.

Hayflick, L. 1977. The cellular basis for biological aging. In C. E. Finch, and L. Hayflick (eds.) Handbook of the Biology of Aging. Van Nostrand Reinhold, New York, pp.159-186.

Hayflick, L. 1991. Aging under glass. Mut. Res. 256:79-80.

Hayflick, L., and Moorhead, P. S. 1961. The serial cultivation of human diploid cell strains. Exp. Cell Res. 25:585-621.

Holloszy, J. O., and Smith, E. K. 1987. Effects of exercise on longevity of rats. Fed. Proc. 46:1850-1853.

Hood, L. E., Weissman, I. L., and Wood, W. B. 1982. Immunology. Second edition. Benjamin-Cummings, Menlo Park.

Jazwinski, S. M. 1996. Longevity, genes, and aging. Science 273:54-58.

Kay, M. 1985. Aging of cell membrane molecules leads to appearance of an aging antigen and removal of senescent cells. Gerontology 31:215-235.

Kay, M. 1989. Red cell aging: senescent cell antigen, band 3, and band 3 mutations associated with cellular dysfunction. Prog. Clin. Biol. Res. 319:199-217.

Kirkwood, T. B. L. 1989. DNA, mutations and ageing. Mut. Res. 219:1-8.

Kleiber, M. 1947. Body size and metabolic rate. Physiol. Rev. 27:511-541.

Lavie, L., Reznick, A. Z., and Gershon, D. 1982. Decreased protein and puromycinyl-peptide degradation in livers of senescent mice. Biochem. J. 202:47-51.

Luce, M. C., and Bunn, C. L. 1987. Altered sensitivity of protein synthesis to paromycin in extracts from aging human diploid fibroblasts. Exp. Gerontol. 22:165-177.

Luce, M. C., and Bunn, C. L. 1989. Decreased accuracy of protein synthesis in extracts from aging human diploid fibroblasts. Exp. Gerontol. 24:113-125.

Martin, G. M. 1978. Genetic syndromes in man with potential relevance to the pathobiology of aging. Nat. Found. 14:5-39.

Maslansky, C. J., and Williams, G. M. 1985. Ultraviolet light-induced DNA repair synthesis in hepatocytes form species of differing longevities. Mech. Ageing Devel. 29:191-203

Masoro, E. J. 1988. Food restriction in rodents: An evaluation of its role in the study of aging. J. Gerontol. 43,B:59-64.

Maynard Smith, J. 1958. The effects of temperature and of egg-laying on the longevity of Drosophila subobscura. J. Exp. Biol. 35:832-842.

Maynard Smith, J., Bozcuk, A. N., and Tebbutt, S. 1970. Protein turnover in adult Drosophila. J. Insect Physiol. 16:601-613.

McCormick, A., and Campisi, J. 1991. Cellular aging and senescence. Curr. Opin. Cell Biol. 3:230-234.

McKerrow, J. 1979. Nonenzymatic posttranslational amino acid modifications in aging: a brief review. Mech. Ageing Devel. 10:371-377.

Medvedev, Z. A. 1972. Repetition of molecular-genetic information as a possible factor in evolutionary changes of life span. Exp. Gerontol. 7:227-238.

ZS-Nagy, I., and Nagy, K. 1980. On the role of cross-linking of cellular proteins in ageing. Mech. Ageing Devel. 14:245-281.

Nose, K., and Okamoto, H. 1980. Transcriptional activity of nuclei from WI-38 cells at various passages. J. Cell Physiol. 102:51-54.

Orgel, L. E. 1963. The maintenance of accuracy of protein synthesis and its relevance to ageing. Proc. Natl. Acad. Sci. USA 49:517-521.

Pang, H. P., and Chen, K. Y. 1992. A global change of expression of G1/S genes in IMR-90 human diploid cells during cell senescence. FASEB J. 6: A1782. (abstract)

Partdrige, L. 1986. Sexual activity and life span. In K. G. Collatz, and R. S. Sohal (eds.) Insect Aging, Strategies and Mechanisms Springer-Verlag, Berlin, pp 45-54.

Pearl, R. 1922. The Biology of Death, Being a Series of Lectures Delivered at the Lowell Institute in Boston in December 1920. J. B. Lippincott, Philadelphia and London. (quoted by Rose, 1991).

Pearl, R. 1928. The Rate of Living. Alfred A Knopf, New York.

Plisko, A., Gilchrest, B. 1983. Growth factor responsiveness of cultured human fibroblasts. J. Gerontol. 38:513-518.

Powell, J. 1996. Recent advances in Drosophila molecular evolutionary genetics. 42th National Congress of Genetics, Caxambu, Brasil.

Rattan, S. I. S. 1989. DNA damage and repair during cellular aging. Int. Rev. Cytol. 116:47-88.

Reff, M. E. 1985. In C. E. Finch, and E. L. Schneider (eds.) Handbook of the Biology of Aging. New York: Van Nostrand Reinhold, 2nd edition, pp 225-249.

Richardson, A., and Birchenall-Sparks, M. C. 1983. Age-related changes in protein synthesis. Rev. Biol. Res. Aging 1:255-273.

Rittling, S. R., Brooks, K. M., Cristofalo, V. J., and Baserga, R. 1986. Expression of cell cycle-dependent genes in young and senescent WI-38 fibroblasts. Proc. Natl. Acad. Sci. USA 86:3316-3320.

Robertson, O. H. 1961. Prolongation of the life span in kokanee salmon (Oncorhynchus nerka kennerlyi) by castration before beginning of gonad development. Proc. Natl. Acad. Sci. USA 47:609-621.

Rose, M. R. 1991. Evolutionary Biology of Aging. Oxford University Press, New York.

Rosen, R. 1978. Feedforwards and global system failure: A general mechanism for senescence. J. Theor. Biol. 74:579-590.

Roses, A. D. 1993. Molecular genetics of neurodegenerative diseases. Curr. Opin. Neurol. Neurosurg. 6:34-39.

Ross, D. W. 1992. Introduction to Molecular Medicine. Springer-Verlag, New York.

Ross, H. H., Ross, C. A., and Ross, J. R. P. 1982. A Textbook of Entomology. Fourth edition. John Wiley and Sons, New York, Chichester, Brisbane, Toronto, Singapore. pp 286-289.

Rothstein, M. 1982. Biochemical Approaches to Aging. New York: Academic Press.

Rothstein, M. 1983. Enzymes, enzyme alteration, and protein turnover. Rev. Biol. Res. Aging 1:305-314.

Sacher, G.A. 1959. Relation of lifespan to brain weight and body weight in mammals. In G. E. W. Wolstenholme, and M. O'Connor (eds.) CIBA Foundation Colloquia on Ageing, Vol. 5, The Lifespan of Animals. Churchill, London, pp. 115-133.

Sacher, G. A. 1978. Evolution of longevity and survival characteristics in mammals. In: E.L. Schneider (ed.), The Genetics of Aging, Plenum Press, New York and London, pp.151-168.

Sager, R. 1991. Senescence as a mode of tumor suppression. Environ. Health Perspect. 93: 59-62.

Sharma, H. K., and Rothstein, M. 1980. Altered enolase in aged Turbatrix aceta. Results from conformational changes in the enzyme. Proc. Natl. Acad. Sci. USA 77:5865-5868.

Smith, J. R., and Lincoln, D. 1984. Aging of cells in culture. Int. Rev. Cytol. 89:151-177.

Stadtman, E. 1989. Protein modifications in aging. J. Gerontol. 43:112-120.

Starke-Reed, P. E. 1989. The role of oxidative modification in cellular protein turnover and aging. Prog. Clin. Biol. Res. 287:269-276.

Stein, G. H., Drullinger, L. F., Robetorye, R. S., et al. 1991. Senescent cells fail to express cdc2, cycA, and cycB in response to mitogen stimulation. Proc. Natl. Acad. Sci. USA 88:11012-11016.

Strehler, B. L., Hirsch, G., Gusseck, D., Johnson, R., and Bick, M. 1971. Codon-restriction theory of aging and development. J. Theor. Biol. 33:429-474.

Strehler, B. L. 1977. Time, Cells and Aging. Second Edition. Academic Press, New York.

Strehler, B. L. 1986. Genetic instability as the primary cause of human ageing. Exp. Gerontol. 21:283-319.

Tollefsball, T., Gracy, R. W. 1983. Premature aging diseases: cellular and molecular changes. Bioscience 33:634-638.

Tonegawa, S. 1983. Somatic generation of antibody diversity. Nature 302: 575-581.

Van Leeuen, F., van der Beek, E., Seger, M., Burbach, P., and Ivell, R. 1989. Age related development of a heterozygous phenotype in solitary neurons of the homozygous Brattleboro rat. Proc. Natl. Acad. Sci. USA 86:6417-6420.

Voet, D., and Voet, J.G. 1990. Biochemistry. John Wiley & Sons, New York.

Wallace, D. C. 1992. Mitochondrial genetics: a paradigm for aging and degenerative diseases? Science 256:628-632.

Warner, H., and Wang, E. (eds.). 1989. Proceedings of the workshop on 'Control of cell proliferation in senescent cells'. Exp. Gerontol. 24:351-585.

Weindruch, R., and Walford, R. L. 1988. The Retardation of Aging and Disease by Diet Restriction. Springfield, Ill.:Thomas.

Wise, P. M. 1983. Aging of the female reproductive system. Rev. Biol. Res. Aging 1:195-222.

Würgler, F. E., Arni, P., Fahrig, R., et al. 1991. Genetische Endpunkte. Eine Mitteilung der 'GUM Kommission zur Erarbeitung der Richtlinien für die Genotoxizitätsprüfung'. Bioforum 10:376-380.

Yuan, P., Talent, J. M., and Gracy, R. W. 1981. Molecular basis for the accumulation of acidic isozymes of triosephosphate isomerase in aging. Mech. Ageing Dev. 17:151-162.

Yuh, K. M., and Gafni, A. 1987. Reversal of age-related effects in rat muscle phosphoglycerate kinase. Proc. Natl. Acad. Sci. USA 84:7458-7462.

Sergio U. Dani

2

Biophysical Principles of Aging

The First Law of Thermodynamics

The Second Law of Thermodynamics

Irreversible Thermodynamics Takes Time into Account

Steady-state, or the Makeshift Maintenance of Life

Metabolic Control is Attained by the Make-up and Maintenance of Thermodynamic Gradients Through the Regulation of Enzymatic Activity

Aging as a Manifestation of the Progressive Departure of Living Systems from Steady State to Equilibrium

Oxidative Stress is Both Necessary and Detrimental to Life

When did Aging First Obtrude?

Aging, Likewise Evolution, is Inherent in Life

An Overall View

Aging, in the strict sense of the word, means nothing else than 'becoming old' by the passage of time. The notion has been applied to both living and non-living things to imply certain kinds of changes in structure or composition of matter which occur with time: wine is said 'to age' when it is left in barrels for certain periods of time; humans are already 9-month-old (from the moment of the fertilization of the egg) when they are born; iron bars 'become old' as they get oxidation spots; fossils are dated and their 'ages' estimated according to changes in the ratios between carbon isotopes that constitute their matter, and so on.

While differences between biological and non-biological aging are seemingly apparent, and generally acknowledged, similarities are often neglected. For a time, the doctrine termed *Vitalism* frontally rejected the idea that similarities between the principles governing the animate matter and the inanimate matter exist at all. Vitalists stated that biological processes are not bound by the physical laws that govern inanimate objects, but by an immaterial principle: the *entelecheia*, for Aristotle and Hans Driesch; the *élan vital*, for Henri Bergson and Bernard Shaw.

Modern biologists no longer need vitalistic principles to account for biological processes. The view of an immaterial principle governing life has been refuted, both theoretically as well as by careful experimental measurements on living animals and plants that are entirely consistent with the predictions of the laws of physics. That both biological and non-biological aging are governed by the same physical laws surely belongs to the similarities between living and non-living matter, and shall be highlighted in this chapter. More specifically, we shall review the basic principles of thermodynamics which were developed as early as in the second half of the nineteenth century. A knowledge in thermodynamics can help us determine whether a biophysical process like aging is possible, and the conditions under which it occurs spontaneously (by itself). However, the reader should be cautioned that classical thermodynamics does not indicate the rates at which aging or any other process actually occurs in different organisms and conditions; the description of aging rates requires further molecular kinetics and evolutionary models. Yet, thermodynamics is indispensable in formulating such models because the models must conform to thermodynamic principles.

The First Law of Thermodynamics

The first law of thermodynamics, attributed to German physicist and physiologist Hermann von Helmholtz (1821–1894), states that the total energy of a closed system remains constant throughout any transformation: Energy can assume different forms, but can neither be created nor destroyed. The mathematical statement of the first law takes the form of the following equation:

$$\Delta E = E_{final} - E_{initial} = q - w \qquad \text{[Eq. 1]},$$

where ΔE is the variation in energy, i.e., the difference between the final and initial energy, q represents the *heat* absorbed by the system from the surroundings, and w is the *work* done by the system on the surroundings. Heat is a reflection of random molecular motion whereas work, which is defined as force times the distance moved under its influence, is associated with organized motion.

Processes in which the system releases heat, which by convention are assigned a negative q, are known as *exothermic processes* (Greek: *exo*, out of); those in which the system gains heat (positive q) are known as *endothermic processes* (Greek: *endon*, within). Consider, for instance, the transformation of ice into liquid water and steam. This is clearly an endothermic process because heat is absorbed from the surroundings to increase the kinetic energy of water molecules which are initially restrained, thus relatively 'motionless' in the crystal structure of ice. As temperature increases, the random motion of water molecules progressively increases, and the crystal is dismantled as ice melts. Further absorption of heat by the liquid finally causes the water molecules to move more freely in steam. The reverse direction, i.e. from steam to ice, is obviously an exothermic process.

The energy of a system is said to be a *state function* because the energy depends only on the current properties of the system or its state, not on how it reached that state. Consequently, there is no net change in energy ($\Delta E = 0$) for any process in which the system returns to its initial state. A closely related state function known as *enthalpy* (Greek: *enthalpein*, to warm in), is defined

$$H = E + PV \qquad \text{[Eq. 2]},$$

where V is the volume of the system and P is its pressure. P and V are used in Eq. [2] for enthalpy because in many systems work is done by change in pressure and volume, accompanied by the generation or absorption of heat. However, under constant pressure and negligible volume changes, conditions typical of most biochemical processes, the enthalpy change between the initial and final states of a process, ΔH, is the easily measured heat that it generates or absorbs.

We stated earlier in the chapter that thermodynamics serves to indicate whether a particular process like aging occurs spontaneously. Yet, we cannot envisage a way by which the first law of thermodynamics, by itself, provides the basis for such an indication. It is the second law of thermodynamics that provides such a criterion.

The Second Law of Thermodynamics

The second law of thermodynamics states that spontaneous processes occur in directions that increase the overall disorder of the universe, that is, of the system and its surroundings. Since the number of equivalent ways, W, of arranging the components of the universe is usually inconveniently immense, a more manageable quantity known as *entropy* (Greek: *en*, in + *trope*, turning) was defined in 1877 by Austrian physicist Ludwig Boltzmann (1844–1906):

$$S = k_B \, ln \, W \qquad \text{[Eq. 3]}$$

Entropy, S, like enthalpy, is also a state function because it depends only on the parameters that describe a state (k_B is the *Boltzmann constant*). In Boltzmann's equation entropy increases with W in a more manageable way. Yet, in chemical and biological systems, it is nearly impossible to determine the entropy of a system by counting the number of ways, W, it can assume its most probable state. For this matter, a more practical definition of entropy was proposed in 1864 by Rudolf Clausius taking into account the absolute temperature, T, at which a change in heat, q, occurs in a system that remains in equilibrium throughout the change. This is known as a *reversible process*. Although life is not a reversible process (life is only possible as long as a makeshift *nonequilibrium state* is maintained, as we shall see further in this text), Clausius' definition of entropy is still valid for the analysis of entropy in living things. For constant temperature conditions typical of biological processes, Clausius' equation takes the form:

$$\Delta S \geq qT^{-1} \qquad \text{[Eq. 4]}$$

In general, for any constant energy process ($\Delta E = 0$), a spontaneous process is characterized by $\Delta S > 0$ simply because any system of reasonable size will spontaneously adopt its most probable arrangement, the one in which entropy is maximum. Since the energy of the universe is constant, any spontaneous process must cause the entropy of the universe to increase:

$$\Delta S_{system} + \Delta S_{surroundings} = \Delta S_{universe} > 0 \quad [\text{Eq. 5}]$$

Equation [5] is the usual expression for the second law of thermodynamics. It states that the entropy of the universe tends towards a maximum. Since we are born, we live and die in a physical world, aging must conform with this law, too. Yet, it is nearly impossible to monitor the entropy of the entire universe, let alone to predict the spontaneity of a process from a knowledge of the system's entropy change alone.

To overcome these difficulties, a state function that straightforwardly predicts whether or not a given process is spontaneous was formulated by J. Willard Gibbs in 1878. Variations in the *Gibbs free energy* function, G, are described by the formula:

$$\Delta G = \Delta H - T\Delta S \qquad [\text{Eq. 6}]$$

We recall that ΔH, under conditions typical of most biochemical processes, is the measured heat, q, that a process generates or absorbs, and that $T\Delta S \geq q$ for spontaneuos processes, as Eq. [4] suggests. Substituting the terms of Eq. [6] accordingly results that $\Delta G < 0$ is the criterion of spontaneity for the constant T and P conditions that are typical of biochemical processes. Spontaneous processes, i.e., those with negative ΔG values, are said to be *exergonic* (Greek: *ergon*, work); they can be utilized to do work. Processes that are not spontaneous, those with positive ΔG values, are termed *endergonic*; they must be driven by the input of free energy, e.g., through coupling endergonic reactions with sufficiently exergonic processes so that the overall reaction is exergonic. The most important mechanism of coupled reactions in living things is the use of the free energy of ATP hydrolysis, a highly exergonic process, to drive many otherwise endergonic biological processes.

In biochemical systems, work represented by changes in pressure and volume (*P-V* work) is unimportant, and ΔG for a biological process represents its maximum recoverable work. Actually, the work put into any system can never be fully recovered due to the inherent dissipative character of the universe. Also, it is remarkable that a negative value of ΔG does not ensure a chemical reaction will proceed at a biologically significant rate. In the majority of the cases, only with the introduction of the proper enzymes the reaction will proceed at a reasonable pace. Yet a catalyst, which by definition acts by its presence without being changed by the reaction, cannot affect the ΔG of a reaction: An enzyme can only accelerate the attainment of thermodynamic equilibrium; it cannot, for example, promote a reaction that has a positive ΔG. None the less, this subtle function of a catalyst is so remarkable because it helps create and maintain physicochemical gradients upon which biological processes are based.

Irreversible Thermodynamics Takes Time into Account

Whereas the notion that living things obey to the first law of thermodynamics is entirely consistent with calorimetric measurements on living animals, the experimental verification of the second law in living systems proved to be more difficult. The second law of thermodynamics states that there will be a gradual tendency of energy to be distributed uniformly among the discrete units of matter in a closed system, i.e., entropy tends to increase. In such a system, the heat, q, of a reaction at constant T and P is only equal to $T\Delta S$ if the reaction is carried out reversibly, in conditions of equilibrium [Eq. 4].

However, living systems, by definition, can never be at equilibrium. At equilibrium, no gradient-forming process can be directed, no useful work can be performed. Thus, equilibrium is incompatible with the maintenance of the intricate regulatory functions which characterize life. This realization is in the basis of *nonequilibrium* or *irreversible* thermodynamics. In contrast to classical thermodynamics, the theory of irreversible thermodynamics explicit takes time into account. It is ultimately a matter of time to explain, for instance, how spontaneous reactions are maintained at biologically significant rates, and for how long. Also, it is a profound truth that biological processes such as development, maturation, reproduction, death, in a word, aging, only take place when 'time has come'.

Steady-state, or the Makeshift Maintenance of Life

Living systems are open systems that continuously change matter and energy with the environment. Contrarily to any closed system that must inevitably reach equilibrium, living things have to maintain a nonequilibrium state or a *steady-state* as long as they are able to remain alive. In an ideal steady-state, $\Delta S = 0$, so that a positive ΔS is balanced by a negative ΔS, and the system feeds on *negentropy* from the surroundings. To build up and maintain low-entropic states at the expense of a net increase in the entropy of the universe, living organisms continuously acquire free energy from the surroundings in the form of reactants, heat or work. They ingest high-enthalpy, low-entropy nutrients, which they convert to low-enthalpy, high-entropy waste products.

These negentropic properties of living systems were described by French physiologist Claude Bernard (1813–1878) when he proposed that living things are distinguished by a constancy or *homeostasis* in their *milieu interne*. He recognized that biological systems have an intrinsic ability to maintain homeostasis in spite of their continuous relationships of exchange with the *milieu externe*. Bernard went on to conclude that homeostasis is actually the trait that distinguishes the living matter from the non-living. The concept of homeostasis became widely used both in the specialized and in the non-specialized literature. Similarly to what happened to many scientific theories that, once becoming popular, were interpreted according to the 'mores' of the times, also home-ostasis was taken as synonymous with the 'perfectness' or 'equilibrium' of life. This notion has certainly contributed to the popular expression that 'Nature knows best', an idea refuted in the early 1960's by Peter Medawar:

'It is a profound truth - realized in the nineteenth century by only a handful of astute biologists and by philosophers hardly at all (indeed, most of those who held any views on the matter held a contrary opinion) - a profound truth that Nature does not know best; that genetical evolution, if we choose to look at it liverishly instead of with fatuous good humour, is a story of waste, makeshift, compromise, and blunder.'

The principle behind the concept of homeostasis is that slight perturbations from the steady state give rise to changes in flows that counteract these perturbations so as to return the system to the steady state. This is the nonequilibrium analogy to *Le Chatelier's principle*. However, since living systems are no exception to the laws of classical thermodynamics (they invariably and progressively depart from steady state and approach equilibrium, and indeed reach an equilibrium state when they die or become extinct), homeostasis and the related thermodynamical concept of steady state in living systems must be considered under the general scope of makeshift adjustments. Paradoxically, it is precisely this makeshift character of life that gives us individuality (within the time constraint of the lifetime of an individual) and continuity (within the time constraint of species existence and evolution). Thus, differences in life span and longevity between different organisms, or between different stages in the life of an organism (e.g. development, maturation and senescence) are differences of degree only, not of thermodynamical principle. For *all* living things, as we shall see in the next sessions, aging is characterized by the progressive departure from steady state to the more entropic equilibrium state. The differences in the degree of aging between different organisms, and between different stages in the life of a single organism are largely conferred by metabolic regulation, which determines the rate at which an organism will approach equilibrium.

Metabolic Control is Attained by the Make-up and Maintenance of Thermodynamic Gradients Through the Regulation of Enzymatic Activity

The overwhelming majority of chemical reactions in living cells are subject to rate enhancement by protein enzymes, one exception being the recently discovered ribozymes, which are not proteins, but nucleic acids. Almost all metabolic reactions fall into four categories: group-transfer reactions; oxidation-reduction reactions; eliminations, isomerizations, and rearrangements; and reactions that make or brake carbon-carbon bonds. Reactions for which the sign of Gibbs free energy change, ΔG, for the chemical transformation is positive are unfavorable and therefore their rates are unaffected by the presence of a

catalyst. Catalysis by enzymes is thus concerned not with the possibility of a reaction taking place but with the frequency of its occurrence in a unit of time - a matter for kinetic analysis.

Factors affecting the kinetics of a reaction include the free energy of activation of the reactants to their transition states and the relative concentration of reactants and products. It is the role of an enzyme to selectively reduce the free energy of activation of a chemically coupled reaction so that it approaches equilibrium faster than the more thermodynamically favoured uncoupled reaction. One example of such an enzymatic effect is the enhanced rate of the reaction between ATP and glucose (phosphorylation of glucose) in the presence of a suitable enzyme, as compared to the rate of the reaction between ATP and water (ATP hydrolysis): although the hydrolysis of ATP is a more exergonic reaction than the phosphorylation of glucose, the latter reaction is predominant in the presence of a suitable enzyme because it is kinetically favored. In its turn, the activity of an enzyme can be significantly altered. Most enzymes in a metabolic pathway operate near equilibrium and therefore have net rates that vary with their substrate concentrations. However, certain allosteric enzymes operate far from equilibrium. It is the relative insensitivity of the rates of the reactions catalyzed by such enzymes to variations in the concentrations of their substrates that permits the establishment of a steady state flux of metabolites throughout the metabolic pathway. This situation optimizes the pathway's thermodynamic efficiency and allows the flux to be allosterically controlled.

An instructive example of make-up and maintenance of thermodynamic gradients through the regulation of enzymatic activity is the regulation of the *sodium-potassium pump*, an ATP-dependent molecular machine that cares for the osmotic control of the cell's water content, the active transport of glucose and amino acids into some cells, and the maintenance of the transmembrane electrochemical potential required for nerve impulse transmission. The sodium-potassium pump, also called sodium-potassium ATPase, is an integral membrane protein. It is a multimeric complex consisting of two different polypeptides: a 110-kD transmembrane catalytic α subunit and an ~55-kD glycoprotein β subunit (Figure 2–1). The function of the sodium-potassium pump is to balance the passive fluxes of sodium and potassium into and out of the cell by active transport driven in the opposite direction by an ATP-dependent reaction: ATP transfers its terminal phosphate group to the catalytic subunit of the pump forming a covalent intermediate in the presence of sodium. Protein phosphorylation changes the conformation of the complex, which leads to the removal of three sodium ions from the inside of the cell to the outside in exchange for two extracellular potassium ions. The phosphorylated catalytic subunit is hydrolyzed in the presence of potassium ions. The overall reaction results in the hydrolysis of ATP, an exergonic reaction used in this case to perform the work represented by the endergonic pumping of sodium and potassium ions against an

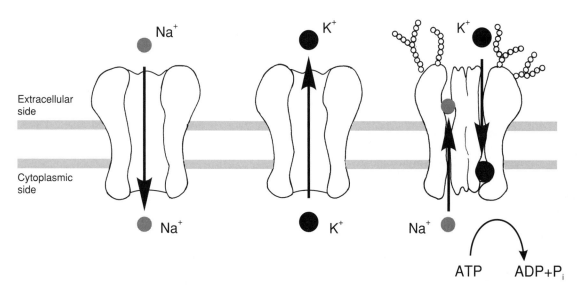

FIGURE 2–1

The passive fluxes of sodium and potassium into and out of the cell are balanced by active transport driven in the opposite direction by the sodium-potassium pump, also called sodium-potassium ATPase. The pump is a multimeric complex consisting of two different polypeptides: a 110-kD transmembrane catalytic α subunit and an $\sim$55-kD glycoprotein β subunit. ATP transfers its terminal phosphate group to the catalytic subunit of the pump forming a covalent intermediate in the presence of sodium. Protein phosphorylation changes the conformation of the complex, which leads to the removal of three sodium ions from the inside of the cell to the outside in exchange for two extracellular potassium ions. The phosphorylated catalytic subunit is hydrolyzed in the presence of potassium ions.

electrochemical gradient. When the cell is at rest, the active fluxes (driven by the pump) and the passive fluxes (due to diffusion) are balanced for sodium and potassium, so that the net flux of each of these two ions is zero. Thus, at the resting membrane potential the cell is not in equilibrium, but rather in a steady state: metabolic free energy must be used to maintain the ionic gradients across a *thermodynamic driving force* (Koester, 1991).

Aging as a Manifestation of the Progressive Departure of Living Systems from Steady State to Equilibrium

Ilya Prigogine, a pioneer in the field of nonequilibrium thermodynamics, postulated that the steady state of an open system is its state of maximum attainable thermodynamic efficiency under the constraints governing such a system. As reviewed above, steady state is largely accomplished by regulating the activity of a number of enzymes in an effort to sustain certain spontaneous reactions at biologically significant rates. While most regulatory processes are highly directed and thus operate far from equilibrium, metabolism is also characterized by a great number of reactions that occur close to or at equilibrium. Whereas these reactions are poorly or not directed, they still have biological significance in the sense that they progressively lead the living organism to departure from the steady state. Living things must then cope with this paradox of life: The means that they are continuously using to produce more of themselves are the very means that have the potential to destroy their lives.

Evidence that this is indeed how things happen is accumulating. The concept of genetic instability as a progressive change in the patterns of gene expression that occurs during aging has gained force in recent years from a number of studies focusing on altered gene expression as a consequence of the gradual deterioration of the covalent structure of proteins, lipids, and above all, DNA. The various forms of molecular damage are generated during the lifetime of an organism by a number of intrinsic or extrinsic reactive agents, and eliminated by a number of ubiquitous repair enzymes. However, due to thermodynamical reasons discussed above, even these enzymatic repair systems cannot be perfect. Thus differences in longevity (defined as the age-specific resistance to metabolic failure or resistance to departure from steady-state), may lie largely on constitutive differences in the efficiency of macromolecular repair and turnover systems. In this context, it is paradigmatic that DNA repair levels correlate with life span, metabolic rates and diet; that repair-defective cells are at higher risk of degeneration; and that genetic diseases causing higher levels of DNA damage or a deficiency in DNA repair also have features of premature aging and senescence. Examples of such conditions will be given in Chapter 3 along with a review on the relationship between mutation, evolution and aging. Here we shall focus on oxidative stress, which is both necessary and detrimental to life.

Oxidative Stress is Both Necessary and Detrimental to Life

Neurons are especially dependent on and vulnerable to, oxidative stress. Nerve cells are the largest cells in the body and also have the highest metabolic rates; up to 70 percent of the ATP produced in neurons is utilized to maintain the functions driven by the sodium-potassium pump, as described above. ATP cannot be stored for a long time and thus must be continuously produced in mitochondria through the mechanism of oxidative phosphorylation (OXPHOS) to attend the cell's demands for free energy. As a result of this high metabolic activity, great amounts of oxidant radicals are produced regularly within mitochondria. Aside the oxidation of lipids, proteins and other molecules, mitochondrial DNA (mtDNA) is especially vulnerable to oxidation because mtDNA not only lacks the protection of histones, but also suffers more directly the burden represented by oxygen free radicals (superoxide anion and hydrogen peroxide). Whereas the high rates of mitochondria replication, and the turnover of damaged molecules, may represent a mechanism to compensate for oxidative stress (all mtDNA replication enzymes are encoded by the nucleus), an extra burden of oxidative stress like that observed in *Down syndrome* might reduce the threshold for cell dysfunction and death. Individuals with Down syndrome carry, in the vast majority of the cases, a trisomy of the chromosome 21 in each of their cells. The extra copy of the *Cu/Zn superoxide dismutase* gene that is physically mapped to chromosome 21 has been associated with the production of an abnormally high level of the DNA damaging agents H_2O_2, the hydroxyl radical and singlet oxygen, all of which are extremely reactive radicals. Down syndrome patients have a number of abnormal phenotypes, the most striking of which are the mental retardation and the short life span. In addition, they characteristically develop degenerative changes in neurons much earlier than in the normal population. One hypothesis to explain this precocious neuronal degeneration in Down syndrome involves the exarcerbation of the generally detrimental, but also life-promoting process of oxidation.

When did Aging First Obtrude?

In the antiquity Aristotle wondered why some animals and plants live longer than others, and whether in a natural structure longevity and a sound constitution are coincident or independent from each other. These are indeed two crucial questions about the origins of the differences in life span and longevity, two indissociable aspects of aging. Life span is simply the life time of an organism, measured in hours, days, months or years. Longevity is the age-related resistance to metabolic failure, in other words, the maintenance capacity of an organism, measured by physiologic parameters indicative of fitness, such as muscular strength and physical activity or the incidence of pathologic events such as cancer or neurodegeneration at any given period in life time. Today we

know that life span is not necessarily a measure of longevity; while in the wild, life span usually corresponds to longevity for a great number of organisms, in domestication, however, life span usually surpasses longevity.

For the German zoologist August Weismann (1834–1914), aging is not inherent in life itself but is rather a later addition due to evolution. Weismann pointed to the example of a dividing amoeba and asked: Does this division end an individual life and do two new individuals emerge from that? Opposing objections that after thousands of cell divisions only a correspondingly small amount of the original substance would be present and thus the original cell would have perished, he asked: Where is the corpse? What is dying?

Weismann's ideas were instrumental to the development of the evolutionary theory of aging, which is largely based on population genetics, and less on the individuals and their constitutive parts. Yet, we can no longer rule out, as he did, that aging is inherent in life, rather than an addition due to evolution. Evolution, by increasing the complexity of organisms, can only increase the probability of dysfunction; however it cannot change the biophysical principles that govern life. A closer view to the problem reveals that there is no difference, in biophysical principles, between a dividing amoeba and a dividing cancer cell in an aged multicellular organism. In both instances, there are molecular forces driving the system to a state of maximum entropy. Such forces are easily observed in the case of tumor cells; they are represented by gross somatic mutations, DNA brakes and chromosomal anomalies that drive the transformed cell to a state of uncontrolled growth, endangering the survival of all cells in the host organism. The forces are less apparent in the case of dividing amoebas. Yet, if one assumes that multicellular organisms evolved from simpler, unicellular living things, one must assume that even free-living cells such as amoebas must be susceptible to mutations, without which they would never evolve to multicellular systems. The corpse, in Weismann's question, is just difficult to see or detect in an unicellular organism. But it is right there. Mutations are intrinsic causes of dysfunction and death and, eventually, of evolution, as we shall discuss in the next chapter. Mutations generate new molecular combinations that can be either life-promoting or life-threatening, depending on the environment.

Aging, Likewise Evolution, is Inherent in Life

If one assumes that living systems we know nowadays are just the sustainable proportion of the total number of living systems that already existed (compare with Stanley, 1987), one may ask what happened to the living forms that no longer exist. Individual organisms can disappear, by means of extinction or evolution, thanks to conservative forces that maintain not only novel sustainable combinations, but also highly entropic, unsustainable ones. Loss of maintenance capacity takes place when the living system is overwhelmed with an amount of changes beyond its capacity of self-repair or adaption. When the critical threshold is achieved, the organism undergoes dysfunction (compare with theoretical reasoning by Mézard, Nadal and Toulouse, 1986). As a consequence, we may note, if living things progressively lose their temporary ability to maintain their homeostasis, the boundaries between the *milieu interne* and the *milieu externe* progressively become erased and the living would get closer and closer to what we call non-living. This progressive loss of maintenance capacity of living things describes what we call biological aging.

Deviations from stability to irreversibility, in the chaos theory, are possible when there is a 'continuous injection of enough energy to drive the system to a high enough excitation that non-linearity becomes appreciable' (Firth, 1991). Purely mathematical reasoning shows that relatively simple systems can develop quite complex behavior even after slight perturbations, if non-linear interactions are involved (Van der Steen and Kamminga, 1991; May, 1976). This phenomenon is regarded as important for empirical research since it is exhibited by certain physical and chemical systems. This brings us back to considerations about conservative forces, loss or changing maintenance capacity, and the beginning of life. Relatively simple instances have been long recognized: protobiotic coacerbation of lipoproteic membranes maintained by weak intermolecular attractive forces of the van der Waals type. More complex systems involve associations between nucleotide sequences and peptides or proteins. Such systems are capable of self replication, modulation and modification. Recently, simple self-replicating molecules have been synthesized that are also capable of 'successful mutation' (Amato, 1992; Hong *et al.*, 1992). Such molecules constitute a strong experimental evidence for the molecular theory of evolution and aging, emphasizing that the machinery of molecular turnover displays, in many respects, some features of evolutionary mechanisms, adaptive and non-adaptive. As the evidence suggests, such mechanisms are invariably determined by the laws of physics, and this is probably the major argument for the general conclusion that aging, likewise evolution, is a progressive, inexorable, process.

An Overall View

A central corollary of thermodynamics is that the direction of time is determined by the direction in which the energy distribution tends to go spontaneously. This is understandable in the sense that, if energy is conserved (first law of thermodynamics), the only way to measure the passage of time is to relate the notion 'time' to the notion 'energy flow'. Since the universe marchs toward a state of higher entropy (second law of thermodynamics), then the direction of time is necessarily determined by the direction in which the energy distribution tends to go spontaneously. Consequently, entropy will increase spontaneously and progressively in any system which is not already in its most stable condition (the equilibrium state) and which possesses sufficient thermal energy to permit reactions to occur.

Whatever difference may exist between the aging of wine, babies, metal bars and fossils, it must be a difference of degree at which equilibrium is attained only, not of principle. Similarly, there is no reason to believe that differences in life span and longevity between different organisms, or between different stages in the life of an organism (e.g. development, maturation and senescence), are differences of principle, and not of degree only. This conclusion, which approaches what could be a thermodynamical definition of biological aging, seems to justify the use of the expression 'makeshift' to describe the steady state that characterizes living systems.

Selected Readings

Elskens, Y., and Prigogine, I. 1986. From instability to irreversibility. Proc. Natl. Acad. Sci. USA 83:5756.

Hart, R. W., and Setlow, R. B. 1974. Correlation between deoxyribonucleic acid excision repair and lifespan in a number of mammalian species. Proc. Natl. Acad. Sci. USA 71:2169–2173.

Lindahl, T. 1993. Instability and decay of the primary structure of DNA. Nature 362:709–715

Prigogine, I., and Stengers, I. 1984. Order out of Chaos: Man's New Dialogue with Nature. Toronto: Bantam.

Strehler, B. L. 1986. Genetic instability as the primary cause of human ageing. Exp. Gerontol. 21:283–319.

References

Amato, I. 1992. Capturing chemical evolution in a jar. A system of self-replicating molecules can now spin off a faster-multiplying 'mutant' form. Science 255:800.

Aristotle. De Longitudine et Brevitate Vitae. Translation by G. R. T. Ross (1908). Clarendon Press, Oxford.

Burnet, F. M. 1974. Intrinsic Mutagenesis: A Genetic Approach to Aging. John Wiley & Sons, Inc. New York, NY.

Firth, W. J. 1991. Chaos - predicting the unpredictable. Br. Med. J. 303:1565–1568.

Hong, J. -I., Feng, Q., Rotello, V., and Rebek, J. Jr. 1992. Competition, cooperation, and mutation: improving a synthetic replicator by light irradiation. Science 255:848.

Koester, J. 1991. Membrane Potential. In Kandel, E.R., Schwartz, J.H., and Jessel, T.M., Principles of Neural Science. Elsevier, NY, p. 87.

May, R. M. 1976. Simple mathematical models with very complicated dynamics. Nature 261:459–67.

Medawar, P. 1960. The Future of Man. BBC Reith Lectures 1959. Methuen.

Mézard, M., Nadal, J. P., and Toulouse, G. 1986. Solvable models of working memories. J. Physique (Paris) 47:1457–1462.

Stanley, S. 1987. Extinction. New York: Freeman.

Van der Steen, W. J., and Kamminga, H. 1991. Laws and natural history in biology. British Journal of the Philosophy of Science 42:445–467.

Voet, D., and Voet, J. G. 1990. Biochemistry. John Wiley & Sons, New York.

Wallace, D. C. 1992. Mitochondrial genetics: A paradigm for aging and degenerative diseases? Science 256:628–632.

Sergio U. Dani
Andrew J.G. Simpson

3

Mutation, Evolution and Aging

The Control of the Mutation Rate is Central to Evolution and Aging
    Mutations Accumulate Exponentially Over Time
    The Efficiency of Repair Systems is Variable

Cancer is by Far the Best Understood Disease Caused by the Accumulation of Mutations
    Cancer Parallels Evolution

Postmitotic Cells Such as Neurons are also Vulnerable to DNA Damage and Genetic Instability

An Overall View

Life has evolved through the slow alteration of genomes over time. The genome alterations responsible for evolution are the result of random mutations that are introduced at every generation. These mutations may or may not become established depending on many variables including their effect on the phenotype of the organism. The majority of mutations will either be neutral, having no effect on phenotype or deleterious. Very few will confer a direct positive advantage. Due to the fact that deleterious mutations will far outnumber advantageous mutations the rate at which mutations are introduced into the germline is crucial. If too many mutations occur the species will face rapid extinction due to the overload of incapacitating errors. On the other hand, if too few mutations occur the species will face extinction over evolutionary time due to its inability to adapt to environmental changes. The ideal level of mutation will depend on the characteristics of the species in terms of population size, generation time and reproductive capacity as well as the rate of change of the environment. These considerations imply that mutation rates must be tightly controlled.

The last few years have seen the elucidation of highly conserved cellular mechanisms responsible for the recognition and correction of DNA mutations which provide a molecular basis for the control of mutation rates (Cleaver, 1994). Evolution has led to the control of mutation rates at low but finite levels through the fine tuning of the efficiency of repair mechanisms. Germline and somatic mutations are controlled by the same intrinsic mechanism (Sommer, 1990). The evidence available suggests that mutation accumulation appears to be an exponential process, and that relatively low levels of germline mutation lead to very much higher levels of somatic mutation later in life resulting in the development of age-associated diseases such as cancer which are thus a direct reflection of the evolutionary process (Crow, 1993; Martin *et al.*, 1996). Thus, the major features of age related diseases can be accounted for by a model in which aging progresses by the acquisition of neutral mutations at normal but exponential rates. In consequence senescence and related conditions can be viewed as phenotypic expressions of preprogrammed somatic evolution.

The Control of the Mutation Rate is Central to Evolution and Aging

In spite of the fact that somatic mutation theories of aging have been formulated almost 40 years ago, by Failla (1958) and Szilard (1959), the role of somatic instabilities in the etiology of aging and age-related diseases has only begun to be revealed. The concept of progressive genetic instability with age has gained force in recent years from a number of studies focusing on changes in gene expression as a consequence of the gradual deterioration of the covalent structure of proteins, lipids, and above all, DNA (Chapter 7). Since it is the DNA molecule that conveys the genetic information for the maintenance of life, DNA damage by a number of intrinsic or extrinsic reactive agents has been proposed as the primary cause of genetic instability. DNA damage involves covalent changes such as methylation, glycosylation, acetylation, oxidation and other changes which may eventually lead to the exchange, insertion, or loss of nucleotides. In addition to these major lesions, several distinct minor DNA lesions called *I-compounds* (from *indigenous*, or *intrinsic*) were identified by Randerath and colleagues. These compounds, like all other types of DNA lesions, are generated during the lifetime of an organism.

While DNA molecules are being continuously damaged even in the very young, the predominant forms of damage are eliminated by a number of repair enzymes (Pacifici and Davies, 1991; Lindahl, 1993; Cleaver, 1994; Radman *et al.*, 1995; Jackson, 1996). In this context, it is paradigmatic that DNA repair levels correlate with lifespan (see Tice and Setlow, 1985; and Bernstein and Bernstein, 1991, for reviews), metabolic rates and diet, that repair-defective cells are at higher risk of degeneration, and that humans with genetic diseases causing higher levels of DNA damage or a deficiency in DNA repair also have features of premature aging. In the context of genetic diseases, individuals with *Down syndrome* have an extra copy of the Cu/Zn superoxide dismutase gene, which probably causes the production of an abnormally high level of the DNA damaging agents H_2O_2, the hydroxyl radical and singlet oxygen. Severe cases of *xeroderma pigmentosum* have repair-defective cells which seem unable to remove a major oxygen radical-induced form of DNA damage, which might accumulate (Satoh *et al.*, 1993). Xeroderma pigmentosum patients suffer from a gradual but massive loss of neurons with accompanying mental deterioration over a period of decades and also exhibit a

significantly increased frequency of internal cancers (Cleaver and Kraemer, 1989). Furthermore, the genetic defect responsible for both *Bloom syndrome* and *Werner syndrome* have recently been identified; the genes affected in both cases are *helicases*, enzymes responsible for unwinding the DNA double helix and thought to play an integral role in some forms of DNA repair (Yu *et al.*, 1996; Rothstein and Gangloff, 1995). In the absence of such repair processes the chromosomes of Werner syndrome patients exhibit multiple chromosome abnormalities and deletions which are correlated with the clinical syndrome of arteriosclerosis, malignant neoplasms, type II diabetes mellitus, osteoporosis and ocular cataracts together with early greying and loss of hair, skin atrophy and generally aged appearance (see Chapter 30). In Bloom syndrome somatic cell mutations are also dramatically increased and affected individuals present a vastly elevated incidence of cancer.

Since some of the minor DNA lesions such as the I-compounds may only become relevant after slow accumulation, it is conceivable that selection pressures relaxed, and no efficient enzymatic system evolved to cope with these minor lesions. As noted by Lindahl, 'even in normal human cells, there would be little or no evolutionary reason to repair accumulating DNA lesions in stem cells or in neurons that might only become affected after 40–100 years'. It might be conceded, however, that efficient systems did evolve as lifespan progressively increased in phylogeny, to handle even those minor lesions in long-lived species like ours. That many patients dying at advanced ages do not show any remarkable psychological or histological changes in their brains, suggests that these individuals are genetically adapted enough to reach old age with a relatively well maintained brain. We can speculate that the frequency of this adaptation in the population is conceivably low due to a still relaxed force of natural selection with aging (early humans seldomly lived longer than 40 years, and reproductive maturity is achieved long before this age). Furthermore, if these highly efficient maintenance systems are inherited in a polygenic fashion, as they probably are, the critical combination of relevant genes is hard to be fixed in a wide population base like ours. It follows that one might expect to find an accumulation of one or several, usual and unusual, DNA base derivatives and abnormal proteins in long-lived human cells such as neurons.

Mutations Accumulate Exponentially Over Time

The internal mutation rate is common both to the germline and somatic lineages so that the rate of accumulation of mutations that occur in the germline is shared by all somatic tissues. Studies of mutation rates in the human population have shown, as we would predict, that the number of mutations passed from one generation to the next is dependent on parental age and sex (Crow, 1993). What is not immediately predictable however is that the number of mutations is not a linear function of the parental age but rather a quadratic function. Thus, the accumulation of mutations appears to be exponential in the germline. The same has been shown to be true for mutations in somatic tissues (Martin *et al.*, 1996). Therefore, the rate of mutation selected to be optimal for species survival has direct implication for the survival of the individual since mutations will continue to accumulate exponentially beyond the reproductive age.

It has been argued that one of the factors that controls the mutation rate over evolutionary time is the development of aging or age-related diseases. If the mutation rate is too high one can assume that age-related dysfunctions may occur before puberty, thus hindering reproduction. In this model, mutation rates would be selected for or against, or simply go unselected, depending on the onset time of age-related diseases. A counter argument is the antagonistic pleiotropy theory of aging, which stands for the condition of a given gene or genes being beneficial during development, though detrimental after reproductive maturity is reached. The theory does not explicitly take somatic mutation rates into account to explain why "good" genes may turn out to be "bad" genes once a certain age or developmental stage is trespassed. Rather, the antagonism seems to be connected with programmed actions of inherited genes which have been selected for or against, or gone unselected, during development and early adulthood over evolutionary time, than with sporadic transformations as somatic mutational events are generally believed to be. Although changes in gene expression are well documented for particular stages during development, when the changes occur in a tightly programmed, cannonical fashion, information on age-dependent alterations in transcriptional and translational activities beyond developmental stages is scanty and conflicting. There is no consensus on any particular gene that could be otherwise termed a 'biological clock'. On the basis of genetic syndromes characterized by dementia or certain types of neurodegenerative conditions G. M. Martin calculated that as many as 2,350 genes could be involved only in brain aging. These include a large number of enzymes involved in metabolic pathways, housekeeping, free-radical scavenging, inter and intra-cellular transport, and DNA, RNA and protein synthesis. This complex situation would render aging of the individual an almost insoluble problem in biology, as once pointed out by Peter Medawar.

We favor the view that aging is largely driven by the accumulation of mutations and thus that aging is the unavoidable result of the method for controlling the mutation rate in evolutionary time. It is tempting to see this as a trade off in that age-related diseases are the cost that has to be paid to ensure the survival of the species. However, it is equally rational to argue that indeed the in built demise of the individual is also to the species' advantage in that it provides a direct and compelling stimulus for reproduction and reduces subsequent competition. Thus, aging and death may have been selected for and the associated diseases are not aberrations but the inevitable consequence of natural selection.

The Efficiency of Repair Systems is Variable

Differences in longevity (defined as age- and organ-specific resistance to failure), may lie primarily in the constitutive structure of DNA and the efficiency of DNA repair. Put in these terms, the interpretation of differences in longevity would favor the idea of a rather deterministic, programmable aging process. However, it is at present not clear whether repair systems may become less effective with age or under special circumstances. For example, the DNA repair process appears to be selective at the gene level (Hanawalt, 1991; Hanawalt *et al.*, 1992), with active genes being much more efficiently repaired than inactive ones (Bohr *et al.*, 1985; Madhani *et al.*, 1986), and at the organelle level. In eucaryotes, nuclear DNA (nuDNA) may be more protected than mitochondrial DNA (mtDNA), which not only lacks the protection of histones, but also suffers more directly the burden represented by oxygen free radicals (superoxide anion and hydrogen peroxide). The former evidence strongly supports the 'use it or loose it' paradigm, whereas the latter evidence favors the 'wear and tear' concept.

The question whether genetic instability is programmed or unscheduled or both is complicated by the observation that the occurrence of deleted mtDNA is apparently low in cardiac tissue of patients dying after the age of 80 (Hattori *et al.*, 1991). In the nuDNA of postmitotic mouse tissues, a twofold increase in the steady-state level of 7-methylguanine (presumably from endogenous sources) was correlated with aging from 11 to 28 months. However, the persistence of additional 7-methylguanines induced by N-methyl-N-nitrosourea did not increase with age (Tan *et al.*, 1990). In a series of normal aging brains, an abrupt decrease in the amount of total neuronal RNA (mostly ribosomal RNA) observed in the entorhinal cortex of patients dying at relatively young ages correlated with an increase in the incidence of abnormal proteins in the form of neuritic plaques (NP) and neurofibrillary tangles (NFT) at those ages, but no comparable change in RNA and incidence of NP and NFT was found at more advanced ages (Dani *et al.*, 1993). One possible interpretation for the above findings is that the level of the changes observed may reflect stages of an ongoing process, in that affected cells and organelles are eliminated if the lesions are irreversible, leaving behind relatively healthy cells which are often taken as an evidence that changes are mild at more advanced ages. If this interpretation is correct, then cell demise during development and senescence is to be viewed under the general scope of a continuum of changes by which a decrease in cell viability only becomes manifest after a threshold of expression is reached.

An important corollary of the above conclusion is that, while all living beings may invariably develop DNA lesions during the course of their lives, they may differ in relation to expression thresholds. Thus, while genetic instability may be a universal feature of life, threshold differences would give rise to differences. All available data are thus consistent with the view that the mutation rate of every species is tightly controlled. Control is at the level or repair of mutations that occur either due to intrinsic replication errors or external mutagens. That this multifactorial system is highly conserved from bacteria to man is a clear indication that repair systems are central to life, evolution, and aging. However, this does not imply that mutation rates are the same in every organism. Probably all organisms have slightly different mutation rates as is suitable for their requirements.

Cancer is by Far the Best Understood Disease Caused by the Accumulation of Mutations

There is increasing evidence that many, if not all, age related diseases are the direct result of the accumulation of mutations in the genome and also in mitochondrial DNA. By far the best understood of such diseases is cancer where the direct link between mutation and disease is irrefutable. Moreover, the disease depends on the accumulation of a series of mutations in the same cell lineage and thus would be expected to be extremely sensitive to fluctuations in mutation rate. Given the direct dependence of the disease on the accumulation of mutations it is entirely consistent that the incidence of the disease also increases exponentially with age (Vogelstein and Kinzler, 1995).

Some aspects of cancer may be worth examining from the viewpoint that it is a phenotypic manifestation of accumulated somatic mutation dependent on intrinsically controlled rates of mutation. Firstly, childhood cancers would immediately seem not to be well explained by this model and indeed do have a distinct etiology. In general childhood cancers are dependent on single genetic alterations and thus do not require the time needed for the accumulation of mutations in various genes. Secondly, many such malignancies are the result of translocations between chromosomes. There is evidence that such translocations are a reflection of a general increase in translocations in children which subsequently declines (Finette *et al.*, 1996). Thus, pediatric tumors are a special case which also conform to the view that cancer incidence reflects the underlying rate of mutation. Inherited predisposition to cancer also appears at first sight not to conform to the model proposed. However, it actually is nicely explained on this basis. As mutation accumulation is exponential, small alterations at the beginning of the process have profound effects later. The inheritance of a single pertinent mutation thus moves the curve of acquisition substantially towards younger ages. Moreover, the genes that are mutated in inherited predisposition may also directly influence the mutation rate and alter the shape of the curve. Thirdly, since the mutation is, in many cases, one that is normally observed in sporadic cancers, then its inheritance is a further factor reducing the age and increasing the probability of cancer in that fewer mutations are required.

The effect of environmental mutagens is also well explained from the point of view being propounded. Smoking for example causes an increased incidence of lung cancer. The massive exposure of lung tissue to the multitude of mutagens in cigarrette smoke will presumably increase the mutation rate in this tissue since the repair processes will not be able to cope with mutational load. In addition, the increased rate of cellular proliferation that results will also increase the accumulation of mutations over time. The effect of smoking can thus be envisaged to be the selective accelerated aging of the lung and the accelerated appearance of age related disease in this tissue with respect to the rest of the body. This manifests itself by an increase in lung cancer since the average age at which malignancy arises is brought forward relative to the age of incidence of other age related diseases.

Cancer Parallels Evolution

The intimate association between cancer and evolution can be extended further. Not only the cause of cancer, the mutation rate required for evolution, but also the disease process itself can be viewed in terms of neo-Darwinian selection. Since mutations are introduced into somatic cells at every division then all cells in the body have different genomes. Since it has been observed that the numbers of mutations increase exponentially with age the genetic differences between cells will also increase accordingly. Many mutations will have no or little effect on the cell's phenotype. Others will be so deleterious that the cell will no longer be functional and the lineage will die out. In other cases small deleterious effects will slow the rate of cell division. In a few instances the mutation will increase the rate of cell division and such cells will have a selective advantage in constantly renewing tissues. Such competition has been directly observed in fibroblasts in culture. Since the cell population is very large and has exponential potential then increased mutation rate will also be selected for indirectly as it increases the probability of producing cells with proliferative advantage. Thus during the life of the individual, the overall number of mutations will be increasing due to the selection of more vigorous lineages and also due to the selection of lineages with higher intrinsic mutation rates. The end point of this selection, due to the probability of the permutations of mutations, will be super cells with high mutation rates and proliferative indexes. We refer to such cells as being malignant. Thus, we can envisage the increasing overall mutation load of the body as going hand in hand with increasing genetic heterogeneity to the point where the average mutation load is no longer of importance as a single lineage has evolved to such a stage of selective advantage that it is distinct from the average. Once the threshold of malignancy has been crossed, lineage competition plays a more important role and defines tumor progression. The rate of mutation and proliferation is now so great that even direct attack in the form of chemotherapy can be adapted to by the selection of resistance clones within the tumor.

An immediate and important implication of the model of cancer as a somatic evolutionary process is that all tumors will be distinct even when they arise in the same tissue. The differences will be due to differences between the genotypes of individuals, the phenotypes of the cells in which they arise and the exact permutation of mutations present in the lineage. It is thus not surprising that tumor progression, morphology and response to therapy are highly variable and we have to talk in terms of risk and averages. Fortunately, some of the major genes that have strong effects have been identified and their mutation can thus provide broad guidelines as to what to expect from a given tumor. Nevertheless, even if two tumors were identical at a given point in time they would not be equally following the next cell division as new mutations will constantly be arising in an unpredictable manner. Thus, prognosis will always be based on probability and would have to be continually updated, as is the weather forecast.

One of the key contributions of the neo-Darwinian theorists was the proposal that overall phenotypic alteration is the composite of many discrete alterations which each having a very minor effect. An allied supposition is that of partial dominance where no genes are seen as being 100 percent dominant or recessive and that all mutations that alter protein structure or expression have some phenotypic effect. We can thus consider the mutations that are associated with cancer and which have been classified as recessive, in tumor supressor genes, and dominant, in oncogenes, in this light. Mutations in the tumor supressor gene *p53* clearly can be considered to have partial dominant effects. The mutation of one allele may produce aberrant proteins which may be necessary and sufficient to trigger cancer. Genes of the mismatch repair system may function in a similar way since there is direct experimental evidence showing an increase in replication error repair in the heterozygotic cells in the normal tissues of individuals carrying a mutation in one of such genes (Parsons *et al.*, 1995). This may function simply at the level of reducing the amount of functional protein in the cell thus reducing the cell's capacity to recognise and repair mismatched bases.

Postmitotic Cells Such as Neurons are also Vulnerable to DNA Damage and Genetic Instability

Neurons seem to be relatively protected against genomic mutations if compared to mitotic cells such as glial cells. However, neurons may be specially vulnerable to major agents of DNA damage such as free oxygen radicals generated within mitochondria. Due to their large sizes and high metabolic rates, neurons have to rely on high rates of oxidative phosphorylation (OXPHOS) to remain alive. OXPHOS genetics is complex because the genes for component peptides are distributed throughout both the nuDNA and the mtDNA. Because all mtDNA replication enzymes are encoded by the nucleus, it has been put forward that the rate of replication of mtDNA is directly proportional to the length of the molecule, so that deleted molecules may have a replicative advantage and consequently increase in number over time (Wallace, 1992a).

This mechanism would provide an explanation why even postmitotic cells such as neurons may be progressively enriched of deleted mtDNAs; as a corollary cell dysfunction and death would ensue after a tissue-specific threshold or limit for the accumulation of defective mtDNA is reached. Since genotypically normal people would start their lives with a high amount of normal mtDNA and die before most tissue thresholds are traversed, and individuals born with deleterious mutations would start with lower levels of normal mtDNA and cross expression thresholds within their life times (op. cit.), it is likely that what we call 'unscheduled changes' may be actually programmed, thus inherited, to a certain extent.

The question whether genetic instability in postmitotic cells is programmed or unscheduled or both is also complicated by evidence indicating that environmental conditions can be associated with increased secondary, thus somatic, damage to DNA. Recent studies suggest that hypertension and hypoxia are likely to increase the incidence of mitochondrial deletion mutations (Merril *et al.*, 1996) and NP and NFT incidences in the brain (Sparks *et al.*, 1993, 1995). The highly metabolically active, large neuronal cells are known to be extremely sensitive to hypoxia, and the evidence suggests that low oxygen is a strong candidate to cause or aggravate genetic instability in the brain. Further evidence for a role of environmental factors arises from the analysis of the pattern of onset of NP and NFT in the brain. An intriguing similarity has been found in the mean age of onset of NP and NFT between ethnically distinct groups of patients, indicating that neurodegeneration may be programmed to some extent (Dani *et al.*, 1994). Notwithstanding, the extent of the pathological changes, i.e., the percent of entorhinal cortex affected with NP and the percent of NFT-bearing neurons varied remarkably in a way suggesting that differences in brain-weight and corresponding differences in neuronal size-distribution may account for much of the differences observed in the extent of neurodegeneration (Chapter 19). Interestingly, that metabolism poses a constraint on brain size (Martin, 1981; Armstrong, 1983) and on longevity (Masoro and McCarter, 1991) has long been held. Furthermore, diet restriction is presently the only reliable model of life span retardation in mammals (Masoro *et al.*, 1991).

An Overall View

The genetics of aging is a complex one, a polygenic one, and highly influenced by environmental factors. Instead of thinking of it as a highly complicated form of simple segregative inheritance (segregative inheritance is surely the case in many syndromes presenting with age-related, though early onset phenotypes), we must study it in its own right. The major tenet here is that damage to DNA and its phenotypic expressions tend to accumulate over time. Thus, all the mutations that occur in the coding or control regions of functional genes may have small and cumulative effects on the complex somatic evolutionary process that is constantly taking place in all organisms, from the unicellular to the multicellular. This process, like evolution itself, is featured by an increasing mutation diversity.

By placing cancer and degenerative diseases firmly in the classification of age related diseases the notion of these conditions being preventable is questionable. Certainly the incidence of particular forms of cancer can be reduced where there is a clear etiological agent responsible for early onset. However, this reduction will be matched by an equal increase in other cancer forms or indeed other age related illnesses. Furthermore, the complexity and inexorable nature of the somatic evolutionary process both as applied to the incidence and progression of age related diseases is a major complicating factor in terms of the probability of successfully treating such diseases by any current methodology. Indeed, the argument put forward here suggests that the only effective way of reducing cancer and other degenerative diseases would be to reduce overall mutation rates by improving DNA repair. Thus, longevity may be linked with the capacity of the molecular-repair and turnover systems to care for the maintenance of a genetic make-up that ensures survivability and fitness to given environmental conditions for a given life span.

Selected Readings

Alexander, P. 1967. The role of DNA lesions in processes leading to aging in mice. Symp. Soc. Exp. Biol. 21:29–50.

Bohr, V. B., Smith, C. A., Okumoto, D. S., and Hanawalt, P. C. 1985. DNA repair in an active gene: removal of pyrimidine dimers from the DHFR gene of CHO cells is much more efficient than in the genome overall. Cell 40:359–369.

Bernstein, C., and Bernstein, H. 1991. Aging, Sex, and DNA Repair. Academic Press, San Diego, pp. 109–113.

Burnet, F. M. 1974. Intrinsic Mutagenesis: A Genetic Approach to Aging. John Wiley & Sons, Inc. New York, NY.

Failla, G. 1958. The aging process and carcinogenesis. Ann. N. Y. Acad. Sci. 71:1124–1135.

Holmes, G. E., Bernstein, C., and Bersntein, H. 1992. Oxidative and other DNA damages as the basis of aging: a review. Mut. Res. 275:305–315.

Lindahl, T. 1993. Instability and decay of the primary structure of DNA. Nature 362:709–715.

Randerath, K., Liehr, J. G., Gladek, A., and Randerath, E. 1989. Age-dependent covalent DNA alterations (I-compounds) in rodent tissues: species, tissue and sex specificities. Mut. Res. 219:121–133.

Roses, A. D. 1993. Molecular genetics of neurodegenerative diseases. Curr. Opin. Neurol. Neurosurg. 6:34–39.

References

Armstrong, E. 1983. Relative brain size and metabolism in mammals. Science 220:1302–1304.

Cleaver, J. E. 1994. It was a very good year for DNA repair. Cell 76:1–4.

Cleaver, J. E., and Kraemer, K. H. 1989. In C.R. Scriver et al. (eds.), The Metabolic Basis of Inherited Disease, 6th ed., pp. 2949–2971. McGraw-Hill, New York.

Crow, J. F. 1993. How much do we know about spontaneous human mutation rates? Environ. Mol. Mutagen 21:122–129.

Dani, S. U., Bergmann, B., Walter, G. F., Pittella, J. E. H., and Hori, A. 1993. A multivariate approach to the relationship between aging, RNA depletion and the incidence of plaques and tangles. Neuropathology (Kyoto) 13:243–249.

Dani, S. U., Pittella, J. E. H., Hori, A., Bergmann, B., Stan, A. C., and Walter, G. F. 1994. Different rates of neuronal degeneration: An exquisite variation of the cascade hypothesis. Dementia 5:110–118.

Finette, B. A., Poseno, T., and Albertini, R. J. 1996. V(D)J recombinase-mediated HPRT mutations in peripheral blood lymphocytes of normal children. Cancer Res. 56:1405–1412.

Gaubatz, J. W., and Cutler, R. G. 1978. Age related differences in the number of ribosomal RNA genes of mouse tissues. Gerontology 24:179–207

Hanawalt, P. C. 1991. Heterogeneity of DNA repair at the gene level. Mutat. Res. 247:203–211

Hanawalt, P. C., Gee, P., Ho, L., Hsu, R. K., and Kane, C. J. M. 1992. Genomic heterogeneity of DNA repair. Role in aging? Ann. N.Y. Acad. Sci. 663:17–25.

Jackson, S. P. 1996. The recognition of DNA damage. Curr. Biol. Genet. Dev. 6:19–25.

Madhani, H. D., Bohr, V. A., and Hanawalt, P. C. 1986. Differential DNA repair in a transcriptionally active and inactive proto-oncogene: c-abl and c-mos. Cell 45:417–423.

Martin, G. M. 1988. Genetics of aging and of disease models. In R.D. Terry, (ed.), Aging and the Brain. New York: Raven Press, p. 1.

Martin, G. M., Ogburn, C. E., Colgin, L. M., Gown, A. L., Edland, S. D., and Monnat, R. J. Jr. 1996. Somatic mutations are frequent and increase with age in human kidney epithelial cells. Hum. Mol. Genet. 5:215–221.

Martin, R. D. 1981. Relative brain size and basal metabolic rate in terrestrial vertebrates. Nature 293:57–60.

Masoro, E. J., and McCarter, R. J. M. 1991. Aging as a consequence of fuel utilization. Aging 3:117–128.

Masoro, E. J., Shimokawa, I., and Yu, B. P. 1991. Retardation of the aging process in rats by food restriction. Ann. N.Y. Acad. Sci. 621:337–352.

Merril, C. R., Zullo, S., Ghanbari, H., et al. 1996. Possible relationship between conditions associated with chronic hypoxia and brain mitochondrial DNA deletions. Arch. Biochem. Biophys. 326:172–177.

Pacifici, R. E., and Davies, K. J. A. 1991. Protein, lipid and DNA repair systems in oxdative stress: The free radical theory of aging revisited. Gerontology 73:166–180.

Parsons, R., Li, G., Longley, M., et al. 1995. Mismatch repair deficiency in phenotypically normal human cells. Science 268:738–740.

Paul, J., and Gilmour, R. S. 1968. Organ specific restriction of transcription in mammalian chromatin. J. Mol. Biol. 34:305–316.

Radman, M., Matic, I., Halliday, J.A., and Taddei, F. 1995. Editing DNA replication and recombination by mismatch repair: from bacterial genetics to mechanisms of predisposition to cancer in humans. Philos. Trans R. Soc. Lond. B. Biol. Sci. 347:97–103.

Rothstein, R., and Gangloff, S. 1995. Hyper-recombination and Bloom's syndrome: microbes again provide clues about cancer. Genome Res. 5:421–426.

Satoh, M. S., Jones, C. L., Wood, R. D., and Lindahl, T. 1993. DNA excision-repair defect of xeroderma pigmentosum prevents removal of a class of oxygen free radical-induced base lesions. Proc. Natl. Acad. Sci. USA 90:6335–6339.

Sommer, S. S. 1990. Mutagen test. Nature 346:22–23.

Szilard, L. 1959. On the nature of the aging process. Proc. Natl. Acad. Sci. USA 45:35–45.

Tan, B. H., Bencsath, F. A., and Gaubatz, J. W. 1990. Steady-state levels of 7-methylguanine increase in nuclear DNA of postmitotic mouse tissues during aging. Mutat. Res. 237:229–238.

Tice, R. R., and Setlow, R. B. 1985. DNA repair and replication in aging organisms and cells. In C. E. Finch and E. L. Schneider (eds.). Handbook of the Biology of Aging, 2nd edn., Van Nostrand Reinhold, New York, N.Y. pp. 173–224.

Vogelstein, B., and Kinzler, K. W. 1995. The multistep nature of cancer. Trends Genet. 9:138–141.

Wallace, D. C. 1992a. Mitochondrial genetics: A paradigm for aging and degenerative diseases? Science 256:628–632.

Wallace, D. C. 1992b. Diseases of the mitochondrial DNA. Ann. Rev. Biochem. 61:1175–1212.

Yu, C., Oshima, J., Fu, Y., et al. 1996. Positional cloning of the Werner's syndrome gene. Science 272:258–262.

Joseph L. Graves, Jr.

4

General Theories of Aging: Unification and Synthesis

'In almost any other important biological field than that of senescence, it is possible to present the main theories historically and to show a steady progression from a large number of speculative ideas to one or two highly probable, main hypotheses. In the case of senescence this cannot be profitably done.'

Alex Comfort, *The Biology of Senescence* (1979)

'The chief purpose of this book is to argue that aging can now be regarded as problem that is well on its way toward a scientific solution.'

Michael Rose, *The Evolutionary Biology of Aging* (1991)

To say that human beings have always been concerned with the causes of senescence and death is probably an understatement. Christian mythology begins with the tale of how human death resulted from the original sin of tasting from the fruit of the tree of knowledge. Genesis describes antediluvian patriarchs that lived for 900 years: Methuselah, Moses, Noah, etc. Western African mythology describes how human death was brought into the world from external sources (Mbiti, 1989). The pre-scientific study of longevity and mortality is also ancient. Egyptian physicians recorded the maximum human life span at 110 years, with specific individuals described as living into their 80's (Wilder-Smith, 1993). Genesis reports the life span for the Generations of Adam in the hundreds of years (Methuselah > 900 years). However, Psalms suggests that the maximum human life span was 70 years (the days of our lives are threescore and ten and if by reason of strength they be fourscore). Records from

relationship of various disease conditions to antagonistic pleiotropy and mutation accumulation mechanisms. It would seem that there will be little or no penalty for the alteration of mutation accumulation systems, while antagonistic pleiotropy on the other hand, may prove to have more difficult and intractable consequences. For example, somatic cell therapy might work well in either case; but if germ line techniques are ever developed to deal with aging phenomena, the early life impacts of genes that have antagonistic pleiotropy would have to be assessed. The study of this problem must begin with the type of large scale evolutionary and quantitative genetic experiments that are now possible utilizing organisms such as *Drosophila, C. elegans,* or *Saccharomyces.*

Aging as a Polygenic Phenomenon

The antagonistic pleiotropy and mutation accumulation hypotheses indicate that there should be a large number of loci involved in aging (Medawar, 1952; Williams, 1957; Hamilton, 1966; Charlesworth, 1980; Rose, 1985; Graves and Rose, 1989; Rose, 1990, 1991). In fact, if aging is defined as the age-specific decline in fitness, then almost every locus has some impact on the process of senescence. Further difficulty arises from the fact that quantitative traits are quite sensitive to gene x environment interactions. This makes practical attempts to identify such loci fraught with experimental difficulties. The key then is to attempt to quantify major and minor effects of various loci on senescence (this might vary greatly phylogenetically and even within the same species due to gene x environment interaction). Having said this I shall briefly review what we currently think about the quantitative genetics of aging.

The work by Luckinbill and colleagues (1987) was an early biometrical attempt to quantify the number of loci involved with the production of postponed senescence in *Drosophila melanogaster* stocks selected for postponed senescence. This study indicated that there was only one or a few major loci involved in the differentiation of these stocks (in violation of the central prediction of the polygenic inheritance pattern observed for aging). The quantitative genetic analysis contained in Luckinbill and colleagues (1988) and Hutchinson and Rose (1990) however strongly contradicted this result. Utilizing the classical genetic technique of constructing chromosome substitution lines, Luckinbill and colleagues (1988) found major effects on longevity arising from chromosome 1, 3 and a significant 2×3 interaction, indicating *epistasis* (epi- + Greek *stasis*, position = the concealing of one hereditary character by another superposed upon it). Further demonstrations of epistatic impacts on the production of the postponed aging phenotype were given by Arking and colleagues (1994). Utilizing the same stocks as did Luckinbill and colleagues (1988), they demonstrated an epistatic effect on the expression of ADH (*alcohol dehydrogenase,* enzyme crucial to fly survival). Stocks that had chromosome 3 derived from the long-lived strain, only showed one band for ADH, while those with a chromo-

some 3 from the short-lived strain showed three. Hutchinson and Rose (1990) utilized conventional quantitative genetic estimators for gene number, for traits including 24-hour fecundity, ovary weight, female and male starvation resistance, and longevity and demonstrated that a large number of loci must be involved in the postponed senescence response.

The polygenic character of aging is also supported by evidence at the molecular level. Fleming and coworkers (1993) examined protein differentiation between control (B) and postponed senescent (O) populations of *D. melanogaster* by use of two-dimensional electrophoresis. This study found that 321 proteins were resolvable per population, but that significantly smaller subset was consistently differentiated between the control and postponed senescence stocks, and that variation within lines was also consistently differentiated. *Maximum parsimony trees* were constructed that separated the populations by control v. selected and demonstrated a *homoplastic pattern.* The antagonistic pleiotropy hypothesis is supported by the fact that only a small fraction of the resolvable proteins was differentiated. This is consistent with the idea that some genes are pleiotropic, that is, having effects on multiple characters in the postponed senescent phenotype. Johnson (1994) suggests that the large number of loci involved in increasing life span in selected stock in *Drosophila* may simply result from increased heterosis in the long-lived strains. In a sense this could be problematic, if one wishes to champion the idea that genetic research should attempt to identify major loci impacting longevity. The importance of epistasis must be recognized, particularly in transgenic studies. I shall return to this discussion below.

Single Alleles with Major Effects: Longevity Assurance Genes

Roundworms

One prediction of classical population and quantitative genetics, would be that single alleles with large positive effects on longevity should be rare. Longevity in almost every species that has been examined follows the classic continuous distribution (as opposed to discrete) which follows from polygenic determination. This is consistent with the general requirement of alleles involved in the determination of quantitative traits. These loci should have small additive effects on the trait in question. The results from selection experiments for postponed senescent in *Drosophila* have tended to confirm that prediction. Johnson and Lithgow (1992) argue for another approach to identifying genes that may contribute to the extension of life span. This approach specifically searches for rare alleles that do seem to have a major impact on extending life span. This research has been mainly carried out in the nematode *Caenorhabditis elegans.* This invertebrate system has shown powerful results and great promise in regard to the analysis of aging (Johnson, 1987; Johnson and Lithgow, 1992; Johnson *et al.,* 1994; Jazwinski,

1996). *C. elegans* has been utilized for over 25 years for studies in development, genetics, and behavior. It has the advantage of possessing 959 somatic cells in hermaphroditic adults and 1031 in the facultative males (Johnson and Lithgow, 1992). Additional advantages for genetic analysis include the fact that they are small, have rapid life cycle, self fertilizing hermaphrodite, and lack inbreeding depression, amongst others. Johnson (1994) discusses some of the theoretical implications of these advantages, relative to other model organisms (in particular *Drosophila*).

Friedman and Johnson (1988) reported that in *C. elegans* the mutant allele *age-1(hx542)* increased the average life span 70 percent, while simultaneously reducing fertility in hermaphrodites (this depression is now known to be the result of a closely linked locus known as *fer-15*). The *hx542* allele was found by exposing strains of *C. elegans* that carried the *fer-15 (b26)* allele (which blocks fertility at 25°C) to the mutagen *ethyl methanosulphonate* (EMS). The effect of the age-1 locus has been shown to be most associated with an increase in post-reproductive life span (Johnson, 1987, 1994). In the *C. elegans* recombinant inbred strains and *age-1* mutants utilized by the Johnson group, developmental periods, and the length of reproductive period are uncorrelated to increased life span (Johnson, 1987). General motor activity is correlated with the increase in post-reproductive life span (Johnson, 1987, 1994). In addition, lipofuscin content and lysosomal enzyme levels are unaltered by *hx542* at *age-1* (Johnson, 1994). Despite that, worms carrying the *age-1 hx542* allele were simultaneously shown to produce elevated levels of anti-oxidants, and resistant to the toxic effects of *paraquat* (a herbicide that leads to generation of superoxide radicals). Johnson (1994) utilizing recombinant inbred strains formed by crossing N2 and Bergerac stocks has reported the mapping of the *age-1* and *fer-15* loci. The map positions on linkage group II in *C. elegans* were determined from left to right, *dpy-10*, *zP1*, *zP6*, *zP2*, *fer-15*, *zP5*, *zP7*, *age-1*, *unc-4*, *zP4*. The locus *dpy-10* is a marker for a dumpy, squat phenotype, and the *unc-4* stands for an uncoordinated rolling behavior. These map positions were determined by a combination of fine structure and deficiency mapping (Johnson, 1994). This confirmed the hypothesis that *age-1* and *fer-15* were separate loci, one impacting longevity and the other fertility.

These results beg interpretation under the two population genetic mechanisms that are consistent with the evolutionary theory of aging, mutation accumulation and antagonistic pleiotropy. The original reporting of the *age-1* locus (Friedman and Johnson, 1988a,b) suggested that the *age-1* locus had both the impact of extending life span and reducing fertility. This was interpreted as the discovery of a single locus that was capable of producing antagonistic pleiotropy. Subsequent analysis of this genetic region however, now reveals that there are two loci *age-1* and *fer-15*, which in the original stocks, happened to have alleles (*age-1, hx542* and *fer-15, b26*), which in combination produced both an increase in life span and a depression in fertility (the pattern predicted by antagonistic pleiotropy). It must be remembered that the alleles were

isolated after treatment with a mutagen, EMS. R. A. Fisher, in *The Genetical Theory of Natural Selection* (1930), pointed out that the vast majority of mutant alleles have deleterious impacts on fitness. Sewall Wright, and Motoo Kimura have modified this thinking slightly by pointing out that some subset of these mutations have neutral impacts on fitness. Taken alone, allele (*b26*) at *fer-15* depresses fertility, with no demonstrated positive impact on survivorship. Its frequency would be determined by simple selection/mutation balance. On the other hand, allele *hx542* at *age-1*, simply increases post-reproductive life span. This is problematic, in that the *hx542* allele is correlated with general motor activity and elevated resistance to anti-oxidants. However, these things seem to have no impact on fitness (reproductive values of *hx542* is equivalent to the wild type allele). Its frequency then would be governed by mutation accumulation, neutral impact on early fitness, and a positive effect on later survival. Thus, neither of these alleles alone would be expected to reside at high frequency in wild type *C. elegans* stocks. In fact, Johnson (1994) concludes from the results of the deficiency analysis that the *hx542* allele may be a null (no function). Here arises an interesting question for the genetic approach to analyzing the phenomenon of life span extension. What kind of genetic systems are we really looking for? Some alleles may extend life span, but do so in ways that only prolong a period of senescent decline. Or do we wish to find genetic systems that actually increase or maintain physiological performance at later age? The *hx542* allele at *age-1* actually is a candidate for both categories. Only subsequent analysis will tell.

Ebert and colleagues (1993) report the mapping of five quantitative trait loci that seem to be associated with aging in *C. elegans*, in at least two different environments, in non-interactive ways. These researchers utilized the same recombinant inbred strains as the Johnson group (Bergerac-BO x Bristol N2). They produced the strains for analysis by allowing an initial cross, followed by random mating for 4 generations, then finally inbreeding for seven generations. The resulting F_{10-12} worms comprised different chromosomal mosaics of the parental strains. The genotypes of young worms v. longest-lived worms were analyzed utilizing PCR (Polymerase Chain Reaction) with strain specific markers. This produced the chromosomal map of life determining genes in these stocks under the environmental conditions surveyed. The regions that were identified as containing longevity enhancing genes were LG-II, 30–42 cm's (area where *age-1* is found); LG-IV, 28–40, and at 44 cm's; LG-V, 26–28 cm's; and LG–X, 40–50.

Interpretation of these results was complicated by the fact that the original N2 and Bergerac BO strains had differential reproductive fitness in the breeding scheme. The hypothetical frequency of alleles originating from both stocks should have been around 50 percent; however regions were found in which the higher reproductive rate of the N2 strain biased the result. Interestingly enough, the authors did not recognize that when such N2 alleles were also regions that showed enhancement of the BO alleles in the longest lived population, that they were observing

analysis of the results relied on the fact that the temperature by treatment interaction term in the analysis of variance model, was not confounded by the effects of position or length of insert. Thus, in experiment 1, they found no significant effect of extra EF-1α on life spans of males with replication, a significant 30 percent increase in life span for females, a -93 percent early life fecundity, -77 percent total life time fecundity, -7.3 percent female eclosion weight, and no effects on time to eclosion or pupation. The second experiment, focusing on the effect of genetic backgrounds found weak significant effects of extra EF-1α on only life span of virgin males (+6.8 percent) and time to eclosion (-1.1 percent). The final experiment, examining the impact of insert position, only found a significant treatment effect for female dry weight at eclosion (-8 percent).

This experiment is of profound importance if we are to understand the general impact of transgenic research on our analysis of the mechanistic basis of aging. Here, the decline of elongation factor activity was correlated with the process of senescence in *Drosophila*. However, attempts to supplement flies with additional EF-1α, lead to contradictory impacts on various features of life history. These contradictory results depended on the nature of the experiment (lack v. adequate replication) or genetic factors (such as genetic background - epistasis, position effects, and gene x environment interaction). Thus extreme care must be taken, with the analysis of data from the use of transgenic manipulations to associate the action of any specific genes, with the postponement of aging.

For example, Seto and colleagues (1990) report that overexpression of Cu-Zn superoxide dismutase did not affect life span in *Drosophila*. P element mediated transformation was used to create five transformant strains of wild type isogenic Oregon R that differed in insert position. Four of these strains had inserts on chromosome 2R (48B, 49BC, 51AB, and 60B) and one on chromosome 3L (67AB). These were compared for SOD (Superoxide Dismutase) specific activity, paraquat resistance, and life span with a SOD null mutant Df(3L)lxd and the wild type strain. The tranformants differed in activity by insert position and were all greater in SOD specific activity than the wild types > nulls. However, despite that, the transformants were not significantly greater (or were worse) than the wild types in paraquat sensitivity and mean life span. The wild types were greater than the nulls, in both these assays. These assays were all conducted at 25°C. On the other hand, Reveillaud and colleagues (1991) utilized bovine Cu-Zn superoxide dismutase, under control of the actin 5C gene promoter, to show transformant lines with slight, but significant increases in life span. Here, the wild type strain was w67C23. Thus, genetic background and insertion effects would have been different from those experienced in the experiment above. Transgenic males showed significantly greater paraquat resistance, and 4 of the 5 transgenic lines showed greater mean life span. Orr and Sohal (1994) reported that overexpression of both Cu-Zn SOD and catalase lead to an increase in paraquat resistance and longevity in transgenic

stocks. The transgenic stocks carried three copies of *Drosophila* Cu-Zn SOD and catalase. They reported that in three of stocks there was an increase in median longevity and mortality rate doubling time. These stocks also showed a decrease in protein oxidative damage and a delay in the loss of physiological performance. However, they based their conclusions on data from the three most successful stocks. They actually report that of the 14 stocks that had a third copy of these genes added, 8 had no effect on longevity, and 3 actually had a negative effect! These results again underscore the types of complications which result from genetic background and insertion type effects as described in Stearns and Kaiser (1994). The differences between stocks may result from the fact that overexpression of these enzymes might cause other metabolic problems (Seto *et al.*, 1990); such as the generation of other forms of toxic free radical compounds ($^{.}OH$; or $^1O_2$). These impacts might be differentially tolerated depending on genetic background. Thus the data suggest that while free radical damage is important in determining some components of longevity, single or limited gene alterations, may not always be enough to ameliorate the impact.

Transgenic organisms have also been constructed to mimic normal facets of senescence in mammalian neural systems. Vickers and colleagues (1994) report results from transgenically constructed mice that express human neurofilament subunits. This study showed that mice from the transgenic line NF(M)27, which express the human midsized neurofilament subunit at low levels (2-25 percent of the endogenous NF-M), develop neurofilamentous accumulations in specific subgroups of neurons that are age dependent, affecting 78 percent of transgenic mice over 12 months of age. Similar accumulations did not occur in age-matched, wild-type litter mates or in 3-month-old transgenic mice. In 12-month-old transgenic mice, somatic neurofilament accumulations resembling *neurofibrillary tangles* (Chapters 19 and 20) were present predominantly in layers III and V of the neocortex, as well as in select subpopulations of subcortical neurons. Intraperikaryal, spherical neurofilamentous accumulations were particularly abundant in cell bodies in layer II of the neocortex, and neurofilament-containing distentions of Purkinje cell proximal axons occurred in the cerebellum. These pathological accumulations contained mouse as well as human NF subunits, but could be distinguished by their content of phosphorylation-dependent NF epitopes. The authors concluded that these cytoskeletal alterations closely resemble the cell-type-specific alterations in neurofilaments that occur during normal human aging and in diseases associated with aging. They thus suggested that these transgenic animals may serve as models of some aspects of the pathologic features of human neurodegenerative diseases. However, the results reviewed above from *Drosophila* research indicate that care must be utilized in suggesting the generality of this result. In particular genetic background effects might readily produce idiosyncratic results. Such results would limit the utility of any transgenic system for the study of 'normal' aging.

Physiology of Aging

Probably the most exciting results that came out of the early *Drosophila* research on postponed senescence, were the physiological performance of the late-life selected flies. It was clear from the examination of longevity and reproductive patterns in these stocks, that they seemed to be postponing senescence, rather than changing the sequence or temporal manifestation of these events (Rose, 1984; Luckinbill *et al.*, 1984; Arking *et al.*, 1994). These postponed senescent organisms showed improved general physiological performance over a range of adult ages (Service *et al.*, 1985; Service, 1987; Graves *et al.*, 1988; Graves and Rose, 1990; Graves *et al.*, 1992). There was also general agreement for the physiological characters that have been assayed in the stocks derived from the original geographic localities (Ives, Massachusetts, and NDCLA, Michigan; Graves and Rose, 1989). These studies found that the lines exhibiting postponed senescence were superior in a number of physiological performance and environmental stress resistance characters; amongst them were starvation, desiccation, and ethanol vapor resistance, and tethered flight duration. In addition, Service (1987) found that later spontaneous activity levels of postponed senescent stocks were greater than controls. This result is of particular importance for research concerning neural aspects of postponed senescence. However, to this point, the mechanistic basis of this result has not been examined. Subsequent genetic analysis showed that these enhanced performance and stress resistance characters have a negative genetic correlation with early-reproduction, as predicted by the antagonistic pleiotropy hypothesis (Service *et al.*, 1988; Graves *et al.*, 1992; Rose *et al.*, 1992).

It is noteworthy that not all the physiological systems examined were involved in postponing senescence. Service and colleagues (1985) and Rose and colleagues (1984) did not find any difference in heat shock tolerance or body weight between early-and late-reproduced selected lines. Arking and associates (1988), working on stocks derived from those used by Luckinbill and colleagues (1984), found no difference in metabolic rates at any point in the life cycle. Service (1987) used 5 replicate lines for both early- (B) and late-reproduced lines (O). He found that metabolic rates of early- (B) lines were higher during early life, 8 days past eclosion, than late-reproduced lines (O). At later ages the metabolic rates of the B and O lines had both declined, with both lines having equal rates at 22 and 35 days. The discrepancy between the Service and Arking results may have arisen from a real differentiation in these stocks, but could also have resulted from the considerably greater replication of the former study. If the differences in response to selection are real, then the absence of a change in early metabolic rate in the former stock argues against the predictions of the rate-of-living theory; argued originally by Pearl (1928). Additional evidence against this idea is supplied by a comparative analysis of Mammalian life histories with metabolic rates (Harvey *et al.*, 1989). When the effects of body size variation are re-

moved, then no consistent correlation between metabolic rate and mammalian life history variation can be discerned (although it has been extensively investigated). Indeed, the results of the *Drosophila* selection studies argue against the primacy of any one of the classic mechanisms of aging (Table 4–1).

Another example of the failure to adhere to classical mechanisms, was the fact that initially postponed senescent stocks showed no mean weight difference as adults (Rose *et al.*, 1984). This directly argues against the generality of the body size to life span hypothesis. Further evidence against this notion is supplied by comparative phylogenetic analysis on mammalian body weights (Harvey *et al.*, 1989). At the level of species variation within genera, only about 3 percent of life history variation is explained by body weight. The amount of variance explained at higher taxonomic levels is more significant (that is about 21 percent of the variance of families with orders, and 69 percent of the variance of orders within classes was explained). These studies show that all such correlations between morphometric or physiological characters, such as: body weight or metabolic rates and life history variables such as mean or maximum life span must be corrected for phylogenetic relatedness.

Comparative Evidence for the Physiological Uniformity of Postponed Senescence

Selection for postponed aging in *D. melanogaster* has revealed physiological systems that are correlated to postponed aging. Amongst these are starvation, ethanol vapor, and desiccation resistance, and flight duration. Subsequent experiments have worked out the discrete character of these physiological suites (Service *et al.*, 1985; Graves *et al.*, 1992). Starvation, desiccation, and ethanol vapor resistance, along with sustained flight duration are directly linked to the utilization of reserve substances. These physiological systems have been studied across the genus, and also throughout the order Diptera (Wigglesworth, 1972; Chippendale, 1978; Downer, 1978). *Drosophila melanogaster* utilizes both glycogen and lipid deposits during starvation (Wigglesworth, 1949). However, *Drosophila* utilizes only glycogen reserves during flight. The energetic basis of flight is thought to be uniform throughout the genus and order. Dipterans utilize glycogen as their primary flight fuel, as they have no anaerobic metabolism in the flight muscles, and thus the exhaustion of glycogen reserves means the end of flight (Wigglesworth, 1949, 1972; Chippendale, 1978). Previous studies on flight duration and physiology of aging carried out with *D. funebris* (Williams *et al.*, 1943) match subsequent studies in other species (*D. melanogaster;* Wigglesworth, 1949, Graves *et al.*, 1988; Graves and Rose, 1990; Graves *et al.*, 1992) and even in a non-Drosophilid, *Musca domestica* (Rockstein and Bhatangar, 1966). Some insect orders use both glycogen and lipid deposits for flight (Orthoptera, Lepidoptera, Hemiptera; Chippendale, 1978). Migratory insects face the problems of flight fuel, economy of weight, and water resources (Downer, 1981). Thus trade-offs are

the average and maximum life span of animals (here we should also include experimental manipulations such as selection for delayed reproduction, or transgenic organisms).

Rose and Graves (1989) presented the view that much could be gained for gerontological research by application of the general evolutionary theory of aging. Clearly, the population genetic mechanisms: mutation accumulation and antagonistic pleiotropy have great potential for explaining the prevalence of aging diseases in human populations. Werner and other progeroid syndromes (Chapter 30) would be governed by mutation/selection balance and be at low frequencies, while diseases like Huntington Chorea or Alzheimer could accumulate at intermediate frequencies due to genetic drift (mutation accumulation). Albin (1994) pointed out that the identification of antagonistic pleiotropy might be more problematic. In his article, he did not consider however, alleles that might have such high selective advantages that they are fixed in human populations. Such genetic systems would not overtly contribute to what we consider aging diseases per se, but might easily be considered part of 'normal aging.' Graves (1993) presented the view that oncogenes might be fixed in human populations, due to their role in normal development. Their expression at later age would be associated with various forms of cancer. Mutations in these systems, such as BRCA1 or BRCA2, or other early onset neoplasms would be expected at low frequencies. In a similar fashion, systems as integral to metazoan function such as oxidative metabolism, can also be understood within the antagonistic pleiotropy framework. The oxygen paradox is described as the fact that oxygen is potentially toxic. Yet it is necessary for aerobes for immediate survival (positive effect on early fitness) and hazardous to their long term survival (deleterious late life effect; e.g., Sohal and Weindruch, 1996). Thus, the population genetic mechanisms, consistent with the evolutionary theory of senescence may also shed light on the nature of specific physiological systems that operate in senescence.

For example, the high metabolic rate of nervous systems, and their reliance on membrane bound phenomena seem to make them primary candidates for damage from oxidative stress through time. There is evidence that oxidative stress is involved in many aspects of neural aging (e.g., Felten et al., 1992; Nixon and Cataldo, 1994; Friedlich and Butcher, 1994; Matteson, 1995). Felten and colleagues (1992) hypothesized that the anatomical and metabolic deterioration of the dopaminergic (DA) nigrostriatal system with age occurred due to autodestruction by reactive oxygen intermediates derived from oxidative metabolites of DA. Fischer 344 rats were treated with a presynaptic agonist to diminish DA turnover and thus confer a protective effect. Pergolide mesylate, a potent D2 agonist with predominantly presynaptic action, when given in the diet (0.5 mg/kg/day) to male Fischer 344 rats from 3 months of age to 26 months of age, preserved the integrity of both cell bodies and terminals of the nigrostriatal system, partially reversed the age-related decline in DA uptake, and had no adverse effects on behavior or

postsynaptic DA receptors on striatal neurons compared with age-matched, pair-fed control rats. Nixon and Cataldo (1994), Friedlich and Butcher (1994) and Matteson (1995) all examined the role that free radicals might be playing in the degeneration of neurons in Alzheimer disease.

There is also strong evidence that oxidative damage is ameliorated by at least two of these experimental treatments: caloric restriction (Sohal and Weindruch 1996), transgenic organisms and selection for delayed reproduction (Reveillaud et al., 1991; Tyler et al., 1993). Graves (1993) has suggested that caloric restriction is simply a phenotypic manipulation that mimics the genetic trade-offs produced by antagonistic pleiotropy (lowers reproductive investments, favoring somatic maintenance).

Graves (1993) also raised the importance of hormonal cues in communicating the reproductive status of organisms. Both the antagonistic pleiotropy and mutation accumulation mechanisms require that the negative late life fitness impacts are accrued after the reproductive values of individuals begin to decline. Therefore, the late life negative impacts of individual loci escape the action of natural selection, by having some means of accessing the organism's reproductive environment. Again this hypothesis suggests that neuroendocrine mechanisms related to reproduction must be playing a crucial role in regulating gene expression responsible for senescence. Mobbs (1994) summarizes an argument for the role of *molecular hysteresis* involving glucose hormones, which is consistent with this scheme for neural systems.

An Overall View

The maturity of any science is judged by the ascendancy of its dominant paradigms. Gerontology, 20 years ago was in its adolescence, dominated by a series of disconnected mechanistic paradigms. The emergence of the evolutionary theory in the last decade has made the unification and thus maturation of this discipline possible. Success in unraveling the proximate mechanisms of senescence now only requires the successful integration of the ultimate paradigm, in the daily implementation of its subsidiary research programs. This synthesis is now well underway in some research arenas. We can anticipate greater progress in gerontology as the influence of the evolutionary paradigm grows.

Selected Readings

Beverly, S. M., and Wilson, A. C. 1984. Molecular evolution in *Drosophila* and the higher Diptera. II. A time scale for fly evolution. J. Mol. Evol. 21:1–13.

Charlesworth, B., and Williamson, J. A. 1975. The probability of the survival of a mutant gene in an age-structured population and implications for the evolution of life-histories. Genet. Res. 26:1–10.

Charlesworth, B. 1990. Natural selection and life history patterns. Chapter 3. in Genetic Effects on Aging II., Telford Press, Caldwell, NJ.

Clare, M. J., and Luckinbill, L. S. 1985. The effects of gene-environment on the expression of longevity. Heredity 55:19–29.

Cohan, M. C., and Hoffman, A. A. 1989. Uniform selection as a diversifying force in evolution: Evidence from *Drosophila*. Am. Nat. 134(4):611–37.

Fleming, J. E., Spicer, G. S., Garrison, R. C., and Rose, M. R. 1993. Two-dimensional protein electrophoric analysis of postponed aging in *Drosophila*. Genetica 91:183–198.

Giesel, J. T. 1979. Genetic covariation of survivorship and other fitness indices in *Drosophila melanogaster*. Exp. Gerontol. 14:323–328.

Jazwinski, S. M. 1996. Longevity, Genes, and Aging. Science 273:54–59.

Kern, M. J. 1986. Brain aging in Insects. In K. G. Collatz and R. J. Sohal (eds.) Insect Aging: Strategies and Mechanisms. Heidelberg: Springer-Verlag. pp. 90–105.

Lerner, I. M. 1954. Genetic Homeostasis. Oliver and Boyd. New York.

Rose, M. R., and Service, P. M. 1985. Evolution of Aging. Rev. Biol. Res. Aging. 2:85–98.

Rose, M. R., and Graves, J. L. 1990. Evolution of Aging. Rev. Biol. Res. Aging. 4:3–14.

Rose, M. R., Graves, J. L., and Hutchinson, E. W. 1991. The use of selection to probe patterns of pleiotropy in fitness characters. Chapter 2. Insect Life Cycles: Genetics, Evolution, and Coordination. Springer-Verlag, Berlin.

Rose, M. R., and Nusbaum, T. J. 1994. Prospects for postponing human aging. FASEB J. 8:925–928.

Service, P. M., and Rose, M. R. 1985. Genetic covariation among life-history components: The effect of novel environments. Evolution 39:943–45.

Sohal, R. S., and Weindruch, R. 1996. Oxidative stress, caloric restriction, and aging. Science vol. 273:59–63.

Stearns, S. C. 1976. Life-history tactics: A review of the ideas. Quart. Rev. Biol. 51:3–47.

Stearns, S. C. 1977. The evolution of life-history traits: A critique of the theory and a review of the data. Ann. Rev. Ecol. Syst. 8:145–77.

Stearns, S. C. 1983. The influence of size and phylogeny on patterns of covariation among life history traits in the mammals. OIKOS 41:173–87.

Stearns, S. C. 1992. The Evolution of Life Histories. Oxford University Press, New York.

References

Abrams, P. 1991. Fitness costs of senescence: the evolutionary importance of events in early adult life. Evolutionary Ecology 5:343–360.

Albin, R. L. 1994. Antagonistic pleiotropy, mutation accumulation, and human genetic disease. In M. R. Rose and C. Finch (eds.), Genetics and Evolution of Aging. Kluwer Academic Press. pp. 307–314.

Aristotle. De Longitudine et Brevitate Vitae. Trans. by G. R. T. Ross (1908), Clarendon Press, Oxford.

Arking, R., Buck, S., Wells, R., and Pretzlaff, R. 1988. Metabolic rates in genetically based long-lived strains of *Drosophila*. Exp. Gerontol. 23:59–76.

Arking, R., Dudas, S. P., and Baker III, G. T. 1994. Genetic and environmental factors regulating the expression of an extended longevity phenotype in a long-lived strain of *Droso-*

phila. In M. R. Rose and C. Finch (eds.), Genetics and Evolution of Aging. Kluwer Academic Press. pp. 145–160.

Ayala, F. J., Powell, J. P., and Dobzhansky, T. 1971. Polymorphisms in continental and island populations of *Drosophila willistoni*. Proc. Natl. Acad. Sci. USA. 68(10):2480–83.

Bacon, Sir Francis. 1645. Historica Vitae et Mortis.

Ball, Z. B., Barnes, R. H., and Visscher, M. B. 1947. The effects of calorie restriction on maturity and senescence with particular reference to fertility and longevity. Amer. J. Physiol. 150:511–519.

Bell, G. 1994. Pathogen evolution within host individuals as a primary cause of senescence. In M. R. Rose and C. Finch (eds.), Genetics and Evolution of Aging. Kluwer Academic Press. pp. 29–44.

Belt, E. 1952. Leonardo da Vinci's study of the aging process. Geriatrics 7:205–210.

Bishop, J. M. 1983. Cellular oncogenes and retroviruses. Biochemistry 50:301–354.

Bodkin, N. L, Ortmeyer, H. K., and Hansen, B. C. 1995. J. Gerontol. 50,B142.

Bozcuk, A. N. 1972. DNA synthesis in the absence of of somatic cell division associated with aging in *Drosophila subobscura*. Exp. Gerontol. 7:147–156.

Breitner, J. C., Murphey, E. A., and Folstein, M. F. 1986. Familial aggregation in Alzheimer dementia - II. Clinical genetic implications of age-dependent onset. J. Psych. Res. 20:45–55.

Carey, J. R. 1993. Applied Demography for Biologists: With Special Emphasis on Insects. Oxford University Press. New York.

Carey, J. R., Liedo, P., Orozco, D., and Vaupel, J. D. 1992. Slowing of mortality rates at older ages in large Med-fly cohorts. Science 258:457–461.

Chambers, K. C., McDonald, J. F., McElfresh, M., and Ayala, F. J. 1978. Alcohol oxidizing enzymes in 13 Drosophila species. Biochem. Genet. 16(7/8):757–67.

Charlesworth, B. 1980. 'Evolution in Age-Structured Populations.' London: Cambridge University Press.

Charlesworth, B. 1994. Evolutionary mechanisms of senescence. In M. R. Rose and C. Finch (eds.) Genetics and Evolution of Aging. Kluwer Academic Press. pp. 13–21.

Chen, J. B., Sun, J., and Jazwinski, S. M. 1990. Prolongation of the yeast life span by the v-Ha-Ras oncogene. Molec. Microbiol. 4:2081–2086.

Cheney, K. E., Liu, R. K., Smith, G. S., *et al.* 1980. Survival and disease patterns in C57BL/6J mice subjected to undernutrition. Exp. Gerontol. 15:237–258.

Chippendale, G. M. 1978. The functions of carbohydrates in insect life processes. In Biochemistry of the Insects. New York: Academic Press.

Chippendale, A. K., Leroi, A. M., Kim, S. B., and Rose, M. R. 1993. Phenotypic plasticity and selection in *Drosophila* life-history evolution. I. Nutrition and the cost of reproduction. J. Evol. Biol. 6:171–193.

Clark, A. G., and Doane, W. W. 1983. Desiccation tolerance of the adipose mutant[60] of *Drosophila melanogaster*. Hereditas 99:165–75.

Comfort, A. 1979. The Biology of Senescence, Third edition. Churchill Livingstone, Edinborough and London.

Crew, M. D. 1994. Genes of the major histocompatibility complex and the evolutionary genetics of life span. In M. R. Rose and C. Finch (eds.) Genetics and Evolution of Aging. Kluwer Academic Press. pp. 256–269.

Curtsinger, J. D. 1995a. Density and age-specific mortality. Genetica 96(3):179–182.

Curtsinger, J. D. 1995b. Density, mortality, and the narrow view. Genetica 96(3):187–189.

Darnell, J., Lodish, H., and Baltimore, D. 1990. Molecular Cell Biology. 2nd. Ed. W. H. Freeman, New York.

De, A. K., Chipalkatti, S., and Aiyar, A. S. 1983. Some biochemical parameters of aging in relation to dietary protein. Mech. Age. Dev. 21:37–48.

D'Mello, N. P., and Jazwinski, S. M. 1991. Telomere length constancy during aging of Saccharomyces cerevisiae. J. Bacteriol. 173:6709–6713.

D'Mello et al. 1994. J. Biol. Chem. 269:15451.

Dorman, J. B., Albinder, B., Shroyer, T., and Kenyon, C. 1995. The age-1 and daf-2 genes function in a common pathway to control the life span of Caenorhabditis elegans. Genetics 141(4):1399–1406.

Downer, R. 1978. Functional role of lipids in insects. In Biochemistry of the Insects. New York: Academic Press.

Downer, R. 1981. Energy Metabolism in Insects. New York: Plenum Press.

Ebert, R. H. II, Cherkasova, V. A., Dennis, R. A., et al. 1993. Longevity-determining genes in Caenorhabditis elegans: Chromosomal mapping of multiple noninteractive loci. Genetics 135:1003–1010.

Edney, E. G., and Gill, R. W. 1968. Evolution of senescence and specific longevity. Nature 220:281–82.

Egilmez, N. K., Chen, J. B., and Jazwinski, S. M. 1990. Preparation and partial characterization of old yeast cells. J. Gerontol. 45:B9–17.

Emlen, J. M. 1970. Age-specificity and ecological theory. Ecology 51:588–601.

Epstein, C. J., Martin, G. M., Schultz, A. L., and Motulsky, A. G. 1966. Werner's syndrome: A review of its symptomology, natural history, pathologic features, genetics, and relationship to the natural aging process. Medicine 45:177–221.

Etges, W. J., and Klassen, C. S. 1989. Influences of atmospheric ethanol on adult Drosophila mojavensis: Altered metabolic rates and increases in fitness among populations. Physiol. Zool. 62(1):170–193.

Felten, D. L., Steece, S. Y., Collier, K., Date, I., and Clemens, J. A. 1992. Age-related decline in the dopaminergic nigrostriatal system: the oxidative hypothesis and protective strategies. Ann. Neurol. 32 Suppl: S133–6

Finch, C. 1990. Longevity, Senescence and the Genome. The University of Chicago Press. Chicago.

Fischer, R. A. 1930. The Genetical Theory of Natural Selection. Dover, New York.

Fischer, R. A. 1958. The Genetical Theory of Natural Selection. Second Revised Edition. Dover, New York.

Friedlich, A. L., and Butcher, L. L. 1994. Involvement of free oxygen radicals in Beta-amyloidosis: An hypothesis. Neurobiol. Aging 15(4):443.

Friedman, D. B., and Johnson, T. E. 1988a. A mutation in the age-1 gene in Caenorhabtis elegans lengthens life and reduces hermaphrodite fertility. Genetics 118:75–86.

Friedman, D. B., and Johnson, T. E. 1988b. Three mutants that extend both mean and maximum life span in the nematode, Caenorhabtis defines the age-1 gene. J. Gerontol. Biol. Sci. 43:B102–109.

Fukui, H. H., Xiu, L., and Curtsinger, J. D. 1993. Slowing of age-specific mortality rates in Drosophila melanogaster. Exp. Gerontol. 28:585–599.

Gardner, M. B. 1994. Genetic control of retroviral disease in mice. In M. R. Rose and C. Finch (eds.) Genetics and Evolution of Aging. Kluwer Academic Press. pp. 232–242.

Geer, B. W., Dybas, L. K., and Shanner, L. J. 1989. Alcohol dehydrogenase and ethanol tolerance at the cellular level in Drosophila melanogaster. J. Exp. Zool. 250:22–39.

Gems, D. L., and Riddle, D. L. 1996. Longevity in Caenorhabditis elegans reduced by mating but not gamete production. Nature 379(6567):723–725.

Graves, J. L. 1993. The costs of reproduction and dietary restriction: Parallels between insects and mammals. Growth, Development, and Aging 57:233–249.

Graves, J. L., Luckinbill, L. S., and Nichols, A. 1988. Flight duration and wing beat frequency in short- and long-lived Drosophila melanogaster. J. Insect. Physiol. 34:1021–26.

Graves, J. L., and Mueller, L. D. 1993. Population density effects on longevity. Genetica 91:99–109.

Graves, J. L. and Mueller, L. D. 1995. Population density effects on longevity revisited. A note in response to 'Density and age-specific mortality' by J. W. Curtsinger. Genetica 96:183–186.

Graves, J. L., and Rose, M. R. 1989. Population genetics of senescence in Drosophila. Genet. (Life. Sci. Adv.) 8:45–55.

Graves, J. L., and Rose, M. R. 1990. Flight duration in Drosophila melanogaster selected for postponed senescence. Chapter 5. in Genetic Effects on Aging II., Telford Press, Caldwell, NJ.

Graves, J. L., Toolson, E., Jeong, C. M., Vu, L. N., and Rose, M. R. 1992. Desiccation, flight, glycogen and postponed senescence in Drosophila melanogaster. Physiol. Zool. 65(2):268–286.

Haines, J. L., St George-Hyslop, P., Polinsky, R., et al. 1990. Linkage Analysis in Alzheimer's Disease. In Genetic Effects on Aging II., Telford Press, Caldwell, NJ. Chapter 31, pp. 557–569.

Haldane, J. B. S. 1941. New Paths in Genetics. Allen and Urwin, London.

Hall, J. M. et al. 1990. Science 250, 1684.

Hamilton, W. D. 1966. The moulding of senescence by natural selection. J. Theor. Biol. 12:12–45.

Harrison, D. E., and Archer, J. R. 1990. Commentary - Natural selection for extended longevity from food restriction. In Genetic Effects on Aging II., Telford Press, Caldwell, NJ. Chapter 16, pp. 275–278.

Harvey, P. H, Read, A. F., and Promislow, D. E. L. 1989. Life history variation in placental mammals: unifying the data with theory. In P. Harvey and L. Partridge (eds.) Oxford Surveys in Evolutionary Biology, Oxford University Press, New York.

Hawking, S. 1988. A Brief History of Time. Bantam Books. New York.

Hirakawa, T., and Ruley, H. E. 1988. Rescue of cells from ras oncogene-induced growth arrest by a second, complementing, oncogene. Proc. Natl. Acad. Sci. USA 85:1519–1523.

Holehan, A. M., and Merry, B. J. 1986. The experimental manipulation of aging by diet. Biol. Rev. Camb. Phil. Soc. 61:329–368.

Holliday, R. 1989. Food, reproduction, and longevity: is the extended life span of caloric restricted animals an evolutionary adaptation? BioEssays 10:125–127.

Holliday, R. 1994. Longevity and Fecundity in eutherian mammals. In M. R. Rose and C. Finch (eds.) Genetics and Evolution of Aging. Kluwer Academic Press. pp. 217–225.

Hovemann, B. S., Richter, S., Walldorf, U., and Cziepluch, C. 1988. Two genes encode related cytoplasmic elongation factors EF-1α in Drosophila melanogaster with continuous and stage specific expression. Nucleic Acid Research 16:3175–94.

Hutchinson, E. W., and Rose, M. R. 1990. Quantitative genetic analysis of postponed aging in *Drosophila melanogaster*. In Genetic Effects on Aging II., Telford Press, Caldwell, NJ. Chapter 6, pp. 65–85.

Ingram, D. K., Cutler, R. G., Weindruch, R. *et al.* 1990. Dietary restriction and aging: The initiation of a primate study. J. Gerontol.: Biol. Sci. 45(5):B148–163.

Jazwinski, S. M. 1993. Genes of youth: Genetics of aging in baker's yeast. ASM News 59:172–178.

Jazwinski, S. M. 1994. The genetics of aging in the yeast *Saccharomyces cerevisiae*. In M. R. Rose and C. Finch (eds.) Genetics and Evolution of Aging. Kluwer Academic Press. pp. 54–70.

Johnson, T. E. 1987. Aging can be genetically dissected into component processes using long-lived of *Caenorhabditis elegans*. Proc. Natl. Acad. Sci. USA. 84:3777–3781. Johnson. 1994

Johnson, T. E., and Lithgow, G. 1992. The search for the genetic basis of aging: The identificatin of gerontogenes in the nematode *Caenorhabditis elegans*. J. American Geriat. Soc. 40:396–945.

Johnson, T. E., Tedesco, P. M., and Lithgow, G. L. 1994. Comparing mutants, selective breeding, and transgenics in the dissection of the aging processes of *Caenorhabditis elegans*. In M. R. Rose and C. Finch (Eds.) Genetics and Evolution of Aging. Kluwer Academic Press. pp. 83–95.

Kemnitz *et al.* 1994. Dietary restriction increases insulin sensitivity and lowers blood glucose in rhesus monkeys. Am. J. Physiol. 266(4):E540.

Kenney, R. A. 1989. The Physiology of Aging: A Synopsis. 2nd. Ed. New York Medical Publishers. Chicago.

Kenyon, C., Chang, J., Gensch, E., Rudner, A., and Tabitang, R. 1993. A *C. elegans* mutant that lives twice as long as wild type. Nature 366:461–464.

Klein, G. 1988. Oncogenes and tumor suppressor genes. Acta Oncol. 27:427–437.

Kuhn, T. 1970. The Structure of Scientific Revolutions. Second Edition. University of Chicago Press. Chicago.

Lane, M. A., *et al.* 1994. Am. J. Physiol. 266.

Lane, M. A., *et al.* 1996. Longevity and the genetic determination of collagen glycoxidation kinetics in mammalian senescence. Proc. Natl. Acad. Sci. USA 93(1):485–490.

Larsen, P. L., Albert, P. S., and Riddle, D. L. 1995. Genes that regulate both development and longevity in *Caenorhabditis elegans*. Genetics 139(6):1567–1583.

Laslett, P. 1985. Societal development and aging. In R. H. Binstock and E. Shanas (eds.), Handbook of Aging and the Social Sciences. Van Nostrand Reinhold, New York. pp. 199–230.

Leroi, A., Chippendale, A. K., and Rose, M. R. 1994. Long-term laboratory evolution of a genetic trade-off in *Drosophila melanogaster* I. The role of genotype x environment interaction. Evolution 48(4):1244–1257.

Lewin, B. 1994. Genes V. Oxford University Press, New York.

Lints, F.A., Stoll, J., Gruwez, G., and Lints, C. V. 1979. An attempt to select for increased longevity in *Drosophila melanogaster*. Gerontology 25:192–204.

Lithgow, G. J., White, T. M., Hinerfield, D. A., and Johnson, T. E. 1994. Thermotolerance of a long-lived mutant of *Caenorhabditis elegans*. J. Gerontol. 49(6):B270.

Lithgow, G. J., White, T. M., Melov, S., and Johnson, T. E. 1995. Thermotolerance and extended life span conferred by single gene mutations and induced by thermal stress. Proc. Natl. Acad. Sci. USA 92(16):7540–7544.

Luckinbill, L. S., Arking, R., Clare, M. J., *et al.* 1984. Selection for delayed senescence in *Drosophila melanogaster*. Evolution 38:996–1003.

Luckinbill, L. S., and Clare, M. J. 1985. Selection for life span in *Drosophila melanogaster*. Heredity 55:9–18.

Luckinbill, L. S., Clare, M. J., Krell, W. L., *et al.* 1987. Estimating the number of genetic elements that defer senescence in *Drosophila melanogaster*. Evol. Ecol. 1:37–46.

Luckinbill, L. S., Graves, J. L., Tomkiw, A., and Sowirka, O. 1988. A qualitative analysis of life-history correlates of longevity in *Drosophila melanogaster*. Evol. Ecol. 2:85–94.

Martin, G. 1990. Segmental and unimodal progeroid syndromes of man. In Genetic Effects on Aging II., Telford Press, Caldwell, NJ. Chapter 28, pp. 493–520.

Matteson, M. P. 1995. Free radicals and disruption of neuronal ion homeostasis in AD: A role for amyloid beta-peptide? Neurobiol. Aging 16(4):679.

Mayer, P. J., and Baker, G. T. 1985. Genetic aspects of *Drosophila* as a model system of Eukaryotic aging. Int. Rev. Cytol. 95:61–102.

Maynard Smith. 1962. The causes of aging. Proc. Roy. Soc. (London) ser B, 157:115–127.

Mbiti, J. S. 1989. African Religions and Philosophy 2nd. ed. Heineman, Oxford.

McCay, C. M., Crowell, M. F., and Maynard, L. A. 1935. The effect of retarded growth upon the lenght of life span and upon the ultimate body size. J. Nutrit. 18:15–25.

Medawar, P. B. 1946. Old age and natural death. Mod. Quart. 1:30–56.

Medawar, P. B. 1952. An Unsolved Problem in Biology. London: H.K. Lewis.

Miner, G. D., Richter, R. W., Blass, JP., *et al.* 1989. Familial Alzheimer's Disease: Molecular Genetics and Clinical Perspectives. Marcel Dekker, Inc. New York.

Miquel, J., Bensch, K. G., Philpott, D. E., and Atlan, H. 1972. Natural aging and radiation induced life shortening in *Drosophila melanogaster*. Mech. Age. Dev. 5:347.

Miquel and Philpot, 1986

Mobbs, C. V. 1994. Molecular hysteresis: residual effects of hormones and glucose on genes during aging. Neurobiol. Aging. Jul-Aug; 15(4):523–34.

Mueller, L. D. 1987. Evolution of accelerated senescence in laboratory populations of *Drosophila*. Proc. Nat. Acad. Sci. USA 84:1974–1977.

Narod, S. A., *et al.* 1991. Familial breast ovarian cancer locus on chromosome 17q-12-923. Lancet 338(8759):82.

Nee, L. E., Polinsky, R. J., Eldridge, R., *et al.* 1983. Family with histologically confirmed Alzheimer's disease. Arch. Neurol. 40:203–23.

Negus, N. C., and Berger, P. J. 1987. Mammalian reproductive physiology: Adaptive responses to changing environments. In H. H. Genoways (ed.) Current Mammalogy Vol. 1. Plenum Press, New York.

Nixon, R. A., and Cataldo, A. M. 1994. Free radicals, proteolysis, and the degeneration of neurons in Alzheimer's disease: How essential is the β-amyloid link? Neurobiol. Aging Vol. 15(4):463.

Orr, W. C., and Sohal, R. S. 1994. Extension of life-span by overexpression of superoxide dismutase and catalase in *Drosophila melanogaster*. Science 263:1128–30.

Parsons, P. A. 1980. Ethanol utilization: Threshold differences among six closely related species of *Drosophila*. Aust. J. Zool. 28:535–41.

Parsons, P. A. 1981. Longevity of cosmopolitan and native Aus-

Alvaro Macieira-Coelho

5

Structural Regulation of Gene Expression: Chromatin Reorganization

Chromatin Structure has Hierarchical Levels of Organization

    Chromatin is Thermodynamically Unstable

    The Nuclear Matrix is a Protein Framework With Which DNA is Associated

    Chromatin Structure is Important to Gene Expression, and Chromatin Structure Changes with Age

Chromatin Studies in Brain Cells Suggest a Loss of Conformational Flexibility of the Chromatin Structure with Age

Modifications in Chromatin may Account for Changes in Gene Expression as a Function of Brain Aging

Studies in Experimental Systems Indicated Reorganization of the Genome During Serial Cell Divisions

    Terminal Differentiation and Aberrant Gene Expression: a Mechanism of Programmed Cell Aging?

    Terminal Differentiation State of Proliferating Cells is Preceded by Chaotic Reorganization of the Chromatin

An Overall View

When the genetic code was deciphered, many biologists thought that DNA had revealed all its secrets. Another code though started to unravel when the elaborate folding of DNA in the nucleus began to be known.

Each diploid human cell contains some 6×10^9 base pairs (bp) of DNA, measuring 1–2 meter when extended, confined in a sphere (the nucleus) with an average diameter of 5–10 μm, depending on the metabolic activity of individual cell types. This implies an elaborate folding which is regulated, *inter alia*, by the structure of DNA (Crothers *et al.*, 1990), by DNA bound proteins, disulfide bonds, enzymes, and by the anchorage of this make-up to a protein matrix. In addition there are glycoproteins present (Zardi *et al.*, 1976) whose role is yet to be determined; since these molecules are highly charged, it is reasonable to think that they must also function as regulators of chromatin conformation.

Chromatin Structure has Hierarchical Levels of Organization

In general, at least three hierarchical levels of nuclear organization resulting from DNA folding are accepted although more have been postulated (Lima-de-Faria, 1983; Nicolini, 1983). The first level corresponds to the 10-nm 'bead-on-a-string' chromatin fiber that results from the repeating unit formed by two superhelical turns of the DNA double helix (145 bp) around a protein core formed by an octamer of two molecules each of H2A, H2B, H3 and H4 histones (Figure 5–1). The unit is called the *nucleosome*. Another histone (H1 in mammalian cells) binds to 20 bp of the linker DNA (DNA filament that connects two nucleosomes) to seal the two superhelical turns, forming a *chromatosome*. H1 is also involved in the maintenance of the higher order structure of chromatin. The number of base pairs of the repeating structure formed by the linker and the nucleosome, is called the DNA repeat length. The DNA repeat length varies, *inter alia*, with gene expression.

The second level of DNA high order organization, results from the folding of the 10-nm fiber into a 30-nm wide solenoid with a helical pitch of 11 nm and 6–8 nucleosomes per turn (Finch and Klug, 1976) (Figure 5–1). There is no complete agreement concerning the organization at this level (Walker and Sikorska, 1987). Finally the third level results from the further folding of the solenoid into supercoiled loops, each with approximately 10,000 bp of DNA, anchored at the periphery of the nucleus (Pardoll *et al.*, 1980).

A higher order of organization of the genome has been proposed at the level of the chromosome (Lima-de-Faria, 1983). According to this proposal 'a chromosomal field is defined as the system of interrelationships existing between the different DNA sequences, which results in the establishment of the order and hierarchy observed within the centromere-telomere segment'. Genes are classified as centrons, medons and telons depending on their position close to centromeres, median region or terminal near telomeres, respectively.

Chromatin is Thermodynamically Unstable

The elaborate packing of the DNA molecule is thermodynamically unstable and thus is in permanent folding and unfolding, movement and variance creating heterogeneity within the whole structure. The flexibility of conformation of this complex structure is crucial for gene expression by exposing to or covering DNA sequences from the action of molecular regulators of transcription. The flexibility depends upon several biochemical events that regulate the binding of proteins to DNA. One of these events is the covalent attachment of branched chains of ADP-ribose to nuclear proteins (*ADP-ribosylation*). It weakens the binding (mainly of histone H1) through an increase in the protein negative charge and probably also by distorting the chromatin structure through the presence of the long branched chain (Kanungo, 1980). *Acetylation* and *methylation* are two other biochemical reactions regulating protein-DNA binding; the former, decreasing the net positive charge, would also dissociate the binding whereas methylation would render the binding stronger through

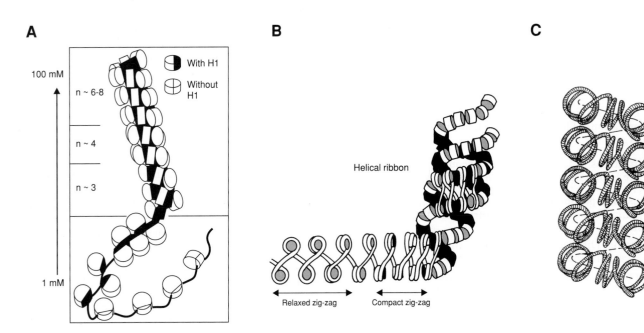

A

B

C

Helical ribbon

Relaxed zig-zag   Compact zig-zag

FIGURE 5–1

Histones are the proteins responsible for packing the DNA molecule in the form of heterochromatin. The histone subclasses H2-H4 form nucleosomes, most of which are packed into a 30-nm chromatin filament or fibre, which is then folded further. The filaments are stabilized by H1 histones, and form loops surrounding a central fibrous protein scaffold to which they are attached. This figure illustrates three models of the 30-nm chromatin filament.

In (**A**) and (**B**) the fully compacted structure is seen at the top of the figure and intermediate steps in the ionic strength-induced compaction are shown in the bottom part. (A) is from Thoma *et al.*, 1979; (B) is from Woodcock *et al.*, 1984.

C. Only the DNA path is shown and chromatosomes on the further side of the solenoid are ommitted for clarity. From McGhee, 1983.

Nuclear Protein Classes and Functions   BOX 5–1

1. Histones - comprise more than one half of chromatin mass, and about 90 percent of chromosomal proteins. They have a large proportion of positively charged residues and are involved in the packing of DNA into nucleosomes. Histone subclasses: H1 (helps pack nucleosomes together to form the 30-nm filaments), H2A, H2B, H3, H4.

2. Non-Histone Proteins:

2.1. Of the Ribonucleoprotein Matrix: *RNA processing proteins*; *RNA polymerases* (500,000 daltons or more), *proteins in hnRNP* (at least 10 different proteins of mass 25,000 to 120,000 daltons, which form a complex with growing RNA transcripts. Except for histones, they are the most abundant proteins in the cell nucleus).

2.2. HMG, *high-mobility group* (high-mobility proteins in electrophoresis); some are transcription factors. *Nu-*

cleoplasmin is a 29,000 daltons protein that acts as a molecular 'chaperone' to bring histones (H2A and B) and DNA together in a controlled fashion. *N1 protein* is present only in neurons, and binds to H3 and H4. *Lamins* are intermediate filaments that make up the nuclear lamina that supports nuclear membrane. *Topoisomerase II* belongs to the group of 'scaffolding' nuclear proteins. It relieves torsional stress and prevents the formation of tangles in the DNA molecule.

2.3. Other Classes of Non-Histone Proteins include structural proteins composing the nuclear matrix; proteins that prevent the binding of histones to DNA; proteins of the pore complex; DNA polymerases; and initiation/elongation factors that bind to polymerases

From: Alberts *et al.*, 1989; Voet and Voet, 1990; and Darnell *et al.*, 1990.

---

an increase of the positive charge. These two reactions seem to act mainly on nucleosomal core histones.

A fourth biochemical reaction controlling protein-DNA binding is *phosphorylation* which is the general mechanism used by the cell to vary the configuration of molecules and thus regulate their potential to intervene in metabolism and their response to different effector molecules. The regulation of molecular shape is fundamental for all cellular processes. The decrease of molecular and cellular conformational flexibility seems to be an important parameter of senescence.

The Nuclear Matrix is a Protein Framework With Which DNA is Associated

It is not only the biochemical modification of the DNA-bound proteins that influences gene expression, a tissue specificity of the proteins seems also required. A positive controlling effect on gene expression of non-histone proteins could be demonstrated when it was found that these proteins from erythropoietic tissue can cause transcription of the globin gene from brain chromatin (Paul and Gilmour, 1968), a tissue where this gene is not normally expressed.

The scaffold upon which chromatin is anchored plays a crucial role in the folding and conformation of DNA and thus on gene expression. There is indeed a protein framework (Box 5–1) called the *nuclear protein matrix* with which DNA is associated (Berezney and Coffey, 1975) (Figure 5–2). Nascent RNA was also found to be associated with the nuclear cage (Jackson *et al*, 1984). The *nuclear lamina*, a filamentous protein meshwork lining the nucleoplasmic surface of the nuclear envelope, seems to provide an anchoring site at the nuclear periphery for interphase chromatin (Gerace, 1985), since when the nu-

clear shell is isolated it contains chromatin structures made of packed nucleosomes 28–32 nm thick that are associated with the three nuclear proteins called lamins that constitute the lamina (Bouvier *et al.*, 1985).

The lamins seem to be intermediary structures between DNA-binding proteins and the cytoskeleton. Indeed on the one hand the lamina is tightly bound to chromatin since it can be dissociated from chromatin only by high salt solution which also extracts the tightly bound histones in the nucleosome cores (Bouvier *et al*, 1985). On the one hand, lamins have a striking sequence homology with *intermediate filaments*, a component of the cytoskeleton (Gerace, 1985) (Figure 5–2). Evidence in favor of the influence of intermediate filaments on chromatin conformation was reported by Hay and Deboni (1991) who showed that the disruption of intermediate filaments induces chromatin motion in neuronal interphase nuclei. So the anchorage of chromatin seems to be fulfilled with the preservation of the continuity with the cytoplasmic scaffold. This way DNA is linked to the cytoskeleton through its anchorage to the nuclear cage and via the former to the cell membrane and the extracellular matrix. This whole structure has to be seen as a tridimensional manifold where the information flows to a great extent through topological constraints. This flow of information is probably altered in the neurons of the aged brain because of the modifications occurring in their cytoskeleton.

Chromatin Structure is Important to Gene Expression, and Chromatin Structure Changes with Age

The control of genetic expression in eukaryotes is primarily exerted at the level of transcription. Because chroma-

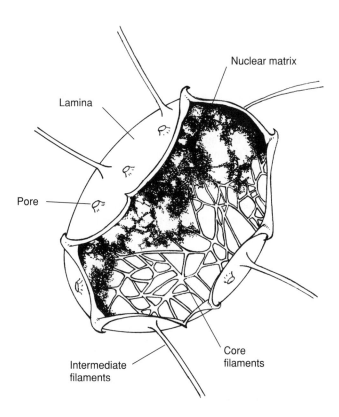

FIGURE   5–2
Schematic representation of the morphology of the nuclear matrix. Nuclear matrix can be prepared from cells directly, using buffers containing detergents, DNase and ammonium sulfate. The complex structure seen in the left hand side of this figure can be extracted with 2 M NaCl to reveal underlying core filaments (right hand side).

tin structure is different between transcriptionally active and transcriptionally inactive regions, it has been generally accepted that chromatin structure is important to gene expression. The chromatin in the transcriptionally active regions, also called *euchromatin* or *active chromatin*, is diffusely packed, as opposed to the densely packed *heterochromatin* or *inactive chromatin* in the transcriptionally inactive regions. Although densely packed chromatin is usually transcription inactive, RNA synthesis can proceed through nucleosomes (Alberts *et al.*, 1989). In order to the polymerase to gain access to DNA, a disruption of the nucleosome packing must be conceded, and therefore an initial chromatin decondensation step might be required before eukaryotic genes can be activated. As a result, the densely packed heterochromatin exists in two forms: The *constitutive heterochromatin*, which is permanently condensed, and the *facultative heterochromatin*, which is variably condensed. The study of the biochemical mechanisms involved in the formation of active and inactive chromatin might provide clues for the mechanisms of activation and inactivation of genes during aging (Box 5–2).

Chromatin Studies in Brain Cells Suggest a Loss of Conformational Flexibility of the Chromatin Structure with Age

The difficulty in studying the changes that occur in the chromatin of brain cells during aging is due not only to the unknowns concerning the exact organization of chro-

matin, but also to the presence of cell types with different functions.

The central nervous system (CNS) is composed of neurons and glial cells which are 10 times more abundant than neurons in the mammalian brain. Glial cell types include oligodendrocytes, astroglial and ependymal cells and microglia. Oligodendrocytes reach a postmitotic terminal differentiation state in the adult brain. Astrocytes retain the potential to divide and progress through the cell cycle at a very slow rate (Fedoroff *et al.*, 1990). Ependymal cells are low columnar ciliated epithelial cells that line the cavities of the CNS; they probably retain proliferative activity. Microglia are derived from precursor cells in the bone marrow and represent the mononuclear phagocytic system in nervous tissue (Junqueira *et al.*, 1995). Since no method has been devised so far to separate the different cell types, most studies, though not all, have been made on whole brain tissue and hence correspond to a very heterogeneous source of material representing not only the CNS cells, but also the cells from the blood vessels and capillaries. A few investigations though have attempted to analyse separately neurons and glial cells. One should not expect the chromatin of these cell types to be in the same state, since they have different functions and age at different rates. Hence it is difficult to ascertain the meaning of most studies performed so far, at most one can only guess.

The disturbance in the metabolism of the cytoskeletal network (Schröder *et al.*, 1983) allows for the assumption that the conformational flexibility of chromatin is decreased during aging, in the cells of the brain. In old brains the protein kinase and the adenosine triphosphatase activities associated with microtubules was found to be decreased. This concerns obviously the very fundamental mechanism of inducing changes in molecular conformation, i.e., phosphorylation. The modifications concerning the cytoskeleton explain also the excentricity of the nucleus frequently observed in the neurons of old brains, which again points to a decreased conformational flexibility of the chromatin.

The first approach used to analyze the state of chromatin (Hahn, 1963) has given repeatedly consistent results regarding the thermolability of DNA. The temperature needed to separate the two DNA strands increases with aging in the brain (Kurtz and Sinex, 1967; Zs-Nagy and Zs-Nagy, 1975). It was interpreted in terms of an increased binding of proteins to DNA. It could also be due to an increased number of cross links due to disulfide bonds which have been observed in other tissues (Tas *et al.*, 1980). The increased binding of proteins to DNA could have various causes among which the decreased phosphorylation of histones observed by Kanungo (1980).

Mechanisms of Formation of Chromatin

BOX 5–2

The total amount of facultative heterochromatin is very different in different cell types: embryonic cells seem to have little, whereas some highly specialized cells like neurons have a great deal. A further increase of the transcriptionally inactive fraction of neuronal chromatin has been reported during aging and degenerative dementia of the Alzheimer type (Crapper *et al.*, 1979), supporting the view that changes in chromatin structure and composition may play an important part in aging and senescence.

All this evidence suggests that, as cells develop and become old, progressively more genes can be packaged in a condensed form in which they are no longer accessible to gene activator proteins (Alberts *et al.*, 1989). In most mature cells about 90 percent of the chromatin is thought to be transcriptionally inactive, in the form of heterochromatin. Presumably the condensation of facultative heterochromatin functions to transcriptionally inactivate large chromosomal blocks. The condensate state renders the genes transcriptionally inactive by making the DNA inaccessible to the proteins mediating transcription. The phenomenon called chromosomal position effect in transgenic animals may be largely due to this property of heterochromatin: Variations on the expression of transferred genes into transgenic animals depend on the exact site where the transgene has inserted into the host animal's chromosome. This effect is thought to be caused not only by the need of specific distant sequences for quantitatively correct expression, but also by the level of neighbouring heterochromatin, which can spread to the transgene, inactivating it.

The mechanisms that form active chromatin - one of them is thought to be the supercoiling of the DNA molecule - are not well understood, but we know that active chromatin is biochemically distinct. Although the 4 nucleosomal histones are present in normal amounts in active chromatin, they appear to be unusually highly acetylated on lysines near their amino terminus. The acetyl groups are constantly being added to these histones by the enzyme histone acetylase and removed by histone deacetylase, and each acetyl group persists on average for only about 10 minutes. In addition, the nucleosomes in active chromatin selectively bind two closely related small chromosomal proteins, HMG 14 and HMG 17. Any of these changes might play an important part in uncoiling the chromatin of active genes, helping to make the DNA available as a template for RNA synthesis, but more direct experiments are needed to test this idea (Alberts *et al*, 1989).

Adapted from Alberts *et al.*, 1989.

Other biochemical reactions playing a role in changes in the conformation of proteins which are modified with age are acetylation and methylation (Kanungo, 1980). A decline of nonhistone chromosomal proteins has also been reported (Kurts and Sinex, 1967), and could also contribute to the lack of conformational flexibility of the chromatin structure.

Price and colleagues analyzed the incorporation of radioactive deoxyribonucleotide monophosphates into nuclei of neurons and astrocytes in sections of fixed mouse brain, in the presence of DNA polymerase. The increased incorporation in old mice brains was interpreted as the accumulation of DNA strand breaks. The same conclusion was reached by Chetsanga and coworkers and Wheeler and Lett with alkaline sucrose gradient; Hartnell and colleagues with alkali-induced DNA unwinding, and by Nakanishi and coworkers with immunofluorescence. In the latter antibodies against cytosine nucleosides were employed to examine DNA single strandness. On the other hand, Su and colleagues, Ono and coworkers, and Mullaart and colleagues could not find any evidence of DNA breaks in total brain preparations of *Mus musculus* and *Peromyscus leucopus* with the same alkaline sedimentation method.

Another work attempting to investigate what takes place in different cell types was performed in rat brain by Berkowitz and colleagues. A method was used that is claimed to separate cerebral cortical nuclei into neuronal and neuroglial. Cerebellar nuclei were used without fractionation since neurons outnumber the other cell types. It was reported that nucleosomal spacing increases dramatically with aging while neuroglial chromatin showed no change. Neuronal preparations were also more susceptible to digestion by micrococcal nuclease. However, Gaubatz and coworkers did not find any change in the size of the DNA repeat unit in whole brain preparations.

Kanungo and coworkers have used different approaches to ascertain the structural modification occurring in brain chromatin during aging (Chaturvedi and Kanungo, 1985; Mishra and Das, 1992; Singh and Kanungo, 1993). Nick translation reaction after digestion with DNase I and restriction enzymes indicated that rat brain chromatin undergoes increasing condensation as a function of age. The rate and extent of digestion by DNase I is lower in the old. Assays of template-engaged RNA polymerase II suggested that the increased condensation results in decreased transcriptional activity. A sharp age related decline of ADP-ribosylation of chromosomal proteins was also observed. Hill, however, could not find a decreased chromatin transcription in murine brain, when a homologous RNA polymerase was used.

So the modifications occurring with age in brain chromatin are as complex as the structure itself, which is not surprising. For the moment they have to be considered with restraint until the different cell types can be analyzed separately and the exact organization of chromatin will be ascertained. It is obvious however, that changes do occur that must reduce the functional capacities of the organ.

Modifications in Chromatin may Account for Changes in Gene Expression as a Function of Brain Aging

Cutler found qualitative changes in mouse brain RNA as a function of age. Certain new species of RNA appear in the old, and other species synthesized in the adult disappear. Ono and Cutler also found evidence suggesting a derepression of certain genes in the brain of old animals. Cytosine methylation could be an explanation for the derepression. An age-dependent loss of hybridizable ribosomal DNA from human cerebral cortex was also detected (Strehler and Chang, 1979). It was interpreted as a loss of ribosomal RNA genes. Gaubatz and Cutler, however, attributed it to the age-related increase in tightly bound proteins, since they could demonstrate a recovery of the hybridization of the probe with genomic DNA, after intense deproteinization of the DNA. Other possible causes of a decreased hybridizability are DNA-DNA cross links due to oxidized SH groups. These works concerning the loss of the hybridization signal have to be viewed under the general scope of the loss of hybridization described for different probes during cellular senescence (see below).

A gene that also seems to be affected in the brain, is the one coding for the calcium-binding protein calbindin-28K; the level of its mRNA and protein decreases with aging in different areas of the brain (Iacopino and Christakos, 1990). Epidermal growth factor mRNA also decreases in the brain of male mice; the decrease is of the order of 75 percent between 12 to 27 months of age (Gresik et al., 1986). Beta-nerve growth factor mRNA level increases up to 47 weeks and then decreases (Whittenmore et al., 1986). The astrocytic specific mRNA for glial fibrillary acidic protein increases with aging but that of glutamine synthetase which is also specific for this cell, does not change (Goss et al., 1991). Pro-opiomelanocortin mRNA levels decrease significantly in old age as well as the number of neurons expressing the gene (Gruenwald and Matsumoto, 1991). On the other hand the expression of beta-actin and beta-tubulin genes does not vary (Wismer et al., 1988).

Rats from various ages were submitted to stress either by exposure to 40°C or through restriction from mobility and the expression of a gene coding for a heat shock protein, the $hsp70$ gene, was analyzed. The expression of the gene was decreased after both stresses in the brain of the old animals (Blake et al., 1991). The expression of two oncogenes, c-fos and c-myc, was also appraised; in both cases the expression was increased (Kanungo, 1995).

Brains of old transgenic mice with segments of the promoter of the human transferrin gene fused to the bacterial CAT gene had a higher activity of this gene (Zakin, 1992).

With all the modifications taking place in chromatin through aging of the organism, it is not surprising that changes in gene expression do take place. The question remains, why are some genes affected and others not. It is reasonable to assume that some chromatin regions that are critical for the functioning of the organ are better preserved than others. It is possible that the chromatin modifications are random and diffuse and related not only to processes intrinsic to the chromatin structure but also to the modifications occurring elsewhere in the cell and in the cell environment. Chromatin, however, could be organized in such a way so that critical regions are protected through localized structural differences that minimize the disturbances in the functioning of the organ and prolong survival. For the moment we can only guess and await the development of new methodologies allowing the study of chromatin structure in situ and the analysis of what happens in the different cell types that constitute the brain.

Studies in Experimental Systems Indicated Reorganization of the Genome During Serial Cell Divisions

In the early 1960's an experimental system was proposed by Hayflick and Moorhead for the studies of aging of dividing cells that could constitute a reference to putative changes occurring in astrocytes. The system consists of human fibroblastic mesenchymal cells proliferating in vitro, which go through progressive modifications during serial divisions. With time the cell population becomes increasingly heterogeneous in the initiation of and in transit time through the division cycle (Macieira-Coelho et al., 1966). It has been suggested that these modifications evolve towards a terminal differentiation (Martin et al., 1974). Astrocytes in vivo evolve in the same fashion (Fedoroff et al., 1990). This evolution of the kinetics of proliferation results from the progressive modifications occurring in the genome during successive cell cycles with subsequent changes in cell function (Macieira-Coelho, 1988).

The first work suggesting a reorganization of the genome during serial cell divisions resulted from the measurement of DNA contents of mother cells and daughter cells at different population doubling levels (Macieira-Coelho et al., 1982). It showed that in a significant fraction of cells, DNA is not distributed symmetrically between daughter cells at each division. These findings were followed by the analysis of the physico-chemical properties of chromatin during serial cell proliferation of the fibroblastic population (Macieira-Coelho, 1991). It was found that chromatin becomes increasingly thermolabile so that the molecular weight of chromosomal DNA decreases in alkaline sucrose gradients when the cells were lysed at 37°C instead of 20°C. Chromatin also becomes more sensitive to strong detergents.

Attempts were made to detect eventual modifications in the different hierarchical orders of DNA structure (Macieira-Coelho, 1991). It was found that at the level of the

30-nm solenoid, the density of the chromatin fibers decreases progressively. The 10-nm fiber was investigated following its rate of digestion by micrococcal nuclease which cuts the fiber at the linker region (Dell'Orco et al., 1986). Digestion becomes faster with increasing population doublings. It could be attributed either to an increased heterogeneity of the DNA repeat length, or to a conformational modification.

Finally a decreased hybridization with chromosomal DNA of the probes for the alpha-globin and beta-actin genes but not for the beta-interpheron gene, could be demonstrated (Icard-Liepkalns et al., 1986).

Terminal Differentiation and Aberrant Gene Expression: a Mechanism of Programmed Cell Aging?

The possibility that a particular gene (or genes) may be activated after a certain number of cell divisions has been envisaged as a mechanism of programmed cell aging and senescence (Comfort, 1979; Finch, 1991). X chromosome inactivation (*Lyonisation*) of specific genes for example may be reversed with aging, with the reexpression of genes on the previously inactivated X (Wareham et al., 1987; Cattenach, 1974). Also a reduction in the methylation of DNA has been found with aging (Wilson and Jones, 1983; Mays-Hoopes, 1985; Goldstein and Shmookler-Reis, 1985), together with the finding that 5-azacytidine, a demethylation inducer, causes a decrease in DNA methylation and reduces the life span of cultured cells (Holliday, 1986; Fairweather et al., 1987). Provided that demethylation of DNA is correlated with increased transcription in eukaryotic cells, these findings suggest the occurence of nonprogrammed, aberrant changes of gene activity during aging (Holliday, 1987). However, this by no means implies that the overall gene expression in aging is always enhanced. Instead, an age-related lack of expression of a number of genes (Rittling et al, 1986; Chang and Chen, 1988; Warner and Wang, 1989; Shepherd et al., 1989; Seshadri and Campisi, 1990; Stein et al., 1991; McCormick and Campisi, 1991; Pang and Chen, 1992) seems to be common.

Terminal Differentiation State of Proliferating Cells is Preceded by Chaotic Reorganization of the Chromatin

Another reorganization taking place in the genome during serial proliferation concerns *telomere shortening*, has to be viewed under the general scope of the loss of hybridization signal described for different probes during cellular senescence. The loss of the hybridization signal can be due to loss of sequences, but can also be attributed to recombinations in the region, which will decrease the efficiency of hybridization. Indeed, telomere-promoted recombination can lead to degeneration of the telomeric sequence and subsequent loss of hybridization ability (Ashley and Ward, 1993). Apparent terminal deletions can in fact be subtelomeric translocations which are not detected by conventional methods (Meltzer et al., 1993).

Hence, although there seems to be a relationship in the human species between aging of proliferative cells and modifications in the telomere regions, the exact nature of these modifications are yet to be determined. They could be part of the reorganization taking place in the genome through proliferation, to which TTAGGG repeats seem particularly prone.

In vitro proliferation of the mesenchymal cell population evolves towards a terminal postmitotic state preceded by chaotic events (Macieira-Coelho, 1995). DNA partition between daughter cells becomes significantly skewed, heterochromatin decondenses, there is a profound disorganization of the 30-nm chromatin fibers mainly at the periphery in their relationship with the *lamina densa* and in the nucleoli, the nucleosomal structure unfolds in the presence of nonionic detergents, and extrachromosomal circular DNA becomes apparent. The structural reorganization of chromatin is accompanied by the repression of the expression of some genes and the derepression of other genes (Hara et al., 1993). This terminal cell observed *in vitro* is found *in vivo* only in pathological states (Macieira-Coelho, 1995).

It would be interesting now to ascertain if cell populations such as astrocytes which evolve similarly from the point of view of the kinetics of proliferation (Fedoroff et al., 1990) also go through the same structural modifications at the molecular level.

An Overall View

Several changes have been described in the chromatin of brain cells and in the expression of different genes, and a relationship of causality between both phenomena most certainly exists. However, due to the complexity of chromatin structure about which much uncertainties persist, and to the difficulty of separating the different types of brain cells, it is not yet possible to establish the specifics of the relationship.

Experimental systems developed *in vitro* allow extrapolations to what may occur in at least one type of brain cell. The coupling of molecular genetics with structural biochemistry may help uncover major mechanisms of macromolecular regulation. Studies on the changes of the nuclear matrix with age may yield important informations about the state of chromatin condensation and its relation to DNA, along with other nuclear features that presumably play a major part in the control of gene expression.

Selected Readings

Berkowitz, E. M., Sanborn, A. C., and Vaughan, D.W. 1983. Chromatin structure in neuronal and neuroglial cell nuclei as a function of age. J. Neurochem. 41:516–523.

Chaturvedi, M. M., and Kannungo, M. S. 1985. Analysis of chromatin of the brain of young and old rats by nick-translation. Bioch. Bioph. Res. Comm. 127:604–609.

Crapper, D. R., Quittkat, S., and De Boni, U. 1979. Altered

chromatin conformation in Alzheimer's disease. Brain 102:483–495.

Cutler, R. G. 1975. Transcription of unique and reiterated DNA sequences in mouse liver and brain tissues as a function of age. Exp. Geront. 10:37–60.

Dell'Orco, R. T., Whittle, W. L., and Macieira-Coelho, A. 1986. Changes in the higher order organization of DNA during aging of human fibroblast-like cells. Mech. Ageing Dev. 35:199–208.

Fairweather, D. S., Fox, M., and Margison, G. P. 1987. The *in vitro* lifespan of MRC-5 cells is shortened by 5-azacytidine-induced demethylation. Exp. Cell Res. 168:153–159.

Fedoroff, S., Ahmed, I., and Wang, E. 1990. The relationship of expression of statin, the nuclear protein of nonproliferating cells, to the differentiation and cell cycle of astroglia in culture and *in situ*. J. Neurosci. Res. 26:1–15.

Foe, V. E., Wilkinson, C. E., Laird, C. D. 1976. Comparative organization of active transcription units in *Oncopeltus fascialis*. Cell 9:131–146.

Fujita, S. 1965. Chromosomal organization as a genetic basis of cytodifferentiation in multicellular organisms. Nature 206:742–744.

Holliday, R. 1987. The inheritance of epigenetic defects. Science 238:163–170.

Kurtz, D. I., and Sinex, F. M. 1967. Age-related differences in the association of brain DNA and nuclear proteins. Bioch. Bioph. Acta 145:840–842.

Macieira-Coelho, A. 1991. Chromatin reorganization during senescence of proliferating cells. Mutat. Res. 256:81–104.

Newport, J. W., Forbes, D. J. 1987. The nucleus: structure, function, and dynamics. Ann. Rev. Biochem. 56:535–566.

Strehler, B., and Chang, M. P. 1979. Loss of hybridizable ribosomal DNA from human postmitotic tissues during aging. II. Age dependent loss in human cerebral cortex-hippocampal and somato-sensory cortex comparison. Mech. Ageing Dev. 11:375–382.

Westerhoff, H. V., and Van Workum, M. 1990. Control of DNA structure and gene expression. Biomed. Biochim. Acta 49:839–853.

Wijgerde, M., Grosveld, F., and Fraser, P. 1995. Transcription complex stability and chromatin dynamics *in vivo*. Nature 377:209–213.

References

Alberts, B., Bray, D., Lewis, J., Raff, M., Roberts, K., and Watson, J. D. (eds.) 1989. Molecular Biology of the Cell. Second edition. Garland Publishing, Inc, New York and London.

Ashley, T., and Ward, D. C. 1993. A 'hot spot' of recombination coincides with an intersticial telomeric sequence in the armenian hamster. Cytogent. Cell Genet. 62:169–177.

Bacon, Sir Francis. 1645. Historia vitae et mortis. Amsterdam, Theatrum Orbis Terrarum; New York, Da Capo Press, 1968.

Berezney, R., and Coffey, D.S. 1975. Nuclear protein matrix: association with newly synthesized DNA. Science 189:291–293.

Blake, M. J., Udelsman, R., Feulner, G. J., Norton, D. D., and Holbrook, N. J. 1991. Stress induced heat shock protein 70 expression in adrenal cortex, an adrenocorticotropic hormone-sensitive age-dependent response. Proc. Natl. Acad. Sci. USA 88:9873–9879.

Bouvier, D., Hubert, A. P., and Bouteille, M. 1985. Characterization of lamina-bound chromatin in the nuclear shell isolated from HeLa cells. Exp. Cell Res. 156:500–512.

Cattenach, B. M. 1974. Position effect variegation in the mouse. Genetics Research 23:291–306.

Chang, Z. -F., and Chen, K. -Y. 1988. Regulation of ornithine decarboxylase and other cell cycle-dependent genes during senescence or IMR-90 human diploid fibroblasts. J. Biol. Chem. 263:11431–11435.

Chetsanga, C. J., Tuttle, M., Jacoboni, A., and Johnson, C. 1977. Age-associated structural alterations in senescent mouse brain DNA. Bioch. Bioph. Acta 474:180–187.

Chrothers, D. M., Haran, T. E., and Nadeau, J. G. 1990. Intrinsically bent DNA. J. Biol. Chem. 265:7093–7095.

Comfort, A. 1979. The Biology of Senescence. Third Edition, Churchill Livingstone, Edinburgh and London.

Darnell, J., Lodish, H., Baltimore, D. 1990. Molecular Cell Biology. Second edition. Scientific American Books, New York.

Finch, C. E. 1991. Longevity, Senescence, and the Genome. Chicago, IL: University of Chicago Press.

Finch, J. T., and Klug, A. 1976. Solenoid model for superstructure in chromatin. Proc. Natl. Acad. Sci. USA 73:1897–1901.

Gaubatz, J., Ellis, M., and Chalkley, R. 1979. Nuclease digestion studies of mouse chromatin as a function of age. J. Geront. 34:672–679.

Gaubatz, J. W., and Cutler, R. G. 1978. Age related differences in the number of ribosomal RNA genes of mouse tissues. Gerontology 24:179–207.

Gerace, L. 1985. Structural proteins in the eukaryotic nucleus. Nature 318:508–509.

Goldstein, S., and Shmookler-Reis, R. J. 1985. Methylation patterns in the gene for the alpha subunit of chorionic gonadotrophin are inherited with variable fidelity in clonal lineages of human fibroblasts. Nucleic Acids Res. 13:7055–7065.

Goss, J. R., Finch, C. E., and Morgan, D. G. 1991. Age-related changes in glial fibrillary acidic protein mRNA in the mouse brain. Neurobiol. Aging 12:165–170.

Gresik, E. W., Wenk-Salamore, K., Onetti-Muda, A., Gubitts, R. M., and Shaw, R. A. 1986. Effect of advanced age on the induction by androgen or thyroid hormone of epidermal growth factor and epidermal growth mRNA in submandibular glands of C57 BL6 male mice. Mech. Ageing Dev. 34:175–182.

Gruenwald, D. A., and Matsumoto, A. M. 1991. Age-related decrease in propiomelanocortin gene expression in the arcuate nucleus of the male rat brain. Neurobiol. Aging 12:113–120.

Hahn, H. P. 1963. Age-dependent thermal denaturation and viscosity of crude and purified DNA prepared from bovine thymus. Gerontologia 8:123–131.

Hara, E., Yamaguchi, T., Tahara, H., Tsuyama, N., Tsurui, H., Ide, T., and Oda, K. 1993. DNA-DNA subtractive cDNA cloning using oligo(dT)-latex and PCR: Identification of cellular genes which are overexpressed in senescent human diploid fibroblasts. Analyt. Bioch. 214:58–66.

Harley, C. B., Futcher, A. B., and Greider, C. W. 1990. Telomeres shorten during aging of human fibroblasts. Nature 345:458–460.

Hartnell, J. M., Storrie, M. C., and Mooradian, A. D. 1989. The tissue specificity of the age-related changes in alkali-induced DNA unwinding. Mutat. Res. 219:187–192.

Hay, M., and Deboni, U. 1991. Chromatin motion in neuronal interphase nuclei - changes induced by disruption of intermediate filaments. Cell Motil. Cytoskeleton 18:63–70.

Hayflick, L., and Moorhead, P. S. 1961. The serial cultivation of human diploid cell strains. Exp. Cell Res. 25:585–621.

Hill, B. T. 1976. Influence of age on chromatin transcription in murine tissues using an heterologous and an homologous RNA polymerase. Gerontology 22:111–123.

Holliday, R. 1986. Strong effects of 5-azacytidine on the in vitro lifespan of human diploid fibroblasts. Cell Res. 166:543–552.

Iacopino, A. M., and Christakos, S. 1990. Specific reduction of calcium-binding protein (28-kilodalton calbindin D) gene expression in neurodegenerative diseases. Proc. Natl. Acad. Sci. USA 87:4078–4084.

Icard-Liepkalns, C., Doly, J., and Macieira-Coelho, A. 1986. Gene reorganization during serial divisions of normal human cells. Bioch. Bioph. Res. Comm. 141:112–123.

Jackson, D. A., McCready, and Cook, P. R. 1984. Replication and transcription depend on attachment of DNA to the nuclear cage. J. Cell Sci. Suppl. 1:59–79.

Junqueira, L. C., Carneiro, J., and Kelley, R. O. 1995. Basic Histology, pp. 162–164. Prentice Hall, Englewood Cliffs, New Jersey.

Kanungo, M. 1980. Biochemistry of Aging, p. 53. Academic Press, New York.

Kanungo, M. 1995. Changes in gene expression during aging of mammals, in A. Macieira-Coelho (ed.) Molecular Basis of Aging. pp. 183–218. CRC Press Inc., Boca Raton, Florida.

Lima-de-Faria, A. 1983. Molecular Evolution and Organization of the Chromosome. p. 376. Elsevier, Amsterdam.

Macieira-Coelho, A. 1988. Biology of Normal Proliferating Cells in Vitro. Relevance for in vivo Aging. pp. 94–134. Karger S. A., Basel.

Macieira-Coelho, A. 1995. The last mitoses of the human fibroblast proliferative life span. Physiopathologic implications. Mech. Ageing Dev. 82:91–104.

Macieira-Coelho, A., Pontén, J., and Philipson, L. 1966. The division cycle and RNA synthesis in diploid human cells at different passage levels in vitro. Exp. Cell Res. 42:673–684.

Macieira-Coelho, A., Bengtsson, A., and VanderPloeg, M. 1982. Distribution of DNA between sister cells during serial subcultivation of human fibroblasts. Histochemistry 75:11–24.

Macieira-Coelho, A. 1991. Dérégulation du flux d'information dans l'organisme. Comptes Rendues de Societ. de Biologie 185:110–120.

Martin, G., Spague, C. A., Norwood, T. H., and Pendergrass, W. R. 1974. Clonal selection, attenuation and differentiation in an in vitro model of hyperplasia. Am. J. Pathol. 74:137–154.

Mays-Hoopes, L. I. 1985. Macromolecular methylation during aging. Rev. Biol. Res. Aging 2:361–393.

McGhee, J. D. 1983. Higher order structure of chromatin: orientation of nucleosomes within the 30 nm chromatin solenoid is independent of species and spacer length. Cell 33:831–841.

McCormick, A., and Campisi, J. 1991. Cellular aging and senescence. Curr. Opin. Cell Biol. 3:230–234.

Meltzer, P. S., Guan, X. Y., and Trent, J. M. 1993. Telomere capture stabilizes chromosome breakage. Nature Genetics 2:252–254.

Mishra, S. K., and Das, B. R. 1992. (ADP-ribosyl)ation pattern of chromosomal proteins during ageing. Cell. Mol. Biol. 38:457–462.

Mullaart, E., Boerrigter, M. E. T. I., Brouwer, A., Berends, F., and Vijg, J. 1988. Age-dependent accumulation of alkali-labile sites in DNA of postmitotic but not in that of mitotic rat liver cells. Mech. Ageing Dev. 45:41–50.

Nakanishi, K., Shima, A., Fukuda, M., and Fujita, S. 1979. Age associated increase of single stranded regions in the DNA of mouse brain and liver cells. Mech. Ageing Dev. 10:273–280.

Nicolini, C. 1983. Chromatin structure: from nuclei to genes. Anticancer Res. 3:63–86.

Ono, T., and Cutler, R. G. 1978. Age-dependent relaxation of gene expression: Increase of endogenous leukemia virus-related and globin-related RNA in brain and liver of mice. Proc. Natl. Acad. Sci. USA 75:4431–4435.

Pang, H. P., and Chen, K. Y. 1992. A global change of expression of G1/S genes in IMR-90 human diploid cells during cell senescence (abstract). FASEB J. 6:A1782.

Pardoll, D. M., Vogelstein, B., and Coffey, D. S. 1980. A fixed site of DNA replication in eucaryotic cells. Cell 19:527–536.

Paul, J., and Gilmour, R. S. 1968. Organ specific restriction of transcription in mammalian chromatin. J. Mol. Biol. 34:305–316.

Price, G. G., Modak, S. P., and Makinodan, T. 1971. Age-associated changes in the DNA of mouse tissue. Science 171:917–920.

Rittling, S. R., Brooks, K. M., Cristofalo, V. J., and Baserga, R. 1986. Expression of cell cycle-dependent genes in young and senescent WI-38 fibroblasts. Proc. Natl. Acad. Sci. USA 86:3316–3320.

Ross, D. W. 1992. Introduction to Molecular Medicine. Springer-Verlag, New York.

Schröder, H. C., Bernd, A., Zahn, R., and Müller, W. E. G. 1983. Age-dependent alterations of microtubule-associated enzyme activities from bovine brain (protein kinase, adenosine triphosphatase). Mech. Ageing Dev. 22:35–50.

Seshadri, T., and Campisi, J. 1990. Repression of c-fos transcription and altered genetic program in senescent human fibroblasts. Science 247:205–209.

Shepherd, J. C. W., Walldorf, U., Hug, P., and Gehring, W. J. 1989. Fruit flies with additional expression of the elongation factor EF-1alpha live longer. Proc. Natl. Acad. Sci. USA 86:7520–7521.

Sing, S., and Kanungo, M. 1993. Changes in expression and CRE binding proteins of the fibronectin gene during aging of the rat. Bioch. Bioph. Res. Comm. 193:440–445.

Stein, G. H., Drullinger, L. F., Robetorye, R. S., Pereira-Smith, O. M., and Smith, J. R. 1991. Senescent cells fail to express cdc2, cycA, and cycB in response to mitogen stimulation. Proc. Natl. Acad. Sci. USA 88:11012–11016.

Su, C. M., Brash, D. E., Turturro, A., and Hart, R. W. 1984. Longevity-dependent organ-specific accumulation of DNA damage in two closely related murine species. Mech. Ageing Dev. 27:239–246.

Tas, S., Tam, C. F., and Walford, R. L. 1980. Disulfide bonds and the structure of the chromatin complex in relation to aging. Mech. Ageing Dev. 12:65–88.

Thoma, F., et al. 1979. Involvement of histone H1 in the organization of the nucleosome and of the salt-dependent superstructures of chromatin. J. Cell Biol. 83:403–427.

Voet, D., Voet, J. G. 1990. Biochemistry. John Wiley & Sons, New York.

Walker, P. R., and Sikorska, M. 1987. Chromatin structure, evidence that the 30-nm fiber is a helical coil with 12 nucleosomes/turn. J. Biol. Chem. 262:1223–1227.

Wareham, K. A., Lyon, M. F., Glenister, P. H., and Williams, E. D. 1987. Age related reactivation of an X-linked gene. Nature 327:725–727.

Warner, H., Wang, E. (eds.) 1989. Proceedings of the workshop on 'Control of cell proliferation in senescent cells'. Exp. Gerontol. 24:351–585.

Wheeler, K. T., and Lett, J. T. 1974. On the possibility that DNA repair is related to age in non-dividing cells. Proc. Natl. Acad. Sci. USA 71:1862–1865.

Whittenmore, S. R., Ebendal, T., Larkfors, L., *et al.* 1986. Proc. Natl. Acad. Sci. USA 83:817–822.

Wilson, V. L., and Jones, P. A. 1983. DNA methylation decreases in aging but not in immortal cells. Science 220:1055–1057.

Wismer, C. T., Sherman, K. A., Zibart, M., and Richardson, A. 1988. In R. Strong, G. Wood, and W. J. Burke (eds.) Central Nervous System Disorders of Aging. Chap. 4. Raven Press, New York.

Woodcock, C. L. F. *et al.* 1984. The higher-order structure of chromatin: evidence for a helical ribbon arrangement. J. Cell Biol. 99:42–52.

Zakin, M. M. 1992. Regulation of transferin gene expression. FASEB J. 6:3253–3261.

Zardi, L., Siri, A., and Santi, L. 1976. A serum protein associated with chromatin of cultured fibroblasts. 191:869–870.

Zs-Nagy, I., and Zs-Nagy, V. 1975. Age dependence of heat induced strand deparation of DNA *in situ* in postmitotic cells of rat brain as revealed by acridine orange microfluorometry. Mech. Ageing Dev. 4:349–360.

Steve Zullo
Carl R. Merril

6

Deletions of the Mitochondrial Genome and Neurodegenerative Diseases

Human mitochondrial DNA (mtDNA) deletion mutations have been found in a number of neurodegenerative diseases, including *Kearns-Sayre syndrome* (KSS), *Leber's hereditary optic neuropathy* (LHON), *Alzheimer disease* (AD), and *Parkinson disease* (PD) (Wallace, 1992; Beal, 1995), and with aging (Wallace, 1992). Abnormalities in mitochondrial metabolism likewise have been associated with neurodegenerative diseases, *e.g., Huntington disease* (HD) (Beal, 1995). In addition, a decline of aerobic energy metabolism in the affected tissue is often associated with the progression of these neurodegenerative diseases. A decline in aerobic metabolism has also been observed in aging tissues (Wallace, 1992), however, the source of these tissues has often been individuals who suffered from conditions associated with chronic hypoxia. The results from a study employing age-comparable individuals, suggest that conditions associated with chronic hypoxia may be an important factor in the occurrence of mtDNA deletion mutations (Merril *et al.*, 1996).

In the first described mitochondrial defect, a mitochondrial myopathy, the patient presented with an increased (150–200 percent of normal) basal metabolic rate despite normal thyroid function (Ernster *et al.*, 1959; Luft *et al.*, 1962). Since this description of *Luft disease*, over 100 diseases have been described in which a primary mitochondrial dysfunction has been implicated (Wallace, 1987). In this regard it should be noted, that as a result of the dual origin of mitochondrial components, diseases with seriously compromised mitochondrial function can be caused by errors in the nuclear genome and/or the mitochondrial genome. Thus, these diseases have been termed 'disorders of two genomes' (Shoffner and Wallace, 1990).

Mitochondrial Proteins are Encoded by both the Mitochondrial and the Nuclear Genomes

The complex mitochondrion contains hundreds of structural and functional proteins, most encoded by the nuclear genome. However, 13 proteins involved in the mitochondrial *electron transport chain* (ETC)-a component of *oxidative phosphorylation* (OXPHOS), are encoded in the maternally inherited mitochondrial genome, a circular 16.5 kilonucleotide pair (knp) molecule (Anderson *et al.*, 1981). The 13 proteins encoded in the mtDNA, are: 7 subunits of the NADH dehydrogenase (OXPHOS complex I); cytochrome b (a component of OXPHOS complex III); 3 subunits of cytochrome oxidase (OXPHOS complex IV); and 2 subunits of ATPase (OXPHOS complex V). The mitochondrial genome also encodes 2 mitochondrial ribosomal RNA subunits and 22 mitochondrial transfer RNA genes (Box 6–1). There are very few noncoding nucleotides, predominantly in the major control region which also serves as the origin of replication of the heavy strand, the strand is so called due to a greater number of adenines and guanines than are present in the complementary light strand. Replication of the light strand commences after 2/3 of the heavy strand has replicated, and the light strand origin has been exposed.

The brain is the body's most dependent organ system on aerobic metabolism, followed in order by the heart, kidney, liver, and muscle (Wallace, 1992). The mtDNA content of this subcellular organelle correlates with this aerobic dependency trend: 4.3 times more mtDNA per organelle in brain than in the heart, 1.86 times more mtDNA per organelle than in the kidney and 1.65 times more mtDNA per organelle than in the liver (Veltri *et al.*, 1990). These mtDNA levels may have evolved for rapid production of mtDNA-encoded OXPHOS subunits to constantly replace those subunits rendered inefficient or useless by oxidative damage and/or to counteract the effect of oxidative damage to mtDNA.

Highly reactive free radicals are often byproducts of mitochondrial metabolism. Free radical damage to the mitochondrial genome has been measured at 16 times the free radical damage to the nuclear genome (Richter *et al.*, 1988), contributing to a point mutation rate in this genome that is 17 times the point mutation rate in the nuclear genome (Wallace *et al.*, 1987). This correspondence suggests that free radical damage is an overwhelming contributor to mtDNA point mutations. In addition, a possible lack of DNA repair mechanisms and continuous replication, the mammalian brain mtDNA turnover rate is about 30 days (Menzies and Gold, 1971), may also contribute to the relatively high mutation rate. Indeed, it has been found that during replication of oxidatively damaged mtDNA by *Xenopus laevis* mtDNA polymerase γ, dA is incorporated opposite an abasic site most of the time and opposite a 7,8-dihydro-8-oxo-2'-deoxyguanosine (8-oxo-dG adduct) 27 percent of the time, thus regularly generating mutations (Pinz *et al.*, 1995).

Deletion mutations of mtDNA can be induced by environmental factors, such as mutagens or anoxia (Mayer and Legator, 1970). In addition, human nuclear gene mutations (Ballinger *et al.*, 1992; Bernes *et al.*, 1993; Ozawa *et al.*, 1988) and the aging process (Cortopassi and Arnheim, 1990; Ikebe *et al.*, 1990; Soong *et al.*, 1992; Corral-Debrinski *et al.*, 1992) have also been implicated in the occurrence of human mtDNA deletion mutations. Some of these deletion mutations may be enhanced via free radical damage as described above. Such free radical damage, resulting in mtDNA deletion mutations, may be enhanced by conditions associated with chronic hypoxia (Merril *et al.*, 1996).

Mitochondrial DNA Deletions and Disorders Affecting the Brain

The mtDNA[4977] Deletion is One of the Most Common of the Human mtDNA Deletion Mutations

Katsumata, *et al.*, (1994), using the polymerase chain reaction (PCR) and 180 primer pairs to detect deletions throughout the entire human mitochondrial genome, described 235 different types of mtDNA deletions. The human mtDNA[4977] deletion is one of the most common of the human mtDNA deletion mutations, occurring in 30–50 percent of the patients with disorders associated with mtDNA deletions (Wallace, 1992). This deletion mutation results from elimination of 4977 np between the directly repeated sequence, ACC TCC CTC ACC A, from np 8470 to np 8482 and from np 13447 to np 13459 in the human mtDNA sequence (Anderson *et al.*, 1981). The direct repeats contain 61.5 percent GC. Including the surrounding 12 np on either side, the regions are 54.1 percent GC, suggesting that these regions are subject to increased guanine adduct formation compared to the entire mitochondrial genome (44.4 percent GC). The mtDNA[4977] deletion encompasses the genes for subunit 6 of the mitochondrial ATPase (OXPHOS complex V), subunit 3 of cytochrome oxidase (OXPHOS complex IV), and subunits 3, 4L, 4 and most of 5 of NADH dehydrogenase (OXPHOS complex I), as well as a number of tRNA genes.

Mitochondrial genomes with the mtDNA[4977] deletion are found in a number of disorders associated with abnormal mitochondrial function (Holt *et al.*, 1988; Moraes *et al.*, 1989; Shoffner *et al.*, 1989; Schon *et al.*, 1989). Specific regions of the human brain have been found to harbor increasing levels of the mtDNA[4977] deletion with advancing age (Cortopassi and Arnheim 1990; Ikebe *et al.*, 1990; Soong *et al.*, 1992; Corral-Debrinski *et al.*, 1992). Although the number of subjects in all of these studies were limited and they suffered from other disease states as well, this increase had been attributed to advancing age. Regions of the brain rich in iron deposition (Corral-Debrinski *et al.*, 1992; Drayer *et al.*, 1986), and those regions having reduced glucose metabolism with aging (Chawluk *et al.*, 1990), appear to be most affected.

The mtDNA[4977] deletion may have a replicative advantage over the nondeleted molecule (Wallace, 1993).

Human mtDNA map showing the location of major disease mutations   BOX 6–1

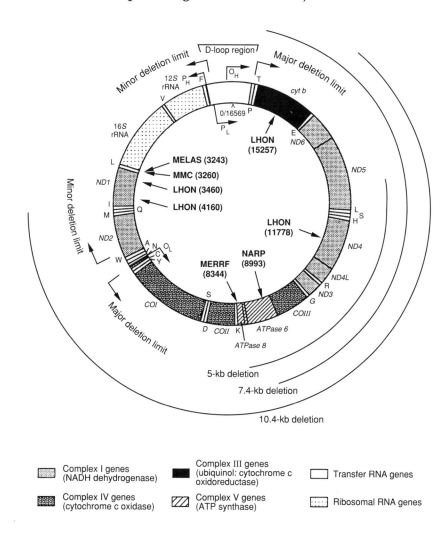

two-thirds of the way around the circle, displacing the parental H-strand. When O_L is exposed, L-strand replication initiates and proceeds counterclockwise back around the free parental H-strand. Transcription initiates at the H-strand and L-strand promoters (P_H and P_L, respectively) within the D-loop. The P_H promoter transcribes all genes but ND6 and eight tRNAs. The PL promoter directs transcription of these genes and synthesizes the primer of H-strand DNA replication.

Disease mutation base substitutions are shown inside the circle: MELAS (mitochondrial encephalopathy, lactic acidosis, and stroke-like symptoms), MMC (maternally inherited myopathy and cardiomyopathy), LHON (Leber's hereditary optic neuropathy), MERRF (myoclonic epilepsy and ragged-red fiber disease), NARP (neurogenic muscle weakness, ataxia, and retinitis pigmentosa). Deletion mutations are shown outside the circle. The nucleotide positions of the base substitution mutations are given in parentheses, and only the four primary LHON

Legend:
- Complex I genes (NADH dehydrogenase)
- Complex IV genes (cytochrome c oxidase)
- Complex III genes (ubiquinol: cytochrome c oxidoreductase)
- Complex V genes (ATP synthase)
- Transfer RNA genes
- Ribosomal RNA genes

Figure 6–1 shows the human mtDNA map. Nucleotides 0 to 16569 of the mtDNA sequence are numbered counterclockwise from the center of the D-loop. Shaded regions indicate the location of rRNA and protein genes (ND1-ND6, NADH dehydrogenase genes; COI-COIII, cytochrome c oxidase genes; ATPase, ATP synthase genes; cyt b, cytochrome b). These genes are punctuated by tRNA genes (clear sectors) whose cognate amino acids are indicated by the adjacent amino acid abbreviations: A, Ala; C, Cys; D, Asp; E, Glu; F, Phe; G, Gly; H, His; I, Ile; K, Lys; L, Leu; M, Met; N, Asn; P, Pro; Q, Gln; R, Arg; S, Ser; T, Thr; V, Val; W, Trp; and Y, Tyr. H-strand replication starts at O_H and proceeds clockwise

mutations are shown. The regions removed by the 5-kb (4977-np), 7.4-kb (7436-np) and 10.4-kb (10423-np) deletions are indicated by the external arcs. The outer limits for CEOP (chronic external ophtalmoplegia plus), KSS (Kearns-Sayre syndrome), and Pearson syndrome deletions are encompassed by the arcs bracketed by O_H and O_L. Most deletions occur within the major deletion limit, which extends clockwise in the direction of H-strand replication from O_H to O_L (positions 16085 through 5786). The remainder of the deletions occur within the minor deletion limit, which extends from O_L to O_H (positions 5448 through 470) and which can remove P_H but not P_L. From Wallace, 1992.

The deletion continues to possess both origins of replication (O_H, O_L) and is about 2/3 the size of the nondeleted mitochondrial genome. Due to the decreased size, along with the possible deletion of genetic down-regulation elements (Shoubridge *et al.*, 1990), replicative efficiency of the mtDNA[4977] deletion molecule may be increased over its non-deleted counterpart. The mtDNA deletion mutation may also metabolically compromise the mitochondria, leading to the activation of mitochondrial proliferation (Shoubridge et al., 1990).

We have chosen to highlight the association of mtDNA deletions in the brain and in neurodegenerative diseases with chronic hypoxia in this review. In addition, the reader is encouraged to consult recent excellent reviews concerning associations of functional and structural abnormalities of mitochondria with numerous diseases for further insight into mtDNA mutations and disease (e.g., Beal, 1995; DiMauro et al., 1990; Shoffner and Wallace, 1990; Wallace, 1987; Wallace, 1992; Wallace et al., 1995; Zeviani et al., 1989a). Some of the most common disease mutations are highlighted in the Box 6–1.

Kearns-Sayre Syndrome

Kearns-Sayre syndrome (KSS) is a disorder affecting organs highly dependent on OXPHOS, i. e., nervous tissue (cerebellar syndrome and high cerebral spinal fluid protein content), inner ear (deafness), retina (retinal pigmentary degeneration), external ocular muscles (external ophthalmoplegia), heart (complete heart block), skeletal muscle weakness, ataxia and diabetes (Kearns and Sayre, 1958; Kearns, 1965; Zeviani et al., 1988). Multiple mtDNA deletions that have been found in KSS include deletions from 2.0 to 7.0 knp (Zeviani et al., 1988), a 7767 np deletion from np 7669 to np 15437 between 8 np direct repeats (Heddi et al., 1994); a 7521 np deletion from np 7983 to np 15504 between 8 np direct repeats (Nakase et al., 1990; Mita et al., 1990; Zupanc et al., 1991); as well as the mtDNA^{4977} deletion (Nakase et al., 1990; Shoffner and Wallace, 1990; Shoffner et al., 1989). These mtDNA deletions are sporadic mutations. The mtDNA^{4977} deletion exhibited an autosomal dominant inheritance pattern in 7 KSS patients of 15 members in two generations of a family (Leveille and Newell, 1980). Additionally, a 9-year-old girl and an unrelated 11-year-old Chinese boy both presented with KSS compounded with mitochondrial encephalomyopathy, lactic acidosis, and stroke-like episodes, or MELAS (Zupanc et al., 1991). These examples exhibit the often complex manifestations of mtDNA deletions.

It is not known what proportion of deleted mtDNA can be tolerated before pathophysiological effects of these mtDNA deletions are manifest. Hybrids created from mtDNA-less HeLa EB8 cells and enucleated skin fibroblasts of a 14 year-old patient with clinical KSS exhibited mitochondrial dysfunction only when the mtDNA^{4977} deletion represented > 60 percent of the total mtDNA (Hayashi et al., 1991). Transcripts of genes within a 7767 np mtDNA deletion of a KSS patient were reduced in relation to the percentage of deleted mtDNA present in the tissue (Heddi et al., 1994). Although fusion transcripts were observed in lymphoblasts containing 30 percent deleted mtDNA from this patient, no apparent fusion proteins were detected. Either the fusion transcript was not translated, or post-translational enzymatic degradation eliminated the fusion protein. However, as cells in tissue culture are classically known to have abnormal OXPHOS

characteristics, it should not be assumed that this is a minimal level of mtDNA deletions needed for organ dysfunction to occur in vivo.

Alzheimer Disease

Wallace's group utilized PCR to reveal the levels of mtDNA^{4977} deletions in patients with or without Alzheimer disease (AD), under the age of 75 years and over the age of 75 years (Corral-Debrinski et al., 1994). While levels of mtDNA^{4977} deletions were 15 times higher in the cortical brain tissue from patients under the age of 75 years with AD than the levels found in age matched controls, the levels of mtDNA^{4977} deletion in cortical brain tissue from patients over the age of 75 years with AD was one-fifth the level found in controls (Corral-Debrinski et al., 1994). The levels of mtDNA^{4977} deletions in younger AD patients were fourfold higher than the levels in older AD patients. The implications of the higher levels of mtDNA^{4977} deletions found in the younger patients may be that the mtDNA^{4977} deletions are associated with an active phase of the disease process. If accumulation of mtDNA deletions impairs aerobic metabolism and cell survival, the accumulation of mtDNA deletions will lead to loss of the affected cells early in the disease process. Blanchard and colleagues (1993), in a study of 6 elderly (71–95 years old) AD and 6 age-matched individuals, also found that a slight increase in the mtDNA deletion levels from 0.12 percent mtDNA^{4977} in control brain tissue to 0.14 percent mtDNA^{4977} in AD brain tissue was not statistically significant. The results of these studies corroborate the conclusion of Merril and colleagues (1996) that factors other than aging, such as conditions associated with chronic hypoxia, may be important to the mtDNA deletion process.

Oxidative damage to both nucDNA and mtDNA in postmortem AD brain tissue was increased over that found in normal brain tissue, as measured by the guanine adduct, 8-oxo-dG (Mecocci et al., 1994). The mtDNA from the AD brain contained 3-fold more 8-oxo-dG than the mtDNA from the normal brain, while the nucDNA values demonstrated slight significance. This suggests that mitochondrial dysfunction, indicated by the oxidative damage to mtDNA, may be an important factor in AD complications.

Parkinson Disease

Ozawa and colleagues (1990) found that the mtDNA^{4977} deletion level increased over 10-fold in the striatum of a 73 year old female Parkinson disease (PD) patient when compared with the mtDNA^{4977} deletion level in the striatum of a 38 year old male who died an accidental death, 5 percent of the total mtDNA versus 0.3 percent, respectively. Ozawa's group expanded their study (Ikebe et al., 1990), including 5 PD striata and 6 control striata, finding the mtDNA^{4977} deletion increased in the PD striata relative to normal striata. However, the increase in the frontal cortex was smaller, implicating a relationship between the degeneration of the nigrostriatal pathway in the brain of PD sufferers and the mtDNA^{4977} deletion level in PD striata.

Chronic Hypoxia and Central Nervous System Disease

There is increasingly convincing evidence that chronic hypoxia and CNS disease are strongly linked. Neuropsychological performance deficits were strongly correlated with the severity of hypoxemia in patients with chronic obstructive pulmonary disease (Grant et al., 1982; Pritgatano et al., 1983). In addition, Sparks and colleagues (1993) observed that senile plaques, one of the most consistent features of AD (Chapter 19), increased in patients who had greater than 75 percent obstruction of a coronary artery or occlusion of at least one major coronary artery. Likewise, women suffered a five-fold increase in the occurrence of dementia if they had a history of myocardial infarction (Aronson et al., 1990). Sparks and colleagues (1994) fed rabbits a diet high in cholesterol, commonly thought to increase arterial occlusions and thus chronic hypoxia downstream of the occlusions, and elicited 'Alzheimer-like β-amyloid' immunoreactivity in their brain tissue. In this vein, the plasma protein apolipoprotein E-4 has been clearly associated with higher plasma cholesterol levels and an increased risk of heart disease in population studies (Strittmatter et al., 1993; Davignon et al., 1988; Hallman et al., 1991; Cumming & Robertson, 1984; Kuusi et al., 1988). Indeed, search for a critical role for apolipoprotein E-4 in the CNS has been encouraged by the apparent linkage of apolipoprotein E-4 with AD (Strittmatter et al., 1993). The association of the apolipoprotein E-4 with heart disease may influence the actions of the E-4 gene product in neurodegenerative processes as well. Alternatively, the E-4 gene product may directly interact in neurodegenerative processes.

Observations of increased levels of mtDNA deletion mutations in specific regions of the brain of patients with conditions associated with chronic hypoxia, namely significantly increased levels of mtDNA^{4977} deletions observed in both the frontal cortex and rostral putamen of 42 age-comparable (ages 34 to 73) individuals (Merril et al., 1996), are consistent with the relationships between cardiovascular problems and neurodegenerative changes in the CNS cited above. Although previous studies, inferred from small numbers of individuals (6 to 12), that aging may be responsible for the mtDNA deletions found in specific areas of the brain (Blanchard et al., 1993; Corral-Debrinski et al., 1992; Cortopassi and Arnheim, 1990; Ikebe et al., 1990; Soong et al., 1992), the large sample size examined by Merril and colleagues permitted age-comparable statistical analyses to determine that the mtDNA^{4977} deletion levels observed were not age-driven.

An increase in mtDNA deletions with hypoxia was initially found in yeast by Mayer and Legator (1970), and later in human heart tissue by Wallace's group (Corral-Debrinski et al., 1991). Mayer and Legator (1970) found

that a greater number of mtDNA deletion petite mutants were induced by either N-methyl-N'-nitro-N-nitrosoguanidine (MNNG) or UV irradiation under anaerobic conditions than when the cells were maintained in aerobic conditions. Corral-Debrinski and colleagues (1991) found mtDNA deletions increased 8 to 2200 fold in human cardiac tissue from individuals suffering from ischemic heart disease, compared with age matched controls.

High concentrations of dopaminergic neurons in the putamen and the generation of oxygen radicals by monoamine oxidase in these neurons (Soong et al., 1992; Corral-Debrinski et al., 1992) may be involved in processes which have resulted in the high level of mtDNA^{4977} deletion mutations found there. The high levels of nonhaemin (ferrous) iron of the putamen, half of which is located in the mitochondria and microsomes, may also affect the formation of mtDNA^{4977} deletion mutations. Hydrogen peroxides which can react with ferrous ions to form highly reactive hydroxyl radicals (Halliwell and Gutteridge, 1985), may also further damage the mitochondria through interference with the ETC.

Mechanisms Involved in the Origin of mtDNA Deletions

Mendelian Inheritance of mtDNA Deletions

Ophthalmoplegia and mitochondrial myopathy were distinguishing characteristics of all mtDNA deletion syndromes until a report by Wallace's group in 1992. In this report Ballinger and colleagues (1992) described an apparently maternally-inherited 10.4 knp mtDNA deletion in a small pedigree, without ophthalmoplegia and mitochondrial myopathy, but associated with diabetes and premature deafness. The deleted mtDNA molecule comprised 69 percent of the total mtDNA, as judged by Southern blotting of muscle biopsy DNA from the proband with radiolabeled HeLa mtDNA probe. All family members of the maternal line possessed from 38 percent to 44 percent deleted mtDNA. However, autosomal inheritance of some factor leading to the increased mtDNA deletion levels could not be ruled out. Autosomal dominant mutations associated with mtDNA deletions have been suggested in other studies (Cormier et al., 1991; Yuzaki et al., 1989; Suomalainen et al., 1995; Zeviani et al., 1989b; Zeviani et al., 1990).

While Southern blot analysis was first used to reveal mtDNA deletions in a CNS disorder, KSS (Zeviani et al., 1988), Southern blotting is capable of quantifying mtDNA deletion levels only if the proportion of deleted mtDNA molecules is relatively large in comparison with the undeleted mtDNA molecules. The relative proportion of hybridization signal from full-length and deleted molecules was estimated by densitometry to range from 45 percent to 75 percent in the study by Zeviani and colleagues (1988). Shoffner and associates (1989) likewise revealed a 50 percent relative level of deleted mtDNA molecules in KSS patients using densitometry of Southern blots. Yuzaki and colleagues (1989) also found a 30–70 percent level of mtDNA deletions via Southern blotting in cases of familial mitochondrial myopathy. We are unaware of any study detecting mtDNA deletion levels below 30 percent utilizing Southern blot technology.

Recombination as a Mechanism Leading to mtDNA Deletions

Poulton and colleagues (1993) observed that mtDNA duplications may be intermediates in the rearrangement of mtDNA leading to mtDNA deletions. Poulton's group utilized an elaborate series of restriction enzyme digests and 2-dimensional gel electrophoresis of DNA from a patient with KSS and diabetes mellitus, to demonstrate that mtDNA duplications decreased as the mtDNA deletions increased in both muscle and brain. The duplications also decreased in clonal tissue culture cell lines supplemented with uridine and pyruvate (Hayashi et al., 1991). The results of Poulton's group strongly implicate homologous recombination as one mechanism leading to mtDNA deletions in human mitochondria.

Evidence for probable recombinational events in the generation of large-scale mtDNA deletions in patients with *progressive external ophthalmoplegia* (PEO) and *ragged red fibers* (RRF) have also been found by other groups (Mita et al., 1990; Holt et al., 1988; Zeviani et al., 1989b). Two classes of deletions were defined by Mita and colleagues (1990), who sequenced the breakpoints of deletions from 28 patients. Direct repeats precisely flank class I deletions, while class II deletions are not precisely flanked by direct repeats. Imperfect repeats are present near the deletion breakpoints in some class II deletions, suggesting that short distance slippage may be occurring in these cases. Additionally, Katsumata and colleagues (1994) observed 235 types of deletions via PCR analysis of the entire human mitochondrial genome with 180 pairs of primers. Their data must be interpreted with caution, as some of the apparently deleted mtDNAs contained both origins of replication while other apparently deleted mtDNAs lacked one or both origins of replication. Their data may represent not only replicating forms of deleted mtDNAs, but examples of recombination products as well.

Potential Gene Products Involved in mtDNA Deletions

Disruption of the yeast *LON* protein gene, a homologue of the bacterial ATP-dependent protease *Lon* gene, yielded cells phenotypically similar to a respiration-deficient mutant with extensive deletions of the mtDNA (ρ^-) or without mtDNA (ρ^0) (Suzuki et al., 1994). The bacterial Lon protease apparently eliminates abnormal or damaged proteins from the bacterial cytoplasm, and the human and yeast homologues may function similarly. The yeast mutants generated by Suzuki and colleagues (1994) still contained mtDNA as demonstrated by *4,6-diamino-2-phenylindole* (DAPI) staining, suggesting that disruption of *LON* led to a ρ^- mutant, *i. e.*, mtDNA deletions. Thus,

generation of mtDNA deletions in yeast may involve an enzymatic process in which the *LON* gene product plays a role. As the human *LON* gene product is highly homologous to the bacterial Lon protease (Wang et al., 1993) and to the yeast *LON* gene, the human *LON* may be involved in the generation of mtDNA deletions in humans. Oxidatively damaged DNA processing enzymes may accumulate in the presence of a disrupted *LON* gene or damaged *LON* gene product, leading to creation of deleted mtDNA molecules through intramolecular recombination. Additional enzymes and transcription factors may be involved in the formation of deleted mtDNA molecules including mtDNA polymerase γ, damage to which may result in slip-replication (Shoffner et al., 1989); mtDNA topoisomerase II, inhibition of which in trypanosome kinetoplasts results in DNA minicircle concatamers (Shapiro, 1994); mtDNA endonuclease G (Cote and Ruiz-Carrillo, 1993), that preferentially cleaves mtDNA at GC-rich tracts; mtDNA ligase (Levin and Zimmermann, 1976); mtDNA endonuclease (not mtDNA endonuclease G) (Tomkinson et al., 1988); or glycosylases (Domena and Mosbaugh, 1985).

Suomalainen and colleagues (1995) found linkage in a Finnish pedigree of an autosomal locus on 10q23.3–24.3 to *autosomal dominant progressive external ophthalmoplegia* (adPEO), a condition in which multiple mtDNA deletions accumulate in the patients' tissues. One mtDNA-associated nuclear-encoded protein gene has been assigned to 10q, the gene for mitochondrial transcription factor A (TCF6, nee mtTF1) (Tiranti et al., 1995), making *TCF6* a candidate gene for adPEO in this Finnish family. Two additional Italian families, with adPEO, did not show linkage to 10q23.3–24.3 in this study, accentuating the heterogeneity of mtDNA disorders.

Comparison of Common Deletions in Humans and Other Mammals May Facilitate Studies on Mechanisms Leading to mtDNA Deletions

Competitive PCR has been used by Edris and colleagues (1994) to quantify a reportedly age-related increase in a 4.8 knp rat mtDNA deletion from rat liver; and from rat brain (Filburn, personal communication). This deletion can be considered an 'animal model' of the human 'common' mtDNA deletion (Table 6–1). The rat and human mtDNA molecules are similar in size, 16295 np and 16569 np, respectively; additionally, the human mtDNA^{4977} deletion occurs between two 13 np repeats and the rat mtDNA^{4834} occurs between two 16 np repeats. The gene order and content are the same in both organellar genomes, thus the rat mtDNA^{4834} deletion affects nearly all of the same genes as the human mtDNA^{4977} deletion. The competitor PCR products were generated by site-directed mutagenesis of the original deletion and light-strand origin (non-deletion) PCR products by the method described by Higuchi (1990). Mismatch primers were constructed which eliminate the *Rsa*I site from the light-strand origin fragment, and a *Ban*II site from the deletion fragment. The two partial PCR products

TABLE **6-1.**   Comparison of common deletions in humans and other mammals, with sequences and positions of direct repeats indicated.

Species	Deletion Size (np)	Sequence of Direct Repeats*
Human *Homo sapiens*	4977	ACC TCC CTC ACC A | | 8470 8482 13447 13460
Rhesus Monkey *Macaca mulatta*	~8000	CCCCA | | 7572 7576 15598 15602
Rat *Rattus norvegicus*	4834	CCT GAG CCC TAA TAA T | | 8103 8118 12937 12952
Mouse *Mus domesticus*	3868	AGC CCT ACT AAT TAC | | 9089 9103 12956 12970
Mouse *Mus domesticus*	3727	AAG CAA ATC CAT AT | | 9553 9566 13279 13292

* Data are from Mita *et al.*, 1990 (Human); Lee *et al.*, 1993 (Rhesus Monkey); Edris *et al.*, 1994 (Rat); Brossas *et al.*, 1994 (Mouse). Numbering for Rhesus Monkey mtDNA sequence, based on Human mtDNA sequence, is approximate.

utilizing each original rat mtDNA PCR product as templates were then combined and PCR commenced with the original PCR primers. The resultant PCR products had been mutagenized, and PCR products derived from the 'mutagenized' targets could be differentiated by restriction digest from products derived from the mtDNA template. Prior to amplification, the DNA sample was digested with *Sau*3A which digests outside the 16 np direct repeats in both deleted and nondeleted genomes, and between the direct repeats in the nondeleted genomes. This approach decreased the competition from nondeleted mtDNA molecules for the deletion primers. Graded amounts of the competitor PCR product were added to the rat brain DNA followed by PCR. Restriction digestion and subsequent agarose gel electrophoresis revealed a pattern of three bands; the undigested product from the mutant template, and the two fragments from the mtDNA template. The three bands were analyzed densitometrically and the ratio of mutant mtDNA product:normal mtDNA product versus the copies of mutant template added revealed a straight line with a slope of 1 on a log-log plot. With this approach, the determined ratio of deletion:total mtDNA in 6 month old rats ranged from 5×10^{-6} to 3×10^{-5}, while in 24 month old rats, the ratio varied from 8×10^{-4} to 5×10^{-3}, indicating a mean 100 fold increase with age.

Three mtDNA deletions in rhesus monkey skeletal muscle mtDNA appear to increase with age (Lee *et al.*, 1993). The deletions appear in the same region of the mitochondrial genome as the human mtDNA[4977] deletion, offering another potential animal model for the investigation of the human mtDNA[4977] deletion consequences and mechanism as one deletion is bounded by a short, 5 np, direct repeat (Table 6-1).

Finally, multiple mouse mtDNA deletions bounded by direct repeats have also been recognized that delete an analogous region as the human common deletion (Table 6-1). Generally, the mtDNA deletions in mammals other than humans have been correlated with aging. Aging is a parameter that can be easily evaluated in non-human mammals. Our laboratory is currently developing both rat and mouse models to evaluate factors affected by chronic hypoxia that could lead to mtDNA deletions.

Chronic Hypoxia and Components of the Central Nervous System

Effects of Chronic Hypoxia on Neurons

Depression of synaptic potential is seen during hypoxia at all nerve junctions (Somjen, 1993). Aerobic mitochondrial metabolism is essential to satisfy the continual en-

voke this OXPHOS dysfunction. This mitochondrial catastrophe foments free radical production, leading to mtDNA, protein, and phospholipid free radical oxidative damage. This free radical damage leads to further free radical damage, augmenting the oxidative destruction of mitochondrial components already present. The mitochondrial membrane can then become pervious to free radicals, leading to oxidative damage of cytoplasmic components, as well as nuclear components, including nucDNA. Actively transcribed genes, exposed to the alien free radicals, can be mutated, amplifying the damage again (Ozawa, 1995). Naturally occurring mutagens, such as nitric oxide and ethylene may further aggravate the situation. Tissue vascularization differences and metabolic rate variations along with tissue specificity of such mutagens may be instrumental in the regional localization of neurodegenerative diseases.

An Overall View

Since neuronal cells are some of the most aerobic and metabolically active cells in the body, deficits in aerobic energy metabolism may have a particularly adverse effect on these cells, resulting in many acute and chronic diseases affecting the central nervous system (CNS). These adverse effects may be region specific. For example, individuals with conditions associated with chronic hypoxia often display relatively high levels of molecular lesions, such as mtDNA deletions, in the putamen even though such mtDNA deletions are rarely found in the cerebellum. Variations in regional blood flow, metabolic rates, aging and the presence of known mutagens, such as nitric oxide and ethylene may be partially responsible for the regional distribution of the mtDNA deletions. These mtDNA mutation events may be secondary disease events or they may initiate disease processes, particularly if such deletion mutations become predominant, lowering the oxidative phosphorylation potential of affected cells. As neurons require considerable amounts of energy to restore transmembrane potentials following each depolarization, this loss of critical mitochondrial function is particularly deleterious to the CNS. In addition, mitochondrial dysfunction can lead to a metabolic catastrophe, free radicals can be produced in large concentrations, compounding the damage to a cell's aerobic capacities. Such adverse effects of mitochondrial dysfunction may be related to a number of reports linking mitochondrial mutations to diseases affecting the CNS.

Additional studies into the underlying mechanisms of neurodegenerative diseases are needed to elucidate the contribution of the mitochondrial genome to neurodegenerative diseases; clinical studies can only counsel us of the possible role of mitochondrial catastrophes in neurodegenerative diseases. Animal model systems, and to a lesser extent tissue culture systems, are essential to understanding the complex interactions between mtDNA deletions, the cardiovascular and pulmonary systems, and the CNS in neurodegenerative diseases.

Selected Readings

Corral-Debrinski, M., Horton, T., Lott, M. T., et al. 1992. Mitochondrial DNA deletions in human brain: regional variability and increase with advanced age. Nature Genet. 2:324–329.

Corral-Debrinski, M., Horton, T., Lott, M. T., et al. 1994. Marked changes in mitochondrial DNA deletion levels in Alzheimer brains. Genomics 23:471–476.

Gupta, K. P., van Golen, K. L., Randerath, E., and Randerath, K. 1990. Age-dependent covalent DNA alterations (I-compounds) in rat liver mitochondrial DNA. Mutat. Res. 237:17–27.

Levin, C. J., and Zimmerman, S. B. 1976. A DNA ligase from mitochondria of rat liver. Biochem. Biophys. Res. Commun. 69:514–520.

Merril, C. R., Zullo, S., Ghanbari, H., et al. 1996. Possible relationship between conditions associated with chronic hypoxia and brain mitochondrial DNA deletions. Arch. Biochem. Biophys. 326:172–177.

Mita, S., Rizzuto, R., Moraes, C. T., et al. 1990. Recombination via flanking direct repeats is a major cause of large scale deletions of human mitochondrial DNA. Nucleic Acids Res. 18:561–567.

Ozawa, T. 1995. Mechanism of somatic mitochondrial DNA mutations associated with age and diseases. Biochim. Biophys. Acta. 1271:177–189.

Pinz, K. G., Shibutani, S., and Bogenhagen, D. F. 1995. Action of mitochondrial DNA polymerase gamma at sites of base loss or oxidative damage. J. Biol. Chem. 270:9202–9206.

Poulton, J., Deadman, M. E., Bindoff, L., Morten, K., Land, J., and Brown, G. 1993. Families of mtDNA re-arrangements can be detected in patients with mtDNA deletions: duplications may be a transient intermediate form. Hum. Molecular Genet. 2:23–30.

Schon, E. A., Rizzuto, R., Moraes, C. T., et al. 1989. A direct repeat is a hotspot for large scale deletion of human mitochondrial DNA. Science 244:346–349.

Shoubridge, E. A., Karpati, G., Hastings, K. E. M. 1990. Deletion mutants are functionally dominant over wild-type mitochondrial genomes in skeletal muscle fiber segments in mitochondrial disease. Cell 62:43–49.

Suomalainen, A., Kaukonen, J., Amati, P., et al. 1995. An autosomal locus predisposing to deletions of mitochondrial DNA. Nature Genet. 9:146–151.

Tiranti, V., Rossi, E., Ruiz-Carrillo, A., et al. 1995. Chromosomal localization of mitochondrial transcription factor A (TCF6), single-stranded DNA-binding protein (SSBP), and endonuclease G (ENDOG), three human housekeeping genes involved in mitochondrial biogenesis. Genomics 25:559–564.

Wallace, D. C., Shoffner, J. M., Trounce, I., et al. 1995. Mitochondrial DNA mutations in human degenerative diseases and aging. Biochim. Biophys. Acta 1271:141–151.

Zeviani, M., Bresolin, N., Gellera, C., et al. 1990. Nucleus-driven multiple large-scale deletions of the human mitochondrial genome: a new autosomal dominant disease. American J. Hum. Genet. 47:904–914.

References

Anderson, S., Bankier, A. T., Barrell, B. G., et al. 1981. Sequence and organization of the human mitochondrial genome. Nature 290:457–465.

Aronson, M. K., Ooi, W. L., Morgenstern, H., et al. 1990. Women, myocardial infarction, and dementia in the very old. Neurology 40:1102–1106.

Ballinger, S. W., Shoffner, J. M., Hedaya, E. V., *et al.* 1992. Maternally transmitted diabetes and deafness associated with a 10.4 kb mitochondrial DNA deletion. Nature Gen. 1:11–15.

Beal, M.F. 1995. Mitochondrial dysfunction and oxidative damage in neurodegenerative disease. R. G. Landes Co. Austin, TX.

Beck, I., Weinmann, R., and Caro, J. 1993. Characterization of hypoxia-responsive enhancer in the human erythropoietin gene shows presence of hypoxia-inducible 120-Kd nuclear DNA-binding protein in erythropoietin-producing and non-producing cells. Blood 82:704–711.

Bernes, S. M., Bacino, C., Prezant, T. R., *et al.* 1993. Identical mitochondrial DNA deletion in mother with progressive external ophthalmoplegia and son with Pearson marrow-pancreas syndrome. J. Pediatrics 123:598–602.

Blanchard, B. J., Park, T., Fripp, W. J., Lerman, L.S., and Ingram, V.M. 1993. A mitochondrial DNA deletion in normally aging and in Alzheimer brain tissue. Neuroreport 4:799–802.

Brossas, J. Y., Barreau, E., Courtois, Y., and Treton, J. 1994. Multiple deletions in mitochondrial DNA are present in senescent mouse brain. Biochem. Biophys. Res. Commun. 202:654–659.

Chawluk, J. B., Dann, R., Alavi, A., *et al.* 1990. The effect of focal cerebral atrophy in positron emission tomographic studies of aging and dementia. Nucl. Med. Biol. 17:797–804.

Cormier, V., Rötig, A., Tardieu, M., *et al.* 1991. Autosomal dominant deletions of the mitochondrial genome in a case of progressive encephalomyopathy. American J. Hum. Genet. 48:643–648.

Corral-Debrinski, M., Horton, T., Lott, M. T., *et al.* 1994. Marked changes in mitochondrial DNA deletion levels in Alzheimer brains. Genomics 23:471–476.

Corral-Debrinski, M., Horton, T., Lott, M. T., *et al.* 1992. Mitochondrial DNA deletions in human brain: regional variability and increase with advanced age. Nature Genet. 2:324–329.

Corral-Debrinski, M., Stepien, G., Shoffner, J. M., *et al.* 1991. Hypoxemia is associated with mitochondrial DNA damage and gene induction. J. Amer. Med. Assoc. 266:1812–1816.

Cortopassi, G. A., and Arnheim, N. 1990. Detection of a specific mitochondrial DNA deletion in tissues of older humans. Nucl. Acids Res. 18:6927–6933.

Cote, J., and Ruiz-Carrillo, A. 1993. Primers for mitochondrial DNA replication generated by endonuclease G. Science 261:765–769.

Cumming, A. M., and Robertson, F. 1984. Polymorphism at the apoprotein-E locus in relation to risk of coronary disease. Clin. Genet. 25:310–318.

Davignon, J., Gregg, R. E., and Sing, C. F. 1988. Apolipoprotein E polymorphism and atherosclerosis. Atherosclerosis 8:1–21.

DiMauro, S., Bonilla, E., Lombes, A., Shanske, S., Minetti, C., and Moraes, C. T. 1990. Mitochondrial encephalomyopathies. Pediat. Neurol. 8:483–506.

Domena, J. D., and Mosbaugh, D. W. 1985. Purification of nuclear and mitochondrial uracil-DNA glycosylase from rat liver. Identification of two distinct subcellular forms. Biochemistry 24:7320–7328.

Drayer, B. P., Burger, P., Darwin, R., *et al.* 1986. MRI of brain iron. Amer. J. Radiol. 147:103–110.

Edris, W., Burgett, B., Stine, O. C., and Filburn, C. R. 1994. Detection and quantitation by competitive PCR of an age-associated increase in a 4.8-kb deletion in rat mitochondrial DNA. Mutat. Res. 316:69–78.

Ernster, L., Ikkos, D., and Luft, R. 1959. Enzymatic activities of human skeletal muscle mitochondria: A tool in clinical metabolic research. Nature 184:1851–1854.

Grant, I., Heaton, R. K., McSweeny, A. J., Adams, K. M., and Timms, R. M. 1982. Neuropsychologic findings in hypoxemic chronic obstructive pulmonary disease. Arch. Intern. Med. 142:1470–1476.

Gupta, K. P., van Golen, K. L., Randerath, E., and Randerath, K. 1990. Age-dependent covalent DNA alterations (I-compounds) in rat liver mitochondrial DNA. Mutat. Res. 237:17–27.

Halliwell, B., and Gutteridge, J. M. C. 1985. Oxygen radicals and the nervous system. Trends Neurosci. 8:22–26.

Hallman, D. M., Boerwinkle, E., Saha, N., *et al.* 1991. The apolipoprotein E polymorphism: a comparison of allele frequencies and effects in nine populations. Am. J. Hum. Genet. 49:338–349.

Hardy, J. A., Wester, P., Winblad, B., *et al.* 1985. The patients dying after long terminal phase have acidotic brains; implications for biochemical measurements on autopsy tissue. J. Neural Transm. 61:253–264.

Hattori, K., Tanaka, M., Sugiyama, S., *et al.* 1991. Age-dependent increase in deleted mitochondrial DNA in the human heart: possible contributory factor to presbycardia. Am. Heart J. 121:1735–1742.

Hayashi, J.-I., Ohta, S., Kikuchi, A., Takemitsu, M., Goto, Y.-I., and Nonaka, I. 1991. Introduction of disease-related mitochondrial DNA deletions into HeLa cells lacking mitochondrial DNA results in mitochondrial dysfunction. Proc. Natl. Acad. Sci. USA 88:10614–10618.

Heddi, A., Lestienne, P., Wallace, D. C., and Stepien, G. 1994. Steady state levels of mitochondrial and nuclear oxidative phosphorylation transcripts in Kearns-Sayre syndrome. Biochim. Biophys. Acta. 1226:206–212.

Higuchi, R. 1990. Recombinant PCR, In M. A. Innis, D. H. Gelfand, J. J. Snisky, and T. J. White (Eds.), PCR Protocols. pp. 177–183. Academic Press, San Diego, CA.

Holt, I. J., Harding, A. E., and Morgan-Hughes, J. A. 1988. Deletions of mitochondrial DNA in patients with mitochondrial myopathies. Nature 331:717–719.

Hutchin, T., and Cortopassi, G. 1995. A mitochondrial DNA clone is associated with increased risk for Alzheimer disease. Proc. Natl. Acad. Sci. USA 92:6892–6895.

Ikebe, S. -I., Tanaka, M., Ohno, K., *et al.* 1990. Increase of deleted mitochondrial DNA in the striatum in Parkinson's disease and senescence. Biochem. Biophys. Res. Commun. 170:1044–1048.

Katsumata, K., Hayakawa, M., Tanaka, M., Sugiyama, S., and Ozawa, T. 1994. Fragmentation of human heart mitochondrial DNA associated with premature aging. Biochem. Biophys. Res. Commun. 202:102–110.

Kearns, T. P., and Sayre, G. P. 1958. Retinitis pigmentosa, external ophthalmoplegia, and complete heart block. Arch. of Ophthalmol. 60:280–289.

Kearns, T. P. 1965. External ophthalmolplegia, pigmentary degeneration of the retina, and cardiomyopathy: A newly recognized syndrome. Trans. Am. Ophthalmol. Soc. 63:559–625.

Kuppuswamy, M. N., Hoffmann, J. W., Kasper, C. K., *et al.* 1991. Single nucleotide primer extension to detect genetic diseases: experimental application to hemophilia B (factor IX) and cystic fibrosis genes. Proc. Natl. Acad. Sci. USA 88:1143–1147.

Kuusi, T., Nieminen, M. S., Ehnholm, C., *et al.* 1988. Apoprotein E polymorphism and coronary artery disease: increased prevalence of apolipoprotein E-4 in angiographically verified coronary patients. Atherosclerosis 9:237–241.

Lee, C. M., Chung, S. S., Kaczkowski, J. M., Weindruch, R., and Aiken, J.M. 1993. Multiple mitochondrial DNA deletions associated with age in skeletal muscle of rhesus monkeys. J. Gerontol. 48:B201–B205.

Leveille, A. S., and Newell, F. W. 1980. Autosomal dominant Kearns-Sayre syndrome. Ophthalmology 86:99–108.

Levin, C. J., and Zimmerman, S. B. 1976. A DNA ligase from mitochondria of rat liver. Biochem. Biophys. Res. Commun. 69:514–520.

Levy, A. P., Levy, N. S., Wegner, S., and Goldberg, M. A. 1995. Transcriptional regulation of the rat vascular endothelial growth factor gene by hypoxia. J. Biol. Chem. 270:13333–13340.

Lin, F. -H., Lin, R., Wisniewski, H. M. 1992. Detection of point mutations in codon 331 of mitochondrial NADH dehydrogenase subunit 2 in Alzheimer's brains. Biochem. Biophys. Res. Commun. 182:238–246.

Luft, R., Ikkos, D., Palmieri, G., Ernster, L., and Afzelius, B. 1962. A case of severe hypermetabolism of nonthyroid origin with a defect in the maintenance of mitochondrial respiratory control: A correlated clinical, biochemical, and morphological study. J. Clin. Invest. 41:1776–1804.

Mayer, V. W., and Legator, M. S. 1970. Induction by N-methyl-N'-nitro-N-nitrosoguanidine and UV light of petite mutants in aerobically and anaerobically cultivated Saccharomyces cerevisiae. Mutat. Res. 9:193–198.

Mecocci, P., MacGarvey, U., and Beal, M. F. 1994. Oxidative damage to mitochondrial DNA is increased in Alzheimer's disease. Ann. Neurol. 36:747–751.

Menzies, R. A., and Gold, P. H. 1971. The turnover of mitochondria in a variety of tissues of young adult and aged rats. J. Biol. Chem. 246:2425–2459.

Merril, C. R., Zullo, S., Ghanbari, H., et al. 1996. Possible relationship between conditions associated with chronic hypoxia and brain mitochondrial DNA deletions. Arch. Biochem. Biophys. 326:172–177.

Mita, S., Rizzuto, R., Moraes, C. T., et al. 1990. Recombination via flanking direct repeats is a major cause of large scale deletions of human mitochondrial DNA. Nucl. Acids Res. 18:561–567.

Moraes, C. T., DiMauro, S., Zeviani, M., et al. 1989. Mitochondrial DNA deletions in progressive external ophthalmoplegia and Kearns-Sayre syndrome. N. Engl. J. Med. 320:1293–1299.

Nakase, H., Moraes, C. T., Rizzuto, R., Lombes, A., DiMauro, S., and Schon, E.A. 1990. Transcription and translation of deleted mitochondrial genomes in Kearns-Sayre syndrome: Implications for pathogenesis. Am. J. Hum. Genet. 46:418–427.

Ozawa, T., Yoneda, M., Tanaka, M., et al. 1988. Maternal inheritance of deleted mitochondrial DNA in a family with mitochondrial myopathy. Biochem. Biophys. Res. Commun. 154:1240–1247.

Ozawa, T., Tanaka, M., Ikebe, S.-I., Ohno, K., Kondo, T., and Mizuno, Y. 1990. Quantitative determination of deleted mitochondrial DNA relative to normal DNA in parkinsonian striatum by a kinetic PCR analysis. Biochem. Biophys. Res. Commun. 172:483–489.

Ozawa, T. 1995. Mechanism of somatic mitochondrial DNA mutations associated with age and diseases. Biochim. Biophys. Acta. 1271:177–189.

Pinz, K. G., Shibutani, S., and Bogenhagen, D. F. 1995. Action of mitochondrial DNA polymerase gamma at sites of base loss or oxidative damage. J. Biol. Chem. 270:9202–9206.

Poulton, J., Deadman, M. E., Bindoff, L., et al. 1993. Families of mtDNA re-arrangements can be detected in patients with mtDNA deletions: duplications may be a transient intermediate form. Hum. Mol. Genet. 2:23–30.

Prigatano, G. P., Parsons, O., Wright, E., Levin, D. C. and Hawryluk, G. 1983. Neuropsychological test performance in mildly hypoxemic patients with chronic obstructive pulmonary disease, J. Consult. Clin. Psychol. 51:108–116.

Pulsinelli, W. 1995. The ischemic penumbra in stroke. Sci. Am. Sci. and Med. 2:16–25.

Richter, C., Park, J.-W., and Ames, B.N. 1988. Normal oxidative damage to mitochondrial and nuclear DNA is extensive. Proc. Natl. Acad. Sci. USA 85:6465–6467.

Rosenbaum, D. M., Michaelson, M., Batter, D. K., Doshi, P., and Kessler, J. A. 1994. Evidence for hypoxia-induced, programmed cell death of cultured neurons. Ann. Neurol. 36:864–870.

Schon, E. A., Rizzuto, R., Moraes, C. T., et al. 1989. A direct repeat is a hotspot for large scale deletion of human mitochondrial DNA. Science 244:346–349.

Schurr, A., and Rigor, B. M. 1987. The mechanism of neuronal resistance and adaptation to hypoxia. FEBS Letters 224:4–8.

Shapiro, T. A. 1994. Mitochondrial topoisomerase II activity is essential for kinetoplast DNA minicircle segregation. Mol. Cell. Biol. 14:3660–3667.

Shoffner, J. M., and Wallace, D. C. 1990. Oxidative phosphorylation diseases. Disorders of two genomes. Adv. Hum. Genet. 19:267–330.

Shoffner, J. M., Brown, M. D., Torroni, A., et al. 1993. Mitochondrial DNA variants observed in Alzheimer disease and Parkinson disease patients. Genomics 17:171–184.

Shoffner, J. M., Lott, M. T., Voliavec, A. S., et al. 1989. Spontaneous Kearns-Sayre/chronic external ophthalmoplegia plus syndrome associated with a mitochondrial DNA deletion: a slip-replication model and metabolic therapy. Proc. Natl. Acad. Sci. USA 86:7952–7956.

Shoubridge, E. A., Karpati, G., and Hastings, K. E. M. 1990. Deletion mutants are functionally dominant over wild-type mitochondrial genomes in skeletal muscle fiber segments in mitochondrial disease. Cell 62:43–49.

Somjen, G. G. 1993. Effects of hypoxia on neuronal membranes. In S. T. Ohnishi, and T. Ohnishi (eds.) Cellular Membrane: a key to disease processes. pp. 181–207. CRC Press, Boca Raton, FL.

Soong, N. -W., Hinton, D. R., Cortopassi, G., and Arnheim, N. 1992. Mosaicism for a specific somatic mitochondrial DNA mutation in adult human brain. Nature Genet. 2:318–323.

Sparks, D. L., Liu, H., Scheff, S. W., Coyne, C. M., and Hunsaker, J. C. 1993. Temporal sequence of plaque formation in the cerebral cortex of non-demented individuals. J. Neuropathol. Exp. Neurol. 52:135–142.

Sparks, D. L., Scheff, S. W., Hunsaker, J. C., Liu, H., Landers, T., and Gross, D. R. 1994. Induction of Alzheimer-like β-amyloid immunoreactivity in the brains of rabbits with dietary cholesterol. Exp. Neurol. 126:88–94.

Strittmatter, W. J., Saunders, A. M., Schmechel, D. E., et al. 1993. Apolipoprotein E: high-avidity binding to β-amyloid and increased frequency of type 4 allele in late-onset familial Alzheimer's disease. Proc. Natl. Acad. Sci. USA 90:1977–1981.

Suomalainen, A., Kaukonen, J., Amati, P., et al. 1995. An autosomal locus predisposing to deletions of mitochondrial DNA. Nature Genet. 9:146–151.

Suzuki, C. K., Suda, K., Wang, N., and Schatz, G. 1994. Requirement for the yeast gene *LON* in intramitochondrial proteolysis and maintenance of respiration. Science 264:273–276; (correction):891.

Terada, L. S., Guidot, D. M., Leff, J. A., *et al.* 1992. Hypoxia injures endothelial cells by increasing endogenous xanthine oxidase activity. Proc. Natl. Acad. Sci. USA 89:3362–3366.

Tiranti, V., Rossi, E., Ruiz-Carrillo, A., *et al.* 1995. Chromosomal localization of mitochondrial transcription factor A (TCF6), single-stranded DNA-binding protein (SSBP), and endonuclease G (ENDOG), three human housekeeping genes involved in mitochondrial biogenesis. Genomics 25:559–564.

Tomkinson, A.E., Bonk, R.T., and Linn, S. 1988. Mitochondrial endonuclease activities specific for apurinic/apyrimidinic sites in DNA from mouse cells. J. Biol. Chem. 263:12532–12537.

Tuder, R. M., Flook, B. E., and Voelkel, N. F. 1995. Increased gene expression for VEGF and the VEGF receptors *KDR/Flk* and *Flt* in lungs exposed to acute or to chronic hypoxia. J. Clin. Invest. 95:1798–1807.

Veltri, K. L., Espiritu, M., and Singh, G. 1990. Distinct genomic copy number in mitochondria of different mammalian organs. J. Cell. Physiol. 143:160–164.

Wallace, D. C. 1987. Maternal genes: Mitochondrial diseases. In V. A. McKusick, T. H. Roderick, J. Mori and N. W. Paul (eds.) Medical and experimental mammalian genetics: a perspective, Birth Defects Original Article Series. 23:137–190.

Wallace, D. C. 1992. Diseases of the mitochondrial DNA. Ann. Rev. Biochem. 61:1175–1212.

Wallace, D. C. 1993. Mitochondrial diseases: genotype versus phenotype. Trends Genet. 5:9–13.

Wallace, D. C., Shoffner, J. M., Trounce, I., *et al.* 1995. Mitochondrial DNA mutations in human degenerative diseases and aging. Biochim. Biophys. Acta. 1271:141–151.

Wallace, D. C., Ye, J., Neckelmann, S. N., Singh, G., Webster, K. A., and Greenberg, B. D. 1987. Sequence analysis of cDNAs for the human and bovine ATP synthase β subunit: mitochondrial DNA genes sustain seventeen times more mutations. Curr. Genet. 12:81–90.

Wang, G. L., Jiang, B. -H., Rue, E. A., and Semenza, G. L. 1995. Hypoxia-inducible factor 1 is a basic-helix-loop-helix-PAS heterodimer regulated by cellular O_2 tension. Proc. Natl. Acad. Sci. USA 92:5510–5514.

Wang, N., Gottesman, S., Willingham, M. C., Gottesman, M. M., and Maurizi, M. R. 1993. A human mitochondrial ATP-dependent protease that is highly homologous to bacterial Lon protease. Proc. Natl. Acad. Sci. USA 90:11247–11251.

Yuzaki, M., Ohkoshi, N., Kanazawa, I., Kagawa, Y., and Ohta, S. 1989. Multiple deletions in mitochondrial DNA at direct repeats of non-D-loop regions in cases of familial mitochondrial myopathy. Biochem. Biophys. Res. Commun. 164:1352–1357.

Zeviani, M., Bonilla, E., DeVivo, D.C., and DiMauro, S. 1989a. Mitochondrial diseases. Neurol. Clin. 7:123–156.

Zeviani, M., Bresolin, N., Gellera, C., *et al.* 1990. Nucleus-driven multiple large-scale deletions of the human mitochondrial genome: a new autosomal dominant disease. Am. J. Hum. Genet. 47:904–914.

Zeviani, M., Moraes, C. T., DiMauro, S., *et al.* 1988. Deletions of mitochondrial DNA in Kearns-Sayre syndrome. Neurology 38:1339–1346.

Zeviani, M., Servidei, S., Gellera, C., Bertini, E., DiMauro, S., and DiDonato, S. 1989b. An autosomal dominant disorder with multiple deletions of mitochondrial DNA starting at the D-loop region. Nature 339:309–311.

Zupanc, M. L., Moraes, C. T., Shanske, S., Langman, C. B., Ciafaloni, E., and DiMauro, S. 1991. Deletion of mitochondrial DNA in patients with combined features of Kearns-Sayre and MELAS syndromes. Ann. Neurol. 29:680–683.

7

Sergio U. Dani

Molecular Turnover and Aging

The Turnover Rate of a Molecule is Determined by the Rates of its Synthesis and Degradation

Distinct Molecular Species Turn Over at Different Rates

Nuclear DNA Turnover is Incomplete

Protein Turnover Constitutes a Way Through Which General Molecular Turnover is Controlled in the Cell

Decreased Molecular Turnover with Age Correlates With Increased Post-Translational Modifications of Proteins

Regulation of Protein Synthesis is Accomplished by the Regulation of Gene Expression

The Transcriptional Control is Paramount to Eukaryotic Gene Expression

Transcription Activators and DNA Binding Sites

Regulation by the RNA Polymerases

Accumulation of Negative Gene Regulatory Proteins may Account for the Progressive Reduction of Gene Expression with Aging

Alternatively hnRNA Splicing: a Flexible Mechanism Allowing a Single Gene to Make Different Proteins

mRNA and Proteins are Actively and Selectively Transported From the Nucleus to the Cytoplasm and Vice-versa

Regulation of Gene Expression at the Level of Translation

Feedback Mechanisms Can Regulate Protein Synthesis

Protein Synthesis may be Increased by Gene Dosage and Gene Up-regulation

Regulation of Protein Degradation

The ATP-dependent Proteolytic Pathway may Require or not Ubiquitin

The Calpain System is Activated by Ca^{2+} and is Thought to be Involved in Regulatory Cleavages of Specific Proteins

The Lysosomal Proteolytic Pathway is Non-Selective

The Fine Control of Proteolysis

Large Molecular Weight Proteins and Abnormal or Denatured Proteins are More Promptly Degraded than Small Proteins

Chemical Composition and Conformation Determine a Protein's Susceptibility to Degradation

Increased Cellular Protein Content and the Accumulation of Abnormal Proteins in Senescent Cells may be Explained by Reduced Rates of Proteolysis

The Turnover Kinetics of Nuclear Proteins may Regulate Development and Aging

Protein Synthesis and Degradation May be Integrated According to Feed-back and Chaotic Models

Heat Shock Response, Cytosolic Targetting and Proteolysis: Ecological Modelling

Reduced Molecular Turnover with Aging is a Common Feature of Different Neurodegenerative Conditions

An Overall View

An appraisal of the daily whole body protein synthesis and the daily dietary protein requirements of a man discloses this astonishing picture: Whereas the daily nutritional protein requirement of an adult is estimated to range between 60 to 70 grams, the amount of total protein synthesized in the adult's whole body is estimated to average 280–320 grams per day (Waterlow *et al.*, 1978), i. e., four- to five-fold the daily protein intake! The conclusion must be that, additionally to dietary protein, constitutive body proteins are constantly being degraded and used as source of amino acids for the synthesis of new protein in the body. This is possible as, in the words of McDonald and Barret (1986), 'a synergistic, proteolytic mechanism has evolved in cells which is especially effective in catalyzing the release for subsequent reuse of amino acids from dietary proteins, and from intracellular proteins that are degraded as part of the dynamic process of protein turnover'.

Molecular turnover stands for replacement or recycling of molecular species. However, the role of molecular turnover is not restricted to purely nutritional aspects in the cell's economy. In the last few years it has become clear that metabolic defects affecting crucial proteins such as those involved in the transfer of genetic information, signal transduction, cytoskeletal organization and the removal of abnormal or damaged proteins may have multiple and far-reaching effects on gene expression, cell proliferation, cellular responsiveness and general maintenance and survival of the cell. As it shall be pointed out throughout this chapter and the chapters to follow, controlling molecular turnover rates profoundly affects the rates of development and aging. This principle holds true not only for proteins, but for all biomolecules which are produced and metabolized in the organism, as the hallmark of aging is precisely a progressive deteriorative process of nonreplenishing structures.

The Turnover Rate of a Molecule is Determined by the Rates of its Synthesis and Degradation

The pioneering work by Henry Borsook and Rudolf Schoenheimer demonstrated in the early 40's that the components of living cells are constantly turning over. Involved in this dynamics are the coupled mechanisms of molecular synthesis and degradation. Turnover is sometimes taken as synonym with degradation (proteolysis, in the case of proteins). However this is only partly true as degradation must be coupled to synthesis in order to fully account for the recycling and replenishing of molecular structures.

If we define 'D', the complex function that describes *degradation* of a given molecular species 'M', and 'S', the function that describes *synthesis* of the same molecular species, then D could be depicted as the general function which decreases the amount of the assembled molecule M by releasing free-subunits 'm' from the molecule:

$$D : m \leftarrow M \qquad \text{[Eq. 7–1]}$$

Conversely, the function 'S' could be depicted as the general function which increases the amount of the assembled molecule M by the reverse path, i.e., the incorporation of free subunits m in the molecule:

$$S : m \rightarrow M \qquad \text{[Eq. 7–2]}$$

The rate of change in the cellular level of the molecule M, (d[M]/dt), can be calculated from the difference between its measured rates of synthesis and degradation:

$$(d[M]/dt) = K_S[M] - K_D[M] \qquad \text{[Eq. 7–3]}$$

Thus, the balance between synthesis and degradation of the molecule M can be defined as the composite function 'T' (T, from *turnover*), as:

$$T(M) = f[S(M), D(M)] \qquad \text{[Eq. 7–4]}$$

In the *steady state*, the levels of the molecule M being turned over in a given cell or tissue are maintained constant because M is being replaced by synthesis at the same rate as it is being broken down by degradation. As a consequence, the rate of its synthesis (d[S]/dt, or K_S) equals the rate of its degradation (d[D]/dt, or K_D):

$$K_S \approx K_D \qquad \text{[Eq. 7–5]}$$

and there is no net change of the function T over time. The integral ($\int$) of the function T is defined geometrically as the area below the graphic shown in Figure 7–1. The area below the graphic represents the total amount of the molecule M being turned over in a given interval of time. In the steady state condition, the amounts of the molecule M being replaced is constant over time:

$$\int_{t0}^{t1} T(M)dt \approx \int_{t1}^{t2} T(M)dt \qquad \text{[Eq. 7–6]}$$

However, conditions other than steady state are more common in cells. These conditions are featured by dynamic fluctuations in the amounts of the molecule M being replaced. A net *decrease* in the amounts of the molecule may be caused by the rate of synthesis being smaller than the rate of degradation in a given period of time:

$$K_S[M] < K_D[M] \qquad \text{[Eq. 7–7]}$$

The number of molecules being replaced per unit time during this same period is also reduced. This condition is illustrated in Figure 7–1 as a decrease in the area below the graphic of T (M):

$$\int_{t0}^{t2} T(M)dt > \int_{t2}^{t4} T(M)dt \qquad \text{[Eq. 7–8]}$$

A net *increase* in the amounts of the molecule being replaced may be caused by the rate of synthesis being greater than the rate of degradation:

$$K_S[M] > K_D[M] \qquad \text{[Eq. 7–9]}$$

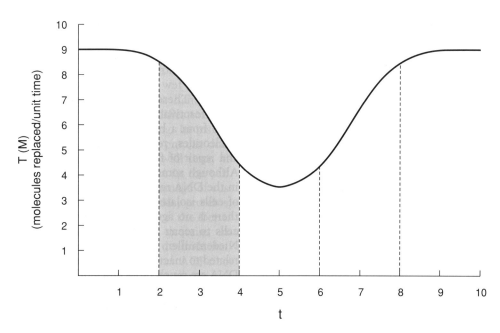

FIGURE 7–1

Molecular turnover (T) of a molecule (M) over time (t). Molecular turnover is determined by the balance between molecular synthesis and degradation. The graphic shows the turnover rate T (M), expressed as molecules replaced per unit time. Within the interval t_2-t_4 the molecule is broken down faster than it is replaced; in interval t_6-t_8 the molecule is replaced faster than it is broken down. The integral ($\int$) of the function T (M) is defined geometrically as the area below the graphic of T (M), which gives the total number of molecules being replaced. During the interval t_2-t_4 (shaded area), 14 molecules are turned over or replaced, as calculated from the area below the graphic. During the interval t_2-t_8, a total of 36 molecules have been replaced. Steady state is observed in the intervals t_0-t_1 and t_9-t_{10}. Note that the amount of the molecule in the interval t_0-t_2 is twice that seen in the interval t_4-t_6.

Accordingly, the area below the graphic of T (M) increases with time (Figure 7–1):

$$\int_{t4}^{t6} T(M)dt < \int_{t6}^{t8} T(M)dt \qquad \text{[Eq. 7–10]}$$

After these considerations, we come to the conclusion that molecular turnover, or the rate at which molecules are replaced and their pools are replenished, depend on both the rates of molecular synthesis and degradation. The rate of molecular turnover is not generally constant, however, but depends very much on the physiological state of the cell.

Distinct Molecular Species Turn Over at Different Rates

The distinct classes of biomolecules in the brain can be listed according to a series of increasing turnover rates: Nuclear DNA < myelin lipids < histone proteins < mitochondrial DNA < microsomal lipids < RNAs and proteins (Table 7–1). Thus, while DNA turnover rates are typically low, RNA and protein turnover rates are the highest. The physiological consequences of decreased turnover include the accumulation of altered and abnormal molecules in the cell, due to increased dwell time, and as a consequence, a disruption of the organization and function of the cell. We shall discuss such effects as regards to DNA and protein turnover, and their consequences to aging.

Nuclear DNA Turnover is Incomplete

Nuclear DNA is duplicated during the S-phase of the cell cycle, when a new DNA strand is synthesized having the old strand as a template. Strictly speaking, the duplication of DNA must be classified as a copying process, not an actual turnover, as the duplication process does not involve the degradation of the template- or old strand, which is passed to the daughter cells together with the newly synthesized strand.

However during most of the time when the cell is not replicating, which varies from minutes or hours in mitotic cells such as epithelial cells, to several years or the whole organism's life, in postmitotic cells such as neurons, the nuclear DNA molecule does turn over, though incompletely. DNA turnover occurs when damaged stretches of the molecule are repaired by DNA-repair enzymes. Thus the dwell time of nuclear DNA is very high, and the molecule is continuously exposed to damage. Major DNA-damaging agents include solar UV radiation, background ionizing radiation, a wide range of chemicals in food and in the environment, and several endogenous agents such as aldehydes, active oxygen species and other free radicals which are the result of metabolic pathways. In addition,

TABLE 7–3.   Average age of onset and main abnormally turned over structures found in several neurodegenerative diseases[*]

Disease	Age of onset (mean, years)	Main abnormally turned over structures in the brain
AD	55–65 (and later)	NP and NFT (GVD, HB and LB in some cases)
Pick	55–65 (and later)	Masses of straight fibrils; densely packed spherical aggregates (PB)
PD	middle or late life	LB
ALS	50 and later	Lipofuscin (excessively accumulated); 'spheroids' containing accumulations of neurofilaments
CJD	55–75	Vacuoles; protease resistant fibrils, PrP, amyloid
GSS	40–50	Vacuoles; plaquelike deposits of amyloid, PrP

[*] Abbreviations: AD, Alzheimer disease or degenerative dementia of the Alzheimer type; Pick, Pick disease; PD, idiopathic parkinsonismus or Parkinson disease; ALS, amyotrophic lateral sclerosis; CJD, Creutzfeldt-Jacob disease; GSS, Gerstmann-Sträussler-Scheinker disease; NP, neuritic plaque; NFT, neurofibrillary tangle; GVD, granulovacuolar degeneration; HB, Hirano body; LB, Lewy body; PB, Pick body; PrP, prion protein. The participation of infective agents referred to as slow virus or unconventional agents (prions) whose viral nature has not yet been excluded is ascertained in CJD. GSS is considered to be an inherited form of CJD.

dence that a cellular PrP gene is transcribed at similar levels in both normal and scrapie-infected tissue, and that PrPs in normal and infected tissues appear to have identical amino acid sequences, the difference between them probably lying on post-translational modification such as glycosylation. Scrapie-derived PrP, but not its normal homolog, aggregates into helically twisted rods and is less susceptible to protease degradation than is normal PrP. In order to effectively infect a hamster, about 10^{15} molecules of the pathological PrP form directly injected into brain is necessary - an impressive figure, taken into account that one single molecule of certain virus is able to infect a whole organism. In addition, incubation times for PrPs are usually prolonged. Since PrP of BSE, for instance, may be contracted orally, great resistance of this protein against proteolytic breakdown in the gastrointestinal tract, in serum and finally in brain, must be assumed. Moreover, although cases of early onset of PrP-related conditions CJD and GSS are observed, late onset seems to be the rule, maybe indicating that age-related changes such as decreased proteolytic capacity favor the appearance of the symptoms of the diseases (Table 7–3).

The study of the patterns of expression and activity of proteases thus constitutes a worth testing approach in aging research.

An Overall View

The molecular turnover concept provides a plausible explanation for the age-related accumulation of abnormal macromolecules within cells, thus offering a valuable insight to the phenomenon of progressive aging and associated diseases. The rates of molecular synthesis and degradation continuously change in a given cell or organism. In a situation of sustained stress as life itself, it would be detrimental if the overall pattern of molecular turnover remained unchanged. The progressive loss of the ability of individual cells and of the organism to reset their rates of macromolecular synthesis and degradation according to environmental signals is decidedly an important mechanism underlying the loss of maintenance capacity. Thus the most promising research strategies to unravel the molecular basis of aging and modulate the process will include an analysis of the formation and maintenance of macromolecular repair processes at all levels of the organization of life: stability of the nuclear and mitochondrial genome, accuracy and efficiency of transcription and translation of nucleic acids into proteins, and degradation of damaged macromolecules.

Selected Readings

Barinaga, M. 1995. A new twist to the cell cycle. Science 269:631–632.

Bernstein, C., and Bernstein, H. 1991. Aging, Sex, and DNA Repair. San Diego, CA: Academic Press. pp. 109–113.

Buccala, R., Model, P., and Cerami, A. 1984. Modification of DNA by reducing sugars: a possible mechanism for nucleic acid aging and age-related dysfunction in gene expression. Proc. Natl. Acad. Sci. USA 81:105–109.

Carney, D. H., Crossin, K. L., Ball, R., Fuller, G. M., Albrecht, T., and Thompson, W. C. 1986. Changes in the extent of MT assembly can regulate initiation of DNA synthesis. Ann. N.Y. Acad. Sci. 466:919–932.

Chopp, M. 1993. The roles of heat shock proteins and immediate early genes in central nervous system normal function and pathology. Curr. Opin. Neurol. Neurosurg. 6:6–10.

Dani, S. U., Bergmann, B., Walter, G. F., Pittella, J. E. H., and Hori, A. 1993. A multivariate approach to the relationship between aging, RNA depletion and the incidence of plaques and tangles. Neuropathology (Kyoto) 13:243–249.

Dice, J. F. 1993. Cellular and molecular mechanisms of aging. Physiol. Rev. 73:149–159.

Driscoll, J., and Goldberg, A. L. 1990. The proteasome (multicatalytic protease) is a component of the 1500-kDa proteolytic complex which degrades ubiquitin-conjugated proteins. J. Biol. Chem. 265:4789–4792.

Goldberg, A. L. 1992. The mechanism and functions of ATP-dependent proteases in bacterial and animal cells. Eur. J. Biochem. 203:9–23

Goodison, K. L., Parhad, I. M., White, C. L., Sima, A. A. F., and Clark, A. W. 1993. Neuronal and glial gene expression in neocortex of Down's syndrome and Alzheimer's disease. J. Neuropathol. Exp. Neurol. 52:192–198.

Gurley, W. B., and Key, J. L. 1991. Transcriptional regulation of the heat-shock response: a plant perspective. Biochemistry 30:1–12.

Hanawalt, P.C. 1991. Heterogeneity of DNA repair at the gene level. Mutat. Res. 247:203–211.

Jentsch, S., and Schlenker, S. 1955. Selective protein degradation: a journey's end within the proteasome. Cell 82:881–884.

Kettelhut, I. C., Pepato, M. T., Migliorini, R. H., Medina, R., and Goldberg, A. L. 1994. Regulation of different proteolytic pathways in skeletal muscle in fasting and diabetes mellitus. Brazilian J. Med. Biol. Res. 27:981–993.

Khasigov, P. Z., and Nikolaev, A.Ya. 1987. Age-related changes in the rates of polypeptide chain elongation. Biochem. Int. 15:1171–1178.

Kyriazis, M. 1991. Applications of chaos theory to the molecular biology of aging. Exp. Gerontol. 26:569–572.

McQuarrie, I. G., Brady, S. T., and Lasek, R. J. 1989. Retardation in the slow axonal transport of cytoskeletal elements during maturation and aging. Neurobiol. Aging 10:359–365.

McKerrow, J. 1979. Nonenzymatic posttranslational amino acid modifications in aging: a brief review. Mech. Ageing Dev. 10:371–377.

Pacifici, R. E., and Davies, K. J. A. 1991. Protein, lipid and DNA repair systems in oxydative stress: The free radical theory of aging revisited. Gerontology 73:166–180.

Prusiner S. B. 1993. Genetic and infectious prion diseases. Arch. Neurol. 50:1129–1153.

Raes, M. 1991. Involvement of microtubules in modifications associated with cellular aging. Mutat. Res. 256:149–168.

Rattan, S. I. S. 1991. Protein synthesis and the components of protein synthetic machinery during cellular ageing. Mutat. Res. 256:115–125.

Rattan, S. I. S. 1995. Ageing - a biological perspective. Molec. Aspects Med. 16:439–508.

Schmidt, A. M., Yan, S. D., and Stern, D. M. 1995. The dark side of glucose. Nature Medicine 10:1002–1004.

Walter, G. F. 1996. Prion diseases: Should neurosurgeons be concerned? Clin. Rev. Neurosurg. 6:323–333.

References

Alberts, B., Bray, D., Lewis, J., Raff, M., Roberts, K., and Watson, J. D. 1989. Molecular Biology of the Cell. Second edition. New York and London: Garland Publishing, Inc.

Ananthan, J., Goldberg, A. L., and Voellmy, R. 1986. Abormal proteins serve as eukaryotic stress signals and trigger the activation of heat shock genes. Science 232:522–524.

Aw, T. Y., Nicotera, P., Manzo, L., and Orrenius, S. 1990. Tributylin stimulates apoptosis in rat thymocytes. Arch. Biochem. Biophys. 283:46–50.

Baudry, M., DuBrin, R., and Lynch, G. 1987. Subcellular compartmentalization of calcium-dependent and calcium-independent neutral proteases in brain. Synapse 1:506–511.

Bekkers, J. M., and Stevens, C. F. 1990. Two different ways evolution makes neurons larger. Prog. Brain Res. 83:37–45.

BeMiller, P. M., Baker, U. A., and Schmit, J. C. 1985. Cellular aging and ribosome RNA. In R. S. Sohal, L. S. Birnbaum, and R. G. Cutler (eds.) Molecular Biology of Aging: Gene Stability and Gene Expression. New York: Raven, pp. 223–228.

Bohr, V. A., and Anson, R. M. 1995. DNA damage, mutation and fine structure repair in aging. Mutat. Res. 338:25–34.

Boycott, B. B. 1974 In R. Bellairs, and E. G. Gray (eds.) Essays on the Nervous System. Oxford: Claredon Press.

Branconnier, R. J., Branconnier, M. E., Walshe, T. M., McCarthy, C., and Morse, P. A. 1992. Blocking the Ca(2+)-activated cytotoxic mechanisms of cholinergic neuronal death: a novel treatment strategy for Alzheimer's disease. Psychopharmacol. Bull. 28:175–181.

Brandhorst, B. P., and McConkey, E. H. 1974. J. Mol. Biol. 85:451–563.

Cantor, C. R., Smith, C. L. 1993. In R. N. Rosenberg et al. (eds.) The Molecular and Genetic Basis of Neurological Disease. Butterworth, Boston, pp. 977–987.

Carney, J. M., Starke-Reed, P. E., Oliver, C. N., Landum, R. W., Cheng, M. S., Wu, J. F., and Floyd, R. A. 1991. Reversal of age-related increase in brain protein oxidation, decrease in encyme activeity, and loss in temporal and spatial memory by chronic administration of the spin-trapping compound N-tert-butyl-alpha-phenylnitrone. Proc. Natl. Acad. Sci. USA 88:3633–3636.

Chopp, M. 1993. The roles of heat shock proteins and immediate early genes in central nervous system normal function and pathology. Curr. Opin. Neurol. Neurosurg. 6:6–10.

Croall, D. E., and DeMartino, G. N. 1991. Calcium-activated neutral protease (Calpain) system: Structure, function and regulation. Physiol. Rev. 71:813–847.

Dani, S. U. 1993. The turnover criterion for selection between normal aging or degenerative diseases. Clin. Neuropathol. 12:241 (Abstract).

Dani, S. U. 1994a. Larger neuronal size overwhelms maintenance capacity with aging. Med. Hypotheses 42:208–210.

Dani, S. U. 1994b. Spatial Patterns of Plaques and Tangles in Alzheimer's Disease. Dementia 5:53.

Dani, S. U., Pittella, J. E. H., Hori, A., Bergmann, B., Stan, A. C., and Walter, G. F. 1994. Different rates of neuronal degeneration: an exquisite variation of the cascade hypothesis. Dementia 5:110–118.

Darnell, J., Lodish, H., and Baltimore, D. 1990. Molecular Cell Biology. Second edition. Scientific American Books, New York.

Dice, J. F. 1987. Molecular determinants of protein half-lives in eukaryotic cells. FASEB J. 1:349–357.

Dice, J. F. 1989. Altered protein degradation in aging: a possible cause of proliferative arrest. Exp. Gerontol. 24:451–459.

Dice, J. F. 1990. Pathways of intracellular proteolysis. Semin. Cell Biol. 1:411–413.

Dice, J. F., and Walker, C. D. 1978. The general characteristics of intracellular protein degradation in diabetes and starvation. In H. L. Segal, and D. J. Doyle (eds.) Protein Turnover and Lysosome Function. New York, San Francisco, London: Academic Press. pp 105–118.

Driscoll, D. M. 1971. The relationship between weather and mortality in the major metropolitan areas in the United States, 1962–1965. Int. J. Biometeorol. 15:23–39.

Firth, W. J. 1991. Chaos - predicting the unpredictable. Br. Med. J. 303:1565–1568.

Goedert, M., and Spillantini, M. G. 1990. Molecular neuropathology of Alzheimer's disease: In situ hybridization studies. Cell. Mol. Neurobiol. 10:159–174.

Goldberg, A. L. 1992. The mechanism and functions of ATP-dependent proteases in bacterial and animal cells. Eur. J. Biochem. 203:9–23

Goldberg, A. L., Kowit, J., Etlinger, J., and Klemes, Y. 1978. Selective degradation of abnormal proteins in animal and bacterial cells. In H. L. Segal, and D. J. Doyle (eds.) Protein Turnover and Lysosome Function. New York, San Francisco, London: Academic Press. pp 171–196.

Goldberg, A. L., Olden, K., and Prouty, W. F. 1975. Studies of the mechanisms and selectivity of protein degradation in *E. coli*. In R. T. Schimke, and N. Katunuma (eds.) Intracellular Protein Turnover. Academic Press, Inc, New York, pp 17–55.

Goldberg, A. L., and St. John, A. C. 1976. Intracellular protein degradation in mammalian and bacterial cells. Ann. Rev. Biochem. 45:747–803.

Goldspink, D., and Kelly, F. 1984. Protein turnover and growth in the whole body, liver, and kidney of the rat from foetus to senility. Biochem. J. 217:507–516.

Graves, R. A., Pandey, N. B., Chodchoy, N., and Marzluff, W. F. 1987. Translation is required for regulation of histone mRNA degradation. Cell 48:615–626.

Grube, K., and Bürkle, A. 1992. Poly(ADP-ribose) polymerase activity in mononuclear leukocytes of 13 mammalian species correlates with species-specific life span. Proc. Natl. Acad. Sci. USA 89:11759–11763.

Gurley, W. B., and Key, J. L. 1991. Transcriptional regulation of the heat-shock response: a plant perspective. Biochemistry 30:1–12.

Harpold, M. M., Wilson, M., and Darnell, J. E. 1981. Mol. Cell Biol. 1:188.

Hershko, A., and Ciechanover, A. 1982. Mechanisms of intracellular protein breakdown. Ann. Rev. Biochem. 51:335–364.

Hershko, A., and Ciechanover, A. 1986. The ubiquitin pathway for the degradation of intracellular proteins. Prog. Nucleic Acid Res. Mol. Biol. 33:19–56.

Hightower, L. 1980. Cultured animal cells exposed to amino acid analogs of puromycin rapidly synthesize several polypeptides. J. Cell Physiol. 102:407–427.

Holzer, H. 1978. Control of proteolysis in yeast. In H. L. Segal, and D. J. Doyle (eds.) Protein Turnover and Lysosome Function. New York, San Francisco, London: Academic Press. pp 305–314.

Ihara, Y. 1989. What mediates between β-amyloid and paired helical filaments? Neurobiol. Aging 10:573–574.

Ivy, G. O., Kitani, K., and Ihara, Y. 1989. Anomalous accumulation of tau and ubiquitin immunoreactivities in rat brain caused by protease inhibition and by normal aging: a clue to PHF pathogenesis? Brain Res. 498:360–365.

Iwamoto, N., Thangnipon, W., Crawford, C., and Emson, P. C. 1991. Localization of calpain immunoreactivity in senile plaques and in neurones undergoing neurofibrillary degeneration in Alzheimer's disease. Brain Res. 561:177–180.

Iwatsubo, T., Hasegawa, M., Esaki, Y., and Ihara, Y. 1992. Lack of ubiquitin immunoreactivities at both ends of neuropil threads. Possible bidirectional growth of neuropil threads. Am. J. Pathol. 140:277–282.

Johnson, S. A., Pasinetti, G. M., May, P. C., Ponte, P. A., Cordell, B., and Finch, C. E. 1988. Selective reduction of mRNA for the β-amyloid precursor protein that lacks a Kunitz-type protease inhibitor motif in cortex from AD. Exp. Neurol. 102:264–268.

Khasigov, P. Z., and Nikolaev, A. Ya 1987. Age-related changes in the rates of polypeptide chain elongation. Biochem. Int. 15:1171–1178.

Kyriazis, M. 1991. Applications of chaos theory to the molecular biology of aging. Exp. Gerontol. 26:569–572.

Lazaris-Karatzas, A., Montine, K. S., and Sonenberg, N. 1990. Malignant transformation by a eukaryotic initiation factor subunit that binds to mRNA 5' cap. Nature 345:544–547.

Li *et al.* 1992. Targetted mutation of the DNA methyltransferase gene results in embryonic lethality. Cell 61:915–926.

Lindahl, T. 1993. Instability and decay of the primary structure of DNA. Nature 362:709–715.

Liu, A. Y. -C., Choi, H. -S., Lee, Y. -K., and Chen, K. Y. 1991. Molecular events involved in transcriptional activation of heat shock genes become progressively refractory to heat stimulation during aging of human diploid fibroblasts. J. Cell. Physiol. 149:560–566.

Lowe, J., R. J. Mayer, and Landon, M. 1993. Ubiquitin in neurodegenerative diseases. Brain Pathol. 3:55–65.

McConkey, D. J., Hartzell, P., and Duddy, S. K. 1988. 2,3,7,8-tetrachlorodibenzo-p-dioxin kills immature thymocytes by Ca²⁺-mediated endonuclease activation. Science 242:256–259.

McDonald, J. K., and Barret, A. J. (ed.) 1986. Mammalian proteases: A Glossary and Bibliography. Vol. 2. Exopeptidases. Academic Press, London. pp 207–210.

Medvedev, Z. A. 1986. Age-related changes of transcription and RNA processing. In D. Platt (ed.) Drugs and Aging. Springer-Verlag, Berlin. pp. 1–19.

Millward, D. J., and Garlick, P. J. 1976. In H. Hanson and P. Bohley (eds.) Intracellular Protein Catabolism. Barth, Leipzig. pp 158–164.

Mori, H., Kondo, J., and Ihara, Y. 1987. Ubiquitin is a component of paired helical filaments in Alzheimer's disease. Science 235:1641–1644;

Müller, W. E. G., Agutter, P. S., and Schröder, H. C. 1995. Transport of mRNA into the cytoplasm. In A. Macieira-Coelho (ed.), Molecular Basis of Aging. CRC Press, Boca Raton. pp. 353–388.

Munro, H. N. 1970. (ed.) Mammalian Protein Metabolism, Vol. 4, Academic Press, New York.

Murachi, T. 1990. [Calpain and calpastatin] (in Japanese). Rinsho Byori 38:337–346.

Neurath, H. 1984. The evolution of proteolytic enzymes. Science 224:350–357.

Niedermüller, H. 1995. DNA repair during aging. In A. Macieira-Coelho (ed.) Molecular Basis of Aging. CRC Press, Boca Raton. pp. 137–182.

Nilsson, E., Alafuzoff, I., Blennow, K., Blomgren, K., Hall, C. M., Janson, I., Karlsson, I., Wallin, A., Gottfries, C. G., and Karlsson, J. O. 1990. Calpain and calpastatin in normal and Alzheimer-degenerated human brain tissue. Neurobiol. Aging 11:425–431.

Oechsli, F. W., and Bueckley, R. W. 1970. Excess mortality associated with three Los Angeles september hot spells. Environ. Res. 3:277–284.

Oyama, F., Shimada, H., Oyama, R., Titani, K., and Ihara, Y. 1992. A novel correlation between the levels of β-amyloid protein precursor and tau transcripts in the aged human brain. J. Neurochem. 59:1117–1125.

Oyama, F., Shimada, H., Oyama, R., Titani, K., and Ihara, Y. 1993. β-amyloid protein precursor and tau mRNAs levels versus β-amyloid plaque and neurofibrillary tangles in the aged human brain. J. Neurochem. 60:1658–1664.

Oyama, F., Cairns, N. J., Shimada, H., Oyama, R., Titani, K., and Ihara, Y. 1994. Down's Syndrome: Upregulation of β-amyloid protein precursor and tau mRNAs and their defective coordination. J. Neurochem. 62:1062–1066.

Pagano, M., Tam, S. W., Theodoras, A. M., Beer-Romero, P.,

Del Sal, G., Chau, V., Yew, P. R., Draetta, G. F., and Rolfe, M. Role of the ubiquitin-proteasome pathway in regulating abundance of the cyclin-dependent kinase inhibitor p.27. Science 269:682–685, 1995.

Pitt, D. 1975. Lysosomes and Cell Function. Longman.

Perlmutter, L. S., Siman, R., Gall, C., Seubert, P., Baudry, M., and Lynch, G. 1988. The ultrastructural localization of calcium-activated protease 'calpain' in rat brain. Synapse 2:79–88.

Rattan, S. I. S. 1989. DNA damage and repair during cellular aging. Int. Rev. Cytol. 116:47–88.

Rattan, S. I. S. 1991. Protein synthesis and the components of protein synthetic machinery during cellular ageing. Mutat. Res. 256:115–125.

Rattan, S. I. S. 1995. Translation and post-translational modifications during aging. In A. Macieira-Coelho (ed.) Molecular Basis of Aging. CRC Press, Boca Raton. pp. 389–420.

Rechsteiner, M. 1990. PEST sequences are signals for rapid intracellular proteolysis. Semin. Cell. Biol. 1:433–440

Richardson, A., Birchenall-Sparks, M. C. 1983. Age-related changes in protein synthesis. Rev. Biol. Res. Aging 1:255–273.

Riis, B., Rattan, S. I. S., Clark, B. F. C., and Merrick, W. C. 1990. Eukaryotic protein elongation factors. TIBS 15:420–424.

Rothstein, M. 1983. Enzymes, enzyme alteration, and protein turnover. Rev. Biol. Res. Aging 1:305–314.

Schimke, R. T. 1975. On the properties and mechanisms of protein turnover. In R. T. Schimke, and N. Katunuma (eds.) Intracellular Protein Turnover. Academic Press, Inc., New York, pp. 173–186.

Seïte, R., Mei, N., and Couineau, S. 1971. Modification quantitative des bâtonnets intranucléaires des neurones sympathiques sous l'influence de la stimulation électrique. Brain Res. 34:277–290.

Seïte, R., Mei, N., and Vuillet-Luciani, J. 1973. Effect of electrical stimulation on nuclear microfilaments and microtubules of sympathetic neurons submitted to cycloheximide. Brain Res. 50:419–423.

Shall, S. 1995. ADP-ribosylation reactions. Biochimie 77:313–318.

Shepherd, J. C. W., Walldorf, U., Hug, P., and Gehring, W. J. 1989. Fruit flies with additional expression of the elongation factor EF-1a live longer. Proc. Natl. Acad. Sci. USA 86:7520–7521.

Sherr, C. J. 1994. G1 phase progression: cycling on cue. Cell 79:551– 555.

Shock, N. M. 1980. Physiological and chronological age. In A. A. Dietz (ed.) Aging - Its Chemistry. American Assoc. Clin. Chem., Washington, DC. p. 3.

Silar, P., and Picard, M. 1994. Increased longevity of EF-1a high-fidelity mutants in Podospora anserina. J. Mol. Biol. 235:231–236.

Sohal, R. S., Agarwal, S., Dubey, A., and Orr, W. C. 1993a. Protein oxidative damage is associated with life expectancy of houseflies. Proc. Natl. Acad. Sci. USA 90:7255–7259.

Sohal, R. S., Ku, H. -H., and Agarwal, S. 1993b. Biochemical correlates of longevity in two closely related rodent species. Biochem. Biophys. Res. Commun. 196:7–11.

Stadtman, E. R. 1992. Protein oxidation and aging. Science 257:1220–1224.

Steitz, J. A. 1988. 'Snurps'. Sci. Amer. 258:56–63.

Tanzi, R. E., McClatchay, A. I., Lamperti, E. D., Villa-Komaroff, L., Gusella, J. F., Neve R. L. 1988. Protease inhibitor domain encoded by an amyloid protein precursor mRNA is associated with Alzheimer's disease. Nature 331:528–530.

Van Remmen, H., Ward, W. F., Sabia, R. V., and Richardson, A. 1995. Gene expression and protein degradation. In E. Masoro (ed.) Handbook of Physiology: Aging. Oxford University Press, Oxford. pp. 171–234.

Vitto, A., and Nixon, R. A. 1986. Calcium-activated neutral proteinase of human brain: subunit structure and enzymatic properties of multiple molecular forms. J. Neurochem. 47:1039–1051.

Voet, D., and Voet, J. G. 1990. Biochemistry. John Wiley & Sons, New York.

Waterlow, J. C., Garlick, P. J., and Millward, D. J. 1978. Protein Turnover in Mammalian Tissues and in the Whole Body. North-Holland Pub. Co., Amsterdam - New York - Oxford. pp 461–471.

Ashley I. Bush
Rudolph E. Tanzi

8

The Molecular Biology of Aβ Deposition in Alzheimer Disease

Most Cases of Alzheimer Disease are Sporadic but About Half of the Familial Cases are Mediated by Hereditary Factors

Gene Defects Responsible for Familial Alzheimer Disease Have Been Localized to Loci on Four Chromosomes

The Contribution of Environmental Factors to the Generation of the Alzheimer Disease Phenotype is Still Unclear

Aβ Amyloid is the Pathological Hallmark of Alzheimer Disease

The Amyloid Protein Precursor and Aβ are Soluble Secretion Products

Insoluble Amyloid Forms From Soluble Aβ

Elevated Concentrations of Aβ Alone are Insufficient to Induce Cortical Aβ Precipitation

Interaction of Aβ with Pathological Chaperones is a Possible Mechanism of Amyloidogenesis

Elevated Concentrations of Some Cationic Species are Amyloidogenic

Zinc Ions are the Most Potent Inducer of Aβ Amyloid Formation *in vitro*

Abnormal Zinc Metabolism in the Brain May be Linked with Amyloid Formation

The Effects of Genetic Lesions Upon Aβ and APP Metabolism

An Overall View

Alzheimer disease (AD) is the major form of dementia and is a devastating problem for mankind. The incidence of AD is increasing with the growth of the elderly population, creating a major public health problem as the disorder is neither curable nor preventable. Approximately 10 percent of individuals in their 60's, and 25 percent of individuals in their 80's, are symptomatic with AD. There may be a large subclinical prevalence of AD in the general population as Aβ amyloid deposition in the brain, a pathological hallmark of AD (Glenner *et al.*, 1984; Masters *et al.*, 1985), is found in 45 percent of individuals in their sixth decade (Davies *et al.*, 1988).

Most Cases of Alzheimer Disease are Sporadic but About Half of the Familial Cases are Mediated by Hereditary Factors

Most cases of AD are sporadic, however 10 percent of cases suffer from familial AD (FAD), an aggressive form of the disease with a clinical onset two to three decades earlier than the sporadic disorder, and possessing an autosomal dominant inheritance pattern. Overall estimates of life-time risk of developing AD in first-degree relatives of probands with AD suggest that ≈50 percent of AD cases are mediated by hereditary factors (Breitner *et al.*, 1988). Meanwhile, a relatively low concordance rate of 40 percent in monozygotic twins (Rapoport *et al.*, 1991) implicates non-genetic factors in the expression of the disease. Importantly, AD is also an invariable complication in Down syndrome (DS) where histopathological changes become evident as early as the second decade of life (Rumble *et al.*, 1989).

Gene Defects Responsible for Familial Alzheimer Disease Have Been Localized to Loci on Four Chromosomes

Genetic studies of kindreds with a history of familial AD have led to the localization of responsible gene defects to loci on chromosomes 1, 14, 19 and 21. A variety of pathogenic mutations cause an aggressive form of early-onset (<60 years) familial AD (FAD) that is characterized by *presenile dementia* and premature cerebral Aβ amyloid deposition. Mutations of the Presenilins – *Presenilin-1* (PS-1, formerly S182) on chromosome 14 (Sherrington *et al.*, 1995; Wasco *et al.*, 1995), and *Presenilin-2* (PS-2, previously STM2) on chromosome 1 (Levy-Lahad *et al.*, 1995) – account for over 90 percent of early-onset FAD. These two genes encode novel proteins that share high structural homology in possessing a predicted six- to nine-transmembrane domains and a large, acidic loop domain. The predicted gene products have 24–37 percent identity over 3 groups of >50 residues to a *C. elegans* sperm integral membrane protein (SPE-4) that appears to stabilize the fibrous body-membrane organelle complex during spermatogenesis (L'Hernault *et al.*, 1992), but have even greater (48 percent) identity over a sequence of 460 amino acids to SEL-12 (Levitan *et al.*, 1995), whose function is unclear but appears to facilitate signal transduction mediated by lin-12 and glp-12, members of the *Notch family* of receptors for intercellular signals that specify cell fate.

Forms of early-onset FAD, as well as *hereditary cerebral hemorrhage with angiopathy-Dutch variant* (HCHWA-D) are caused by mutations of the *Aβ amyloid protein precursor* (APP) gene on chromosome 21 (discussed later, and in Chapter 9). These mutations induce amino acid substitutions in regions of the molecule associated with the Aβ domain (van Broeckhoven *et al.*, 1990; Levy *et al.*, 1990; Goate *et al.*, 1991; Chartier-Harlin *et al.*, 1991; Naruse *et al.*, 1991; Murrell *et al.*, 1991; Hendricks *et al.*, 1992). Clinically, these mutations account for a minority (3 percent) of FAD cases (Tanzi *et al.*, 1992). Trisomy 21 (Down syndrome, DS) is a far more common condition and is invariably complicated by premature AD cerebral pathology. Duplication of the APP gene is a plausible explanation for accelerated cerebral Aβ amyloid deposition. But the possibility that duplication of other chromosome 21 genes impacts upon the development of the AD phenotype has not yet been excluded.

The *APOE-e4* allele has been well characterized as a genetic risk-factor for late-onset AD (Corder *et al.*, 1993). 34–65 percent of individuals affected by AD carry the APOE-e4 allele, while it is present in only 24–31 percent of the non-affected adult population (Saunders *et al.*, 1993; Jarvik *et al.*, 1995). The APOE gene on chromosome 19 encodes *apolipoprotein E*, a plasma protein also present in the brain that is involved in the transport of cholesterol and other hydrophobic molecules. Mutations of APP, PS-1 and PS-2 are deterministic for AD. In contrast, APOE genotype is not deterministic since only 25–50 percent of e4 heterozygotes, who account for

88 percent of people having at least one e4 allele, will develop AD (Corder *et al.*, 1993). Also the presence of an e4 allele is not necessary for the development of AD (Roses *et al.*, 1994) since at least 35–50 percent of individuals with AD do not carry an APOE-e4 allele. The identification of the APOE-e4 allele as a genetic risk-factor for late-onset AD has apparently underscored the relevance of the interaction of inherited biological vulnerabilities with environmental or developmental events in generating the AD phenotype.

The Contribution of Environmental Factors to the Generation of the Alzheimer Disease Phenotype is Still Unclear

The contribution of environmental and developmental stressors to the generation of the AD phenotype is more contentious. Head injury appears to be likely to increase the risk of Alzheimer disease in later life (Roberts *et al.*, 1990; Gentleman *et al.*, 1993). Environmental exposure to aluminum (Klatzo *et al.*, 1965; Terry *et al.*, 1965; Perl *et al.*, 1980; Mantyh *et al.*, 1993), iron (Dyrks *et al.*, 1992; Mantyh *et al.*, 1993), or zinc (Mantyh *et al.*, 1993; Bush *et al.*, 1994a) have been put forward as potential pathogens in the evolution of the disorder. Mitochondrial dysfunction, which could be caused by age-related mitochondrial DNA damage (Beal, 1994) or due to an inherited mutation (Hutchin *et al.*, 1995), may play an important role in the pathogenetic sequence of events in AD (Chapter 6).

Aβ Amyloid is the Pathological Hallmark of Alzheimer Disease

The variety of genetic lesions associated with AD indicates that the biochemical etiologies of the sporadic disorder are also likely to be heterogeneous. However, each of these lesions induces increased cerebral Aβ amyloid deposition, suggesting that the amyloidogenic processing of APP may be the final common pathway for the pathogenesis of AD.

The most striking neuropathological change in AD is amyloid deposition in the cerebral cortex, accompanied by gliosis, and neuronal death. Aβ, a 39–43 amino acid peptide, is the major component of AD amyloid and polymerizes in a β pleated sheet conformation (Figure 8–1) within extracellular deposits in the neuropil (*senile plaques*, SP, or *neuritic plaques*, NP) (Masters *et al.*, 1985) and cerebral blood vessels (*amyloid congophilic angiopathy*, ACA) (Glenner *et al.*, 1984). Little or no amyloid deposition occurs in the white matter of the brain or in peripheral tissue. Neuronal and synaptic loss occur most prevalently in the hippocampus and temporal cortex (Price *et al.*, 1991), which may explain the dysmnesia that occurs in AD although clinical correlation with plaque pathology is still contentious (Terry *et al.*, 1991).

The relationship of Aβ amyloid deposition to neurotoxicity and dementia is still unclear. Several studies have demonstrated that aggregated Aβ synthetic peptides are

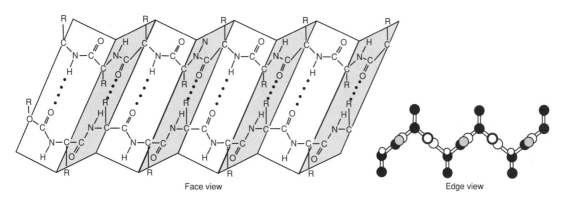

Face view   Edge view

FIGURE 8–1

A regular structural conformation of many proteins including Alzheimer's disease Aβ protein is the β pleated sheet. The β pleated sheet is created by a series of hydrogen bonds between polypeptide strands. A side view of a β pleated sheet shows how the R groups protrude from the faces. Substitutions of hydrophobic amino acids reduce the amyloidogenicity of Aβ peptides (Hilbich et al., 1992) probably by weakening the hydrogen bonding between the peptide strands. (Redrawn from Alberts et al., 1989.)

more capable of inducing neurotoxicity in cell culture than the soluble peptide (Pike et al., 1993), and also can induce the accompanying features of AD neuropathology such as hyperphosphorylation of tau (Busciglio et al., 1995a) (Chapter 9). However, injection of Aβ amyloid into the brains of laboratory animals has not consistently induced AD-like neuropathology or cognitive decline, leaving some doubt as to the position of amyloid deposition in the cascade of events in the development of AD dementia. Nevertheless, the striking association of the heterogeneous genetic lesions that cause and predispose to AD with increased cerebral Aβ deposition argues that the abnormal metabolism of Aβ cannot be separated from the pathogenesis of AD.

However, the mechanisms by which Aβ metabolism may be abnormal are still to be clarified. In this chapter, we argue that the mere production or overproduction of Aβ species alone is unlikely to explain the features of AD. We postulate that although the pathogenic events in AD cannot be separated from abnormal Aβ metabolism, alternative cerebral pathology might impact upon constitutive Aβ metabolism to induce amyloid formation. Some genetic lesions that cause familial AD appear to induce specific changes in Aβ metabolism. We theorize that these changes potentiate and may maximize the amyloidogenic effects of an undetermined stochastic disease process of the brain, so inducing a more aggressive form of a Aβ amyloidosis that would otherwise appear much later in life. In other words, we argue that the explanation for AD pathology is not to be found solely in the abnormal production of Aβ, and that further work is required to study the interaction of the background cerebral pathology in AD upon Aβ metabolism and solubility.

The composition, morphology and neuroanatomical distribution of Aβ amyloid yield important clues about the pathophysiological events that precede the peptide's precipitation. Aβ amyloid composition varies in SP amyloid compared to ACA. The main component of ACA is an Aβ species that terminates at residue 39 [$A\beta_{1-39}$, (Prelli et al., 1988)] or 40 [$A\beta_{1-40}$, (Roher et al., 1993; Miller et al., 1993)], whereas $A\beta_{1-42}$ is enriched in SP amyloid (Kang et al., 1987; Prelli et al., 1988; Roher et al., 1993; Miller et al., 1993), which is surprising since it is a minor species in cerebrospinal fluid (CSF). A longer species, $A\beta_{1-43}$, as well as several carboxyl- and amino- terminal attenuated species, have been described as minor components of SP amyloid (Kang et al., 1987; Mori et al., 1992; Roher et al., 1993).

The Amyloid Protein Precursor and Aβ are Soluble Secretion Products

The discovery of Aβ as a normal secretion product of neuronal cell cultures, and a soluble component of CSF at concentrations in the low ng/ml range (Haass et al., 1992; Seubert et al., 1992; Shoji et al., 1992) has propelled the enquiry into the molecular mechanisms that drive the generation of Aβ from APP. Aβ is generated from its large, transmembrane parent molecule, the amyloid protein precursor (APP) (Kang et al., 1987; Goldgaber et al., 1987; Robakis et al., 1987; Tanzi et al., 1987) by the combined action of proteases whose identities are still unknown. APP is a family of alternatively-spliced proteins that are ubiquitously expressed and whose function is still unclear, although the presence of APP in platelets (Bush et al., 1990) and in synapses (Schubert et al., 1991) suggests an adhesive role in cell-cell connectivity. The major cut that generates the amino-terminus of Aβ occurs 28 residues from the membrane surface by the action of an endopeptidase termed 'β-secretase'. 'γ-secretase' generates the carboxyl terminus of Aβ by an unusual cleavage that presumably occurs within the lipid bilayer. APP is also processed by 'α-secretase' (Sisodia et al., 1990; Esch et al., 1990; Sisodia, 1992), which may be a zinc-metalloproteinase (Roberts et al., 1994), that cleaves the precursor at residue 16 of the Aβ domain rendering a non-amyloidogenic secretion product, APPs, that is found in plasma, platelets and cerebrospinal fluid.

APPs and Aβ are both secreted from neuronal cell cultures, and neurons are presumed to be the major source of these polypeptides in the brain. The generation of APPs and Aβ occurs through constitutive and independent mechanisms that appear to involve the endosomal-lysosomal system (De Strooper et al., 1993; Koo et al., 1994). APP processing yields Aβ fragments with heterogeneous N- and C-termini. The major Aβ species in cell culture (Dovey et al., 1993) and in human CSF (Vigo-Pelfrey et al., 1993) are 1–40 and 1–34.

The APP gene on chromosome 21 codes for 18 exons, and is expressed as a family of at least 8 transmembrane isoforms derived from alternative splicing of exons 7, 8 and 15 (Tanzi et al., 1988; König et al., 1992). Exon 15 codes for a region that is closely upstream to the amino terminus of the Aβ domain. A chondroitin sulfate attachment site is formed when exon 15 is spliced out of APP, and it is proposed that this may have an effect upon β-secretase attachment and the generation of the amino terminus of Aβ (Pangalos et al., 1995).

Insoluble Amyloid Forms From Soluble Aβ

In vitro, synthetic Aβ_{1-42} is relatively insoluble in neutral aqueous solutions (Hilbich et al., 1991), compared to Aβ_{1-39} (Burdick et al., 1992) or Aβ_{1-40} (Tomski et al., 1992) which are both soluble at millimolar concentrations. One in vitro study of amyloid formation with synthetic Aβ peptide solutions reported that kinetically soluble A$\beta_{1-39/40}$ can be destabilized by seeding with Aβ_{1-42} fibrils (Jarrett et al., 1993). This has lead to a hypothesis that Aβ_{1-42} is enriched in SP amyloid because it is a 'pathogenic' species whose production is a feature of AD, whereas Aβ_{1-40} is a constitutive secretion product destabilized by the presence of Aβ_{1-42} in AD. There are several problems with this hypothesis. Firstly, it is based on experimentation with the Aβ_{1-42} peptide in vitro, at concentrations that are several orders of magnitude greater than those found physiologically (Hilbich et al., 1991; Jarrett et al., 1993). Until in vitro studies of the seeding phenomena and aggregation kinetics of Aβ peptides are accomplished at physiological (pM-nM) concentrations, the interpretation of the physiological relevance of the in vitro findings are disadvantaged by amplification artefacts caused by the excessive peptide concentration. A further problem with the 'pathogenic Aβ_{1-42}' hypothesis is that there are no data to show that Aβ_{1-42} is produced in increased amounts in the sporadic AD-affected brain. Also, the intrinsically greater propensity for Aβ_{1-42} to self-aggregate does not adequately explain all the features of Aβ amyloid pathology. It does not explain why there is a greater ratio of Aβ_{1-40} in ACA, and does not explain the microanatomical distribution of amyloid in the neocortex.

Finally, it has been shown that Aβ_{1-42} is found as a soluble component of normal cerebrospinal fluid. Therefore, the presence of the so-called 'pathogenic' Aβ_{1-42} species alone appears insufficient to produce pathology. Possibly, the solubility of the Aβ_{1-42} peptide is preserved by its low

(pM) concentration or by a *solubility chaperone*. Both apolipoproteins E and J (Ghiso et al., 1993) have been described as binding Aβ in CSF, but their effects on Aβ solubility have yet to be proven.

Nevertheless, recently it has been shown that soluble Aβ_{1-42} is found in increased amounts in the brains of individuals affected by DS throughout their life span. In contrast, Aβ_{1-42} is undetectable in the brains of age-matched controls (Teller et al., 1995). In a similar vein, cerebral Aβ_{1-42} deposition has been shown to precede Aβ_{1-40} deposition in DS (Iwatsubo et al., 1995). Therefore, the presence of this peptide in brain tissue appears to indicate the onset of the AD disease process, but does not mean that the soluble peptide itself is 'pathogenic'.

Elevated Concentrations of Aβ Alone are Insufficient to Induce Cortical Aβ Precipitation

Abundant cerebral interstitial Aβ amyloid deposition has been observed in transgenic mice overexpressing a human genomic DNA APP construct possessing the V717F mutation associated with early-onset FAD, driven by a PDGF-β promoter (Games et al., 1995). These animals developed interstitial amyloid in the cerebral cortex, but there is no evidence yet of accompanying cognitive deterioration. It is likely that species differences in the brain environment, or expression and processing changes caused by the intronic arrangement of the construct, its promoter and the attached mutation, combined to facilitate the expression of amyloid in this transgenic animal, where other overexpressed constructs in other rodent species have failed to produce the amyloid-bearing phenotype. It is notable that the success of the production of the amyloid-bearing phenotype in the successful transgenic animal model seems to hinge upon massive overexpression of APP and Aβ. But overexpression of APP and Aβ species to the same extent has failed to induce cortical amyloid pathology in other attempts at a similar transgenic mice model (Hsiao et al., 1995). Therefore, elevated concentrations of Aβ alone are insufficient to induce cortical Aβ precipitation. Since Aβ in CSF is not increased in sporadic AD cases (Shoji et al., 1992; Nakamura et al., 1994; Nitsch et al., 1995), it seems highly likely that pathogenic mechanisms apart from overproduction inititate Aβ amyloid deposition, and that the abnormal milieu of the diseased Alzheimer brain impacts upon Aβ solubility to cause the peptide to precipitate. Several possible mechanisms have been studied.

Interaction of Aβ with Pathological Chaperones is a Possible Mechanism of Amyloidogenesis

One line of enquiry has proposed that ApoE4 is a 'pathological chaperone' responsible for inducing Aβ amyloidogenesis. The three major alleles of ApoE (e2, e3 and e4) differ in only two residues at position 112 (cysteine in e2 and e3, arginine in e4) and 158 (cysteine in e2, and arginine in e3 and e4), and, based on in vitro data these differences have been proposed to account for altered binding with soluble Aβ leading to fibrillogenesis (Strittmatter *et al.*, 1993). However, these data were achieved under conditions where abundantly supraphysiological concentrations of Apolipoprotein E and Aβ were used, and the results have not been consistently reproducible, with disagreement as to which form of ApoE is fibrillogenic. The mechanism by which the ApoE-e4 allele exerts its neurotoxicity may not involve the direct interaction between Apolipoprotein E and Aβ at all. For example, apolipoprotein E may compete with APP for binding to the LDL receptor related protein, so potentially affecting the metabolism of APP (Kounnas *et al.*, 1995).

In a similar vein, it has been proposed that α1-antichymotrypsin, an acute phase reactant that colocalizes with Aβ in SP amyloid, binds the soluble Aβ peptide and induces fibrillogenesis (Ma *et al.*, 1994; Eriksson *et al.*, 1995).

Elevated Concentrations of Some Cationic Species are Amyloidogenic

For many years the role of aluminum has been studied in engendering the pathology of AD. This has been since the original discovery that aluminum salts injected into the brain can induce *neurofibrillary tangles* (Chapter 19) in laboratory animals (Klatzo *et al.*, 1965; Terry *et al.*, 1965). The presence of aluminum with amyloid has been a contentious finding (Edwardson *et al.*, 1989), and although aluminum salts have been shown to precipitate soluble Aβ *in vitro*, the concentrations of the aluminum have been very far above those that are physiologically possible (Mantyh *et al.*, 1993). Concentrations of soluble aluminum salt that are in the low micromolar range have been shown to have no effect upon Aβ solubility *in vitro* (Bush *et al.*, 1994a). Insoluble aluminosilicate particles rapidly induce Aβ aggregation *in vitro* (Candy *et al.*, 1992; Bush *et al.*, 1994c), but it is difficult to conceive how these particles can enter the brain environment *in vivo*. The presence of this inorganic material in SP amyloid may have been due to contamination with glass, since aluminosilicate is a major component of laboratory glassware.

Oxidative stress has been proposed to be a lesion associated with neurodegeneration, AD-associated mitochondrial dysfunction (Beal, 1994; Hutchin *et al.*, 1995) and Down syndrome (Busciglio *et al.*, 1995b), that can also induce amyloid formation from soluble Aβ. Free radical generation can cause Aβ to cross link *in vitro* (Dyrks *et al.*, 1992), inducing the classic *step-ladder pattern* that is seen on SDS-polyacrylamide gel electrophoresis of Alzheimer plaque amyloid (Masters *et al.*, 1985). Free radical generation by the *Fenton reaction* is likely to be the mechanism by which ferrous iron induces Aβ aggregation (Dyrks *et al.*, 1992; Bush *et al.*, 1995). A systematic appraisal of all cations indicated that zinc ions are the most potent inducer of Aβ amyloid formation *in vitro* (Bush *et al.*, 1994a; Bush *et al.*, 1995).

Zinc Ions are the Most Potent Inducer of Aβ Amyloid Formation *in* vitro

A link between the metabolisms of APP and zinc was first recognized when APP co-purified with a zinc-modulated proteolytic mechanism which appeared to mediate the elevation of plasma APP levels observed in AD subjects (Bush *et al.*, 1992; Bush, 1992). Biochemical dissection of the metabolic associations between zinc and APP subsequently identified a specific and saturable zinc binding site on the ectodomain of the protein that enhances the heparin-binding affinity of APP and the inhibitory properties of the *Kunitz-type protease* inhibitory insert (Bush *et al.*, 1993). This site has strong and functionally preserved homology on all known members of the APP superfamily (Bush *et al.*, 1994b), APP and the amyloid precursor-like proteins 1 and 2, and is preserved to the level of *Drosophila* and *C. elegans*. This indicates that zinc interaction may play an important, evolutionarily conserved role in APP function and metabolism.

Aβ itself specifically and saturably binds zinc, manifesting high affinity binding (K_D = 107 nM) with a 1:1 (zinc:Aβ) stoichiometry, and low affinity binding (K_D = 5.2 μM) with a 2:1 stoichiometry (Bush *et al.*, 1994c). Occupation of the zinc binding site inhibits constitutive alpha-secretase type cleavage and so may influence the production of Aβ from APP, and may increase the biological half-life of the peptide (Bush *et al.*, 1994c). Concentrations of zinc above 300 nM rapidly destabilize human $Aβ_{1-40}$ solutions, inducing amyloid formation (Bush *et al.*, 1994a). Zinc-induced Aβ amyloid formation, confirmed by a variety of techniques, is highly specific for zinc, although both copper and iron(II) can induce partial aggregation but not amyloid formation (Bush *et al.*, 1995). Meanwhile, rat $Aβ_{1-40}$ (with substitutions of Arg->Gly, Tyr->Phe and His->Arg at positions 5, 10 and 13, respectively) binds zinc less avidly (K_A = 3.8 μM, with 1:1 stoichiometry) and is unaffected by zinc at these concentrations, perhaps explaining the scarcity with which these animals form cerebral Aβ amyloid (Johnstone *et al.*, 1991; Shivers *et al.*, 1988). In the absence of zinc, the solubilities of the rat and the human Aβ species are indistinguishable (Bush *et al.*, 1994a).

The assembly of zinc-induced human $Aβ_{1-40}$ aggregates is near instantaneous. In comparison, human $Aβ_{1-40}$ (20 μM) has been reported to be stable for 10 days, and seeding the solution with $Aβ_{1-42}$ (2 μM), the more insoluble Aβ species, induced aggregation of this solution which was half-maximal only after 5 days (Jarrett *et al.*, 1993). Thus, the effects of zinc upon $Aβ_{1-40}$ represent a significantly accelerated reaction for inducing amyloid formation *in vitro*. Previous reports of tinctorial Aβ amyloid formation or fibrillogenesis have not been achieved with peptide concentrations less than 0.5 mg/ml (Hilbich *et al.*, 1991), and reports of *in vitro* amyloidogenesis with other APP fragments and other proteins have generally used peptides at concentrations of 2–10 mg/ml (Hilbich *et al.*, 1992; Turnell *et al.*, 1992). In contrast, rapid zinc-induced Aβ aggregation was achieved with a concentration of only 3.5 μg/ml (Bush *et al.*, 1994a).

receptor-related protein, a multifunctional apolipoprotein E receptor, binds the β-amyloid precursor protein and mediates its degradation. Cell 82:331–340.

Ma, J., Yee, A., Brewer, H. B., Jr., Das, S., and Potter, H. 1994. Amyloid-associated proteins alpha 1-antichymotrypsin and apolipoprotein E promote assembly of Alzheimer beta-protein into filaments [see comments]. Nature 372:92–94.

Roher, A. E., Lowenson, J. D., Clarke, S., *et al.* 1993. Structural alterations in the peptide backbone of β-amyloid core protein may account for its deposition and stability in Alzheimer's disease. J. Biol. Chem. 268:3072–3083.

Strittmatter, W. J., Saunders, A. M., Schmechel, D., *et al.* 1993. Apolipoprotein E: high avidity binding to β-amyloid and increased frequency of type 4 allele in late-onset familial Alzheimer disease. Proc. Natl. Acad. Sci. USA 90:1977–1981.

Tanzi, R. E., McClatchey, A. I., Lamperti, E. D., Villa-Komaroff, L., Gusella, J. F., Neve, R. L. 1988. Protease inhibitor domain encoded by an amyloid protein precursor mRNA associated with Alzheimer's disease. Nature 311:528–530.

References

Alberts, B., Bray, D., Lewis, J., Raff, M., Roberts, K., and Watson, J. D. 1989. Molecular Biology of the Cell. Second edition. New York and London: Garland Publishing, Inc., pp. 50.

Assaf, S. Y., and Chung, S.-H. 1984. Release of endogenous Zn2+ from brain tissue during activity. Nature 308:734–736.

Backstrom, J. R., Miller, C. A., and Tökés, Z. A. 1992. Characterization of neutral proteinases from Alzheimer-affected and control brain specimens: identification of calcium-dependent metalloproteinases from the hippocampus. J. Neurochem. 58:983–992.

Beal, M. F. 1994. Energy, oxidative damage, and Alzheimer's disease: clues to the underlying puzzle. Neurobiol. Aging 15:171–174.

Breitner, J., Siverman, J. S., Mohs, R. C., and Davis, K. L. 1988. Familial aggregation in Alzheimer's disease:comparison of risk among relatives of early- and late onset cases, and among male and female relatives in successive generations. Neurology 38:207–212.

Burdick, D., Soreghan, B., Kwon, M., *et al.* 1992. Assembly and aggregation properties of synthetic Alzheimer's A4/β amyloid peptide analogs. J. Biol. Chem. 267:546–554.

Busciglio, J., Lorenzo, A., Yeh, J., and Yankner, B. A. 1995a. β-amyloid fibrils induce Tau phophorylation and loss of microtubule binding. Neuron 14:879–888.

Busciglio, J., and Yankner, B. A. 1995b. Apoptosis and increased generation of reactive oxygen species in Down's syndrome neurons *in vitro*. Nature 378:776–779.

Bush, A. I., Martins, R. N., Rumble, B., *et al.* 1990. The amyloid precursor protein of Alzheimer's disease is released by human platelets. J. Biol. Chem. 265:15977–15983.

Bush, A. I. 1992. Aspects of the pathophysiology and pathogenesis of Alzheimer's disease. Melbourne: University of Melbourne.

Bush, A. I., Whyte, S., Thomas, L. D., *et al.* 1992. An abnormality of plasma amyloid protein precursor in Alzheimer's disease. Ann. Neurol. 32:57–65.

Bush, A. I., Pettingell, W. H., Paradis, Md., Tanzi, R. E., and Wasco, W. 1994b. The amyloid β-protein precursor and its mammalian homologues: Evidence for a zinc-modulated heparin-binding superfamily. J. Biol. Chem. 269:26618–26621.

Bush, A. I., Pettingell, W. H., Jr., Paradis, Md., and Tanzi, R. E. 1994c. Modulation of Aβ adhesiveness and secretase site cleavage by zinc. J. Biol. Chem. 269:12152–12158.

Cai, X.-D., Golde, T. E., and Younkin, S. G. 1993. Release of excess amyloid β protein from a mutant amyloid β protein precursor. Science 259:514–516.

Candy, J. M., Oakley, A. E., and Edwardson, J. A. 1992. Amorphous aluminosilicates promote nucleation of amyloid β protein and tachykinins. Biochem. Soc. Trans. 21:53S. (Abstract.)

Chartier-Harlin, M., Crawford, F., Houlden, H., *et al.* 1991. Early-onset Alzheimer's disease caused by mutations at codon 717 of the β-amyloid precursor protein gene. Nature 353:844–846.

Choi, D. W., Yokoyama, M., and Koh, J. 1988. Zinc neurotoxicity in cortical cell culture. Neuroscience 24:67–79.

Choi, D. W. 1990. Possible mechanisms limiting N-Methyl-D-Aspartate receptor overactivation and the therapeutic efficacy of N-Methyl-D-Aspartate antagonists. Stroke 21(suppl III):20–22.

Citron, M., Oltersdorf, T., Haass, C., *et al.* 1992. Mutation of the β-amyloid precursor protein in familial Alzheimer's disease increases β-protein production. Nature 360:672–674.

Constantinidis, J. 1990. Maladie d'Alzheimer et la théorie du zinc. L'Encephale 16:231–239.

Corder, E. H., Saunders, A. M., Risch, N. J., *et al.* 1994. Protective effect of apolipoprotein E type 2 allele for late onset Alzheimer's disease. Nat. Genet. 7:180–184.

Davies, L., Wolska, B., Hilbich, C., *et al.* 1988. A4 amyloid protein deposition and the diagnosis of Alzheimer's disease: prevalence in aged brains determined by immunocytochemistry compared with conventional neuropathologic techniques. Neurology 38:1688–1693.

De Strooper, B., Umans, L., Van Leuven, F., and Van Den Berghe, H. 1993. Study of the synthesis and secretion of normal and artificial mutants of murine amyloid precursor protein (APP): cleavage of APP occurs in a late compartment of the default secretion pathway. J. Cell Biol. 121:295–304.

Deng, Q. S., Turk, G. C., Brady, D. R., and Smith, Q. R. 1994. Evaluation of brain element composition in Alzheimer's disease using inductively-coupled plasma mass spectrometry. Neurobiol. Aging 15(suppl. 1), S113. (Abstract.)

Dovey, H. F., Suomensaari-Chrysler, S., Lieburg, I., Sinha, S., and Keim, P. S. 1993. Cells with a familial Alzheimer's disease mutation produce authentic β-peptide. NeuroReport 4:1039–1042.

Dyrks, T., Dyrks, E., Hartmann, T., Masters, C., Beyreuther, K. 1992. Amyloidogenicity of βA4 and βA4-containing amyloid protein precursor fragments by metal-catalyzed oxidation. J. Biol. Chem. 267:18210–18217.

Edwardson, J. A., Candy, J. M. 1989. Aluminium and the pathogenesis of senile plaques in Alzheimer's disease, Down's syndrome and chronic renal dialysis. Ann. Med. 21:95–97.

Esch, F. S., Keim, P. S., Beattie, E. C., *et al.* 1990. Cleavage of amyloid β peptide during constitutive processing of its precursor. Science 248, 1122–1124.

Frederickson. C. J., Klitenick. M. A., Manton, W. I., and Kirkpatrick, J. B. 1983. Cytoarchitectonic distribution of zinc in the hippocampus of man and the rat. Brain Res. 273:335–339.

Frederickson, C. J. 1989. Neurobiology of zinc and zinc-containing neurons. Int. Rev. Neurobiol. 31:145–328.

Friedman, B., and Price, J. L. 1984. Fiber systems in the olfactory bulb and cortex: a study in adult and developing rats, using the Timm method with the light and electron microscope. J. Comp. Neurol. 223:88–109.

Games, D., Adams, D., Alessandrini, R., et al. 1995. Alzheimer-type neuropathology in transgenic mice overexpressing V717F β-amyloid precursor protein. Nature 373:523–527.

Gentleman, S. M., Graham, D. I., and Roberts, G. W. 1993. Molecular pathology of head trauma: altered beta APP metabolism and the aetiology of Alzheimer's disease. Prog. Brain Res. 96:237–246.

Ghiso, J., Matsubara, E., Koudinov, A., et al. 1993. The cerebrospinal-fluid form of Alzheimer's amyloid beta is complexed to SP-40,40 (apolipoprotein J), an inhibitor of the complement membrane-attack complex. Biochem. J. 293:27–30.

Glenner, G. G., and Wong, C. W. 1984. Alzheimer's disease: initial report of the purification and characterization of a novel cerebrovascular amyloid protein. Biochem. Biophys. Res. Commun. 120:885–890.

Goate, A., Chartier-Harlin, M., Mullan, M., et al. 1991. Segregation of a missense mutation in the amyloid precursor protein gene with familial Alzheimer's disease. Nature 349:704–706.

Goldgaber, D., Lerman, M. I., McBride, O. W., Saffiotti, U., and Gajdusek, D. C. 1987. Characterization and chromosomal localization of a cDNA encoding brain amyloid of Alzheimer's disease. Science 235:877–880.

Haass, C., Schlossmacher, M. G., Hung, A. Y., et al. 1992. Amyloid β-peptide is produced by cultured cells during normal metabolism. Nature 359:322–325.

Hendricks, L., van Duijn, C. M., Cras, P., et al. 1992. Presenile dementia and cerebral haemorrhage linked to a mutation at codon 692 of the β-amyloid precursor protein gene. Nat. Genet. 1:218–221.

Hilbich, C., Kisters-Woike, B., Reed, J., Masters, C. L., and Beyreuther, K. 1991. Aggregation and secondary structure of synthetic amyloid βA4 peptides of Alzheimer's disease. J. Mol. Biol. 218:149–163.

Hilbich, C., Kisters-Woike, B., Reed, J., Masters, C. L., and Beyreuther, K. 1992. Substitutions of hydrophobic amino acids reduce the amyloidogenicity of Alzheimer's disease βA4 peptides. J. Mol. Biol. 228:460–473.

Howell, G. A., Welch, M. G., and Frederickson, C. J. 1984. Stimulation-induced uptake and release of zinc in hippocampal slices. Nature 308:736–738.

Hsiao, K. K., Borchelt, D. R., Olson, K., et al. 1995. Age-related CNS disorder and early death in transgenic FVB/N mice overexpressing Alzheimer amyloid precursor proteins. Neuron 15:1203–1218.

Hutchin, T., and Cortopassi, G. 1995. A mitochondrial DNA clone is associated with increased risk for Alzheimer's disease. Proc. Natl. Acad. Sci. USA 92:6892–6895.

Hyman, B. T., Van Hoesen, G. W., Kroner, L. J., and Damasio, A. R. 1986. Perforant pathway changes and the memory impairment of Alzheimer's disease. Ann. Neurol. 20:472–481.

Ibata, Y., and Otsuka, N. 1969. Electron microscope demonstration of zinc in the hippocampal formation using Timm's sulfide-silver technique. J. Histochem. Cytochem. 17:171–175.

Iwatsubo, T., Mann, D. M., Odaka, A., Suzuki, N., and Ihara, Y. 1995. Amyloid β protein (Aβ) deposition: Aβ42(43) precedes Aβ40 in Down Syndrome. Ann. Neurol. 37:294–299.

Jarrett, J. T., Berger, E. P., and Lansbury, P. T. 1993. The carboxy terminus of the β amyloid protein is critical for the seeding of amyloid formation: implications for the pathogenesis of Alzheimer's disease. Biochemistry 32:4693–4697.

Johnstone, E. M., Chaney, M. O., Norris, F. H., Pascual, R., and Little, S. P. 1991. Conservation of the sequence of the Alzheimer's disease amyloid peptide in dog, polar bear and

five other mammals by cross-species polymerase chain reaction analysis. Mol. Brain Res. 10:299–305.

Kang, J., Lemaire, H., Unterbeck, A., et al. 1987. The precursor of Alzheimer's disease amyloid A4 protein resembles a cell-surface receptor. Nature 325:733–736.

Klatzo, I., Wisniewski, H., and Streicher, E. 1965. Experimental production of neurofibrillary degeneration. 1. Light microscopic observations. J. Neuropathol. Exp. Neurol. 24:187–199.

Koo, E. H., and Squazzo, S. L. 1994. Evidence that production and release of amyloid β-protein involves the endocytic pathway. J. Biol. Chem. 269:17386–17389.

König, G., Mönning, U., Czeck, C., et al. 1992. Identification and expression of a novel alternative splice form of the βA4 amyloid precursor protein (APP) mRNA in leucocytes and brain microglial cells. J. Biol. Chem. 267:10804–10809.

L'Hernault, S. W., and Arduengo, P. M. 1992. Mutation of a putative sperm membrane protein in Caenorhabditis elegans prevents sperm differentiation but not its associated meiotic divisions. J. Cell Biol. 119:55–68.

Levitan, D., and Greenwald, I. 1995. Facilitation of lin-12-mediated signalling by sel-12, a Caenorhabditis elegans S182 Alzheimer's disease gene. Nature 377:351–354.

Levy, E., Carman, M. D., Fernandez-Madrid, I. J., et al. 1990. Mutation of the Alzheimer's disease amyloid gene in hereditary cerebral hemorrhage, Dutch type. Science 248:1124–1126.

Levy-Lahad, E., Wasco, W., Poorkaj, P., et al. 1995. Candidate Gene for the Chromosome 1 Familial Alzheimer's Disease Locus. Science 269:973–977.

Lui, E., Fisman, M., Wong, C., and Diaz, F. 1990. Metals and the liver in Alzheimer's disease: an investigation of hepatic zinc, copper, cadmium, and metallothionein. J. Am. Geriatr. Soc. 38:633–639.

Mantyh, P. W., Ghilardi, J. R., Rogers, S., et al. 1993. Aluminum, iron, and zinc ions promote aggregation of physiological concentrations of β-amyloid peptide. J. Neurochem. 61:1171–1174.

Masters, C. L., Simms, G., Weinman, N. A., et al. 1985. Amyloid plaque core protein in Alzheimer disease and Down syndrome. Proc. Natl. Acad. Sci. USA 82;4245-4249.

Miller, D. L., Papayannopoulos, I. A., Styles, J., et al. 1993. Peptide compositions of the cerebrovascular and senile plaque core amyloid deposits of Alzheimer's disease. Arch. Biochem. Biophys. 301:41–52.

Mori, H., Takio, K., Ogakawa, M., and Selkoe, D. J. 1992. Mass spectrometry of purified amyloid β protein in Alzheimer's disease. J. Biol. Chem. 267:17082–17086.

Murrell, J., Farlow, M., Ghetti, B., and Benson, M. D. 1991. A mutation in the amyloid precursor protein associated with hereditary Alzheimer disease. Science 254:97–99.

Nakamura, T., Shoji, M., Harigaya, Y., et al. 1994. Amyloid β protein levels in cerebrospinal fluid are elevated in early-onset Alzheimer's disease. Ann. Neurol. 36:903–911.

Naruse, S., Igarashi, S., Kobayashi, J., et al. 1991. Mis-sense mutation Val-Ile in exon 17 of amyloid precursor protein gene in Japanese familial Alzheimer'a disease. Lancet 337:978–979.

Nitsch, R. M., Rebeck, G. W., Deng, M., et al. 1995. Cerebrospinal fluid levels of amyloid beta-protein in Alzheimer's disease: inverse correlation with severity of dementia and effect of apolipoprotein E genotype. Ann. Neurol. 37:512–518.

Pangalos, M. N., Efthimiopoulos, S., Shioi, J., and Robakis, N. K. 1995. The chondoitin sulfate attachment site of appican is

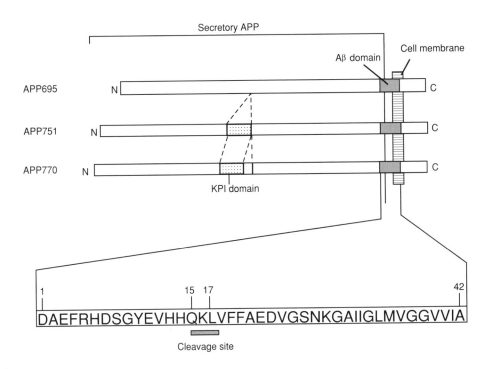

1   15 17   42

DAEFRHDSGYEVHHQKLVFFAEDVGSNKGAIIGLMVGGVVIA

Cleavage site

FIGURE   9–1

Three major APP isoforms (APP$_{695}$, APP$_{751}$, and APP$_{770}$) and the amino acid sequence of Aβ. APP$_{751}$, and APP$_{770}$ contain a Kunitz-type protease inhibitor (KPI) domain. APP$_{695}$, which lacks the KPI domain, is expressed preferentially in postmitotic neurons. The Aβ domain (Aβ) is located at the boundary between extracellular- and transmembrane domains. A proteolytic cleavage occurs in the interior of the Aβ domain (cleavage site), and this cleavage produces secretory types of APP (secretory APP). The proteolytic mechanisms that release intact Aβ from APP have been intensively studied to elucidate the process of extracellular amyloid deposition.

the so called *Kunitz-type protease inhibitors* (KPI) (Figure 9–1). APP mRNAs encoding these isomers are generated by the *alternative splicing* of primary transcripts from one single gene, which is located on chromosome 21. APP mRNAs are ubiquitously and abundantly expressed in neurons of the rat brain (Shivers *et al.*, 1988). APP$_{695}$ mRNA is markedly induced during differentiation of multipotential stem cells into postmitotic neurons (Yoshikawa *et al.*, 1990; Hung *et al.*, 1992; Wertkin *et al.*, 1993). In cerebral neurons *in vivo*, APP is localized to synaptic sites, vesicular elements of neuronal perikarya, dendrites, and axons (Schubert *et al.*, 1991) (Figure 9–2). In peripheral neurons in rat dorsal root ganglia, full-length APP$_{695}$ is rapidly transported anterogradely in axons (Sisodia *et al.*, 1993).

Most Endogenous APP Molecules are Distributed to the Membrane Fractions and Metabolized Within Neurons

The structure of the APP molecule resembles that of membrane-bound receptors (Kang *et al.*, 1987). In APP molecules, the Aβ protein domain is situated at the boundary between the extracellular and transmembrane domains. A proteolytic cleavage occurs physiologically in the interior of the Aβ domain, and the amino (N)-terminal part of APP is secreted into the extracellular space (Esch *et al.*, 1990). However, postmitotic neurons, unlike most of the non-neuronal cell types, do not process significant amounts by secretory cleavage (Hung *et al.*, 1992), suggesting that endogenous APP molecules are physiologically distributed to the membrane fractions and metabolized within neurons. Although the secretory processing produces no intact Aβ peptides, small amounts of intact Aβ_{1-40} have been reported to be released into the extracellular space (Shoji *et al.*, 1992; Seubert *et al.*, 1992).

Two types of abnormalities of the human APP gene suggest a close association of Aβ (or APP) with the pathogenesis of AD: (i) In Down syndrome (trisomy 21), the most common form of mental retardation with a known genetic cause, a gene dosage effect appears to account for high levels of APP mRNA expression in the brain (Tanzi *et al.*, 1988). Since neuropathological features of Down syndrome patients aged over 40 years resemble those of AD, it has been suggested that persistent overexpression of the APP gene gives rise to the development of AD-like neuropathology. (ii) The other important fact is that point-mutations in the APP gene have been found in familial AD (Goate *et al.*, 1991). When a mutant type of APP was overexpressed in transgenic mice, the brain showed AD-like neuropathology including amyloid deposition with neuronal degeneration (Games *et al.*, 1995).

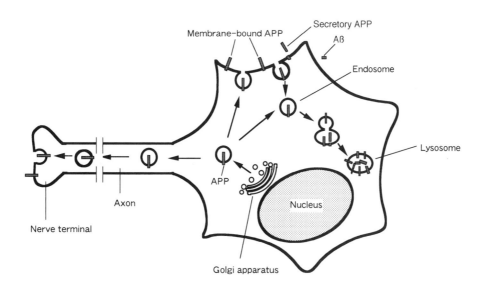

FIGURE   9–2

Synthesis and fate of APP within neurons. APP$_{695}$ is the major APP isoform which is expressed preferentially in differentiated neurons. In neurons, APP is transported to the synaptic sites, endoplasmic reticulum and plasma membranes, and then meta-bolized by secretory and lysosomal pathways. Large amounts of APP may be processed in the endosome-lysosome system after being distributed to internal and plasma membranes of neurons.

These observations favor the proposition that abnormalities of the APP gene generate the AD-like neuropathology that may be linked to the pathogenesis of AD.

Extracellular Aβ May be, or May not be, Cytotoxic in vitro, Depending on Various Factors

Neurotoxicity of an Aβ-containing fragment has been originally demonstrated by Yankner and colleagues (1989) in a cultured cell system of *PC12 pheochromocytoma cells*. They transfected these cells with complimentary DNA (cDNA) encoding a carboxyl (C)-terminal fragment of APP. PC12 cells transfected with cDNA encoding the C-terminal fragment containing the entire Aβ protein region and cytoplasmic domain showed severe degenerative changes when the cells were neurally differentiated by *nerve growth factor* (NGF). In addition, the conditioned medium obtained from the transfected cells was toxic to neurons in primary cultures, suggesting that the secreted APP fragment exerts a neurotoxic effect. After their first report, they found synthetic Aβ$_{1-40}$ to exert trophic effects on immature hippocampal neurons at low concentrations, and neurotoxic effects on the mature neurons at high concentrations (Yankner *et al.*, 1990).

Koh and colleagues reported that exposure of mature cortical neurons to synthetic Aβ$_{1-42}$ increased their vulnerability to excitotoxins such as glutamate, N-methyl-D-aspartate and kainate. Pike and coworkers found that stably aggregated Aβ peptides containing the core sequence Aβ$_{25-35}$ exerted neurotoxic effects on cultured hippocampal neurons. Degeneration was mediated through the activation of an apoptotic pathway (Loo *et al.*, 1993). These observations suggest a relationship between the aggregation state of Aβ and its ability to promote degeneration. It is noteworthy, however, that Aβ$_{25-35}$ (i.e., the core sequence essential for neurotoxicity *in vitro*) is devoid of most of Aβ$_{1-28}$ sequence, which has been shown *in vitro* to exhibit an anti-parallel β-structure, the *β-pleated sheet* (i.e., the basic secondary structure of amyloid fibrils) (Kirchner *et al.*, 1987).

In contrast to the findings supporting the neurotoxicity of Aβ, the lack of evident neurotoxicity of Aβ has been reported in various *in vitro* systems: In high density primary rat hippocampal cultures, there are marked lot-to-lot differences in the neurotoxic properties of synthetic peptide preparations from the same supplier (May *et al*, 1992). Addition of Aβ$_{1-28}$ or Aβ$_{25-35}$ to the medium of hippocampal slice cultures produces no significant changes in dendritic length or the number of branches of the neurons (Malouf, 1992). Aβ$_{1-40}$ and Aβ$_{25-35}$ had negative effects on neuronal survival in low-cell density rat hippocampal cultures in which considerable amounts of neuronal death occurred even in control cultures, but these Aβ peptides did not affect neuronal survival in more stable high density cell cultures where little cell death occurred in control cultures (Mattson and Rydel, 1992), suggesting that Aβ peptides would not cause neuronal damage in stable healthy cultures in which there is no ongoing neuronal death. These results suggest that the neurotoxic effects of Aβ peptides are dependent on var-

embryonal carcinoma cells differentiate into neurons and glial cells when treated with *retinoic acid*. The neural differentiation of P19 cells causes a marked increase in the APP gene expression (Yoshikawa *et al.*, 1990). It has been hypothesized that overproduction of APP in P19 cells by cDNA transfection may induce abnormal production of C-terminal cytotoxic fragments. To test this idea, stable transfectants overexpressing full-length human APP_{695} and APP_{770} were cloned (Yoshikawa *et al.*, 1992). When these transfectants were neurally differentiated by retinoic acid treatment, differentiated postmitotic neurons showed a severe degeneration, and disappeared in a few days (Figure 9–4). Most of the surviving cells in the mixed cultures were degenerating neurons and non-neuronal cells (presumably astrocyte precursors). Part of them had intensely APP immunoreactive materials in lysosome-like structures. The degenerating cells generated N-terminal truncated C-terminal fragments comprising the entire $A\beta$ region as detected by Western blotting. These results suggest that the overexpression of APP induces degeneration of postmitotic neurons and concomitantly generates the abnormally processed C-terminal fragments.

To examine whether the cytotoxicity induced by the abnormal metabolism of APP is specific to neurons, full-length APP cDNAs were transfected into a human glioma cell line, Bu-17 (Hayashi *et al.*, 1992). These APP cDNA transfectants showed a significant cell death accompanied by generation of C-terminal fragments of APP in response to *chloroquine*, an inhibitor of lysosomal functions, at low concentrations which were little toxic to untransfected controls. Thus, it is likely that lysosomal dysfunction in these cells impairs the APP metabolism to generate cytotoxic C-terminal fragments, and concomitantly induces cell degeneration.

The Precise Mechanism of Intracellular Toxicity of Abnormally Metabolized APP is Unknown

The findings in the full-length APP cDNA transfected cell models support the view that neuronal death is due to intracellular abnormal metabolism of APP. Figure 9–5 illustrates a possible mechanism underlying neuronal death and amyloid formation by abnormal metabolism of APP: Under physiological conditions, APP in the neurons is metabolized through both secretory and lysosomal pathways. Since the secretory pathway may not be dominant in terminally differentiated neurons (Hung *et al.*, 1992), it is conceivable that neurons *in vivo* metabolize APP mainly in the lysosomal pathway. If APP is overproduced and/or inadequately metabolized as a result of reduced lysosomal activities, then aberrantly processed APP fragments start to accumulate within the neurons which eventually degenerate and die. Amyloidogenic APP C-terminal fragments in the lysosomes are processed further into smaller amyloidogenic fragments and $A\beta$ peptides. Such conversions from APP C-terminal fragments to $A\beta$ have been experimentally verified using a cDNA transfected cell model (Dyrks *et al.*, 1993). During neuronal degeneration, $A\beta$ may be expelled into the extracellular

space, where amyloid fibrils are formed. This view is compatible with the idea held by some authors that the amyloid mass in senile plaques is not the primary cause of neuronal degeneration but rather an accompanying phenomenon of the APP-associated neuronal death.

The mechanism of neurotoxicity of aberrantly processed fragments is still a speculation: APP-C_{100} overexpressed in COS cells accumulates to form amyloid-like fibrils near or on the nuclear membranes (Maruyama *et al.*, 1990). The C-terminal fragments generated by abnormal metabolism of APP may self-aggregate within the neurons, and the intracellular aggregates eventually impair the viability of the cells. The aggregated fragments may disrupt the organization of intracellular organelles such as the endoplasmic reticulum, endosome and lysosome. Another possibility is that the membrane-bound cytotoxic fragments may interact with other membrane-bound proteins. It is noteworthy that the gene product S182 (*Presenilin-1*) encoded in familial AD genes on chromosomes 14 is a membrane protein with seven transmembrane domains (Sherrington *et al.*, 1995).

Neuropathological Features of Alzheimer Disease May be Explained by a Sequence of Abnormal APP Metabolism

Even though the precise mechanisms of APP-related neurodegeneration are far from being understood, from the evidence reviewed above an association of intraneuronal abnormal APP metabolism and neuronal degeneration can be figured out (Yoshikawa, 1993, 1995) (Figure 9–6): (i) From the early stages of neuronal differentiation, postmitotic neurons express high levels of APP, especially APP_{695}. The neurons may be capable of metabolizing large amounts of APP into non-toxic fragments, and thus maintain the healthy state. (ii) The overproduction of APP (e.g., an increased gene dosage of APP in Down's syndrome), a reduction of lysosomal activity (represented by an age-dependent accumulation of lipofuscin), or missense mutations of the APP gene in familial AD cases lead to an abnormal metabolism of APP in neurons, and aberrantly processed APP fragments start to accumulate within the neurons. (iii) APP fragments and $A\beta$ accumulated along dendritic processes resemble diffuse $A\beta$ deposits ('preamyloid'; type A plaque). This type of $A\beta$ deposition along neuronal membranes has been observed in early stages of senile plaque formation (Allsop *et al.*, 1989, Probst *et al.*, 1991). (iv) When the amounts of these fragments reach critical levels, the neuron starts to degenerate and die. During degeneration, APP fragments are converted into smaller amyloidogenic fragments within the neuron or at the extracellular space. These fragments may contribute to the formation of nascent fibrils (e.g., the 'primordial fibrils'), which eventually develop into mature amyloid structures after undergoing further processing and modification. After the perikarya of degenerated neurons disappear, condensed masses of amyloid fibrils surrounded by dystrophic neurites are left behind at the extracellular space.

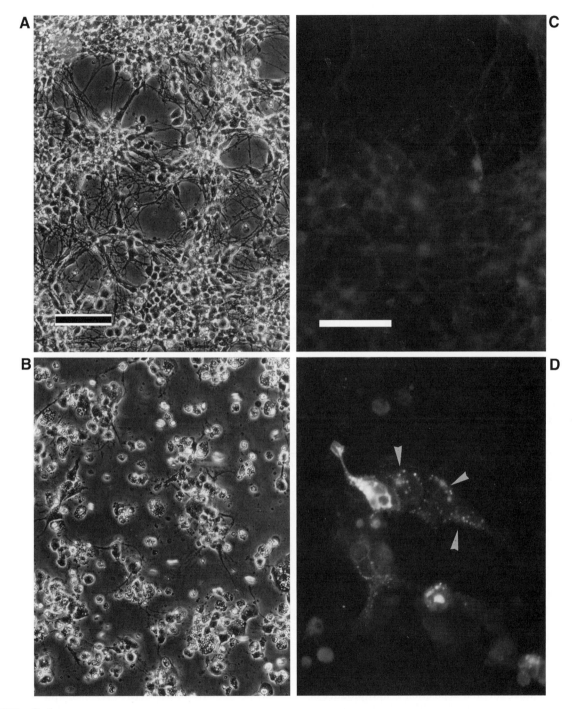

FIGURE   9–4

Degeneration of postmitotic neurons overexpressing APP.
Mouse embryonal carcinoma cells (P19 cells) were stably transfected with cDNA encoding full-length human APP_{695} and differentiated into postmitotic neurons by retinoic acid treatment.

A, C. Control cells transfected with the empty vector.
B, D. Cells transfected with full-length human APP_{695} cDNA.
A, B. Phase-contrast micrography. **C, D.** Fluorescent immunocytochemistry using the anti-C-terminal antibody. When examined
4 days after the treatment, most of the APP_{695} transfectants
show severe degenerative changes (**B**), while control transfectants differentiate normally into neurons (**A**). Note the
accumulation of APP-C-terminal fragments in lysosome-like
organelles (arrowheads in **D**). Scale bars: 100 μm (A, B), and
50 μm (C, D).

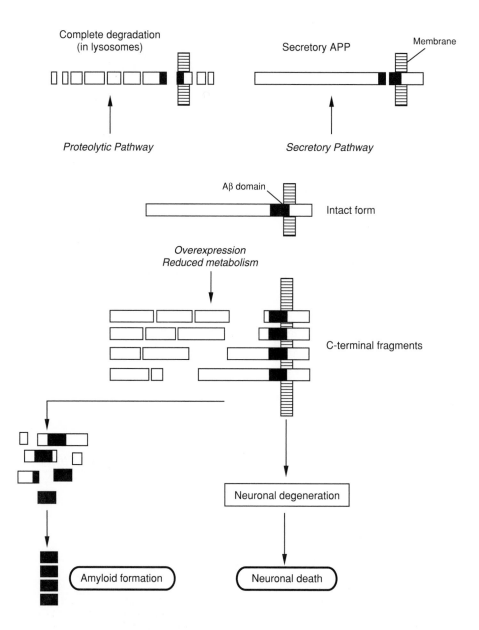

FIGURE 9–5

Possible sequence of events leading to neuronal death and amyloid formation. In this scheme abnormal metabolism of APP induces both neuronal degeneration and generation of Aβ protein deposits. Notice that extracellular amyloid deposition in this model is not a cause but a by-product of neuron death. See text for details.

According to this sequence of neurodegenerative events, extracellular amyloid deposition is a by-product of the abnormal metabolism of APP within the neuron. The reader should be cautioned that this hypothesis cannot account for the genesis of amyloid angiopathy, which has its own etiological background (Chapter 27).

APP May be Abnormally Processed by Lysosomal Enzymes Under the Pathological Conditions Featured by Neuronal Degeneration

Immunocytochemistry using an antibody against the C-terminal sequence of APP revealed punctuated concentrations of APP fragments in pyramidal cells of the neocortex, particularly in associative regions, and intense staining in the CA1 pyramidal cells of the hippocampus (Benowitz et al, 1989). By electron microscopy, this distribution coincided with dense concentrations of APP fragments in secondary lysosomes. In the hippocampus of several AD cases, abnormally dense immunostaining in enlarged intracellular domains is accompanied by a severe atrophy of the CA1 neurons. These observations suggest that the lysosomal accumulation of C-terminal fragments of APP actually occurs within degenerating neurons.

Enzymatically active lysosomal proteases are associated with amyloid deposits in the brain of AD (Cataldo and

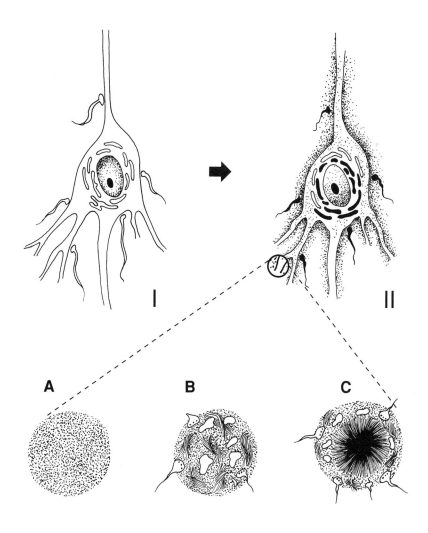

FIGURE   9–6

Internal disintegration of neurons and formation of neuritic plaques in AD. A healthy neuron metabolizes APP completely into non-toxic fragments (phase I). Overproduction of APP, reduction of APP metabolism, or mutation of the APP gene causes abnormal proteolytic processing, which gives rise to intraneuronal accumulation of APP fragments (phase II). In this stage, Aβ-containing fragments are accumulated in the internal and plasma membranes of degenerating neurons. The accumulation in the dendrites may take the shape of extracellular preamyloid plaques (**A**). When the intracellular accumulation of APP fragments reaches a critical level, neurons are internally disintegrated; APP fragments are processed further into Aβ, which eventually form amyloid fibrils; finally, the amyloid deposits and dystrophic neurites are left behind as 'extracellular' plaques (**B, C**), following disappearance of the perikaryon. The plaque in (**C**) has an amyloid core.

Nixon, 1990). High levels of immunoreactivity for the lysosomal enzymes *cathepsins* were localized to extracellular senile plaques in AD brain. At the ultrastructural level, the cathepsin immunoreactivity was localized principally to lysosomal dense bodies and lipofuscin granules in 'extracellular' senile plaques. In more advanced stages of degeneration, cathepsin immunoreactivity was present throughout the cytoplasm. The distribution patterns of these lysosomal proteases in AD brain raise the possibility that the lysosomes are liberated from degenerating neuronal perikarya into the extracellular space. Thus, these findings strongly support the idea that degenerating neurons in the brain with AD actually disintegrate to liberate the lysosomes into the extracellular space. The presence of active lysosomal enzymes in the extracellular space may be responsible for further processing of APP into more dense amyloid fibrils. Cathepsins in lysosomes may play a major role in metabolizing APP into small non-toxic fragments under physiological conditions, whereas they may cleave different sites of APP in unusual pH environments such as the cytoplasm outside the lysosomes and the extracellular space. The abnormally processed fragments of APP can eventually be condensed to form amyloid fibrils within the neurons and the extracellular space.

APP-associated Neuronal Toxicity May Depend on the Level of APP Expression in Different Regions of the Human Brain

APP mRNA, mainly APP_{695} mRNA, is abundant in regions of the association cortices which have been found to be preferentially affected by AD pathology (Tanzi *et al.*, 1988). *In situ* hybridization histochemistry demonstrated that layers III and V of the primate prefrontal cortex contain neurons expressing high levels of APP mRNA, and that signal intensities of APP mRNA are reduced in layer III of the AD brain (Bahmanyar *et al.*, 1987). The cathepsin-laden senile plaques were also localized to layers III and V of the prefrontal association cortex (Cataldo *et al.*, 1990). Taken together, it is conceivable that AD features such as neuritic plaques (Chapter 19) are most numerous precisely in the brain areas where the perikarya of neurons express high levels of the APP gene.

The number of neurons in the association cortices of the human brain has increased during evolution (Chapter 11). In these regions, pyramidal neurons generated at the latest stages of phylogeny had to increase dendritic arborization to receive information from many neurons. These enlarged neurons continuously express high amounts of APP throughout their lifetimes and are thus susceptible to abnormal metabolism of endogenous APP. Therefore, it is likely that a class of neurons created at the latest stages of primate evolution greatly expanded man's intellectual abilities, but simultaneously became vulnerable to Aβ-associated cytotoxicity.

An Overall View

Although it has been widely accepted that amyloid deposition is closely associated with neuronal degeneration in AD, the role, if any, of extracellular amyloid as a cause of neuronal death is controversial. In the light of experimental data it has been possible to demonstrate that intracellularly accumulated Aβ fragments show both aggregation and cytotoxic effects. These findings support the idea that intracellular accumulations of Aβ-containing fragments are the primary cause of neuronal degeneration in AD. Neurons in the most affected brain areas such as the hippocampus and neocortical association cortices are more susceptible to APP-associated toxicity presumably owing to the fact that these neurons express high amounts of APP. Thus, sound strategies for prevention and treatment of AD are likely to include either increasing the degradation of APP or decreasing the production of APP within neurons.

Selected Readings

Bahmanyar, S., Higgins, G. A., Goldgaber, D., *et al.* 1987. Localization of amyloid β protein messenger RNA in brains from patients with Alzheimer's disease. Science 237:77–80.

Games, D., *et al.* 1995. Alzheimer-type neuropathology in transgenic mice overexpressing V717F β-amyloid precursor protein. Nature 373:523–527.

Hung, A. Y., Koo, E. H., Haass, C., and Selkoe, D. J. 1992. Increased expression of β-amyloid precursor protein during neuronal differentiation is not accompanied by secretory cleavage. Proc. Natl. Acad. Sci. USA 89:9439–9443.

Jarrett, J. T., Berger, E. P., and Lansbury, P. T. 1993. The carboxy terminus of the β amyloid protein is critical for the seeding of amyloid formation: implications for the pathogenesis of Alzheimer's disease. Biochemistry 32:4693–4697.

Maruyama, K., Terakado, K., Usami, M., and Yoshikawa, K. 1990. Formation of amyloid-like fibrils in COS cells overexpressing part of the Alzheimer amyloid protein precursor. Nature 347:566–569.

Shoji, M., Golde, T. E., Ghiso, J., *et al.* 1992. Production of the Alzheimer amyloid β protein by normal proteolytic processing. Science 258:126–129.

Tanzi, R. E., McClatchey, A. I., Lamperti, E. D., *et al.* 1988. Protease inhibitor domain encoded by an amyloid protein precursor mRNA associated with Alzheimer's disease. Nature 331:528–530.

Yoshikawa, K., Aizawa, T., and Hayashi, Y. 1992. Degeneration in vitro of post-mitotic neurons overexpressing the Alzheimer amyloid protein precursor. Nature 359:64–67.

References

Allsop, D., Haga, S., Haga, C., Ikeda, S., Mann, D. M. A., and Ishii, T. 1989. Early senile plaques in Down's syndrome brains show a close relationship with cell bodies of neurons. Neuropathol. Appl. Neurobiol. 15:531–542.

Benowitz, L. I., Rodriguez, W., Paskevich, P., *et al.* 1989. The amyloid precursor protein is concentrated in neuronal lysosomes in normal and Alzheimer disease subjects. Exp. Neurol. 106:237–250.

Cataldo, A. M., and Nixon, R. A. 1990. Enzymatically active lysosomal proteases are associated with amyloid deposits in Alzheimer brain. Proc. Natl. Acad. Sci. USA 87:3861–3865.

Cataldo, A. M., Thayer, C. Y., Bird, E. D., Wheelock, T. R., and Nixon, R. A. 1990. Lysosomal proteinase antigens are prominently localized within senile plaques of Alzheimer's disease: evidence for a neuronal origin. Brain Res. 513:181–192.

Clemens, J. A., and Stephenson, D.T. 1992. Implants containing β-amyloid protein are not neurotoxic to young and old rat brain. Neurobiol. Aging 13:581–586.

Dyrks, T., Weidemann, A., Multhaup, G., *et al.* 1988. Identification, transmembrane orientation and biogenesis of the amyloid A4 precursor of Alzheimer's disease. EMBO J. 7:949–957.

Dyrks, T., Dyrks, E., Moenning, U., Urmoneit, B., Turner, J., and Beyreuther, K. 1993. Generation of βA4 from the amyloid protein precursor and fragments thereof. FEBS Letters 335:89–93.

Esch, F. S., Keim, P. S., Beattie, E. C., *et al.* 1990. Cleavage of Amyloid β peptide during constitutive processing of its precursor. Science 248:1122–1124.

Fukuchi, K., Kamino, K., Deeb, S. S., *et al.* 1992a. Mol. Brain Res. 16:37–46.

Fukuchi, K., Kamino, K., Deeb, S. S., Smith, A. C., Dang, T., and Martin, G. M. 1992b. Overexpression of amyloid precursor protein alters its normal processing and is associated with neurotoxicity. Biochem. Biophys. Res. Commun. 182:165–173.

Games, D., Khan, K. M., Soriano, F. G., et al. 1992. Lack of Alzheimer pathology after β-amyloid protein injection in rat brain. Neurobiol. Aging 13:569–576.

Glenner, G. G., and Wong, C. W. 1984. Alzheimer's disease: Initial report of the purification and characterization of a novel cerebrovascular amyloid protein. Biochem. Biophys. Res. Commun. 120:885–890.

Goate, A., Chartier-Harlin, M-C., Mullan, et al. 1991. Segregation of a missense mutation in the amyloid precursor protein gene with familial Alzheimer's disease. Nature 349:704–706.

Haan, J., Hardy, J. A., and Roos, R. A. C. 1991. Hereditary cerebral hemorrhage with amyloidosis-Dutch type: its importance for Alzheimer research. Trends Neurosci. 14:231–234.

Hayashi, Y., Kashiwagi, K., and Yoshikawa, K. 1992. Protease inhibitors generate cytotoxic fragments from Alzheimer amyloid protein precursor in cDNA-transfected glioma cells. Biochem. Biophys. Res. Commun. 187:1249–1255.

Kang, J., Lemaire, H-G., Unterbeck, A., et al. 1987. The precursor of Alzheimer's disease amyloid A4 protein resembles a cell-surface receptor. Nature 325:733–736.

Kirschner, D. A., Inouye, H., Duffy, L. K., Sinclair, A., Lind, M., and Selkoe, D. J. 1987. Synthetic peptide homologous to β protein from Alzheimer disease forms amyloid-like fibrils in vitro. Proc. Natl. Acad. Sci. USA 84:6953–6957.

Kitaguchi, N., Takahashi, Y., Tokushima, Y., Shiojiri, S., and Ito, H. 1988. Novel precursor of Alzheimer's disease amyloid protein shows protease inhibitory activity. Nature 331:530–532.

Koh, J, Yang, L. L., and Cotman, C. W. 1990. β-Amyloid protein increases the vulnerability of cultured cortical neurons to excitotoxic damage. Brain Res. 533:315–320.

Kowall, N. W., Beal, M. F., Busciglio, J., Duffy, L. K., and Yankner, B. A. 1991. An in vivo model for the neurodegenerative effects of β amyloid and protection by substance P. Proc. Natl. Acad. Sci. USA 88:7247–7251.

Kowall, N. W., McKee, A. C., Yankner, B. A., and Beal, M. F. 1992. In vivo neurotoxicity of beta-amyloid [β(1–40)] and the β(25–35) fragment. Neurobiol. Aging 13:537–542.

Loo, D. T., Copani, A., Pike, C. J., et al. 1993. Apoptosis is induced by β-amyloid in cultured central nervous system neurons. Proc. Natl. Acad. Sci. USA 90:7951–7955.

Malouf, A. T. 1992. Effect of beta amyloid peptides on neurons in hippocampal slice cultures. Neurobiol. Aging 13:543–551.

Mattson, M. P., and Rydel, R. E. 1992. β-Amyloid precursor protein and Alzheimer's disease: The peptide plot thickens. Neurobiol. Aging 13:617–621.

May, P. C., Gitter, B. D., Waters, D. C., et al. 1992. β-Amyloid peptide in vitro toxicity: Lot-to-lot variability. Neurobiol. Aging 13:605–607.

Mullan, M., Crawford, F., Axelman, K., et al. 1992. A pathogenic mutation for probable Alzheimer's disease in the APP gene at the N-terminus of β-amyloid. Nature Genetics 1:345–347.

Pike, C. J., Burdick, D., Walencewicz, A. J., Glabe, C. G., and Cotman, C. W. 1993. Neurodegeneration induced by β-amyloid peptides in vitro: The role of peptide assembly state. J. Neurosci. 13:1676–1687.

Podlisny, M. B., Stephenson, D. T., Frosch, M. P., et al. 1992.

Synthetic amyloid β-protein fails to produce specific neurotoxicity in monkey cerebral cortex. Neurobiol. Aging 13:561–567.

Ponte, P., Gonzalez-DeWhitt, P., Schilling, J., et al. 1988. A new A4 amyloid mRNA contains a domain homologous to serine proteinase inhibitors. Nature 331:525–527.

Probst, A., Langui, D., Ipsen, S., Robakis, N., and Ulrich, J. 1991. Deposition of β/A4 protein along neuronal plasma membranes in diffuse senile plaques. Acta Neuropathol. 83:21–29.

Schubert, W., Prior, R., Weidemann, A., et al. 1991. Localization of Alzheimer βA4 amyloid precursor protein at central and peripheral synaptic sites. Brain Res. 563:184–194.

Seubert, P., Vigo-Pelfrey, C., Esch, F., et al. 1992. Isolation and quantification of soluble Alzheimer's β-peptide from biological fluids. Nature 359:325–327.

Sherrington, R., et al. 1995. Cloning of a gene bearing missense mutations in early-onset familial Alzheimer's disease. Nature 375:754–760.

Shivers, B. D., Hilbich, C., Multhaup, G., et al. 1988. Alzheimer's disease amyloidogenic glycoprotein: expression pattern in rat brain suggests a role in cell contact. EMBO J. 7:1365–1370.

Sisodia, S. S., Koo, E. H., Hoffman, P. N., Perry, G., and Price, D. L. 1993. Identification and transport of full-length amyloid precursor proteins in rat peripheral nervous system. J. Neurosci. 13:3136–3142.

Stein-Behrens, B., Adams, K., Yeh, M., and Sapolsky, R. 1992. Failure of beta-amyloid protein fragment 25–35 to cause hippocampal damage in the rat. Neurobiol. Aging 13:577–579.

Wertkin, A. M., Turner, R. S., Pleasure, S. J., et al. 1993. Human neurons derived from a teratocarcinoma cells line express solely the 695-amino acid amyloid precursor protein and produce intracellular beta-amyloid or A4 peptides. Proc. Natl. Acad. Sci. USA 90: 9513–9517.

Yamaguchi, H., Hirai, S., Morimatsu, M., Shoji, M., and Harigaya, Y. 1988. Diffuse type of senile plaques in the brains of Alzheimer-type dementia. Acta Neuropathol. 77:113–119.

Yankner, B. A., Dawes, L. R., Fisher, S., et al. 1989. Neurotoxicity of a fragment of the amyloid precursor associated with Alzheimer's disease. Science 245:417–420.

Yankner, B. A., Duffy, L. K., and Kirschner, D. A. 1990. Neurotrophic and neurotoxic effects of amyloid β protein: Reversal by tachykinin neuropeptides. Science 250:279–282.

Yoshikawa, K., Aizawa, T., and Maruyama, K. 1990. Neural differentiation increases expression of Alzheimer amyloid protein precursor gene in murine embryonal carcinoma cells. Biochem. Biophys. Res. Commun. 171:204–209.

Yoshikawa, K., Maruyama, K., Terakado, K., Usami, M., and Aizawa, T. 1991. A DNA-transfected cell model for Alzheimer amyloidogenesis: Demonstration of primordial amyloid fibrils in COS cells. In T. Ishii, D. Allsop, and D. Selkoe (eds.) Frontiers of Alzheimer Research, pp. 217–227. Elsevier Science Publishers, Amsterdam.

Yoshikawa, K. 1993. Neurotoxicity of β-amyloid. (Scientific correspondence), Nature 361:122–123.

Yoshikawa, K. 1995. Neurotoxicity of amyloid β-protein and the amyloid β-protein precursor. In A. Goate, and F. Ashall (eds.) Pathobiology of Alzheimer disease, pp. 145–165. Academic Press, London.

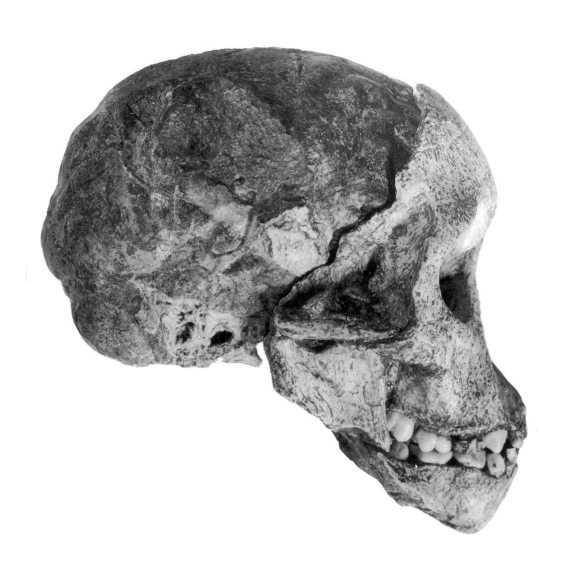

II

Ontogeny, Evolution and Neural Aging

The Taung skull, type specimen of *Australopithecus africanus,*
with its natural endocast in position. Right lateral view.

10

Setsuya Fujita

Cell Differentiation and Ontogeny of the Nervous System

Structural Changes in Chromosomes are the Earliest Events in Neurogenesis

At the Earliest Stage of Development, the Neural Tube is Composed of Multipotent Matrix Cells

Multipotent Matrix Cells Give Birth to Neurons and Glia

   Bundle Formation of Matrix Cells has Important Functions in Corticogenesis

   Neuron Types are Determined at Early Developmental Stages

   The Production of Glial Cells Follows that of Neurons

Major Differentiation is Maintained by the Irreversible Inactivation of Chromosomal DNA

   Major Differentiation Starts in Matrix Cells

   Major Differentiation Directs the Formation of Neurons and Glial Cells

   Reversible Gene Inactivation Accounts for Neural Plasticity

An Overall View

For a long time, the central tenet in the study of the ontogeny and evolution of neural structures was that 'ontogeny recapitulates phylogeny', Haeckel's theory, drawn from his observations that the embryos of more advanced species pass through stages in which they resemble the embryos, but not the adult forms, of simpler species. In 1828, Karl Ernst von Baer, the great embryologist of the 19th century, formulated the four general rules of embryology: (i) the more general features of a great number of animals appear earlier in the embryo than the more specialized features; (ii) less general features develop from the more general ones, until the more specialized features appear; (iii) the embryo of a given species does not repeat the adult stages of other animals during development, rather it distanciates progressively from those stages and, as a corollary, (iv) the embryo of a more advanced animal in the beginning of the development resembles the embryo, but not the adult form, of simpler animals. De Beer proposed that new species evolve because of changes in the embryogenesis of existing species.

Whatever the interpretation it takes, differences in the ontogeny of phylogenetically homologous structures not only have an important bearing on our understanding of the evolution in size and complexity of the brain and other organs; they also have consequences for the aging of the brain and the susceptibility to neurological diseases (Chapters 15 and 16). Since embryonal development is the very starting point of aging, that aging and the susceptibility to age-related diseases follow a phylogenetic path should not be thought too harsh an assumption. On the contrary, ontogeny, evolution and aging are intricately related to each other. Furthermore, ontogeny in the phylogenetically more advanced mammals is by no means over after birth. Instead, prolongation and succession of life periods – fetal, infantile, juvenile, adolescent and adult stages – is a trend in evolution and aging. Thus, it is reasonable to expect that the understanding of neuro-ontogenetical mechanisms shall give us an insight into the mechanisms of neural aging. In this chapter and the following we shall concentrate on such mechanisms, from the early events of cell differentiation to the evolution and development of the human central nervous system.

Structural Changes in Chromosomes are the Earliest Events in Neurogenesis

Neural induction has been regarded as the earliest event in neurogenesis in all the vertebrate ontogeny. However, before the neural competence appears, continuous cellular and chromosomal changes proceed in the cleaving embryo culminating in neural induction.

In aplacental animals, such as amphibians, reptiles and birds, the first 10 or so cleavage divisions following the fertilization of the egg, to the beginning of the blastula stage, are mostly synchronous. The cell cycle is very short, virtually lacking G_1 and G_2 phases. In *Cynops pyrrhogaster* embryos, the metaphase chromosomes remain unchanged in morphology and C-banding pattern (Yamazaki-Yamamoto *et al.*, 1980, 1984) during this phase. However, from blastula to gastrula, chromosomes remarkably shorten to almost half their lengths. This change is accompanied by a prominent decrease in chromosome volume, as the chromosomal width is kept constant. As blastula proceeds to neurula, many C-bands fuse with the neighboring ones and reduce in number. The neural competence appears as early as in the blastula stage, immediately after the shortening of the chromosomes begins. At the same time, dermal differentiation in the embryo is determined, and morphogenetic movements and migration of individual dermal cells begin to take place.

The chromosomal changes that seem to lead to neural induction and neurogenesis are accompanied by a remarkable elongation of S-phase in the cell cycle, from 3 hr in morula stage to 38 hr or more in neurula stage (Yamazaki-Yamamoto *et al.*, 1980, 1984). The time spent for DNA replication is prolonged. The same phenomenon continues in the developing neural tube, as indicated by autoradiographic studies showing remarkable increases in DNA-synthetic times in the structure (Fujita, 1962; Fujita and Kitamura, 1978; Hoshino *et al.*, 1973). Hyodo and Flickinger, studying the early stages of development in the frog *Rana fusca*, found that the velocity of DNA replication is almost constant within each replicon in the frog embryos, being 6 μm/hr. The length of each replicon, however, increases as development proceeds, being estimated at 11, 27 and 29 μm, in gastrula, neurula and tail bud stage, respectively. Obviously, initiation sites of DNA replication in some replicons progressively obliterate or, in other words, many replicons fuse with the neighboring ones as development proceeds. This observation agrees well with the above finding that many C-

bands fuse with the neighboring ones and reduce in number as blastula proceeds to neurula. The obliteration of initiation sites of DNA replication seems to be accompanied by absolute incapability of RNA synthesis on that replicon, while DNA appears to be replicated as a continuation from the neighboring replicons, though taking longer time to complete. At the light microscopic level, the synchrony of the cell division is lost rapidly during this period as a result of progressive elongation of the cell cycles.

At the Earliest Stage of Development, the Neural Tube is Composed of Multipotent Matrix Cells

Analysis of cell proliferation and differentiation of stem cells in the developing vertebrate embryos revealed that there are highly regulated patterns in the genesis of neuronal and glial populations in the vertebrate CNS. At the beginning, there is a stage in which the neural tube is composed solely of multipotent stem cells, also called *matrix* (from the Latin *mater*, mother, and *matrix* = *genetrix*) cells (Fujita, 1962) (Figure 10-1). These cells appear homogeneous in their morphology and behavior. They proliferate steadily and symmetrically to increase the area and thickness of the neural tube (Fujita, 1962, 1963), which at this stage (stage I) is solely composed of a pseudostratified columnar epithelium. Corresponding to the multipotent cell proliferation, the periventricular cell layer expands horizontally and the neural tube grows. While multipotent cells proliferate, they perform an 'elevator' movement synchronous to their mitotic cycle (Fujita, 1960) (Figure 10-2, A). During interphase, the multipotent cells adhere to each other with N-cadherin (Takeichi, 1990). When they enter mitosis, the adhesion is released and the cell body is rounded. Throughout the mitosis, the junctional complex in the apical process remains unchanged so that the cell body is inevitably pulled towards the ventricular surface. F-actin is depolymerized during mitosis, released from linker molecules binding cadherin and F-actin and, as a result, dissociation of the cadherin-mediated adhesion takes place during mitosis (Figure 10-2, B). It is likely that this cyclic modulation of N-cadherin adhesion during mitosis is the mechanism of the elevator movement. N-cadherin, which binds intracytoplasmic F-actin via linker proteins lining the cell membrane, loses homophilic adhesion ability when linker proteins and F-actin depolymerize and dissociate during mitosis (Fujita, 1990). As a result, mitotic multipotent cells are supposed to be released from the neighbors and round up.

Multipotent Matrix Cells Give Birth to Neurons and Glia

After several mitoses during stage I, some multipotent cells begin to differentiate. The ventricular zone from where neurons and glia originate in the developing brain gradually becomes a mosaic of proliferating cells with distinct developmental potentials ranging from the self-renewing, multipotent matrix cell to cells restricted to the

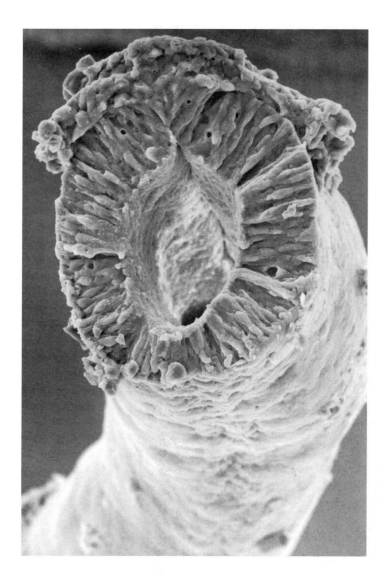

FIGURE   10–1

Scanning electron microscopicy of the neural tube in a chicken embryo of 24 hrs incubation. The neural tube is isolated together with the neural crest. The wall of the neural tube is solely composed of radially arranged matrix cells (primitive neuroepithelial cells).

production of neurons, distinct subtypes of neurons and glial cells (for a review, see McConnel, 1995). The stage of neuron production is sometimes called stage II of cytogenesis (Fujita, 1963), to distinguish it from stage III or the stage of glia production, although some investigators claim that overlap between these stages may exist. It is not yet definitively determined whether neurons and glial cells arise from common progenitors, as we claim, or, sometimes, from distinct and separate progenitors throughout prenatal or postnatal age.

There appears to exist a rigid and close correlation between the time- and place-of-birth and the type of neuron differentiation determined. Neurons are said to have their 'birthday' when, at stage II, a daughter cell produced by a matrix cell division exits the matrix cell pool at the early G_1 phase of the cell cycle and is differentiated into a neuroblast, with absolute repression of DNA replication. The determination of a newly produced daughter cell appears to be a stochastic process taking place independently from each other of the sister cells. To explain the mode of neuroblast differentiation, some investigators propose a mechanism that an asymmetric division of a matrix cell produces a neuroblast. However, it is unlikely that all cortical neurons are generated through asymmetric divisions of matrix cells since clone sizes in the neocortex are much larger than can be accounted for by a purely asymmetric mode of cell division (Reid *et al.*, 1995). While neurons become differentiated from the matrix cells, the matrix cell population still continues to grow, expanding in size in the wall of the neural tube. Differentiation probability (to be determined to become a neuroblast) of a newly born daughter cell during stage II of cytogenesis in human cerebral hemispheres is approximately 0.3. Once a neuron is differentiated from a matrix cell, the destiny (type-differentiation) of the neuron is irreversibly fixed and cannot be altered by subsequent dislocation or environmental changes.

After neuron production has completed, the stage of neuroglia production begins (Fujita, 1964). Matrix cells restricted to produce only non-neuronal cells change into

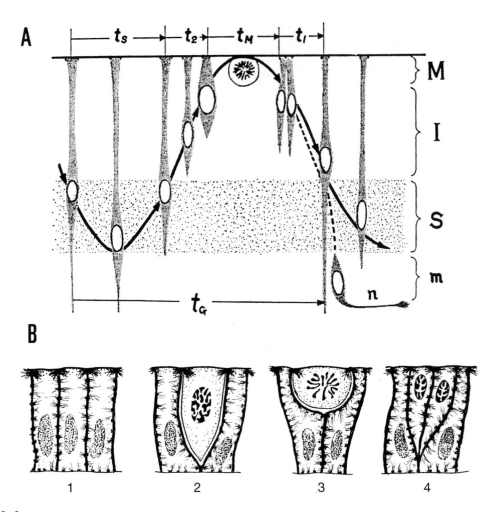

FIGURE   10–2

Elevator movement of matrix cells. **A.** Matrix cells perform an elevator movement synchronous with their mitotic cycle. Adapted from Fujita, 1962.

B. Mechanism of the movement is supposed to be due to cyclic changes of cell adhesion to neighboring cells. During mitosis

(2 and 3), F-actin (fine filaments in cytoplasm) and linker proteins are depolymerized and dissociated and, as a result, N-cadherin loses its ability of homophilic adhesion. From Fujita, 1990.

ependymoglioblasts, which are soon differentiated into ependymal cells and glioblasts. This is stage III of cytogenesis. The glioblast (Fujita, 1965a) is a common progenitor of neuroglial cells of the CNS, and first differentiates into astrocytes, then oligodendroglia and finally microglia (Fujita et al., 1981). Based on this monophyletic theory, cell differentiation in the developing vertebrate CNS is explained with a simple scheme as shown in Figure 10–3, C.

Bundle Formation of Matrix Cells has Important Functions in Corticogenesis

Throughout the stage II of cytogenesis in the cerebral hemisphere of human fetuses, mouse embryos and the optic tectum of the chicken embryos, the outer cytoplasmic processes of matrix cells are found to form bundles that run radially through the entire thickness of the brain wall. Bundle formation occurs due to the fact that the lateral cell membranes of matrix cells in the corticogenetic region can adhere to each other. The bundles, since they are made up of processes of many matrix cells (10–20 in average), can be maintained as stable structures despite the periodic (but asynchronous) withdrawal of individual processes due to the elevator movement described above.

The functions of the bundles are threefold (Figure 10–4) (Fujita, 1986). First, they guide young neurons in their migration into the cortical anlage which lies distant from the matrix cell layer, to form a unit structure of cortical column. For this function, the dynamic adhesion of neurons to matrix cells undoubtedly plays an important role. The second function of the bundle is to guide the processes of matrix cells themselves during their elevator movement. Without these guide rails, smooth perfor-

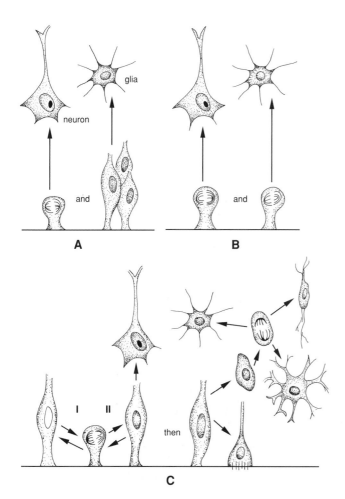

FIGURE 10–3

Theories about the origin of neuronal and glial cell lines.
A. W. His originally proposed about a century ago that neuronal and glial lines were entirely separate: The germinal cell and the spongioblast, respectively. **B.** P. Rakic's radial glia theory is an evolution of His' germinal cell theory. Rakic and coworkers distinguished two committed precursor cells in the wall of the neural tube (the ventricular zone) from the very early stages: elongated radial glia (spongioblast of His) and rounded germinal (or ventricular) cells. They believed that the former are specialized glial precursors and the latter, neuron precursors. They found that many elongated cells in the embryonic brain reacted strongly with anti-GFAP antisera (anti-glial fibrillary acidic protein, a specific glial marker), and concluded that His' spongioblasts are nothing but the radial glia co-existing with neuron-producing ventricular cells. The sole evidence on which they depend, however, is the positive reaction of anti-GFAP antisera in the cells composing embryonic brain vesicles. **C.** The introduction of thymidine autoradiography led Fujita (1963, 1964) to the conclusion that cell proliferation and differentiation proceed through consecutive 3 stages. In stage I, the neural tube is composed soley of matrix cells which perform an elevator movement. In stage II, matrix cells give rise to neurons. When all neurons are produced, matrix cells change into ependymoglioblasts, common progenitors of ependyma and neuroglia. This is the beginning of stage III of cytogenesis. The ependymoglioblasts are rapidly differentiated into ependymal cells and glioblasts. The latter give rise to astrocyte, oligodendrocyte, in sequence, and finally microglia. Adapted from Fujita et al, 1981.

mance of the elevator movement in so thick a wall like cerebral hemispheres or optic tectum would be extremely difficult. The third function of the bundles of progenitor cell processes becomes manifest at the end of stage II of cytogenesis. When the bulk of neuron production is completed in the corticogenetic area, the matrix cells are differentiating into ependymogliobasts (common ependymal and glial precursors), which rapidly change into ependymal cells and gliobasts, as shown in Figure 10–3. The differentiation into these glial cells is characterized by rapid reduction or loss of the long bipolar processes which have spun between pial surface and ventricle, running perpendicularly through the cortical plate.

When the processes of the matrix cells are withdrawn, they leave empty spaces or channels running perpendicularly through the cortical plate into which thalamic fibers or other input axons, having come and waited at the entrance of the cortical plate, penetrate and form synapses with cortical neurons in the column replacing the matrix cell processes. This is why everywhere in the central nervous system, rapid increase of synapse formation coincides with the beginning of stage III of cytogenesis. The same mechanism works in the corticogenetic area to form the functional column in the cortical plate.

Neuron Types are Determined at Early Developmental Stages

In the CNS, modification of neuronal fate can occur only at early stages of matrix cell differentiation, in response to environmental influences and following genetic switches such as the activation of position-specifying genes (see section IV). However, when stage II of neurogenesis starts, neuronal fate is already sealed. This kind of irreversible differentiation is confirmed (Cavines, 1982) in a mutant mice in which the locations of the cortical neurons are drastically disordered, but the type of neuron differentiation remains unchanged. Transplantation into heterotopic sites (Nakamura et al., 1986) or explantation in vitro have failed to change the original type of differentiation of neurons in the CNS once neuronogenesis has started in the transplant. It is likely that type-differentiation of neurons is determined irreversibly when these cells are produced from multipotent cells at stage II, although the same type of neuron retains a remarkable plasticity to adapt to various functional requirements.

The Production of Glial Cells Follows that of Neurons

Several authors (Antanitus et al., 1976; Levitt et al., 1983; Choi, 1986) reported a strong reaction of antiGFAP (Glial Fibrillary Acidic Protein) antisera in matrix cells at an early stage of development, and claimed that neuroglial differentiation proceeds parallel with the production of neurons (Figure 10–3, A, B). If matrix cells produce such a great amount of GFAP, their relationship to neuroglial differentiation would have to be re-examined. Those

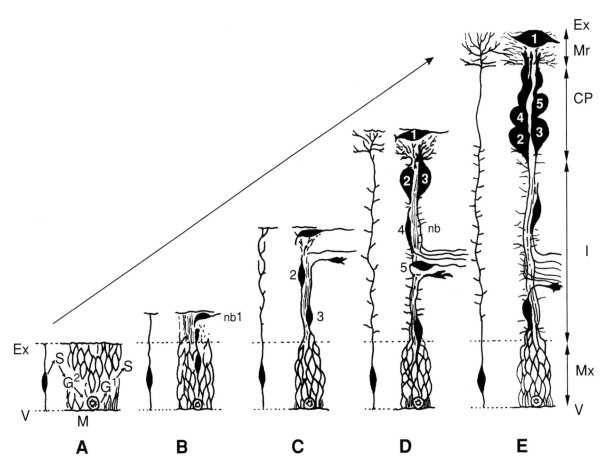

FIGURE   10–4

The generation of cortical neurons in an inside-first, outside-last gradient. Keeping pace with thickening of the wall of the brain (from left to right), matrix cells elongate and their processes tend to adhere to each other and form bundles. **A-B.** The first neurons born in the ventricular zone (*V*) before the bundles are formed (i.e. Cajal-Retzius neurons) migrate to the subpial position and become embedded in the molecular layer (nb1). **C.** Subsequent neurons (n2, n3) produced from the same group of matrix cells that now form a bundle migrate along the bundle to the cortical plate (*CP*) and reach the deepest position adjacent to the molecular layer. **D-E.** Subsequently generated neurons (n4, n5) migrate past the older cells, progressively forming the more superficial cortical layers. The older neurons are schematically illustrated as larger cells. Evidence from cell lineage experiments indicate that clonally related neurons can span several cortical layers, suggesting that precursor cells may often divide to produce a series of neuroblasts within the ventricular zone. Abbreviations: *V*, ventricular zone; *Mx*, matrix cell layer; *I*, intermediate zone; *CP*, cortical plate or cortical anlage; *Mr*, molecular layer; *Ex*, external or pial surface; *n1-n5*, neurons.

investigators who have observed the positive GFAP reaction have used antisera provided by Eng, or by Bignami and Dahl. Eng or Bignami and Dahl themselves, however, have never found any positive GFAP reaction in matrix cells at stages I and II with their own antisera. Critical examination is obviously necessary.

We have investigated using chicken, mouse, rat, bovine and human fetal brains and spinal cords by applying immunohistochemical staining, chemical analysis with SDS-PAGE, and immuno-blotting to detect occurrence of GFAP (Fujita *et al.*, 1981), together with GFAP-encoded mRNA by *in situ* hybridization and Nothern blotting (Fujita *et al.*, 1986), and came to the conclusion that GFAP and its mRNA are not present in stage I and II matrix cells, at least, at the detectable level by the current techni-

ques. Similar observations were made in the mouse by Lewis and Cowan and in chicken brains by Capetanaki and colleagues, using probes for GFAP-mRNA. The authors did not detect any positive signal throughout stage I and II of cytogenesis, but a strongly positive signal appeared when stage III began in those regions. The results reveal that the occurrence of GFAP-encoded mRNA parallels with the appearance of GFAP molecules in the developing CNS (Fujita, 1986).

Summarizing these observations at the protein and mRNA levels, we conclude that GFAP is not present in stage I or stage II of cytogenesis, and hence the matrix cell theory, that matrix cells first proliferate by themselves, then produce neurons and finally change into glial cells, has not been refuted.

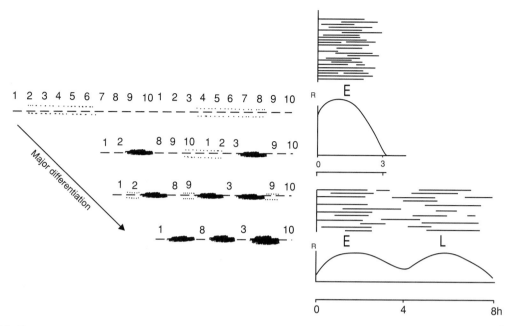

FIGURE   10–5

Changes in chromosomes and DNA synthesis in relation to major differentiation. On the left side of the figure, chromosomal changes during development are illustrated. In an undifferentiated cell (top), all the replicons composing the chromosome are not irreversibly inactivated, although only a few of them are actively transcribing mRNA (dotted segments). All the replicons, as shown in the figure at the top right, are early replicating (**E**) and the rate of DNA synthesis (**R**) is expected to form a simple pulse-shaped curve. The absolute length of the S-phase should be short. While major differentiation proceeds, many replicons are irreversibly inactivated as shown in the condensed state in this diagram (left). They become late replicating (**L**) and make the curve of the rate of DNA synthesis complicated (right, below). The length of the S-phase also becomes longer with additional late replicating segments. The irreversible inactivation of genes is the genetic basis of determination of cell differentiation, and reversible on-off-switching of potentially active genes corresponds to functional modulation of the cell. From Fujita, 1965b.

Major Differentiation is Maintained by the Irreversible Inactivation of Chromosomal DNA

It is generally believed that vertebrate development, when viewed at the cellular level, proceeds by sequential steps in which potencies of progenitor cells become progressively and irreversibly restricted. This type of differentiation has been dubbed *major differentiation* (Fujita, 1965b), as opposed to the reversible expression or repression of genes, the *minor differentiation*. Perhaps the simplest way to explain the mechanism by which cell potencies are restricted is to assume a progressive accumulation of irreversibly inactivated functional subunits (i.e., replicons) of chromosomal DNA (Figure 10–5).

It has been pointed out that the DNA portions that are irreversibly inactivated are characterized by four extraordinary features (Caplan and Ordahl, 1978; Fujita, 1965b; Goldman *et al.*, 1984): (i) incapability of RNA synthesis, (ii) shortened and condensed structure even in the interphase, (iii) replication occurs late in the S-phase, and (iv) the acquired feature of the inactivated DNA is inherited unchanged by the daughter cells through subsequent mitoses. This hypothesis was proposed almost 30 years ago but direct evidence to support it had been lacking since then. However, with the recent introduction of analytical techniques of molecular biology, it has been possible to test the hypothesis by using cDNA probes of specific genes and identifying the timing of their replication in the S-phase in various types of cells, and in the differentiated and undifferentiated states. The results of these experiments now provide strong evidence to support the *major differentiation hypothesis*.

Major Differentiation Starts in Matrix Cells

In the analysis of the elevator movement of matrix cells in various species of animals (Fujita, 1962; Fujita and Kitamura, 1978; Hoshino *et al.*, 1973), an unmistakable tendency of steady elongation of cell cycle and DNA synthetic times during development was found. This tendency has been observed in all animals so far studied. Besides matrix cells of neurectodermal origin, chicken erythroblasts (Holtzer *et al.*, 1977), endodermal cells in the frog *Xenopus laevis*, cells of blastomeres of sea urchin embryo (Dan *et al.*, 1980), etc. have been reported to show the same tendency. The ectodermal cells of *Cynops pyrrhogaster* (Yamazaki-Yamamoto *et al.*, 1984) described above are a typical example. According to the hypothesis of major differentiation (Fujita, 1965b), the length of the S-phase is expected to become longer in differentiated cells in comparison with that of their undifferentiated precursors, as illustrated in Figure 10–5.

At the beginning of the vertebrate ontogenesis, none of the replicons in the zygote are irreversibly inactivated; the cell is accordingly in its maximal totipotent state. DNA replicons in the cell begin to synthesize their DNA synchronously at the onset of the S-phase, at a uniform velocity so that overall rate of DNA synthesis of the cell shows a simple pulse-shaped curve (Figure 10–5, above). The length of the S-phase is expected to be short. As the cell progresses by steps of major differentiation, irreversibly inactivated replicons increase in number and the S-phase becomes longer. The curve of the overall rate of DNA synthesis is now expected to have multiple peaks as shown in the diagram in Figure 10–5.

The tendency toward steady elongation of the S-phase in matrix cells of developing vertebrate embryos (Fujita, 1962; Fujita and Kitamura, 1978) seems to support the notion that matrix cells steadily progress by steps of major differentiation as development proceeds.

Major Differentiation Directs the Formation of Neurons and Glial Cells

If one assumes the above hypothesis that irreversible inactivations of genes determine the differentiation of the cell even when matrix cells are actively proliferating, and that the type of cell differentiation is determined by specific combination of the irreversibly inactivated replicons, one can understand characteristics of matrix cell differentiation and neuron production as follows.

Although matrix cells keep their epithelial morphology unchanged from the very beginning of the neural plate formation to the end of stage II of cytogenesis, they change their state of major differentiation steadily as development proceeds. When they repeat mitoses and enter into G_1 phase, irreversibly inactivated replicons increase in number and the cell accumulates steps of major differentiation. The combinations of the inactivated replicons and their distribution patterns are supposed to be different in different cells; two daughter cells born from the same matrix cell inherit the same pattern of the inactivated replicons but can acquire new inactivations on different additional replicons forming different subclones in terms of major differentiation.

Figure 10–6 shows one branch of the matrix cell subclones. Frames Mx1 to Mx8 represent the magnitudes of differentiation potencies of the matrix cells at given stages of major differentiation. When major differentiation reaches a certain level, matrix cells can differentiate neuroblasts (commencement of stage II). Neuroblast differentiation in the vertebrate CNS is characterized by absolute repression of DNA replication; it is possible that neuroblast differentiation from matrix cells may be determined by an irreversible switching off of a gene or genes directly or indirectly related to DNA duplication for cell proliferation. It has been proposed (Fujita, 1986) that the differentiation of all neurons is commonly determined by one additional inactivation of this kind of replicon in the genome of the matrix cells at a certain state of major differentiation (Mx1 through Mx8). If one can assume this

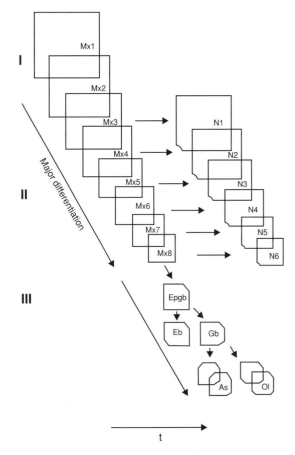

FIGURE 10–6

Schematic diagram showing progression of irreversible differentiation (major differentiation) of matrix cells during development of the CNS. The state of major differentaion of matrix cell population is progressively changing (from Mx1 to Mx8). From each state of major differentiation, specific neuroblasts (N1 to N6) are produced. Their specific states of differentiation are predetermined by those of their immediate precursors, i.e., the matrix cells. What determines the transition from matrix cells to neurons may be a common inactivation of one replicon that contains genes essential for DNA replication. Sizes and shapes of the frames of differentiating cells in this figure represent potency of cells at respective stages of major differentiation. I, II, III correspond to stages of cytogenesis. Abbreviations: *Epgb*, ependymoglioblast; *Eb*, ependymoblast; *Gb*, glioblast; *As*, astrocyte; *Ol*, oligodendrocyte; *t*, time. From Fujita *et al.*, 1986.

mechanism, it is easily understood why highly specialized neurons in the CNS are produced at given times and places during stage II of cytogenesis and their principal fates are irreversibly fixed at their birthdates.

If one assumes that differentiation of neurons and neuroglia is determined by the irreversible repression of replicons during neurogenesis as discussed above, many important problems of cell differentiation in the CNS such as transition of stage II of cytogenesis into stage III can be explained in a simple way. Namely, if major differentiation of matrix cells progresses and neuron-essential genes, without which no neuronal activity can be realized, are irreversibly inactivated in a matrix cell, it can no longer produce neurons. What the matrix cell can differentiate are nothing else but non-neuronal cells, i.e., neuroglial cells. Phenotypically, this signifies the beginning of stage III of cytogenesis.

The progressive gene inactivation hypothesis or the major differentiation hypothesis would explain the sequential occurrence of stage I, II and III, and production of specific cells in the development of the vertebrate CNS. Not only would it explain the cytogenesis but also it would enable us to analyze genetic mechanisms of cellular differentiation in the developing CNS in molecular terms: when, where, and what kind of specific gene or genes are inactivated to determine the differentiation of various kinds of neurons or neuroglia may be analyzed on this hypothesis. An extremely complicated pattern of cell differentiation in CNS, as it would appear at first glance, might turn out to be the result of simple hierarchical repressions of certain classes of essential genes. Some of these genes, of which *NeuroD* and *GliasMissing* are two remarkable examples, have been discovered recently.

Reversible Gene Inactivation Accounts for Neural Plasticity

We have proposed a hypothesis that cellular differentiation in the CNS is realized by progressive and irreversible inactivations of replicons that accumulate during ontogeny. According to this hypothesis, cells in the CNS are characterized by very rigid cytodifferentiation. Paradoxically, it is well-known that the vertebrate CNS, particularly that of the primate, is highly plastic at least in functional aspects. How comes it that neural plasticity is related to the irreversible differentiation of matrix cells in the CNS? According to the hypothesis, the major differentiation of a cell is determined by irreversible inactivation of some replicons. The inactivated replicons are supposed to be minority in number among all the replicons of the genome. The rest, or the majority of replicons are in a potentially active state, and can be switched on and off in response to the signals of intra- and extracellular environment. This type of reversible expression of cellular differentiation which has been called *minor differentiation* is characterized by reversible synthesis of mRNA and protein, and provides neurons with highly plastic potency.

An Overall View

At the beginning of ontogeny, structural changes accumulate in the chromosomes of multipotent matrix cells that direct their differentiation into neurons or glia. While major differentiation is maintained by the irreversible inactivation of chromosomal DNA, reversible gene activation and inactivation accounts for neural plasticity. Neuron types are determined at early developmental stages, and although the question whether glial cell differentiation occurs at the same time of, or following neuronal differentiation is not yet finally resolved, the latter hypothesis seems to be the most plausible.

Selected Readings

Anderson, D. J. 1995. A molecular switch for the neuron-glia developmental decision. Neuron 15:1219–1222.

Caviness, V. S., Jr., Takahashi, T., and Nowakowski, R. S. 1995. Numbers, time and neocortical neurogenesis: a general developmental and evolutionary model. Trends Neurosci. 18:379–383.

McConnell, S. K. 1995. Strategies for the generation of neuronal diversity in the developing central nervous system. J. Neurosci. 15:6987–6998.

References

Antanitus, D. S., Choi, B. H., and Lapham, L. W. 1976. The demonstration of glial fibrillary acidic protein in the cerebrum of the human fetus by indirect immunofluorescence. Brain Res. 103:613–616.

Capetanaki, I. G., Ngai, J., and Lazarides, E. 1984. Regulation of the expression of genes coding for the intermediate filament subunits vimentin, desmin, and glial fibrillary acidic protein. In Borisy, G.G., Cleveland, D.W., Murphy, D.B., (eds.) Molecular Biology of the Cytoskeleton. pp.415-434, New York, Cold Spring Harbor Lab.

Caplan, A. I., and Ordahl, C. P. 1978. Irreversible gene repression model for control of development. Science 201:120–130.

Cavines, V. S., Jr. 1982. Pattens of cell and fiber distribution in the neocortex of a the reeler mutant mouse. J. Comp. Neurol. 170:435–448.

Choi, B. H. 1986. Glial fibrillary acidic protein in radial glia of early fetal cerebrum: A light and electron microscopic immunoperoxidase study. J. Neuropath. Exp. Neurol. 45:408–418.

Dan, K. S., Tanaka, K., Yamazaki, K., and Kato, Y. 1980. Cell cycles during sea urchin development. Dev. Growth Differ. 22:589–598.

DeBeer, G. 1958. Embryos and Ancestors. 3rd. edition, Oxford Universtiy Press, London.

Fujita, S. 1960. Mitotic pattern and histogenesis of the central nervous system. Nature 185:702–703.

Fujita, S. 1962. Kinetics of cellular proliferation. Exp. Cell Res. 28:52–60.

Fujita, S. 1963. Matrix cell and cytogenesis of the central nervous system. J. Comp. Neurol. 122:311–328.

Fujita, S. 1964. Analysis of neuron differentiation in the central nervous system by tritiated thymidine autoradiography. J. Comp. Neurol. 122:311-328.

Fujita, S. 1965a. An autoradiographic study on the origin and fate of the subpial glioblast in the embryonic chick spinal cord. J. Comp. Neurol. 124:51–59.

Fujita, S. 1965b. Chromosomal organization as a genetic basis of cytodifferentiation in multicellular organisms. Nature 206:742–744.

Fujita, S. 1966. Application of light and electron miroscopic autoradiography to the study of cytogenesis of the forebrain. In R. Hassler and S. Stephan (eds.) The Evolution of the Forebrain., Georg Thieme, Stuttgart, pp. 180–196.

Fujita, S. 1986. Transitional differentiation of matrix cells and its functional role in the morphogenesis of the developing vertebrate CNS. In T.S. Okada (ed.) Current Topics of Developmental Biology, Academic Press,New York, pp. 223–242.

Fujita, S. 1990. Confocal microscopy, theory and practice. Protein, Nucleic Acid, and Enzyme 36:2779–2786. (In Japanese).

Fujita, S., Tsuchihashi, Y., and Kitamura, T. 1981. Origin, morphology and function of the microglia. In: Vidrio, E. A. and Fedroff, S. (eds.), Glial and Neuronal Cell Biology, pp.141-169, New York, Alan Liss.

Fujita, S., Fukuyama, R., Nakanishi, K., Kitamura, T., and Watanabe, S. 1986. Development of the CNS and regulations of gene expression in cellular differentiation of neurons and neuroglia. Progr. Neurosci. 30:1044-1060 (In Japanese).

Fujita, S., and Kitamura, T. 1978. Cytogenesis of the CNS. Hdb. Psychiatry, vol. 19A. Neuropathology, p. 79–114, Nakayama Publ. Co., Tokyo (In Japanese).

Goldman, M. A., Holmquist, G. P., Gray, M. C., Caston, L. A., and Nag, A. 1984. Replication timing of genes and middle repetitive sequences. Science 224:686–692.

Haeckel, E. 1866. Generelle Morphologie der Organismen. Berlin.

Haeckel, E. 1875. Ziele und Wege der heutigen Entwicklungsgeschichte. Jena.

Holtzer, H., Weintraub, H., Mayne, R., and Mochan, B. 1977. Cell cycle and erythroblast differentiation. In: Moscona, A.A. and Monroy, A. (eds.), Current Topics of Developmental Biology, 7, pp. 251–265, New York, Academic Press.

Hoshino, K., Matsuzawa, T., and Murakami, U. 1973. Characteristics of the cell cycle of matrix cells in the mouse embryo during histogenesis of telencephalon. Exptl. Cell Res. 77:89–94.

Hyodo, M., and Flickinger, R. A. 1973. Replicon growth rates during DNA replication in developing frog embryos. Biochim. Biophys. Acta 299:24–33.

Levitt, P., Cooper, M. L., and Rakic, P. 1983. Early divergence and changing properties of neuronal and glial precursor cells in the primate cerebral ventricular zone. Dev. Biol. 96:472–484.

Lewis, S. A., and Cowan, N. J. 1985. Temporal expression of mouse glial fibrillary acidic protein mRNA studied by a rapid *in situ* hybridization procedure. J. Neurochem. 45:913–939.

McConnell, S. K. 1995. Constructing the cerebral cortex: neurogenesis and fate determination. Neuron 15: 761–768.

Nakamura, H., Nakano, K. E., Igawa, H. H., Takagi, S., and Fujisawa, H. 1986. Plasticity and rigidity of differentiation of brain vesicles studied in quail-chick-chimeras. Cell Differ.19:187–193.

Reid, C. R., Liang, I., and Walsh, C. 1995. Systematic widespread clonal organization in cerebral cortex. Neuron 15: 299–310.

Takeichi, M. 1990. Cadherins: A molecular family important in selective cell-cell adhesion. Annu. Rev. Biochem. 59:237–252.

Yamazaki-Yamamoto, K., Takata, K., and Kato, Y. 1984. Changes of chromosome length and constitutive heterochromatin in association with cell division during early development of *Cynops pyrrhogaster* embryo. Dev. Growth Differ. 26:295 -302.

Yamazaki-Yamamoto, K., Yamazaki, K., and Kato, Y. 1980. Changes of chromosomes during the early development of a Japanese newt, *Cynops pyrrhogaster*. Dev. Growth Differ. 22:79–92.

Setsuya Fujita

11

Ontogeny and Evolution of the Vertebrate Central Nervous System

The Neural Tube Appeared for the First Time in a Cambrian Protochordate

What Kind of Genomic Evolution Might Have Led to the Creation of the Neural Tube?

The Basic Design of the Vertebrate Brain did not Change over Hundreds of Million Years of Evolution

Evolution of the Brain as Viewed from Progression of Brain Size

Progression in Brain Size was Slow in Fishes, Amphibians and Reptiles

For each Vertebrate Group There is a Characteristic Brain-Body Allometric Relationship

Neocortical Subclones Appeared with the Emergence of Mammals

Regional Specificities in the Cerebral Cortex had their Origins Early in Mammalian Evolution

Brain Shaping (Reorganization) in Evolution

The Growth of the Mammalian Neocortex is a Model to Study the Cellular Mechanisms of Encephalization and Differential Longevity

Positional Influences in the Ontogenesis of the Cortex

Brain Development and Behavior in Primates

The Remarkable Growth of the Primate Brain During Rather Short Periods was Realized by Prolongation of Cytogenesis

The Evolution of Human Brain May be Explained by Additional Mitoses in Matrix Cell Populations

An Overall View

K nowledge of both the anatomical, cellular and molecular similarities and differences between the central nervous system (CNS) of extinct and extant species has improved, and attempts have been made to reconstruct the probable sequence of the evolution of the brain. The diversity of forms of brains found among living animals as well as fossils has been a major source of inspiration to help figure out the possible steps towards the evolution of our own brain. Planarians or flatworms (phylum Platyhelminthes) for example, are thought to provide the simplest example of living animals with mature neuronal forms of nerve cells, and are also the lowest phylum to organize such cells into a cephalic organ fulfilling the criteria of a brain (Sarnat and Netsky, 1985). Platyhelminthes is also the phylum preceding the great divergence in the subsequent evolution of animal life into more complex phyla of invertebrates on the one hand and chordates, including vertebrates, on the other.

The Neural Tube Appeared for the First Time in a Cambrian Protochordate

Most modern paleontologists believe that tadpole-like animals which lived some 550–500 million years ago (Mya) in the Cambrian era had been the ancestors of the vertebrates. These ancestors which were actually very similar to the larvae of the present day tunicate, did not leave any fossil evidence since they had no hard tissues. Their structure and function, therefore, must be inferred from the present day tunicate larva. Ascidians are, indeed, the most simple forms of tunicates and their larvae (Figure 11–1, A) show several characteristics reminiscent of the

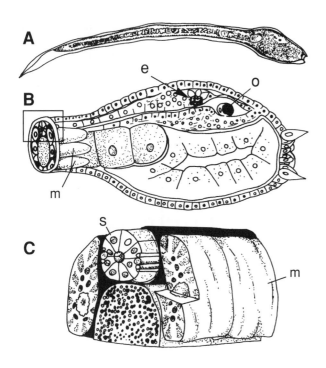

FIGURE   11–1

Ascidian larva. **A.** Tadpole-like larva of a tunicate, Ascidia, immediately after hatching. **B.** Cut surface of the head. **C.** Larger magnification of the frame shown in (**B**). Abbreviations: *m*, muscle cell; *e*, eye; *o*, otolith (mechano-receptor of sounds and acceleration movements); *s*, medullary tube, presumably corresponding to the spinal cord of the vertebrate; in the middle in (**C**), cut surface of a notochordal cell is shown.

most ancient forms of the vertebrate ancestors. Unlike the adult sessile forms of the tunicate, the ascidian larva possesses a muscular tail and a notochord running along the longitudinal body axis, thereby enabling a sigmoid or undulating movement of the body to swim freely in the sea. The ascidian most important innovation, in respect to vertebrate neurogenesis, is the creation of a neural tube (Figure 11-1, B, C).

An ascidian egg, when fertilized, performs within 1 hr the first cleavage that divides the egg into prospective right and left half of the embryo. At 7 hr, the neural plate is induced from the dorsal ectoderm and soon folds and invaginates to form a neural tube, in a manner reminiscent of the induction in amphibian embryogenesis. Meanwhile, a notochord composed of a tandemly arranged row of 40–44 notochordal cells is formed and flanked by 3 rows of 18–20 muscle cells (m) on each side (Figure 11-1, A, B). The rostral end of the neural tube is slightly enlarged, forming a small vesicle. In most ascidian larvae, the vesicle contains 3 lens cells, one pigmented cell and several visual, retinal cells (e), and a unicellular pigmented otolith (o). In the posterior part of this sensory vesicle, several hundreds of neural cells aggregate to form the presumable associate and motor center. This nerve center

has been called 'cerebral ganglion'. There are no peripheral neurons nor definitive peripheral nervous system.

The development *in ovo* of the larva is completed within 24 hr and the tadpole swims out on breaking the egg shell. In the medullary tube (s, in Figure 11-1, C), the roof plate and the floor plate are composed of 2 matrix cells each and the lateral plate, of 2 matrix cells of which the dorsal one corresponds to the alar plate and the ventral one, to the basal plate. In contrast to the cerebral vesicle, the medullary tube that presumably corresponds to the spinal cord is solely composed of epithelial (matrix) cells without neuron differentiation and it is comparable to the neural tube at stage I of cytogenesis in other vertebrate embryos. Between the lateral surface of the medullary tube and the surrounding basal membrane, 4 to 7 axons run down bilaterally from the cerebral ganglion to terminate at the surface of the tail muscle cells. Obviously each axon innervates several muscle cells via cholinergic synapses since 18 to 20 muscle cells are driven by 4 to 7 axons to generate well coordinated S-shape movement of the body. It is interesting for neurologists that the ascidian larval brain shows distinct left-right asymmetry. In the ascidian, larval brain development occurs only in the right half of the brain vesicle and the left remains undeveloped as a matrix cell tube. The latter commences neural development when metamorphosis into adult form begins at the time of the settlement on a rocky substrate at the bottom of the sea (Berrill, 1950).

The larva starts to perform a sigmoid movement of the tail already in the egg shell, even without light or any external stimulus. It is a spontaneous and innate movement of the larva. This type of spontaneous S-shape movement has been noted in a variety of vertebrate embryos *in ovo* and *in utero* at an early stage of development. The larval brain is already equipped with 'the will to move' when it is born out in the world. Vertebrate ancestors in the Cambrian should have also had the will to move when they were first evolved on the earth. Ascidian larvae, when they swim out from the shell, are positively phototactic and negatively geotactic (Berrill, 1975). They swim to the surface of the sea and are dispersed widely on the horizontal direction. However, during the latter half of their larval life, the tadpoles become negatively phototactic and positively geotactic so that they escape from the surface of the sea filled with the sun light, diving down for permanent settlement in the bottom of the sea to spend postlarval sessile life. Undoubtedly, the mode of regulation of motor activities through sensory reactions become different at the beginning and the end of larval life, thereby enabling the dispersal of the larvae to increase the survival ability of the species.

From the study of the present day tunicate larvae, we can infer what took place, with the creation of the neural tube, in Cambrian ancestors of the vertebrate. Contrary to the general belief, no accumulation of peripheral reflex arcs contributed to the creation of the nervous system of the vertebrate but the central nervous system was created from the very beginning. There were neither spinal ganglions nor sympathetic and parasympathetic nervous systems that might have built peripheral nerves. Axons of motor nerves did not exit out of the spinal cord but form multiple cholinergic synapses with the adjacent muscle cells while the axons are running on the lateral surface of the medullary tube. No axons ran out of the medullary tube to form peripheral nerves.

What Kind of Genomic Evolution Might Have Led to the Creation of the Neural Tube?

Ascidian chromosomes are small in size and their number is reported to be 18. The nuclear DNA content is approximately 0.3 pg which is about 1/20 of mammalian DNA. Most of this small amount of DNA should have been occupied by genetic codes of their Precambrian and Cambrian ancestors. Only a small portion of their genome would have been allocated to create matrix cells that could produce the sensory vesicle and the cerebral ganglion for the larva to move spontaneously and coordinatively. Already before creation of the primitive tunicates with larval formation, their ancestors of the Coelenterate family should have developed ectodermal cells that can adhere to each other and to other cells with certain specificity, enabling proper morphogenesis. Functionally the ectodermal cells of their ancestors should have been ionically coupled with neighboring cells and possessed excitable membranes so that they could evoke purposeful movement in effector cells such as muscle cells, cilliated or flagellated cells, in response to incoming signals from the marine environment.

Since the genome of this marine animal had already the blueprint to perform the functions of the ectodermal cells, it seems that it was qualified enough to accomplish the creation of matrix cells. It had only to perform a little step to acquire the blueprint for 'induction'. This step of genomic evolution, however, took place in the Cambrian era, more than 550 Mya, and it is almost impossible to study it directly now. Detailing this evolutionary step is a matter of speculation. Nevertheless, from the discussions made above it can be stated clearly that, when the central nervous system was created in the tadpole-like larva of tunicate ancestors in the Cambrian era, the following phenomena should have been perfected during ontogenesis of the protochordate, the early vertebrate ancestors that lived in the Cambrian, some 550–500 Mya: (i) at the end of gastrula phase, the dorsal ectodermal cells are induced by the notochord to the matrix cells (neuroepithelial stem cells of the central nervous system); (ii) the neural plate which is composed of matrix cells invaginates to form the neural tube; (iii) regional differences appear and are fixed in the neural tube, corresponding to fields that differentiate motor neurons, sensory cells and associate neurons in the brain and spinal cord; (iv) the matrix cells differentiate, with time and locus specificities, sensory, motor and associate neurons that possess specific potentials to form preprogrammed networks to perform purposeful tasks; (v) these neurons are interconnected to form an output system that may be regarded as an equivalent of the *fasciculus longitudinalis internus* running from brain to spinal cord in the vertebrate embryos. The output signals flow out through this system to realize spontaneous S-shape movement of the body; (vi) motor neurons make synapses with proper target muscle cells in a specific, predetermined manner, and (vii) neurons in the brain produce spontaneously excitatory burst to drive body muscle cells to perform S-shape movement.

It is beyond doubt that a blueprint for the perfect accomplishment of the tasks from (i) to (vii) must have been written in the chromosomes of the most simple ancestors of the chordate before definitive vertebrate lineage was established in the sea waters of the Cambrian era. Therefore, if we wonder why and how the matrix cell is induced from the primitive ectoderm; the matrix cell can form the neural tube; the 4-dimensional fields of cell differentiation develop in the neural tube; the 4-dimensional fields determine specificities of neuronal differentiation; axons elongate toward certain preprogrammed directions to reach their target neurons; motor neurons can establish connections with their partner muscle cells specifically, and sensory and associate neurons with their specific target neurons, with their specific types of synapses, all these questions must be directed toward the ancestral forms of the Cambrian era. This is because all the progeny down the vertebrate lineage, including humans, have continuously borrowed the programs of neurogenesis from these ancestral protochordates, reediting and reproducing the blueprint, with slight modifications, generation by generation.

The Basic Design of the Vertebrate Brain did not Change over Hundreds of Million Years of Evolution

During evolution of the vertebrate CNS, stage I of matrix cell proliferation (Chapter 10) prolongs gradually, and the size of neural tube becomes larger and larger, thereby elaborating larger brains and increasing the complexity of the 4-dimensional fields of matrix cell differentiation. Progression along this process of evolution has not only increased brain size, but also created the basic design of the present day vertebrate brain. Surprisingly enough, it was fixed quite early in the evolutionary history.

In the Silurian (440–410 Mya), jaw-bearing marine fishes, the ancestors of sharks and bony fishes, developed from their *agnatha* (jawless) precursors, the *cyclostomata, ostracoderms*, etc. At this time, cranial nerves that controlled eyes and jaw were fully equipped and their arrangement, in respect to the site of exit, running course outside the brain and innervation of muscles and other targets, attained the same pattern as in the present day vertebrate brain. Stensiö (1963) succeeded in reconstructing the external morphology of Silurian and Devonian fish brains by grinding heads of fossil fishes on whetstone. Figure 11–2 shows a brain of Devonian (410–360 Mya) crossopterygian fish, *Eustenopteron foordi*, as reconstructed by Stensiö. Amazingly enough, the layout of various parts of the brain is the same as that of present day vertebrates. The most rostal part of the brain is the olfac-

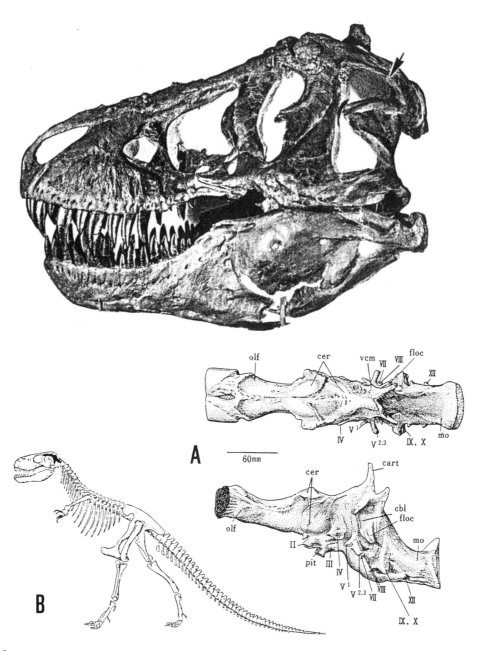

FIGURE 11–3

Cretaceous dinosaur, *Tyrannosaurus* and its endocranial cast. **Top.** Head bones of the huge carnivorous dinosaur. Its brain was entirely encapsulated in the small cranium indicated by the arrow.

A. Above and lateral views of the cranial cast. *olf* indicates olfactory lobe of the brain; *cer*, cerebrum; *cbl* and *floc*, cerebellum;

pit, pituitary gland; *mo*, medulla oblongata. Roman numerals indicate numbers of cranial nerves.

B. The gigantic skeleton. Its body height frequently reached 15 m but its brain was small as shown in black in its skull.

viewed by Jerison (1994), encompassing more than 650 species. From this simple analysis it is possible to conclude that (i) the general relationship between brain volume and body mass is a fundamental principle of the body plan among all vertebrate groups, and that (ii) the mammals polygon is vertically shifted in relation to the polygons of the remainder vertebrate groups, reflecting larger p value. Taking into account that the mammals developed from the reptiles, the shift of the mammals' polygon supports the idea that the increase in the size of the brain was one of the specific adaptations of mammals as compared to their reptile ancestors. This phenomenon of increasing the brain size over the presumable necessities of the body is called 'encephalization'.

Spinal cord

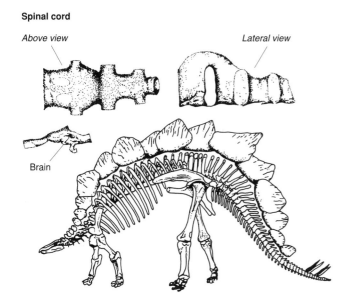

Above view   *Lateral view*

Brain

FIGURE 11-4

Stegosaurus and its spinal cord and brain. **Top.** Above and lateral views of lumbar ampulla of the spinal cord. **Middle.** Lateral view of the endocranial cast at the same magnification as the lumbar ampulla of the spinal cord. Note that the brain is much smaller than the lumbar segments of the spinal cord.

Bottom. Skeleton of *Stegosaurus*. Body height was 8 m, body weight 2 tons, but the brain weighted only 70 g.

Neocortical Subclones Appeared with the Emergence of Mammals

Anatomically this increase in size of the mammalian brain is realized by the creation of a new matrix cell subclone in the cerebral vesicle between the paleocortex (= piriform cortex, rhinencephalon) and the archicortex (hippocampus) (Figure 11–6). The new subclone (represented in thin lines in Figure 11–6) was endowed with a special feature of cell proliferation. In the stage I of cytogenesis (Chapter 10), period of proliferative activity of the new subclone matrix cells was longer so that the cerebral vesicles bulged out on both sides of the brain prominently already at an early stage of neurogenesis. In the stage II of cytogenesis also, matrix cells of the new subclone sustained proliferative activity longer than those of the other brain parts and gave birth to more neurons over a longer period so that 5-layered neocortex was constructed over an extended area of the cerebrum.

As years of evolution passed by, the size of the neocortex continued to increase and the value of p rose to an average of 0.12 (1424p = 170) in present day mammals. Although remarkable, the increase in size of the neocortex in mammals is an extremely slow process; doubling of p-value from 0.06 to 0.12 takes 25 million years or more and in some animals, like the hedge hog, *Erinaceus europaeus*, the p-value remained unchanged for a long period since the Oligocene (25 Mya). These data indicate that (i) creation of a new matrix cell subclone succeeds only

rarely, and (ii) the mode of proliferation and differentiation of matrix cells is an exceedingly conservative process.

Regional Specificities in the Cerebral Cortex had their Origins Early in Mammalian Evolution

Since the electrophysiological experiments by Fritsch and Hitzig (1870), and the histological mapping of Brodmann (1909) revealed the presence of regional differentiation in cerebral cortex, homogenously looking neocortex has been known to be locally specialized, in close correlation with the body map. This regional specialization of the cortex is doubtless derived from the reproducible cortical organization of neurons arranged horizontally and vertically within the cortex. The horizontal differentiation is determined by major differentiation of matrix cells that constitute the cerebral vesicle and transmitted to the neurons they produce. The young neurons migrate along the fascicles of matrix cell processes and reach their final destination in the cortical plate (Fujita, 1986). Thus regional differentiation in the cerebral cortex may be regarded as a kind of decalcomania of differentiation map in the matrix cell layer spreading on the ventricle.

A question may arise as when, during evolution, did the regional specialization, or basic pattern of matrix cell differentiation, first appear in the cerebral cortex? It is well known that the same basic pattern of regional specialization as seen in the human cerebral cortex appeared, though in more simplifed states, also in the monkey, dog, cat, rabbit, rat, mouse, and even in the hedgehog and marsupials (Brodmann, 1909) (Figure 11–7). Surprisingly enough, the same basic pattern occurred in the marsupials that had diverged from mammals in the Mesozoic, about 200–180 Mya. This fact indicates that the spreading of regional pattern of differentiation in the matrix cell population should have been intrinsically determined already at the level of mammal-like reptile, pantotheria, and been conserved over 200 million years of evolution.

Brain Shaping (Reorganization) in Evolution

The complex shape of the nervous system and particularly the brain is assumed to be accomplished by the differential growth (Fujita, 1962, 1986) of various parts of the sheet of precursor cells forming this simple tubular structure expanding at different rates at different parts at different times. The regulation of the final number of nerve cells in the developing brain is a compound function involving mitosis, which is a mechanism for the generation of new cells, and programmed cell death (PCD), e.g., by apoptosis (Chapter 17) which is a mechanism to get rid of excess or surplus nerve cells (for a review, see Oppenheim, 1991). Both mechanisms are active at the embryonal stages of brain development, but the peak of mitosis appears to precede the peak of apoptosis.

The peak of neuronal birthdays in a neural structure is a measure of the duration of cytogenesis for that structure: the longer the termination of neurogenesis is de-

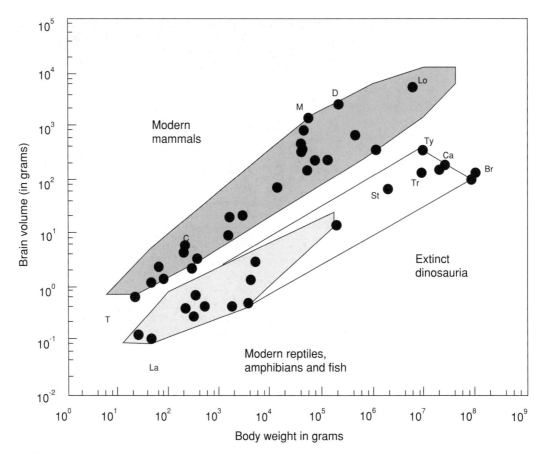

FIGURE   11–5

Brain-body relationships in recent and extinct vertebrates in a logarithmic scale, with minimal convex polygons outlined. The polygons are based on the data used to prepare Table 11-1 and work reviewed by Jerison (1994), encompassing data from more than 650 species. Key to the abbreviations: M, modern man;

D, delphin; Lo, *Loxodonta africana*; C, *Cavia culteri*; T, toad (*Phrynosoma coronatum*); La, *Lacerta viridis*; Ty, *Tyrannosaurus*; Ca, *Camarasaurus*; Br, *Brontosaurus*; Tr, *Triceratops*; St, *Stegosaurus*.

layed, the more precursor cells can be formed and the larger the structure that results. Using a 3-D computer graphics simulation, Fujita (1989) found that larger brains start their development at much slower growth rates in comparison with other animals of smaller brains. In this context, larger brains or, more generally, larger segments in a brain are created by slower decay of the growth rate of the segment. In contrast, small brains are formed by faster growth at the beginning followed by faster decay of the growth rate, so that smaller and simpler brains are produced within a shorter gestational period. An inference was made that the important changes of brain development during primate evolution must have been due to the changing kinetics of precursor cells; a decrease in the proliferation velocity of these cells and a prolonged proliferative period have doubtless played a decisive role in creating larger brains in the later stages of primate evolution.

The same conclusion has been reached in a recent study by Finlay and Darlington (1995), who reviewed

data collected on 131 species of primates, bats, and insectivores. The rash increase in relative brain-size in early hominids might have been the result of an increased rate at which neuronal precursors are produced, an increased lenght of time over which they are produced, a decreased rate of neuronal death, or any combination thereof. However, because a given structure may be thousands of times larger in one species than in another, the authors of the study concluded that the only factor that can plausibly produce differences of this magnitude is the duration of neurogenesis, thus the duration of the mitotic activity in the developing brain. The authors also found that the highly predictable relation between isocortex size and total brain size described by M. A. Hofman applies to all major brain subdivisions except the olfactory bulb. The neocortex, a phylogenetically and ontogenetically late generated structure, quickly expands in volume relative to other structures as brain size increases. Large primates were located on the neocortex curve where small relative changes in brain size were associated with large relative

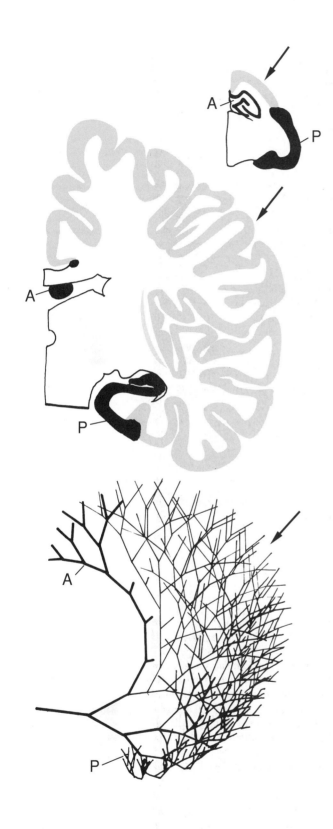

FIGURE 11–6

Germination and expansion of neocortex in the mammalian brain. Top, cross section of brain of hedgehog, regarded as the most similar to the earliest mammalian. **A**, archicortex (= hippocampus); **P**, paleocortex (= piriform cortex or rhinencephalon). Neocortex (shown in gray) which culminates in human brain was created by a new subclone of matrix cells (arrow) between the archicortex (**A**) and the paleocortex (**P**) immediately before the mammalian evolved from reptilian ancestors. In hedgehog, the neocortex occupies only a small area in the cerebral hemisphere. Middle: In the human cerebral cortex, the neocortical subclone propagates itself to cover the entire brain. Paleocortex and archicortex are now pushed behind and almost invisible in the human brain from outside. **A**, in this scheme, indicates the fornix. The bottom of the picture illustrates schematically the germination and propagation of the new subclone of matrix cells giving rise to the neocortex.

The Growth of the Mammalian Neocortex is a Model to Study the Cellular Mechanisms of Encephalization and Differential Longevity

The growth of the mammalian neocortex is a promising system for the analysis of the mechanism of disproportionate brain growth underlying encephalization. Forming in the dorsal telencephalic wall, the cortex is a laminated structure in which the neurons of each layer not only share characteristic morphologies and projection patterns but are born during the same periods of development. The laminar architecture is built up progressively, in an inside-out sequence, so that cells contributing to later-formed, superficial laminae are born later and migrate through earlier-formed laminae on their migration route from the ventricular surface (Fujita,1986, Lumsden, 1994).

Although there appears to be a critical period when commitment to the laminar identity takes place, only the radial extent of cell migration seems to be fixed during this period. Recent recombinant retroviral marking studies of Walsh and Cepko (1992, 1993) suggest that tangential migration is widespread and variable in extent, in cases of rat brains, approaching the entire length of the cerebral cortex. It is, however, important to note that this kind of extensive tangential migration has not been observed in primate or human cerebral cortex in which regional differentiation is the most advanced and precise. It is well known since Lashley's extensive behavioral experiments with rats (1922, 1930) that, in contrast to primate and human brain injuries, regional destruction experiments in rat cerebral hemispheres do not produce well defined regional symptoms; in rat cerebral cortex, overlap between sensory and motor area is extensive and destruction of visual cortex does not result in overt defect of visual behavior. Reid and colleagues (1995) claim that migratory multipotential progenitors may divide asymmetrically at intervals defined by cell cycle length, producing single cells or clusters of cells in different cortical regions. Heterotropic grafting experiments of Schlagger and O'Leary, (1991) have showed that area-specific fates in

changes in isocortex size. Thus, structures that grow disproportionately large as brain size increases have late birthdates, what presumably allows for a longer period for generation of the precursor cell pool.

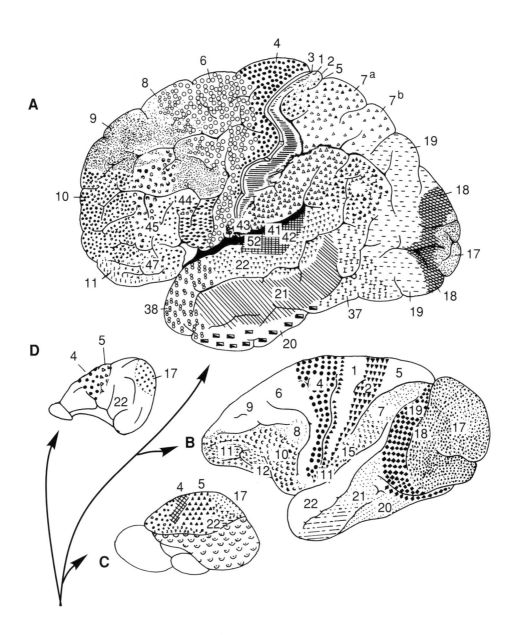

FIGURE   11-7

Development of regional specificities in the brain cortex.

A. Cytoarchitectonics of human brain. Numbers 1, 2, 3, 5 indicate primary somatic sensory areas, and 4, 6, primary motor areas. Areas 17, 18 and 19 constitute the visual cortex.

B. Brain map of rhesus monkey. A striking resemblance is apparent with the human brain map shown in (A).

C. Hedgehog brain. It retains the most ancient features of the mammalian brain organization. Nevertheless, areas 4 (primary

motor cortex), 5 (primary sensory cortex), 17 (primary visual cortex), 22 (primary acoustic cortex) occur in almost the same topical relationship as monkey and human brain.

D. Brain map of a Marsupial, kangaroo. The same topical relationship is detected in marsupials which have evolved separately from the mammalian stock since the time of the Pantotheria in the Mesozoic (200 Mya).

From Brodmann, 1909 (A, C, D), and Vogt and Vogt, 1919 (B).

the visual cortex seem to be decidedly much later in cortical development.

As for a beautiful positive correlation between size of the brain and longevity found in mammals, it is worthwhile mentioning that larger brains are produced, during ontogeny, with initial slower growth and longer cytogenetic period, whereas development of smaller brains starts

with faster growth and the neuronogenesis terminates earlier (Fujita, 1989). These facts indicate that cell cycles of matrix cells in animals with smaller brains are shorter and total number of repeats of the cell cycles is fewer during the neurogenesis. Actually we could estimate lengths of generation times of matrix cells in early neural tubes of mouse, rat, monkey and human embryos at 5, 6, 20 and

22.4 hr, respectively (Fujita, 1989). Repeats of the cell cycle of mouse, rat, monkey and human matrix cells, as counted from the beginning of the neural tube formation to the end of neuronogenesis (stage II of cytogenesis) were estimated at 9, 10, 18 and 20 times, respectively. It is obvious that, in animals with larger brains, the biological clock rhythm that regulates the cell cycle metabolically proceeds much slower than in animals with smaller brains. If one can view aging in mammals as regulated by rhythms of internal clock, we may infer that aging in animals with smaller brains proceeds faster, and in animals of larger brains, to which we humans belong, slower. If one takes this fact into consideration, it is no wonder to find that close correlation exists between size of the brain and longevity among mammals.

Positional Influences in the Ontogenesis of the Cortex

Thus it appears clear that the key determinant of disproportionate increase of neocortex in primates is the overall prolongation of period of active mitotic activity increasing the precursor cell pool in the brain. Increases in the size of the cortex might be regulated by factors that prolong the period of proliferative expansion in the ventricular zone or, conversely, by those that delay the onset of differentiation, allowing the expansion of the precursor pools. The inside-out positional influences, by determining an earlier differentiation of neurons in the deeper gray matter, determine that it is the neocortex, and not the deeper structures of the brain, that incorporates the greater part of late-maturing neurons, and thus it is the cortex that increases most in size and complexity. That the neocortex is largely made up of late-generated neurons might have important consequences for the pattern of cell longevity in this relatively more vulnerable structure.

A prolonged period of active mitotic activity in the precursor lines can be accounted for by a delay in the onset of neuronal and glial cell differentiation, in other words, the resistance of precursor cells to differentiate, reflected in the total number of cell cycles that produce neurons and glia during the period of neurogenesis (Fujita, 1989; Caviness *et al.*, 1995). Such a delay in taking decisions is consistent with the idea of an altricial or protracted development (Chapter 15). Thus, understanding the mechanisms by which the developmental potential and the longevity of a cell are maintained or progressively restricted is in great part a matter of understanding the metabolic regulation of the cell cycle, i.e. the regulation of cell replication and growth.

Brain Development and Behavior in Primates

It is generally agreed that branching of primate lineage from other mammals took place at latest in the Cretaceous (approximately 130 Mya). Paleontologists believe the most primitive primates were small insectivore-like animals very similar to modern tree shrews (*Tupaia gliis*) (LeGros Clark, 1965). They were small arboreal nocturnal animals with a squirrel-like appearance. This mode of life has been responsible for the development of many primate characteristics, such as the acuity of vision, the ability of climbing trees and grasping branches, the high degree of development of the brain to realize highly coordinated sensory and motor functions to support vision, limb movements and body balance.

Viewed from volume increase of the brain during evolution, the primate stock far distinguished itself from other mammals. In modern *Tupaia*, to which the most primitive form of the primate should have bear similar characteristics, the neocortex almost hides the piriform cortex (rhinencephalon), and the visual center is particularly large in comparison with that in the brain of the basic mammalian, hedgehog. Starting with the primitive tree-shrew-like ancestors, the primate stock developed into a lemuroid animal then into tarsius-like forms (in the Eocene). During this evolutionary process, the sense of olfaction was greatly reduced together with reduction of the nose and the olfactory lobes (rhinencephalon) in the brain. This is because olfaction was unreliable in finding the exact direction of food and enemy in the arboreal life. In contrast, the visual cortex of the brain was enlarged and the eye-sight highly developed. The arboreal life provided a particularly suitable environment to select individuals with more developed cortical areas bearing visual functions and manual controls. Primate brain needed to process information coming from the visual center in order to instruct motor center of limbs and body very rapidly and efficiently. Development of the sensory, motor and associative activities is reflected in the enlargement of the primate brain. The tendency of remarkable increase in brain size continued into the higher level of primate evolution represented by *Dryopithecus* (p = 0.255), *Australopithecus africanus* (p = 0.41), *Homo habilis* (p = 0.6), *Homo erectus* (p = 0.7–0.85), and *Homo sapiens* (p = 0.96). The rate of increase was exceedingly high.

The Remarkable Growth of the Primate Brain During Rather Short Periods was Realized by Prolongation of Cytogenesis

The remarkable growth of the primate brain during rather short periods was realized by prolongation of stage I and II of cytogenesis of matrix cells in the cerebral vesicles of the primate stock. If stage I or II elongates by 1 generation time of the matrix cell, the number of neurons produced doubles; if it elongates by 2 generation times, the final output of neurons quadruplicates (Fujita, 1990). Elongation of the stages I and II enables not only to increase the number of cells produced in the cerebrum but also contributes to the more diversified regional (horizontal) differentiations of the matrix cell population and, as a result, more variegated (horizontal and vertical) differentiations of neurons produced therefrom. Genetic changes that enabled the elongation were preferentially fixed in primate stock and the development of the brain goes hand in hand with the development of the arboreal behavior.

12

Phillip V. Tobias

Evolution of Brain Size, Morphological Restructuring and Longevity in Early Hominids

Brains and Braincases

> The Absolute Size of the Endocranial Cavity Reveals that the Human Trend Toward a Dramatic Cerebral Expansion Began with *Homo habilis*

Estimates of the Body Size of the Apemen are Used to Provide Measures of Relative Brain Size or Indices of Encephalization

> Encephalization in Hominids is a Dramatic Example of Non-Conservative Scaling in the Evolution of Brain Size/Body Size

> Encephalization may Enhance Adaptability while Permitting Organisms to Maintain Adaptation

> The Peak of Increase in Cranial Capacity Seems to Have Been Surmounted in *Homo sapiens*

Morphological Reorganization was of Greatest Importance for the Evolution of the Brain and Behavioral Patterns

> Important Brain Morphological Traits Indicate that *Homo habilis* was the First Language-Bound hominid

It is Possible to Estimate the Age at Death of Fossils by the Study of Their Crania

> A Majority of Early Hominid Fossils fall into the Putative Age Category of 20 and Under when Gyral and Other Impressions are Most Manifest

> The Gradual Slight Thickening of the Cranial Bones that Occurs During Adult Life may be Related to the Erasing of Endocranial Impressions with Aging

> The Phylogenetic Meaning of Cranial Thickening in Hominid Evolution is Not Well Understood

The Dramatic Increase in Brain Size may have been Initially a Challenge in the Evolution of Hominid Longevity

> The Deterioration of Africa's Ancient Climate Would Have had a Seriously Deleterious Effect on the Chances of Highly Encephalized Children Surviving to Procreative Age

An Overall View

'You will find something more in woods than in books. Trees and stones will teach you that which you can never learn from masters.'

St. Bernard, 850 years ago.

The subject of paleontology is the search for the signs left in stones and bones from which we are able to read, or infer, indications of ancient happenings where time is measured in hundreds of thousands and even millions of years. Hence, to search for the signs of the evolution of the brain, its morphological restructuring, particularly that underlying the emergence of spoken language, and the repercussions of these changes on longevity, we will pursue the faint echoes of those words in William Shakespeare's *As you Like it:*

'And this our life, exempt from public haunt, Finds tongues in trees, books in the running brooks, Sermons in stones, and good in everything.'

The brain qualifies as one of Charles Darwin's 'organs of extreme perfection and complication'. He admitted that it was most difficult to explain, on 'his' theory, how such organs of astonishing complexity could have evolved gradually and by natural selection. Not less astonishing, the human language capacity is another evolutionary achievement of extraordinary perfection and complexity. Like other human skilled activities, it involves both central (neural) and peripheral (vocal and respiratory) complexes. It is staggeringly difficult to reduce these to simpler building-stones to which evolutionary principles may be applied. It is a far more formidable task to reconstruct

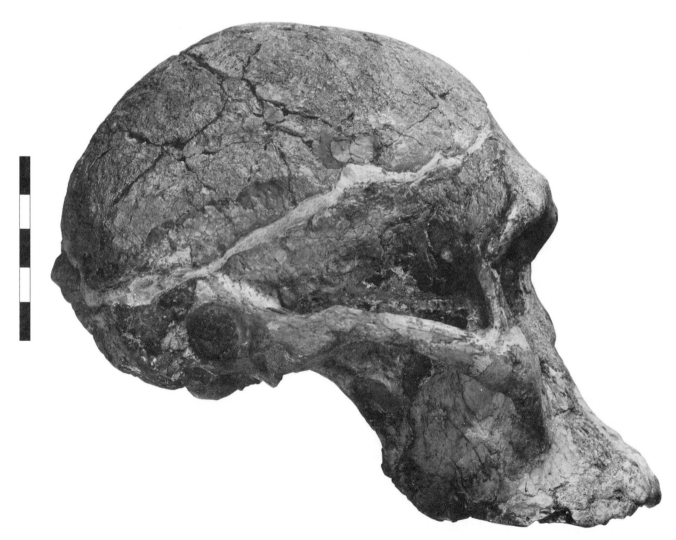

FIGURE   12–1
Right lateral view of the splendidly preserved cranium of Sts 5 ('Mrs. Ples'): a specimen of *Australopithecus africanus* discovered by R. Broom and J. T. Robinson on 18th April 1947 in Member 4 of the Sterkfontein Formation.
Like the other australopithecines, this specimen was possessed

of a small cranium with a capacity of 485 cm^3. However, no natural endocast had formed, probably because the cranium landed in the deposit the right way up, so sandy matrix could not gain access to the inside of the calvaria through the foramen magnum.

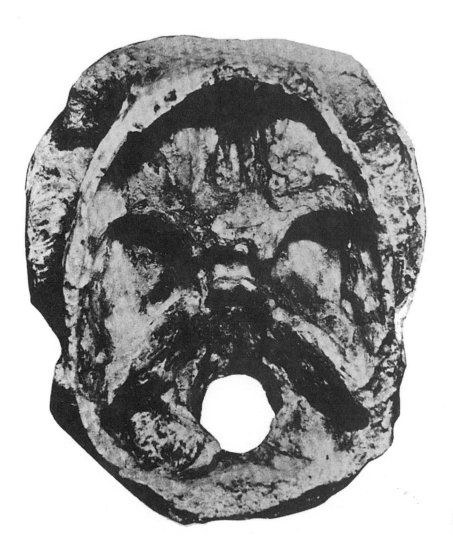

FIGURE   12–2

The well-preserved base of the interior of the braincase of an *Australopithecus africanus* cranium (Sterkfontein Hominid 5). The calvaria was empty, no natural endocast having formed.

the evolution of the brain than, say, that of the bones and the teeth.

Brains do not fossilize. Where then do we find the evidence from which we may infer how brains have evolved? One source of information is the comparative anatomy of the brains of living species. For one thing, modern human brains are, in absolute size, about three times as large as those of living great apes. Human brains permit us to use spoken language and to read and write, whereas so far as is known the brains of no other living animals contain the neurological bases of these functions. Comparative neuro-anatomy has taught us a great deal about the brains of living mammals and, especially, the primates. From such comparative data, it is possible to discern which areas of the brain of humans differ from the corresponding parts of ape brains. In turn, we may infer that, if we and the great apes have in the past had common ancestors, the features which are peculiar to the human brain must have emerged and developed after the lineage lead-

ing to *Homo sapiens* diverged from the lines of descent leading to chimpanzees and gorillas. We are able to supplement such information on brain structure by studies on brain function and on behavior in living primates including humans. Very advanced new techniques such as *PET-scanning* (positron emission tomography, Chapter 29) enable us to locate functions in the brain in living subjects. The fossil record enables us to confirm these inferences from studies on living creatures about the brains of ancient members of the human lineage. Yet, as I said earlier, brains do not fossilize. The key to this brain-teaser is to be found in the curious and unique relationship between the brain and the *braincase* or *calvaria*.

Brains and Braincases

The anatomist reads and interprets the markings and impressions of ligamentous and muscular attachments to bones, as well as the grooves, notches, foramina and

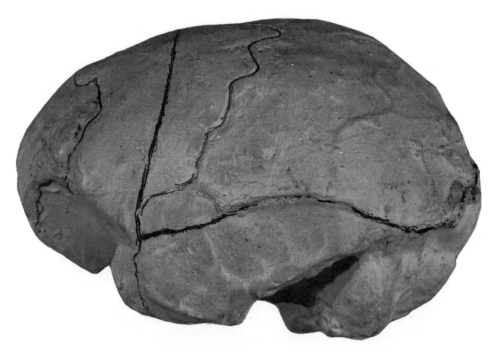

FIGURE   12–3
Artificial endocast of the type specimen of *Australopithecus*
(Paranthropus) boisei: left lateral view.

smoothings owing to the impingement on bones of other
structures such as arteries, veins, nerves, ligaments, and
tendons in transit. In the same way, much information
on functionally important soft tissue anatomy may be gar-
nered from the careful study of even the most ancient fossilized bones.

Of no structure has this proved more valid than the
brain, because it is the only organ that is totally enclosed
in a hollow bony box, the calvaria, which in life is faith-
fully moulded upon the contents. These contents are the
brain, meninges, blood vessels, blood, cerebrospinal fluid
and the stumps of emerging cranial nerves. The brain
makes up the bulk of the contents, varying between 66
percent and 95 percent of the capacity. There is a fine reciprocal relationship between brain and braincase during
the development of an individual. Under conditions of
normal development, a larger brain dictates the growth of
a larger calvaria and a smaller brain is housed in a smaller
calvaria. A broad brain is accommodated in a broad brain-
box. A subject with a relatively small cerebellum has a
proportionately small posterior cranial fossa. If the superior sagittal venous sinus passes to the left, instead of to
the right as is more common, the print of the corresponding groove likewise passes to the left. If a particular gyrus
or convolution on the surface of the cerebrum is well developed and protrudes, there is a matching hollow on the
endocranial surface (Figures 12–1 and 12–2).

All such features of the soft tissue contents of the calvaria may readily be confirmed in modern cadavera.
Hence, from the inner surface of a calvaria, one may draw
conclusions about the brain and blood vessels that once
occupied that braincase. We may facilitate the study by
filling an empty braincase with a plaster or plastic medium and making an artificial *endocranial cast* or *endocast*
(Figure 12–3). In size and form, such an endocast faith-
fully reproduces the size and form of the endocranial cavity. Hence, from the surface of an endocast one may read
the sulcal, gyral and vascular impressions directly.

Sometimes a natural endocast forms during fossiliza-
tion. This is especially likely to happen if the cranium
comes to rest in a protected site such as a cave, and particularly when the cranium lies upside down – since the
cave earth gains access to the calvaria mainly through the
foramen magnum, the large opening on the base through
which, in life, the brain joins the spinal cord. If a cement-
ing agent such as lime is present in the surrounding rocks,
the sandy filling of the braincase becomes calcified. There
results a natural endocast. An example is the beautifully
developed endocast of the Taung skull that Raymond
Dart revealed to the world more than seventy years ago
(Figure 12–4). Details of brain and vessels may be read
from a natural endocast, as from an artificial endocast.
Thus, endocranial surfaces and endocasts provide raw
data for paleoneurobiological research.

The Absolute Size of the Endocranial Cavity Reveals
that the Human Trend Toward a Dramatic Cerebral
Expansion Began with Homo habilis

The most obvious results of endocranial studies are the
endocranial capacities of various hominoids. One is careful to speak of capacities and not brain sizes, for the rea-

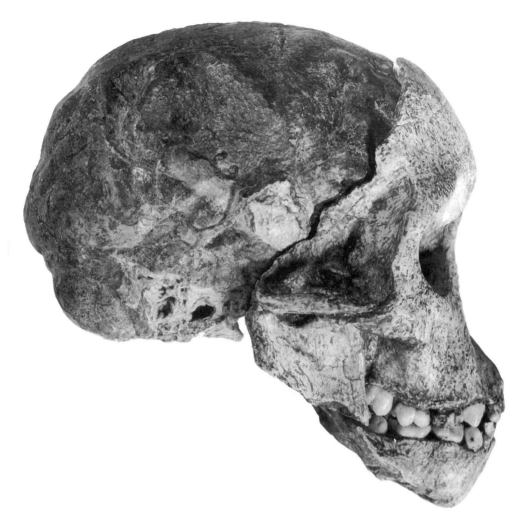

FIGURE 12–4
The Taung skull, type specimen of *Australopithecus africanus*,
with its natural endocast in position. Right lateral view.

sons mentioned earlier, though where data for actual brain size are available, there is a very high correlation between the two sets of measures. Because of difficulties in the measuring of actual brain size and because of the availability of thousands of dried crania of recent humans and apes, far more studies have been devoted to endocranial capacities than to brain volume or weight as such.

From such studies it has been estimated that the average modern human, interethnical, combined-sex capacity is of the order of 1350 cm^3 (Tobias, 1968, 1970, 1971, after Saller, 1959:1211). Since the fossil samples are most likely to include male and female specimens, we may compare their means with pooled male-plus-female data for the apes and the modern human capacity as listed in Table 12–1. In compiling the data for this table, the author has not followed a recent 'splitting' tendency evinced by some investigators who would revive the long-sunk *Paranthropus* as a distinct genus and even *Paran*-

thropinae as a separate subfamily, and who have claimed to recognize additional species, for example *Australopithecus crassidens* and *A. aethiopicus*. The same school of thought tends to recognize *Homo ergaster* and *Homo rudolfensis* as distinct from *H. habilis*, and *Homo neanderthalensis* rather than *H. sapiens neanderthalensis*. This extreme splitting tendency, in the author's view, is not helpful in biological or phylogenetic studies, nor does it take sufficient cognizance of intraspecific variation which, in extant higher hominoids, is marked.

From the data listed in Table 12–1 we conclude that the modern human average brain capacity (irrespective of sex) is roughly three times that of the *australopithecines* (a family of fossils initially found in South Africa – hence the name), 2.68 times the gorilla mean, 3.33 times the orangutan (*Pongo pygmaeus*) value, 3.52 times the chimpanzee (*Pan troglodytes*) average, and 3.93 times the bonobo (*Pan paniscus*) mean. The values cited in Table 12–1

TABLE 12–2.   Mean endocranial capacity, estimated body mass, and coefficients of encephalization for a series of hominoids

Species	Mean endocranial capacity (cm³)	Estimated body mass (kg)	EQ (actual value)	EQ (as % of H. sapiens value)	CC (actual value)	CC (as % of H. sapiens value)
P. troglodytes	395.0	45.0	2.6	34	33.6	31
A. afarensis	413.5	37.1	3.1	41	36.8	34
A. africanus	441.2	35.3	3.4	45	39.7	36
A. robustus	530.0	44.4	3.5	46	45.2	42
H. habilis	640.2	48.0	4.0	53	53.6	49
H. e. erectus (PVT)	895.6	53.0	5.3	70	73.4	67
H. e. erectus (RLH)	929.8	53.0	5.5	72	76.2	70
H. erectus (Asia and Africa)	937.2	53.0	5.5	72	76.8	71
H. e. pekinensis	1043.0	53.0	6.1	80	85.4	78
Homo sapiens	1350.0	57.0	7.6	100	108.8	100

Note: EQ, encephalization quotient; CC, constant of cephalization; PVT, the author's estimate for *H. erectus erectus*; RLH, Holloway's (1981b) estimate for *H. erectus erectus*. McHenry's value of 53.0 kg for *H. erectus* has been used in the above table for all the subsets of *H. erectus*. Although mass is given in kilograms in the table, it is expressed in grams for the calculations.
Source: Modified after McHenry, 1982.

would then not necessarily have favored correlated, uneconomical, increased body sizes: 'If the genetic correlation between brain and body size within populations in the human lineage was... low as suggested by the data on primates, hominids would have been enabled to rapidly increase brain size in response to selection for more complex behaviour without the cost of antagonistic selection to prevent the evolution of gigantism' (Lande, 1985:30).

A number of different techniques have been proposed to determine the degree of encephalization, when body size is taken into account. *EQ* stands for Jerison's *Encephalization Quotient*, which is the ratio of actual brain size to expected brain size (a kind of average for living mammals that takes body size into account) (Jerison, 1970, 1973). As obtained by Jerison, expected brain size is derived from body weight by the formula:

$$\text{expected brain size} = 0.12 \ (\text{body weight})^{0.667}.$$

The scaling coefficient of 0.667 has been claimed to fit the relationship between brain weight and body weight in a large sample of living mammals (Jerison, 1973; Gould, 1975; McHenry, 1982). On a much larger sample of species, however, Martin (1982) has obtained an exponent closer to 0.75, rather than 0.67. A scaling coefficient of about 0.75 has been found to apply to primates (Bauchot and Stephan, 1969), though within the primates these authors report coefficients ranging in various groups from 0.58 to 0.80 in round figures, as cited by Holloway and Post. *CC* is Hemmer's *Constant of Cephalization* and it is derived by dividing the endocranial capacity by the body weight scaled to the power of 0.23.

Table 12–2 gives results for two estimates of relative brain size. The values obtained by the two equations used here for EQ and CC confirm that (i) the various aus-

tralopithecine species were slightly more encephalized than the chimpanzee; and (ii) *H. habilis* was clearly more encephalized than any of the australopithecine series and represented a major step, indeed the first such, in brain aggrandizement: Its values reveal that it had attained some 50 percent of the *H. sapiens* degree of encephalization. More marked encephalization followed from *H. habilis* to *H. erectus*, the latter species reaching some 70 to 80 percent of the degree of encephalization shown by *H. sapiens*.

These coefficients, like Jerison's *Nc*, reveal that *H. habilis* is appreciably advanced in its degree of encephalization as compared with the *Hadar hominids* (Hadar is the name of the locality in Ethiopia where many australopithecine fossils were found) and with *A. africanus*. Since the estimated body size is built into the formulae for EQ and CC, it is clear that the larger endocranial capacity of *H. habilis* is not to be explained solely as the result of its larger estimated body mass nor, for that matter, of a higher estimated stature (Grüsser *et al.*, cited by Grüsser and Weiss, 1985): It clearly represents an advance in encephalization over the small-brained hominids, the australopithecines.

The data presented here, on relative brain size, show that, while the australopithecines were encephalized slightly more than the chimpanzee, *H. habilis* had unequivocally begun the remarkably 'uncoupled' or disproportionate enlargement of the brain that is a critical hallmark of humankind (Figure 12–5). The increase of brain size, whether absolute or relative to body size, is the most dramatic change to have occurred in hominid evolution in the last 3 million years. In that period, spanning some 200,000 generations, brain-size trebled along the human lineage. The advantages of the larger size have been much speculated upon and over a dozen hypotheses have been advanced to explain the sustained tendency in our

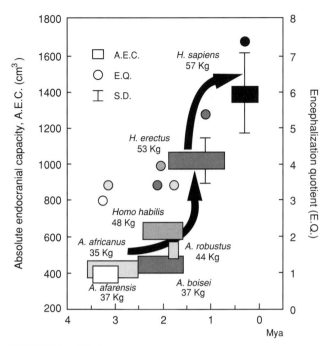

FIGURE 12–5

The encephalization trend in the hominid lineage, as indicated by Jerison's E.Q., Encephalization Quotient (circles). The trend towards marked encephalization clearly initiated with *H. habilis* and persisted in the heyday of *H. erectus* and early days of *H. sapiens*. Absolute endocranial capacity and mean body size are indicated for each taxon.

lineage towards increased encephalization (see reviews of Gabow, 1977, and Tobias, 1981).

The encephalizing trend connotes not only that a bigger percentage of one's bodily bulk is occupied by brain tissue. For size change is only a gross, external indicator of encephalization. In modern animal groups, when comparisons are made between smaller-brained and larger-brained species, it is found that, with larger brain-size, more neurons, more dendrification and connectivity of nerve-cells, and a higher glia-neuron ratio occur – and, with the latter, a decreased packing density of the neurons. It is reasonable to infer that changes in these features must have occurred during hominid encephalization. In addition, direct observations on fossil endocasts tell us what reorganisation of the surface of the brain, mainly of the cerebrum, has occurred during encephalization.

In comparisons among different animals, K. S. Lashley suggested that the total amount of brain material, expressed as a fraction of total body size, 'seems to represent the amount of brain tissue in excess of that required for transmitting impulses to and from the integrative centres' (Lashley, 1949:33). Following up this notion, Jerison (1963) demonstrated that brain size may be considered as two separate components: The first is directly related to the size of the body, and it is bigger in Primates with bigger body size; the second comprises the 'surplus' nerve cells that are present over and above those required for

the satisfaction of immediate bodily needs. These 'surplus' nerve cells, Jerison suggested, are available for response to the challenge of the environment through a wider range of brain-behavior mechanisms; that is, for intelligent adjustment. On the basis of cell counts in a variety of Primates and, given certain assumptions, he developed a series of equations for the calculation of these neuronal values, given the size of the brain and the size of the body. While the African great apes can be shown by Jerison's equations to possess 2.4 to 3.6 billion excess neurons, modern man has 8 billion.

Encephalization may Enhance Adaptability while Permitting Organisms to Maintain Adaptation

What advantages were conferred by increasing encephalization during hominid phylogeny? Many selection pressures have been proposed (see summaries in Gabow, 1977; Tobias, 1981). The most recent and perhaps the most elegant analysis of the meaning and the evolutionary benefits of brain size is that of Jerison (1991) in his James Arthur Lecture in 1989. This work, added to his significant earlier book on *Evolution of the Brain and Intelligence* (1973), provides evidence that brain size 'estimates the total information processing capacity of the brain in a species' (1991:53). In the first Andrew Abbie Memorial Lecture (1979), I listed no fewer than ten selective advantages of enlarged brain size that various workers had hypothesized. At the same time, attention was drawn to two features of hominid encephalization, namely its rapidity and its persistence (Tobias, 1981).

The rapidity of hominid brain evolution had been a source of controversy between Charles Darwin and Alfred Russel Wallace (Eiseley, 1956). In that oft-overlooked disputation, Darwin adhered rigidly to natural selection as an adequate explanation of the rise of humans and their brains. Wallace held that 'some more rapid process of evolution than that envisaged in the Darwinian philosophy must have been at work in the production of man' (op. cit., p. 69). Seven years before Darwin published *The Descent of Man* (1871), Wallace had asserted that evolution in cultured humans was largely mental. However, he did not take the further step of postulating that this very culture had come to dominate the selective processes in humans. Instead, since he could envisage no other force to account for the rapid rise of the human brain, Wallace invoked a directive spiritual force that could not be accounted for in purely mechanistic terms.

An hypothesis I offered earlier (Tobias, 1961) was that, under the peculiar conditions of human social and cultural life, evolution would be expected to occur most rapidly when natural selection, and cultural or social selection drive evolutionary change in the same direction. I had been led to this view in an earlier attempt to explain the evolution of *steatopygia*, or the accumulation of fat in the gluteal region, in the Kalahari Bushmen. It had seemed to me that, under the conditions of Bushman life, both natural and cultural selection had favored the development of steatopygia. I speculated that the same might have obtained with the Bushman's shortness of stature and with the evolution of the large brain and articulate speech of humans.

A second mechanism for rapid evolutionary change was offered, namely the genetic consequences of domestication, since the evolution of the human line resembled the domestication of animals in some respects, including the rapidity of evolution. Closely related was Gabow's (1977) suggestion that the evolving human species – he was thinking especially of *H. erectus* – constituted a subdivided population. Such a model had been proposed by Sewall Wright (1969), and this type of population structure, it was inferred, would have had an accelerating effect on evolutionary change.

Any new explanation that may be offered on hominid encephalization must cover not only the inferred rapidity of the change that has occurred, but also the persistence of encephalization. The enlargement and reorganization of the brain were not once-off responses, but were sustained over several million years. The processes of brain change were undoubtedly involved in the evolution of the earliest hominids, the australopithecines. Further encephalization carried the lineage across a generic boundary into *Homo* and continued through consecutive chronospecies, *H. habilis*, *H. erectus* and *H. sapiens*. Thus, the brain changes transcended systematic categories, geographical dispersal, cultural diversification, ecological radiation and ethological variegation. Whatever selective and other causal agencies were operating, they must have continued influencing the hominid brain throughout the assumption of a bewildering array of new life-styles and environments. The suggestion offered to account for the sustained duration of encephalization was an autocatalytic positive feedback system (cf. Mayr, 1963; Bielicki, 1964, 1969; Tobias, 1971, 1981).

The questions one needs to answer are these: Does the occurrence of a greater relative brain size in humans connote advantages that might have been favored by natural selection? If so, what manner of advantage did the larger brain size confer?

On Lashley's (1949) and Jerison's (1963, 1970, 1973) approaches, 'improved adaptive capacities' provide the key to the selective advantage conferred by increased encephalization. In Jerison's (1991) newest work this view is maintained: He places hominid encephalization in the context of a specific environmental niche, namely the shrinking of the African wet forest and spread of the savanna region at the forest's edge. These conditions were believed to accompany the emergence of the hominids about 5 or 6 Mya. In this setting, he suggests, adaptive changes occurred in the nervous systems of the ancestors of the hominids.

We may paraphrase 'improved adaptive capacities' as increased adaptability or greater evolutionary flexibility. Is this the advantage of greater encephalization? The problem is more exacting than it might seem. Long ago, K. Mather (1943) showed that adaptedness and adaptability in evolution were inversely proportional to each other. In other words the more highly adapted the animal is to

its present environment, the less evolutionary plasticity it has retained for adaptation to a new environment should conditions change. If the attainment by humankind of maximal encephalization implies that humans have attained maximal adaptability, we might expect that, on Mather's analysis, present adaptedness had been sacrificed. It is doubtful whether this deduction would stand up to close scrutiny. Moreover, encephalization is present in a number of other mammalian lineages, for example, the cetaceans, some New and Old World monkeys, tree shrews or Tupaioidea, and certain rodents: The maximally encephalized end-products of these evolutionary lineages certainly appear to be highly adapted in their respective econiches.

The author suggested (Tobias, 1994) that increased encephalization provided a means by which the organisms concerned could rise above the constraints suggested by Mather's paradox. I have hypothesized that the relative enlargement of the hominid brain was a mechanism by which enhanced adaptability might be furnished and on which natural selection could go to work, while adaptation, that is, concurrent adaptedness, was not sacrificed and could even have been improved. In a word, it was proposed that encephalization enhanced adaptability while permitting organisms to maintain adaptation, or even to manifest more efficient adaptation.

This general proposition should have applied to all mammalian lineages characterized by progressive encephalization. In the hominid lineage it has perhaps attained its pinnacle of evolution, as reflected by modern humanity's remarkable degree of encephalization. Along this lineage, the particular property 'secreted' by the expanding brain was the cognitive faculty, of such quality and degree as to generate culture (Figure 12–6). Probably no more puissant force has yet appeared on earth in its capacity to potentiate adaptation and to widen dramatically the evolutionary flexibility of its possessors. In the hominid line, particularly, culture may provide the means by which Mather's paradox has been addressed and surmounted. In this situation, adaptability and adaptedness are *not* inversely proportional.

The Peak of Increase in Cranial Capacity Seems to Have Been Surmounted in Homo sapiens

One provocative factor that arises on contemplation of the data on increasing capacity is that the selective pressures that led to the emergence and further development of the brain size of *Homo erectus* did not lapse. They did not lead to a graphical plateau in the heyday of *H. erectus*. The trend of rising mean endocranial capacities during the earlier stages of Pleistocene hominization undoubtedly continued into the upper Pleistocene; it is reflected by a further increase in brain size in the early stages of *H. sapiens*. (cf. Figure 12–5).

Then the selective pressures seem to have relaxed somewhat, a few score thousand years ago (Von Bonin, 1934, Weidenreich, 1946). Skulls of that date from Neandertal men of Europe, and also those of fossil men from

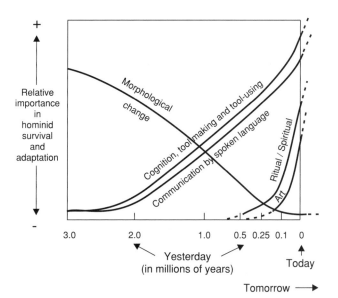

FIGURE 12–6

The relative importance in hominid adaptation and evolution, of certain broad modalities of change, between 3 million years ago and the present. The diagram suggests that morphological changes, though still occurring, have played a decreasingly important role in hominid survival and adaptation during the last 3 million years, whereas functional, cognitive and linguistic behaviour has come to dominate hominid evolutionary adaptation in the last 2.5 million years. A close correlation in time is indicated between tool-using and linguistic communication. The possible nature of future hominid evolution is suggested by the extrapolation of the curves beyond the 0 point towards 'Tomorrow'.

Africa, had bigger braincases on the average than those of their present-day descendants. The graph of rising brain size flattened out to a plateau and then began to drop somewhat. Although no attempt will be made here to review the evidence for this latest phase of hominization, some examples of upper Pleistocene endocranial capacities from Africa may be quoted: Hopefield (Saldanha) ca. 1225 c.c.; Broken Hill 1280 c.c.; Gamble's Cave 1470 c.c. and 1530 c.c.; Naivasha 1453 c.c.; Taforalt 1376 c.c. and 1647 c.c.; Boskop 1650 c.c.; Fish Hoek 1550 c.c.; Matjes River crania 1230 to 1660 c.c.; and Asselar 1520 c.c. Most of the crania cited have high capacities, probably well above the mean for most present-day populations. This underlines the general statement that modern humans – whether in Africa or Europe – would seem to have somewhat lower mean brain sizes than forebears of the early upper Pleistocene.

It seems that the trend toward increased brain size, which marked the first 2 or 3 million years of human evolution, had spent itself – and had done so as recently as the late Pleistocene. The wave of brain expansion had passed its peak. Some of our Stone Age people carried the twin processes of reduction of teeth and jaws, on the one hand, and expansion of brain, on the other, so far that they seem to represent an ancient foreshadowing of the popular idea of *the man of the future*. When one takes a

long-term evolutionary look at this problem, it seems that a larger brain size may once have been vitally important in aiding survival – for instance, in a world teeming with wild animals and devoid of harnessed fire. The further development of man would seem to have placed less and less of a premium on the size of his brain. For culture and the benevolence of social life have taken the place of nimble wits as an insurance policy against extinction. Beyond a certain stage in the increase of brain size, we have no evidence that further increase in any way improved man's adaptive abilities.

Morphological Reorganization was of Greatest Importance for the Evolution of the Brain and Behavioral Patterns

The second part of this chapter is devoted to the morphological restructuring of the brain in hominid evolution. Here we will concentrate on the australopithecine and the habiline brains.

Apart from the size, only five morphological characters distinguish *Australopithecus* endocasts from East and South Africa from the brain of extant apes:

(i) In gross pattern, on the base of the endocranial cast the impression of the australopithecine brainstem is situated further anteriorly than in the apes, and more so in *A. robustus* and *A. boisei* than in *A. africanus*, though in all three species it shows anterior advancement toward the position that pertains in later humans.

(ii) The parietal lobe of the cerebrum appears well developed (Holloway, 1988).

(iii) The cerebellar hemispheres are underslung (Tobias, 1967), so that the occipital poles of the cerebrum form the most posterior part of the endocast (to which generalization, the oldest *A. boisei* endocast (that of KNM-WT 17000) and the second oldest, that of Omo L338y-6, may be exceptions – see Holloway, 1981a, 1988).

(iv) Most of the australopithecine endocasts show the combination of *right fronto-petalia* (that is, the frontal pole of the right cerebral hemisphere protrudes further anteriorly than that of the left hemisphere), with *left occipito-petalia* (the occipital pole of the left cerebral hemisphere protrudes further posteriorly than that of the right hemisphere). This combination A. M. Galaburda describes as the most common in modern man, while Holloway (1988) declares it is not found in the apes, 'even the highly asymmetrical endocasts of *Gorilla*' (op. cit.:98). As in modern humans, there are exceptions to this combination among the early hominids (LeMay, 1976, 1984; LeMay et al., 1982; Holloway and De LaCoste-Lareymondie, 1982; Holloway, 1988; Tobias, 1987).

(v) There is a modest bulbous protrusion in the posterior third of the inferior frontal convolution, corresponding to Broca's cap (Schepers, 1946).

Some investigators, most notably Schepers and later Holloway (1974, 1975, 1985, 1988), have urged a sixth set of criteria upon us, namely the pattern of sulci, especially with regard to the position of what is taken to represent the lunate sulcus: Holloway sees this in early homi-

environmental conditions pertaining to those three earlier hominid species, *A. africanus*, *A. robustus* and *H. habilis*. Much evidence has accumulated recently on the palaeo-ecology of the later Pliocene and the early Pleistocene, the time-periods within which these three species lived. It is now clear that critical changes occurred in the climate and the physical geography of Africa, between the time of *A. africanus* (about 3.5 to 2.5 Mya), and that of the synchronic robust australopithecines (1.8–1.7 Mya) and *H. habilis* (2.3–1.6 Mya). *A. africanus* lived at a time when Africa was more mesic, with a heavier mean annual rainfall, and more wooded and forested conditions. Even the sub-tropical zone where *A. africanus* lived in the Transvaal, several degrees south of the Tropic of Capricorn, was wetter, more forested and frankly more tropical than it is today.

Later, from about 2.5 Mya, about the time when the earlier *A. africanus* lineage was giving way to the lines of the robust (*A. robustus*) and hyper-robust (*A. boisei*) australopithecines, and co-existing line of *Homo*, there is evidence of a wave of tectonic uplift of the African continent, with cooling and desiccation, retreat of the wet forest, opening of the woodland and spread of the savannah (Shackleton and Kennett, 1975; Vrba, 1985a, 1985b; Partridge, 1985; Partridge *et al.*, 1991). Thus, at this momentous period in hominid evolution, when modest brain-size increase was occurring in the robust ape-men and appreciable increase in early *Homo*, environmental challenges to survival were far more exacting. Not only were the climate and physical geography changing, but the fossil record reveals that conspicuous changes were occurring in the flora and the non-hominid fauna of Africa. It was a time of vigorous biological evolution and extinctions, conditions which, when added to the physical worsening, enhanced the competitive element in the struggle for survival.

In other words, *A. africanus* lived in more temperate times; *A. robustus* and *H. habilis* in more arid and more challenging times. We have already seen that *A. africanus* was characterized by greater survival to reproductive age; *A. robustus* and *H. habilis* by appreciably lessened chances of survival to procreate. Hence, the palaeo-ecological evidence corroborates the hypotheses on the influence of more favourable and of more exacting environmental conditions on the demographic pattern and age structure of the hominid populations, in a word on longevity.

The 'lower risk' demographic pattern manifested by *A. africanus* depended upon the more moderate conditions prevailing in Africa at the time, while the 'higher risk' demographic pattern shown by *A. robustus* and by *H. habilis* was determined by the deteriorating climatic, physical and biotic environment of the terminal Pliocene and early Pleistocene. This dependence of demographic patterns on the relative favorableness or adversity of the environment has a further interesting and testable corollary. If the conditions of life to which a population is subject undergo change, it would be a reasonable deduction that the demographic patterns would change, in accordance with the direction of the environmental change. Hence, if con-

ditions changed from unfavourable to more propitious, a secular trend from a 'high risk' to a 'low risk' demographic pattern should take place. An environmental shift from more mesic to more malign circumstances, on the other hand, would be expected to lead from a 'low risk' *A. africanus*-like pattern, to a 'high risk' *H. habilis* -like demographic mode.

Let us now feed into the equation the extra demands which increasing brain size or encephalization might be expected to have made upon the body's nutritional reserves and the population's resource base. It might be postulated that, at a time of minimal encephalization, a population's demands on the resource base would be minimal; during a phase of greater encephalization, these demands would be enhanced, whilst a population undergoing strong encephalization would be subject to appreciable exacerbation of its nutritional demands. We may test this hypothesis by reference to the three early hominid species we have been examining: *A. africanus* was only slightly encephalized as compared with chimpanzee; this would have made small extra demands on the resource base. Moreover, the resource base was presumably adequate at this mesic period. Only 35 percent of individuals died in the 20 and under age category. *A. robustus* was moderately more encephalized than *A. africanus* (CC 42 percent as against 36 percent of adult modern human value); it lived in the cooler, drier and more demanding environment of Africa after 2.5 Mya; so survival was at a premium. The remains of 60 percent of individuals fall into the 20 and under group. *H. habilis* was appreciably more encephalized than *A. africanus* and had passed the 50 percent mark in relation to the mean value in modern humans; it lived in the same cooler, more arid conditions as did *A. robustus*, but its greater encephalic nutritional demands placed it at a decided disadvantage in the struggle for survival. No fewer than 73 percent of the age-determinable individuals are 20 years and under.

These figures appear to show that the differential longevity among these three early hominid species had two principal determinants: one was the circumambient climate which could explain part of the differences, but could not distinguish between the two later synchronic species, the robust australopithecine and *H. habilis*; the other was the intensity of encephalizing pressures to which the various taxa were exposed and this appears to elucidate the difference between the *A. robustus* and *H. habilis* populations.

Thus, while the increased metabolic burden of a larger brain would be a restrictive handicap under any circumstances, its presence in the face of an adverse environment would make survival even more difficult and might be expected to lower the expectation of life. Not only did the burst of encephalization in *Homo habilis* take them by surprise, but it happened at the worst possible time!

An Overall View

In the stages by which the presumably apelike brain of the last common ancestor of humankind and chimpanzee was made over into the human brain, it seems that relatively small changes accompanied the emergence of the earliest available and analyzable hominids, the australopithecines. These changes comprised a minimal increase in absolute and relative size and some limited reorganization of the overall anatomical structure of the brain. As for neurologically important changes in the brain, there is scarcely any evidence of surface alterations in the sulcal and gyral patterns. What differences have been claimed, especially in regard to the expansion of the prestriate area of the cerebral hemispheres, are to say the least problematical.

However, major expansion of the brain and critical cortical reorganization were striking features of the change from *A. africanus* to *H. habilis*. These changes included notable augmentation of the cerebrum, strong lateral expansion of the parieto-occipital region, the appearance of a human-like sulcal pattern and the emergence for the first time of protuberances interpreted as the anterior and posterior speech cortices. That these homologues of Broca's and Wernicke's areas were used by a speaking and language-using ancestor, *H. habilis*, was proposed by Tobias (1980, 1981, 1983), and this claim has subsequently been supported by Falk (1983), Eccles (1989), Andrews and Stringer (1993), Deacon (1994) and Wilkins and Wakefield (1995). Thus, it is with the appearance of *H. habilis* that a gigantic step was taken to a new level of organization in hominid brain evolution.

The maximum life span has doubled from the earliest hominids to modern *Homo sapiens*, but the curve of change has not been a smooth and uninterrupted one. There seems to have been a decided drop in longevity with the emergence of *Homo habilis* and this was sustained through *Homo erectus*. The critical determinants of this drop were twofold: the dramatic and surprising increase in brain size with its enhanced metabolic demands; secondly, the untimeliness of this brain burst when the climate of Africa showed, after 2.5 Mya, a marked deterioration. Only after the stage of *H. erectus*, when encephalization had attained 70–80 percent of that of modern humans, does human longevity increase. In the late stage of hominid evolution, increases in brain size and longevity appear to go hand in hand, to reach their pinnacles in the last hundred thousand years.

Selected Readings

Armstrong, E. 1983. Relative brain size and metabolism in mammals. Science 220:1302–1304.
Conroy, G. C., Vannier, M. W., and Tobias, P. V. 1990. Endocranial features of *Australopithecus africanus* revealed by 2- and 3-D computed tomography. Science 247:838–841.
Gabow, S. L. 1977. Population structure and the rate of hominid brain evolution. J. Hum. Evol. 6:643–645.
Gould, S. J. 1975. Allometry in primates, with emphasis on scal-

ing and the evolution of the brain. In F.S. Szalay (ed.), Approaches to Primate Paleobiology, pp. 244–292. Basel: Karger.
Hofman, M. A. 1982. Encephalization in mammals in relation to the size of the cerebral cortex. Brain Behav. Evol. 20:24–96.
Holloway, R. L. 1966. Cranial capacity, neural reorganization and hominid evolution. A search for more suitable parameters. Am. Anthrop. 68:103–121.
Holloway, R. L. 1983. Cerebral brain endocast pattern of *Australopithecus afarensis* hominid. Nature 303:420–422.
Jerison, H. J. 1991. Brain Size and the Evolution of Mind. New York: American Museum of Natural History.
Martin, R. D. 1980. Adaptation and body size in primates. Z. Morph. Anthropol. 71:115–124.
Martin, R. D. 1981. Relative brain size and basal metabolic rate in terrestrial vertebrates. Nature 293:57–60.
Sacher, G. A. 1978. Evolution of longevity and survival characteristics in mammals. In E.L. Schneider (ed.), The Genetics of Aging. New York and London: Plenum Press, pp.151–168.
Tobias, P. V. 1971. The Brain in Hominid Evolution. New York: Columbia University Press.
Tobias, P. V. 1991. The age at death of the Olduvai Homo habilis population and the dependence of demographic patterns on prevailing environmental conditions. In H. Thoen, J. Bourgeois, P. Vermeulen, P. Crombé, and K. Verlaeckt (eds.), *Studia Archaeologica: Liber Amicorum, Jacques Nenquin*, pp. 57–65. Gent: University of Gent.

References

Acsadi, G., and Nemeskeri, J. 1970. History of Human Life Span and Mortality. Budapest.
Adeloye, A., Kattan, K. R., and Silverman, F. N. 1975. Thickness of the normal skull in the American blacks and whites. Am. J. Phys. Anthropol. 43:23–30
Andrews, P., and Stringer, C. 1993. The primate's progress. In S. J. Gould (ed.) The Book of Life, pp. 219–251. New York: Ebury Hutchinson.
Armstrong, E. 1981. A look at relative brain size in mammals. Neurosci. Lett. 34:101–104.
Armstrong, E. 1983. Relative brain size and metabolism in mammals. Science 220:1302–1304.
Armstrong, E. 1984. Allometric considerations of the adult mammalian brain with special emphasis on primates. In W. L. Jungers (ed.) Size and Scaling in Primate Biology, pp. 115–147. New York: Plenum.
Baer, M. J., and Harris, J. E. 1969. A commentary on the growth of the human brain and skull. American J. Phys. Anthropol. 30:39–44.
Bauchot, R., and Stephan, H. 1969. Encephalisation et niveau evolutif chez les simiens. Mammalia 33:225–275.
Bear, D., Schiff, D., Saver, J., Greenberg, M., and Freeman, R. 1986. Quantitative analysis of cerebral asymmetries: fronto-occipital correlation, sexual dimorphism and association with handedness. Arch. Neurol. 43:598–603.
Bielicki, T. 1964. Evolution of the intensity of feedbacks between physical and cultural evolution from man's emergence to present times. UNESCO Expert Meeting on Biological Aspects of Race, pp. 1–3. UNESCO, Moscow, August 1964.
Bielicki, T. 1969. Deviation-amplifying cybernetic systems and hominid evolution. Mater. Pr. Anthropol. 77:57–60.

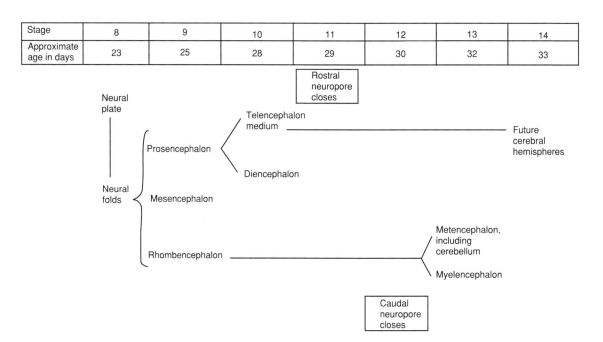

Stage	8	9	10	11	12	13	14
Approximate age in days	23	25	28	29	30	32	33

FIGURE   13–2
Developmental sequence of major parts of the brain.

Proliferative Phase 1

The production of neurons and radial glial cells. Stem cells divide asymmetrically, one daughter cell usually remaining in the proliferative unit, whereas the other leaves the ventricular layer (Rakic, 1991). The first neurons in the neopallial wall migrate into the marginal layer as future Cajal-Retzius cells. Together with afferent nerve fibers they form the primordial plexiform layer (Figure 13–4, B), in which the cells of future cortical layer 1 and of the subplate mature first. Here is where the first synapses develop (Molliver *et al.*, 1973; Larroche, 1981; Choi, 1988). The postmitotic cells that will become the neurons of layers 2–6 migrate to the intermediate layer and later (stage 21) into the cortical plate (Figure 13–4, D).

Proliferative Phase 2

The production of most of the glial cells in the subventricular and intermediate layers. The cells that take part in phase 2 arise in the ventricular layer, but move into the subventricular layer and the intermediate layer when the cortical plate begins to form at 7 weeks (stage 21). In these two strata, interkinetic nuclear migration does not occur, possibly because the dividing cells are not attached to each other. Almost no neurons are produced in these two strata (except in the olfactory bulb). Production of glial cells, which was minimal during phase 1, begins at 7 weeks (about stage 21) and (according to studies of the mouse) increases greatly at 8 weeks (about stage 23). Phase 2 continues throughout the fetal period, and the production of both glial and neural cells is believed to end

together. A secondary proliferative population is lacking in the archipallium (the subiculum, hippocampus, and dentate gyrus).

During and after migration, the neurons that arise in the ventricular layer differentiate. The progression from a

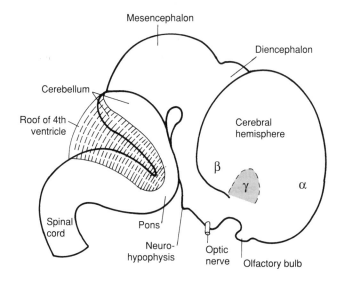

FIGURE   13–3
Right lateral view of the human brain (stage 23) at the end of the embryonic period (8 postfertilizational weeks). The cerebral hemispheres usually cover the diencephalon already, although not in the brain illustrated here. The three poles (frontal, occipital, and temporal) are marked α, β, and γ. The interrupted line indicates the area of the insula. The roof of the fourth ventricle has been shaded.

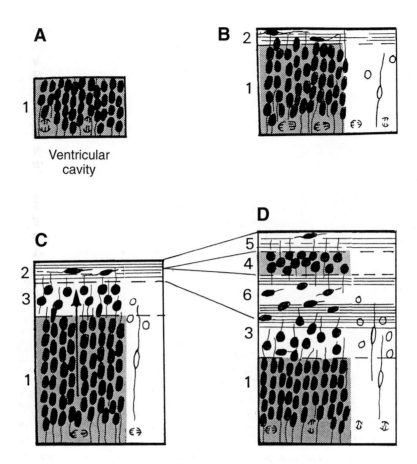

FIGURE 13–4

The production of neurons, glial cells, and fibers in the neopallium.

A. The ventricular layer (1) with mitotic figures near the ventricular cavity (as far as about stage 14).

B. The primordial plexiform layer (marginal zone, 2) at the pial surface (stages 15–17).

C. The intermediate layer (3) between the ventricular and primordial plexiform layers (stage 18).

D. The cortical plate (4) representing future layers 2–6 of the cerebral cortex (stage 21). Future layer 1 is superficial (5), the subplate is deeper (6). Some radial glial cells are shown at the right-hand side in B-D, where the neurons have been omitted for clarity. The fibers in the primordial plexiform layer in B and C, and in the intermediate layer in D, are discussed in the text.

neuroepithelial cell to a specific neuron is programmed (at least in mammals) by specific genes, and different types of receptors of a neuron respond to different transmitters. Thyroid hormone receptors are important for normal development of the brain.

Fibers

The development of axons depends on adhesion, guidance, migration, and growth to reach appropriate targets. Three phases have been distinguished: (i) Initial elongation, (ii) collateral sprouting, and (iii) pruning of extraneous connections.

The earliest afferent (probably catecholamine) fibers in the human embryo can be detected in the primordial plexiform layer of the future temporal cortex at 6 weeks (stage 17). This is the neopallial wall overlying the primordium of the amygdaloid area. Such fibers can easily be identified in silver-impregnated sections (Figures 13–5, A; 13–6, B). Catecholamine fibers may perhaps participate in early synaptogenesis within the subplate in the human embryo (Larroche, 1981). The following is the usual pattern later in development. As the cortical plate forms within the primordial plexiform layer, the latter is separated by the cortical plate into two parts: Future layer 1 and the subplate (Figures 13–4, C and D; 13–5, B and D). Accordingly the fibers are also separated into two sets: a group in future layer 1 and a group in the subplate. Both sets may be cholinergic as found by Bayer and Altman (1991) in the rat, and the early monoamine projection into the subplate is permanent (Bayer and Altman, 1990). According to these authors the primary sources of dopamine axons in the neocortex are the substantia nigra, ventral tegmental area, locus caeruleus, and raphe nuclei. Thalamocortical fibers arrive at 7 weeks (about stage 20) and settle in the subplate (Bayer and Altman, 1991, in

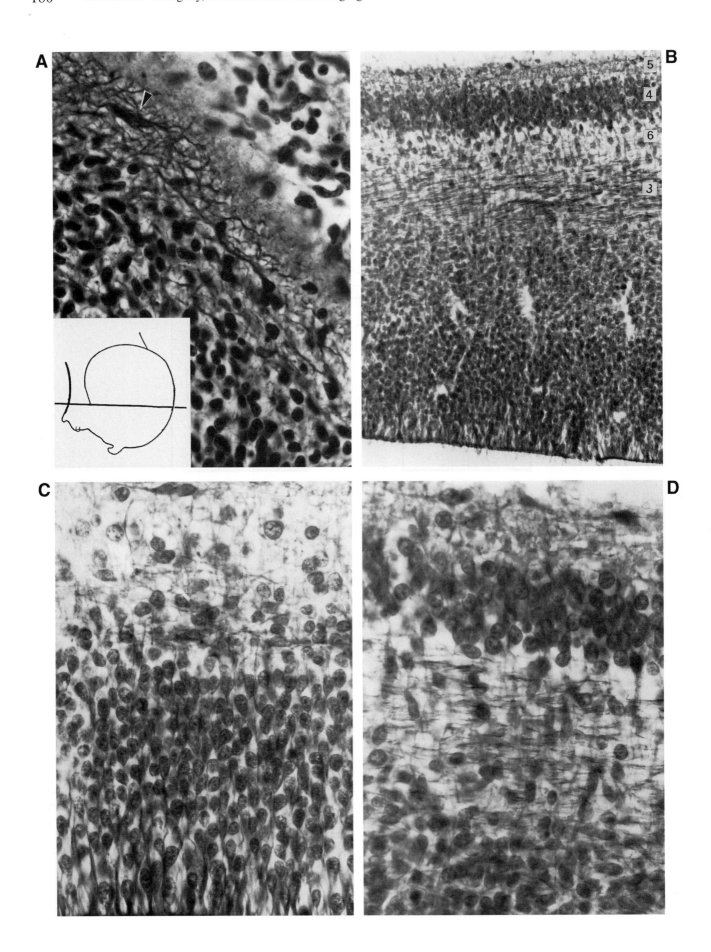

the rat) and in the intermediate layer (Miller, Chou, and Finlay, 1993, in the hamster). Penetration of monoamine fibers of the cortical plate occurs at the end of trimester 1. The highest density is found in the subplate and in the deep part of the cortical plate (Verney *et al.*, 1993).

The Archipallium and the Paleopallium

An intermediate form of cortex develops in the hippocampus, where a condensation of postmitotic cells forms a plate during the fetal period, i.e., after that in the neocortex. The designations archi-, paleo-, and neo-, therefore, are not an ontogenetic sequence (whatever the situation may be in reptiles). Nevertheless, the terms are useful in regard to histogenetic differences, which is not true of the terms archistriatum, paleostriatum, and neostriatum. In the paleopallium, aggregations of postmitotic cells form nuclei in the intermediate layer. A marginal layer is not present.

The Corpus Striatum and other Basal Nuclei

Both the diencephalon and the telencephalon contribute to the complicated formation of the corpus striatum (Figure 13–7). The diencephalon has a relatively short, the telencephalon a long proliferative phase, which seems to extend postnatally (Brana *et al.*, 1995).

The first component of the corpus striatum is initially diencephalic. The medial ventricular eminence (formerly called ganglionic), which is mostly archistriatal, arises early (stage 14) as a thickening rostral to the optic stalk. It represents the ventral part of the *torus hemisphericus*, which separates the developing telencephalic hemispheres from the diencephalon. The medial eminence is then shifted rostrally (because of growth gradients). The lateral ventricular eminence (formerly called ganglionic), which is purely telencephalic and neostriatal, appears as a discrete internal swelling in the neopallial wall (stage 15).

←————————————————————

FIGURE 13–5

Silver-impregnated sections of the cortical layer in the neopallium.

A. Future temporal cortex in a sagittal section (stage 17). The dense net of fibers of the primordial plexiform layer and some Cajal-Retzius cells (arrowhead) are visible.

B. Shows (5) future cortical layer 1, (4) cortical plate, (6) subplate, (3) intermediate layer (containing numerous fibers), and (1) ventricular layer.

C. An area without cortical plate. Many cells of the ventricular layer are attached to the ventricular surface (below).

D. From the section shown in B, at a higher magnification and focused on a different level. The subplate (in the middle of the photomicrograph) shows many fine fibers.

B, C, and **D** are from the same embryo (stage 23) and the plane of section is shown in the inset. From O'Rahilly and Müller, *The Embryonic Human Brain*, Wiley-Liss, New York, 1994, reproduced with permission.

Cell production occurs in the ventricular layer and later also in the subventricular layer. Migration from the matrix begins at 9 mm (Kahle, 1969), i.e., at 5 weeks.

The eminences are characterized by their large size and by the exceptional persistence of their subventricular layer (Figure 13–8). At the end of the embryonic period, the medial and lateral eminences lie along the floor of the lateral ventricle, separated from each other by a faint intereminential sulcus. Exhaustion of the matrix begins during trimester 2 and takes place caudorostrally (Sidman and Rakic, 1982).

The *claustrum* (Figure 13–8, B) arises (at stage 22) shortly before the internal capsule enters the telencephalon and before the fibers of the external capsule are present.

In the archistriatum the amygdaloid body appears as four nuclei consisting of postmitotic cells in the intermediate layer. They arise from rapid cell production in the ventricular layer of the medial eminence (stages 17 and 18). Also related to the medial eminence are probably the *nucleus accumbens* (Sidman and Rakic, 1982), as well as the tail of the caudate nucleus and the caudal part of the putamen (Hewitt, 1958).

In the paleostriatum the *globus pallidus* appears as an agglomeration of postmitotic cells in the intermediate layer (at stages 18 and 19) initially at the di-telencephalic junction. The *globus pallidus internus* (entopeduncular nucleus) develops similarly (stage 21). In the neostriatum the neuronal population may arise from one or several progenitor types (Brana *et al.*, 1995; Halliday and Cepko, 1992), which are defined chemically by the end of trimester 1. The timing and the end-point of mitotic activity in the human neostriatum are unknown (*ibid.*).

It has been suggested that optimal grafting in the treatment of *Huntington disease* (Chapter 32) would result when transplants are derived from the lateral ventricular eminence and when the donors range from stages 19–23. During this developmental period the largest precursor pool of medium-sized projection neurons is present and these would enable long axonal fibers to develop (Freeman *et al.*, 1995a).

The Cerebellum

Cell production occurs in two germinal layers (as also in the remainder of the rhombencephalon), namely the ventricular layer and the rhombic lip (Figure 13–9, B and C). Cell production begins early in the ventricular layer, which forms part of the cerebellar plate here and later gives origin to the piriform (Purkinje) cells and the deep cerebellar nuclei. The term rhombic lip (the germinal trigone of Altman and Bayer, 1985) refers to only the most lateral part of the alar neuroepithelium, which is continuous with the roof plate (Ellenberger *et al.*, 1969) and represents subventricular layer. The rhombic lip begins its mitotic activity after that in the ventricular layer (approximately at stage 16). Its cells participate mainly in the formation of the external germinal layer (stage 23), although

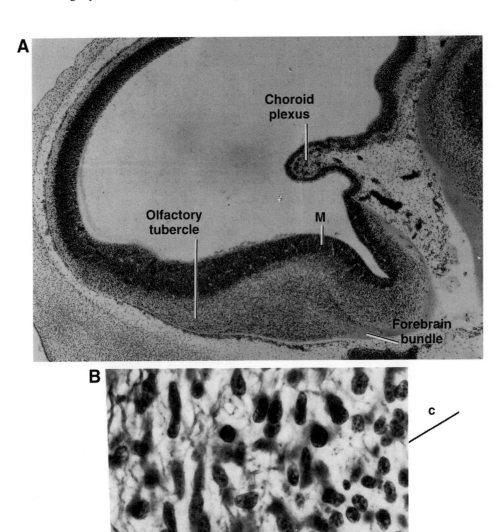

FIGURE   13–6

Area of the amygdaloid nuclei at the future temporal pole.

A. Sagittal section through a cerebral hemisphere (stage 19) showing the medial ventricular eminence containing the amygdaloid nuclei, from which fibers of the forebrain bundle emerge. The olfactory tubercle of the forebrain septum is nearby.

B. Tangential section through the future temporal neopallial wall overlying the amygdaloid nuclei (stage 17). A trilaminar cortex is present here earlier than in any other neopallial area. It shows (a) columns of cells in the ventricular layer, (b) rounded and more loosely arranged neurons in the intermediate layer, and (c) tall, horizontally arranged cells and fibers in the primordial plexiform layer. M, medial ventricular eminence.

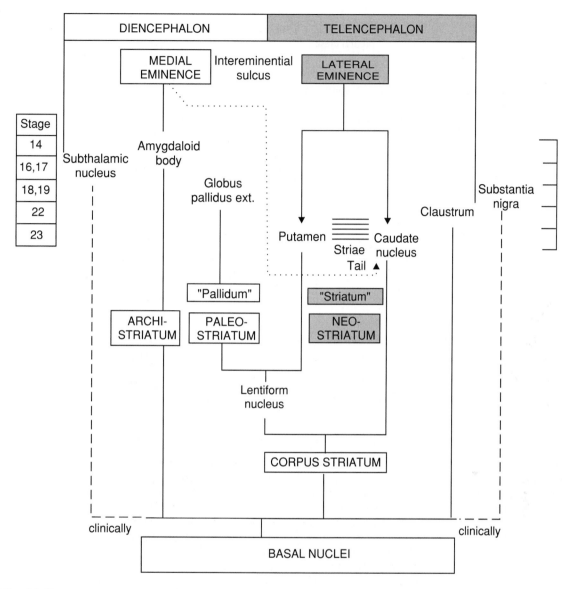

FIGURE   13–7
Scheme of the basal nuclei showing the development of
their diencephalic and telencephalic components.
Stages of appearance are also included.
Late in the embryonic period, the amygdaloid body as well as

the globus pallidus externus move into telencephalic territory.
From O'Rahilly and Müller, *The Embryonic Human Brain*,
Wiley-Liss, New York, 1994, redrawn and reproduced with
permission.

they may also be involved in the development of the dentate nucleus (stage 18).

The cells of the external germinal (or granular) layer divide *in situ*, and proliferation here lasts much longer than
in the ventricular layer, perhaps continuing for several
months after birth (Friede, 1989). The production of the
piriform (Purkinje) cells (Müller and O'Rahilly, 1990b) begins at 7 weeks (stage 21, Figure 13–9, C) rather than at 9
weeks (Sidman and Rakic, 1973). These cells migrate
from the subventricular layer. The formation of the external germinal layer in the material studied by the present
authors occurs at 8 weeks, which is two to three weeks
earlier than in other publications (Sidman and Rakic,

1973; Zecevic and Rakic, 1976). Fibers that are mostly trigeminal develop between the ventricular and intermediate layers (stage 15), and vestibulocerebellar fibers enter
the marginal layer (stage 17) (Müller and O'Rahilly,
1989).

The Remainder of the Rhombencephalon

The floor plate of the rhombencephalic neural tube
(Figure 13–10, B) is induced by the notochord and it controls the pattern of cellular types that appear along the
dorsoventral axis. By releasing chemo-attractrants it acts

TABLE **13–2.** Developmental sequence of features of rhombencephalon

Stage	Age, in weeks	Neural discs	Neural crest	Ganglia	Nuclei	Nerve fibers
9	3½	9 (otic)				
10	4	10 (arch 4)	5, 7, 9, 10 (-11?)			
11			7–8	5, 7–8		
11–12					(5, 7, 9, 10–11, 12 eff.)*	
12				9 superior & 10 superior		5, 7, 9, 11 SVE; 12 GSE
12–13		7, 9 (arches 2 & 3)		9 inferior & 10 inferior	3, 4 eff.	5, 7 eff. 5, 7 GVA
13	4½	5 (arch 1)				3 GSE
13–14					6 eff.	
14						4 GSE; 5 mesenc. root; 8v eff.; 9, 10–11 aff.
14–15	5					6 GSE
15–16					Sup. & inf. salivatory	
16	5½					8 c
17	6				5 motor	
18					5 main sensory	
19	6½				8c ventral & dorsal	
20	7				10 dorsal eff.	
21					8v lateral	
22	8				8v superior	

Abbreviations: aff., afferent; eff., efferent; GSE, general somatic efferent; GVA, general visceral afferent; SVE, special visceral efferent; 8c, 8v, cochlear and vestibular parts of cranial nerve 8, respectively. All the data are based on the authors's studies. *Provisional location.

as an intrinsic organizer of axons in the developing brain and spinal cord.

Throughout the rhombencephalon, cells are produced in the ventricular layer and in the rhombic lip (Figure 13–9, A). Cells that migrate from the ventricular layer settle in the intermediate layer and form nuclei of the cranial nerves (Table 13–2), as well as groups of catecholamine neurons (discussed later). It is not generally appreciated that early in development both somatic efferent (stage 12) and visceral efferent (stage 13) neurons are arranged in two longitudinal columns on each side of the median plane (where the median raphe forms at stage 15). The visceral efferent cells, which are situated medial to those of the somatic column, then migrate laterally and settle as the definitive nuclei (at approximately stages 16 and 17). Hence the original position of the nuclei differs considerably from their definitive site (O'Rahilly et al., 1984; Müller and O'Rahilly, 1990a). The afferent nuclei develop later than the somatic and visceral types of efferent nuclei.

The subventricular layer of the rhombic lip gives rise to postmitotic cells that migrate along the external surface of the brain stem, where they form the transient corpus pontobulbare (reconstructed and described by Müller and O'Rahilly, 1990a). Two streams of cells migrating from the rhombic lip are visible (stages 20–23). A site of origin of the rhombic lip that has been largely ignored in the literature is in the region of the vestibulocochlear nerve (Shaner, 1934; Müller and O'Rahilly, 1990a) and is represented schematically here (Figure 13–9, A).

With regard to fibers and tracts in the rhombencephalon, the lateral longitudinal fasciculus begins to form early (stage 12) adjacent to the sulcus limitans and later reaches from the hindbrain to the isthmus rhombencephali. A few days later than the lateral, the ventral longitudinal fasciculus begins to appear, as does also the common afferent tract, which consists of afferent fibers of the cra-

FIGURE 13–8

Corpus striatum and ventricular eminences.

A. medial (M) and lateral (L) ventricular eminences are separated from each other by a very faint indentation (stage 21). The subventricular layer is as thick as the ventricular layer. The fibers of the internal capsule have not yet arrived. The cortical plate, choroid plexus, and interventricular foramen (arrow) are also visible. Part of the dorsal thalamus (Th.) can be seen at the right, with the stria medullaris thalami (SM) at its periphery.

B. At 8 weeks (stage 23) the internal capsule has arrived and its fibers are probably mostly thalamocortical. They become dispersed in the intermediate layer of the neopallium. The internal capsule separates the future caudate nucleus (C) from the putamen (P) (both derived from the subventricular layer of the lateral eminence). The globus pallidus (GP) is visible at the di-telencephalic junction. The insula is clearly developing. The claustrum is marked by an asterisk. From O'Rahilly and and Müller, *The Embryonic Human Brain*, Wiley-Liss, New York, 1994, reproduced with permission. C, caudate nucleus. GP, globus pallidus. L and M, lateral and medial ventricular eminences. P, putamen. SM, stria medullaris thalami. Th., thalamus.

nial nerves. It will become subdivided later into trigemi-nospinal, vestibulospinal, and solitary tracts (stage 17). The numerous rhombencephalic tracts present at the end of the embryonic period resemble closely those found in the newborn (Müller and O'Rahilly, 1990a).

The Spinal Cord

The trilaminar structure of the neural tube is conserved in the spinal cord of the adult as the ependyma, the gray and the white matter. Neurogenesis and gliogenesis are more complicated in the spinal cord than would appear at

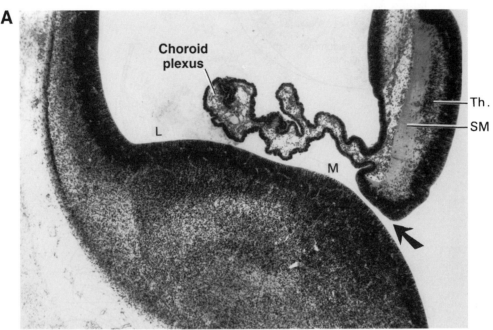

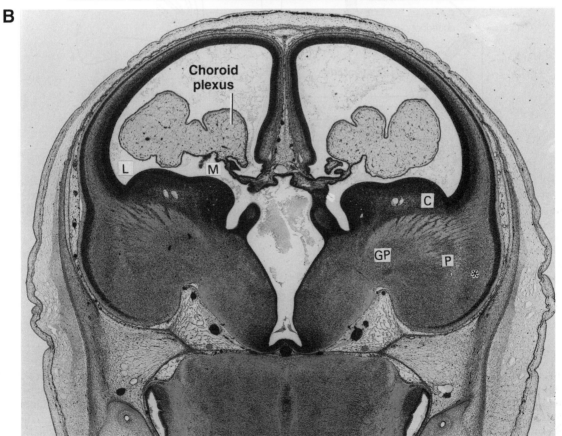

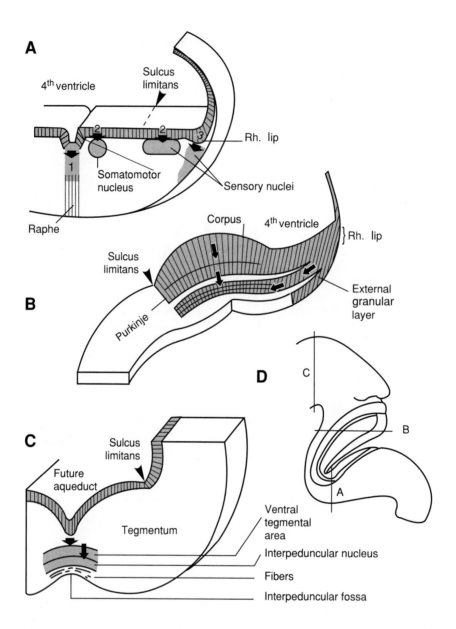

FIGURE 13–9

Production of neurons and their migration in (A) rhombencephalon, (B) the cerebellum, and (C) the mesencephalon.

A. Block from the hindbrain showing (1) early migration from the floor plate to the raphe, (2) migration from the ventricular layer for motor and sensory (e.g., vestibular) nuclei, (3) migration from the rhombic lip, e.g., for cochlear nuclei. The sensory areas are lateral to the sulcus limitans.

B. Migration in the cerebellum from the ventricular layer and the rhombic lip for the primordium of the dentate nucleus (stage

21). Cells from the ventricular layer give rise also to the Purkinje cells, and those from the rhombic lip form the external germinal (or granular) layer (stage 23). From O'Rahilly and Müller, *The Embryonic Human Brain*, Wiley-Liss, New York, 1994, redrawn and reproduced with permission.

C. Migration in the mesencephalic tegmentum from the ventricular layer, producing at first the interpeduncular nucleus and later the ventral tegmental area. The plane of section is shown in **D.**

first glance (Toyhama *et al*, 1991). The transition from a replicating stem cell to a committed precursor is controlled by a number of specific genes (Chapter 4). In the human spinal cord, the acquisition of the neuronal phenotype is exclusively postmigratory (*ibid.*).

The alar or dorsal lamina and the basal or ventral lamina of the neural tube (Figure 13–10, A) are separated by the sulcus limitans, which is present in the midbrain and hindbrain. The alar laminae, which are essentially afferent in function, are united by the roof plate. The basal laminae, essentially efferent, are joined by the floor plate (Figure 13–10, B), which is induced by the notochord. At 6 weeks the spinal cord shows ventricular, intermediate, and marginal layers (Figure 13–10, B). The portion to which a set of spinal roots is attached on each side is termed a myelomere (Figure 13–10, C). From studies of the human embryo (Marti *et al*, 1987), the sequence of appearance is: (i) Cells of the floor plate (which arise before motoneurons), (ii) motoneurons (which are formed in rostrocaudal and ventrodorsal gradients), (iii) cells of the *nucleus proprius*, (iv) sensory neurons in the *substantia gelatinosa* (for pain afferents). The above sequence has been confirmed in the macaque (Knyihar-Csillik, Csillik, and Rakic, 1995).

Motoneurons are the first neural cells to demonstrate expression of neuronal antigens, and synapses are found there very early (stage 15) in the human (Okado, 1981). Moreover, synapses representing connections between primary afferents and interneurons of the *substantia gelatinosa* are also present early (stage 17). The first movements (Okado, 1981; de Vries, 1992) observed in ultrasonic studies occur at about 5½ postfertilizational weeks (probably stage 16).

Afferent fibers reach the dorsal horn well before their peripheral field (e.g., skin) expresses sensory peptides, indicating that peripheral tissue may not direct the formation of central terminations (Marti *et al.*, 1987). The trigeminospinal tract invades the cervical region of the cord already at 6 weeks (stage 17), and the dorsal funiculus is prominent. The *tractus solitarius* soon reaches the thorax (stage 19). By the end of the embryonic period (stage 23), the *funiculi gracilis et cuneatus*, medial lemniscus, corticospinal tracts, and lateral spinothalamic tract are all present (Müller and O'Rahilly, 1990a).

Apoptosis

Apoptosis, which is a morphologically distinct form of programmed cell death (Chapter 17), is an essential feature of normal development, including that of the nervous system. Apoptosis is believed to affect half of the neurons formed. The function of neuronal apoptosis seems to be the removal of excess neurons and the establishment of appropriate synaptic connections. The process occurs in the brain in such regions as the cortical subplate, in the granular cells of the cerebellum, in pyramidal cells of the hippocampus, and others. It takes place in the olfactory epithelium throughout life. The apoptotic zones of the embryonic human nervous system have been studied and tabulated by Ilieş (1969). From studies of the mouse it appears that certain genes and assorted agents are capable of decreasing the extent of apoptosis and hence increasing neuronal survival, whereas other show a contrary effect (Chapter 17).

Neurotrophins, such as nerve growth factor, have been studied chiefly in the peripheral nervous system. They influence the proliferation and differentiation of neuronal progenitor cells (Davies, 1994) and they promote the survival of developing neurons (Johnson and Oppenheim, 1994). In the central nervous system, however, the rela-

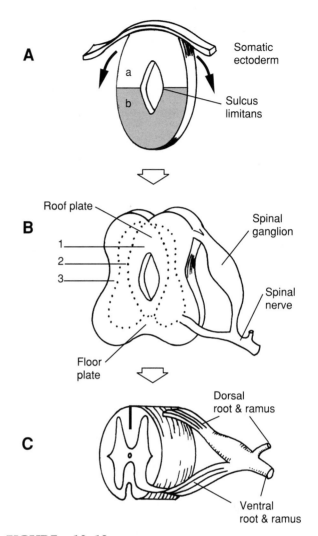

FIGURE   13–10

Cell production in the spinal cord.

A. Neural tube after fusion of the neural folds, showing alar and basal laminae. Neural crest from the neurosomatic ectodermal junction is indicated by arrows and commences early (stages 10 and 11). Migration takes place through the rostral half of the sclerotome. Formation of spinal ganglia then begins (stage 12).

B. At approximately 6 weeks, ventricular (1), intermediate (2), and marginal (3) layers are present. The intermediate layer contains migrating unipolar neurons and glial cells.

C. A myelomere, showing attachment of nerve roots of one spinal nerve.

From O'Rahilly and Müller, *Human Embryology and Teratology*, Wiley-Liss, New York, 1996, reproduced with permission.

tionship of neurons to neurotrophins is more complex than previously thought (*ibid.*). Much of the recent work is based on studies of transgenic mice. A major cause of apoptosis is a lack of neurotrophic factors such as nerve growth factor (NGF) and brain-derived neurotrophic factor. Receptors with a strong affinity for such factors are characterized by tyrosine kinase activity (Onteniente, 1995).

TABLE 13–3.   Development of tracts

Tract	Stage
Lateral longitudinal	12
Ventral longitudinal	13
Common afferent[1]	13
Medial longitudinal*	13
Dorsal funiculus	14
Preoptico-hypothalamic[2]	14
Hypothalamotegmental	14,15
Mamillotegmental	15
Medial forebrain bundle*	15,16
Tractus solitarius separates	
from common afferent tract	15,16
Hypothalamothalamic	15,16
Tract of posterior commissure	15,16
Crossed tectobulbar	16
Fibers from olfactory tubercle	
to amygdaloid body	16,17
Habenulo-interpeduncular*	16,17
Fibers from olfactory bulb	
to olfactory tubercle[4]	17
Mamillothalamic	18
Stria medullaris thalami*	18,19
Lateral lemniscus	18,19
Thalamostriatal[5]	19
Tract of zona intrathalamica	19
Central tegmental*[6]	19

[1]Containing fibers of the future tractus solitarius.
[2]Part of the basal forebrain bundle
[3]Containing striatosubthalamic fibers
[4]Part of the medial forebrain bundle
[5]Synonyms: lateral forebrain bundle; Stammbündel (of His)
[6]Zecevic and Verney (1995)
*Pathways concerned with the transportation of monoamines

Monoamine-Producing and Related Regions

Monoamines are important in the early development of the brain, they are transported by tracts that arise early (Table 13–3), and are significant for synaptic transmission. It is postulated that they have a regulatory or trophic role on target neurons. The regions described below (Figure 13–11) have been studied morphologically in the human by the present authors, particularly in reconstructions made from silver-impregnated sections. The details have been largely confirmed experimentally in rodents and the macaque, and more recently in immunological studies of the human embryo (Freeman *et al.*, 1991; Verney *et al.*, 1991; Zecevic and Verney, 1995).

Locus Caeruleus

The cells of the future locus caeruleus, which are present early (stage 13), are situated in the intermediate layer of rhombomeres 1 and 2, ventral to the sulcus limitans. Cells in a similar location have been found in the rat (Sievers *et al.*, 1981). In the human, brightly fluorescent processes have later (at about stages 19 and 20) been traced into the telencephalic wall (Zecevic and Verney, 1995), and dopamine and adrenergic fibers reach the tectum.

Raphe Nuclei of the Rhombencephalon

These nuclei are essential for the development of the brain, their importance lying in their neurotransmitters. They are related to the *locus caeruleus*, the *substantia nigra*, and the red nucleus. The raphe nuclei arise in the *septum medullae* (which is evident at stages 15 and 16) and their tall cells spread out from the rhombencephalic floor plate (stage 16) (Figure 13–9, A). The *septum medullae* becomes a raphe, into which fibers from cranial nerve nuclei penetrate and reach the raphe nuclei. Connections to the forebrain develop later (at about stages 21–23), probably by the central tegmental tract. Two distinct nuclei at 8 weeks (stage 23) have been reconstructed (Figure 23–25 in O'Rahilly and Müller, 1994).

Interpeduncular Nucleus and Ventral Tegmental Area

The three main dopamine areas of the midbrain are the *substantia nigra*, the interpeduncular nucleus, and the ventral tegmental area. The interpeduncular nucleus is situated immediately dorsal to the interpeduncular fossa, and the ventral tegmental area is dorsal to that nucleus (Figure 13–9, D). The tegmental area begins to develop early (stage 13) and marginal and intermediate layers appear (stage 14). The future interpeduncular nuclear area contains some cells that leave the ventricular layer, and these become traversed (stage 20) by fibers that probably belong to the rubrocerebellar tract. Then the connection with the habenular nuclei by the *fasciculus retroflexus* (habenulo-interpeduncular tract) is completed (stage 21). The ventral tegmental area is probably also present at this time. The various features discussed above are illustrated in the author's Atlas of 1994 (Figures 20–4 and 20–8).

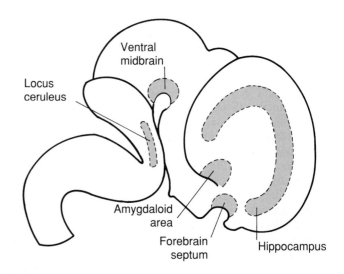

FIGURE   13–11

Some catecholamine-producing areas. Because they are not at the surface, their outlines are shown by interrupted lines.

The timing is basically comparable in rodents and in the macaque (Levitt and Rakic, 1982).

The ventricular zone and the ventral tegmental area have been shown by immunological methods to be the first region to display TH-immune reactivity in human embryos of about 6½ (Freeman et al., 1991) or 7 weeks (Verney et al., 1991). Nigrostriatal fibers develop at about 7 weeks (ibid.), which agrees well with the survival of human dopamine suspension grafts (Freeman et al., 1995b). Such fibers extend initially to the subventricular zone of the lateral eminence (Freeman et al., 1995a). Grafts of dopamine-producing cells from the ventral part of the midbrain are at their best near the end of the embryonic period (Brundin et al., 1989).

Amygdaloid Area

The amygdaloid nuclei arise almost exclusively in the medial ventricular eminence (Figures 13–6, A, 13–7), which is diencephalic. The overlying cortex, however, belongs to the temporal pole and acquires a primordial plexiform layer early (stage 14). Ascending fibers of the future medial forebrain bundle reach this region rapidly (stage 15) and elongated (probably Cajal-Retzius) cells are found (stage 17) (Figure 13–5a). It seems possible that the early arriving monoamine fibers in the precocious temporal pallium influence the rapid formation of the amygdaloid nuclei. The fibers of the primordial plexiform layer are believed to be afferent (Marín-Padilla and Marín-Padilla, 1982). Four amygdaloid nuclei are detectable and connections with the *stria medullaris thalami* develop (stage 18). The medial forebrain bundle can be recognized by immunological methods at about 7 weeks (Zecevic and Verney, 1995). Early development of the amygdaloid nuclei has been confirmed by tritiated thymidine autoradiography in the macaque (Kordower et al., 1992).

Forebrain Septum

The basal part of the medial telencephalic wall (the *septum verum*) forms as the cerebral hemispheres expand beyond the *lamina terminalis*, and it extends between the olfactory bulb and the commissural plate (Figure 13–11). The earliest part of the septum is the olfactory tubercle (stage 16), which contains cellular clusters and receives the nervus terminalis (stage 17). Connections to the olfactory bulb and the amygdaloid nuclei exist. The first septal nucleus develops caudomedial to the olfactory tubercle and is probably the diagonal nucleus. The septal nuclei are cellular agglomerations at the periphery of the intermediate layer. Connections develop between the nucleus of the diagonal band and the hippocampus (stage 20).

The nucleus of the diagonal band has been identified by the present authors because of the projection of its fibers to the hippocampus. Some cells of the nuclei basales of Meynert may begin to differentiate caudally. Connections between the septum and the hippocampus have been investigated in the rat (Linke and Frotscher, 1993). The production of cholinergic neurons in the septal nu-

clei has been studied in the mouse (Schambra et al., 1989) and in the macaque (Kordower and Rakic, 1990). Neurons of the medial septal nucleus, the nucleus of the diagonal band, and the nucleus basalis of Meynert contain nerve growth factor in the aged human (Mufson et al., 1994). These three cholinergic groups of the base of the forebrain 'are the most outstanding sets of neurons regulating cortical functions' (Toledano, 1992). Each group ends in a specific part of the cortex, and their number and function are diminished statistically in Alzheimer disease (ibid.). The nucleus basalis develops during the fetal period (Kostović, 1986). Cholinesterase-reactive fibers arising from it are distributed to the neocortex and the limbic cortex by the end of trimester 2.

Hippocampus

Although it is not strictly part of the regions being discussed in this section, it is related to them. The hippocampal region (Figure 13–11) can be discerned early (stages 13 and 14), but it develops slowly. A marginal layer can be distinguished dorsomedially in the telencephalic roof. This area extends from the amygdaloid region as far rostrally as the olfactory bulb (stage 16) and shows a discrete thickening near the ventricle. The dentate area becomes visible (stage 17) and the hippocampus can be recognized (stages 18–23) by (i) its bulging into the ventricle, (ii) its broad marginal and intermediate layers, and (iii) its narrow ventricular layer. Cells in the various components of the hippocampal formation begin to appear simultaneously in the monkey (Rakic and Nowakowski, 1981), whereas they develop successively (dentate area, hippocampus, presubiculum) in the rat (Bayer, 1980). More on the development of the hippocampus can be found in the next chapter.

An Overall View

The brain begins to develop very early in the embryonic period. At 8 postfertilizational weeks (stage 23) it is quite complicated and the rhombencephalon resembles closely that of the newborn. In the mesencephalon, dopamine-producing areas are believed to be functional. The most advanced regions of the prosencephalon are the forebrain septum, amygdaloid body, habenular nuclei, and subthalamic and hypothlamic nuclei.

Investigations of the timing and sequence of the development of the brain, as is true of other organs also, require the use of morphological stages. It is frequently not appreciated that a considerable body of precisely staged information concerning the human embryo is now available.

Studies of the developing brain in species other than the human continue to yield valuable information, but great caution needs to be exercized in attempting to extrapolate the results to the human.

Selected Readings

Butler, H., and Juurlink, B. H. J. 1987. An Atlas for Staging Mammalian and Chick Embryos. CRC Press, Boca Raton, Florida.

Friede, R. L. 1989. Developmental Neuropathology, 2nd. Ed., Springer, New York.

O'Rahilly, R., and Müller, F. 1994. The Embryonic Human Brain. An Atlas of Developmental Stages. Wiley-Liss, New York.

O'Rahilly, R., and Müller, F. 1996. Human Embryology and Teratology. 2nd Ed. Wiley-Liss, New York.

Sidman, R. L., and Rakic, P. 1982. Development of the human central nervous system. In Histology and Histopathology of the Nervous System. Haymaker W., and Adams, R.D. (eds.) Thomas, Springfield.

de Vries, J. I. P. 1992. Fetal behaviour. The first trimester. In J. G. Nijhuis (ed.), pp. 19–50. Oxford University Press, Oxford.

References

Altman, J., and Bayer, S. A. 1985. Embryonic development of the rat cerebellum. I. Delineation of the cerebellar primordium and early cell movements. J. Comp. Neurol. 231:1–26.

Bayer, S. A. 1980. Development of the hippocampal region in the rat. J. Comp. Neurol. 190: 37–134.

Bayer, S. A., and Altman, J. 1990. Development of layer I and the subplate in the rat neocortex. Exp. Neurol. 170:48–62.

Bayer, S. A., and Altman, J. 1991. Neocortical Development, pp. 49–152. Raven Press, New York.

Brana, C., Charron, G., Aubert, I., et al. 1995. Ontogeny of the striatal neurons expressing neuropeptide genes in the human fetus and neonate. J. Comp. Neurol. 360:488–505.

Brundin, P., Widner, H., Nilsson, O. G., et al. 1989. Intracerebral xenografts of dopamine neurons: the role of immunosupression and the blood-brain barrier. Exp. Brain Res. 75:195–207.

Caviness, V. S., and Takahashi, T. 1995. Proliferative events in the cerebral ventricular zone. Brain and Dev. 17:159–163.

Choi, B. H. 1988. Developmental events during the early stages of cerebral cortical neurogenesis in man. Acta Neuropathol. 75:441–447.

Davies, A. M. 1994. The role of neurotrophins in the developing nervous system. J. Neurobiol. 25:1334–1348.

Ellenberger, C., Hanaway, J., and Netsky, M. G. 1969. Embryogenesis of the inferior olivary nucleus in the rat: A radioautographic study and a re-evaluation of the rhombic lip. J. Comp. Neurol. 137:71–77.

Freeman, T. B., Sanberg, P. R., and Isacson, O. 1995a. Development of the human striatum: implications for fetal striatal transplantation in the treatment of Huntington's disease. Cell Transplantation 4:539–545.

Freeman, T. B., Sanberg, P. R., Nauert, G. M., et al. 1995b. The influence of donor age and the survival of solid and suspension intraparenchymal human embryonic nigral grafts. Cell Transplantation 4:141–154.

Freeman, T. B., Spence, M. S., Boss, B. D., et al. 1991. Development of dopaminergic neurons in the human substantia nigra. Exp. Neurol. 113:344–353.

Gates, M. A., Thomas, L. B., and Howard, E. M. 1995. Cell and molecular analysis of the developing and adult mouse subventricular zone of the cerebral hemispheres. J. Comp. Neurol. 361:249–266.

Halliday, A. L., and Cepko, C. L. 1992. Generation and migration of cells in the developing striatum. Neuron 9: 15–26.

Hewitt, W. 1958. The development of the human caudate and amygdaloid nuclei. J. Anat. 92: 377–382.

Ilieş, A. 1969. La topographie et la dynamique des zones nécrotiques normales chez l'embryon humain de 11–30 mm. II. Système nerveux central et périphérique. Étude histologique et histochimique. Rev. Roum. Embryol. Cytol., Sér. Embryol. 6:31–44.

Johnston, A., and Oppenheim, R. W. 1994. Keeping track of changing neurotrophic theory. Curr. Biol. 4: 662–665.

Kahle, W. 1969. Die Entwicklung der menschlichen Grosshirnhemisphäre. Springer, Berlin. Schriftenreihe Neurologie 1:1–116.

Knyihar-Csillik, E., Csillik, B., and Rakic, P. 1995. Structure of the embryonic primate spinal cord at the closure of the first reflex arc. Anat. Embryol. 191:519–540.

Kordower, J. H., Piecinski, P., and Rakic, P. 1992. Neurogenesis of the amygdaloid nuclear complex in the rhesus monkey. Develop. Brain Res. 68:9–15.

Kordower, J. H., and Rakic, P. 1990. Neurogenesis of the magnocellular basal forebrain in the rhesus monkey. J. Comp. Neurol. 291:637–653.

Kostović, I. 1986. Prenatal development of nucleus basalis complex and related fiber systems in man: a histochemical study. Neurosci. 17:1047–1077.

Larroche, J-C. 1981. The marginal layer in the neocortex of a 7-week-old human embryo. Anat. Embryol. 162:301–312.

Levitt, P., and Rakic, P. 1982. The time of genesis, embryonic origin and differentiation of the brain stem monoamine neurons in the rhesus monkey. Dev. Brain. Res. 4:35–57.

Linke, R., and Frotscher, M. 1993. Development of the rat septohippocampal projection: tracing with DiI and electron microscopy of identified growth cones. J. Comp. Neurol. 332:69–88.

Marín-Padilla, M., and Marín-Padilla, M. T. 1982. Origin, prenatal development and structural organization of layer I of the human cerebral (motor) cortex. A Golgi study. Anat. Embryol. 164:161–206.

Marti, E., Gibson, S. J., Polak, J. M., et al. 1987. Ontogeny of peptide- and amine-containing neurones in motor, sensory, and autonomic regions of rat and human spinal cord, dorsal root ganglia, and rat skin. J. Comp. Neurol. 266:332–359.

Miller, B., Chou, L., and Finlay, B. 1993. The early development of thalamocortical and corticothalamic projections. J. Comp. Neurol. 335:16–41.

Molliver, M. E., Kostović, I., and van der Loos, H. 1973. The development of synapses in cerebral cortex of the human fetus. Brain Res. 50:403–407.

Mufson, E. J., Conner, J. M., Varon, S., et al. 1994. Nerve growth factor-like immunoreactive profiles in the primate basal forebrain and hippocampal formation. J. Comp. Neurol. 341:507–519.

Müller, F., and O'Rahilly, R. 1989. The human brain at stage 17, including the appearance of the future olfactory bulb and the first amygdaloid nuclei. Anat. Embryol. 180:353–369.

Müller, F., and O'Rahilly, R. 1990a. The human rhombencephalon at the end of the embryonic period proper. Am. J. Anat. 189:127–145.

Müller, F., and O'Rahilly, R. 1990b. The human brain at stages 21–23, with particular reference to the cerebral cortical plate and to the development of the cerebellum. Anat. Embryol. 182:375–400.

Okado, N. 1981. Onset of synapse formation in the human spinal cord. J. Comp. Neurol. 201:211–219.

Onteniente, B. 1995. Mieux comprendre le rôle des neurotrophines dans le système nerveux grâce à l'invalidation génique. Médecine/sciences 11:1141–1143.

O'Rahilly, R., and Müller, F. 1987. Developmental Stages in Human Embryos Including a Revision of Streeter's 'Horizons' and a Survey of the Carnegie Collection. Carnegie Institution of Washington, Washington, D.C. Publication No. 637.

O'Rahilly, R., Müller, F., Hutchins, G. M., et al. 1984. Computer ranking of the sequence of appearance of 100 features of the brain and related structures in staged human embryos during the first 5 weeks of development. American J. Anat. 171:243–257.

Rakic, P. 1991. Development of the primate cerebral cortex. In M. Lewis (ed.) Child and Adolescent Psychiatry, Chapter 2, pp. 11–28. Williams and Wilkins, Baltimore.

Rakic, P., and Nowakowski, R. S. 1981. The time of origin of neurons in the hippocampal region of the rhesus monkey. J. Comp. Neurol. 196:99–128.

Schambra, U. R., Sulik, K. K., Petrusz, P., et al. 1989. Ontogeny of cholinergic neurons in the mouse forebrain. J. Comp. Neurol. 288:101–122.

Shaner, R. F. 1934. The development of the nuclei and tracts related to the acoustic nerve in the pig. J. Comp. Neurol. 60:5–14.

Sidman, R. L., and Rakic, P. 1973. Neuronal migration, with special reference to developing human brain: a review. Brain Res. 62:1–35.

Sievers, J., Lolova, I., Jenner, S., et al. 1981. Morphological and biochemical studies on the ontogenesis of the nucleus locus coeruleus. Bibliotheca Anat. 19:52–130.

Takahashi, T., Nowakowski, R. S., and Caviness, V. S. 1995a. The cell cycle of the pseudostratified ventricular epithelium of the embryonic murine cerebral wall. J. Neurosci. 15:6046–6057.

Takahashi, T., Nowakowski, R. S., and Caviness, V. S. 1995b. Early ontogeny of the secondary proliferative population of the embryonic murine cerebral wall. J. Neurosci. 15:6058–6068.

Tohyama, T., Lee, V., M.-Y., Rorke, L. B., et al. 1991. Molecular milestones that signal axonal maturation and the commitment of human spinal cord precursor cells to the neuronal or glial phenotype in development. J. Comp. Neurol. 310:285–299.

Toledano, A. 1992. Evolution of cholinergic cortical innervation after nbM-lesioning (an experimental Alzheimer model). In I. Kostović, S. Knezevic, H. M. Wisniewski, et al. (eds.) Neurodevelopment, Aging and Cognition. Birkhäuser, Boston.

Verney, C., Milosevic, A., Alvarez, C., et al. 1993. Immunocytochemical evidence of well-developed dopaminergic and noradrenergic innervations in the frontal cerebral cortex of human fetuses at midgestation. J. Comp. Neurol. 336: 331–344.

Verney, C., Zecevic, N., Nikolic, B., et al. 1991. Early evidence of catecholaminergic cell groups in 5- and 6-week-old human embryos using tyrosine hydroxylase and dopamine-3-hydroxylase immunocytochemistry. Neurosci. Lett. 131:121–124.

Zecevic, N., and Rakic, P. 1976. Differentiation of Purkinje cells and their relationship to other components of developing cerebellar cortex in man. J. Comp. Neurol. 167:27–48.

Zecevic, N., and Verney, C. 1995. Development of the catecholamine neurons in human embryos and fetuses, with special emphasis on the innervation of the cerebral cortex. J. Comp. Neurol. 351:509–535.

Irina N. Bogolepova

14

The Limbic System as a Model of Cytoarchitectonical Changes in the Developing Brain

All Embryonic Cell Layers can be Recognized in the Telencephalon in the Entire First Half of Gestation

The Meaning of the Differential Positioning of Migrating Neurons in the Cortex for the Susceptibility to Age-Related Degeneration is Unclear

Different Types of Cortex Emerge during Development

The Development of Isocortical Cytoarchitectonics in the Cingulate Gyrus

The Development of the Limbic Cortex Continues After Birth and During the Infantile Period

The Development of Allocortical Cytoarchitectonics in the Hippocampus

An Overall View

The telencephalic wall in primate embryos contains several cellular zones that do not have counterparts in the adult cerebrum. However, through a series of developmental stages, changes accumulate in these zones which ultimately determine the molding of the complicated neural connections or arrays of neural networks that constitute the cytoarchitectonics of the adult brain.

All Embryonic Cell Layers can be Recognized in the Telencephalon in the Entire First Half of Gestation

The cytological organization of the primate brain during gestation has been studied extensively in monkeys, and also in human fetuses. These studies have indicated that the lining of the cerebral ventricle during the entire first half of gestation consists of proliferative cells that eventually produce all neurons of the cortex. The lateral ventricle in a monkey fetus at this age is still relatively large, and the cerebral vesicles are still smooth and lack characteristic convolutions that will emerge in the second half of gestation. However, at this early stage all embryonic layers can be recognized: The ventricular zone, the subventricular zone, the intermediate zone, the subplate zone, the cortical plate, and the marginal zone. The *ventricular zone*, also called *matrix* (Chapter 10) or *germinal zone*, is formed by neuronal and glial precursor cells. These proliferative cells in the ventricular zone are in different phases of the mitotic cycle and have radial processes that protrude towards the pial surface and form the outer cell-free marginal zone. The neuronal precursors, intermixed with dividing glial cells precursors, are arranged in a pseudostratified manner and are attached to the ventricular surface by their endfeet. Migrating neurons move along radial fibers which span the cerebral wall and accumulate in the subplate zone, where they make transient synapses before entering the cortical plate.

The Meaning of the Differential Positioning of Migrating Neurons in the Cortex for the Susceptibility to Age-Related Degeneration is Unclear

Up to the 40th embryonic day, almost all cells in the monkey ventricular zone are mitotic; symmetric division produces two progenitors during each cycle and causes lateral spread. However, after the 40th embryonic day, asymmetrical division produces one postmitotic neuron which leaves the ventricular zone and another progenitor which remains within the proliferative zone (Rakic, 1990). Postmitotic neurons migrate across the intermediate zone and become arranged in the cortical plate in reverse order of their arrival, i.e., the first cells arriving are placed proximal to the ventricular zone, whereas the cells arriving later are placed distal to the ventricular zone. The meaning of this differential 'age' for the susceptibility of age related degeneration is unclear. We do not know, for example, whether the late-arrived, distal or 'outer' cells differ from the early-arrived, proximal or 'inner' cells in the number of steps of major differentiation (Chapter 10) accumulated by the time of their relative positioning in the cortex. One may speculate, for example, that the late-arrived cells are those produced after a larger number of mitosis in the progenitor cell line as compared to the early-arrived cells which may be produced in an earlier asymmetric division in the progenitor line.

Different Types of Cortex Emerge During Development

Although the basic principles underlying cytoarchitectonical changes during development – cell proliferation, migration, apoptosis, dendritic and axonal sprouting and regression – are followed in all parts of the developing brain, remarkable regional differences do appear, giving rise to distinct cytoarchitectonical maps. There are roughly two distinct types of cortex in the adult brain, namely the *isocortex*, a regular, usually six- to seven-layered neuronal assembly bearing in some regions a number of sublayers, and the *anisocortex* or *allocortex*, an irregular assembly featured by a variable, though lesser number of layers as compared to the first type. The phylogenetically younger region of the mammalian and primate brain, the *neocortex*, is mainly made up of isocortex; allocortex can be found mainly in the *paleo-* or *archicortex*.

There is one system in the brain presenting both types of cortices, and also transitional zones between, namely the limbic system. Details on the anatomy of this complex system can be found in the literature quoted as selected readings at the end of this chapter; here we will concentrate on the description of the most important cytoarchitectonical differences arising during the ontogeny of the limbic cortices of the *cingulate gyrus* (isocortex) and the *hippocampal formation* (allocortex) which have important implications for neuronal aging and degeneration. In the following chapters these limbic structures will be mentioned again, particularly the hippocampus, because this is a preferential site for common types of age-related, neurodegenerative changes.

The Development of Isocortical Cytoarchitectonics in the Cingulate Gyrus

In human embryos at the 10th gestational week (G-10), the telencephalic wall is clearly subdivided into four embryonic cell layers – the ventricular zone, the intermediate zone, the cortical plate and the marginal zone (Figure 14–1). At this developmental stage, it is still impossible to distinguish any cortical region in the brain such as the motor, visual or limbic cortices, because the cortical plate forms an uniform structure in its whole extension. However, as the migration of neuronal cells continues through G-16 to G-20, remarkable changes can be detected: The ventricular zone narrows, the intermediate zone and the cortical plate widen, as the latter starts to divide into two parts, the superior and the inferior, deeper one. Whereas the structure of the superior part is an homogeneous one, that of the inferior part is more laminar (Figure 14–2). At this stage the cortex of the cingulate gyrus can be clearly distinguished. In addition, for the first time in ontogeny, anterior limbic cortex differentiates and separates from the posterior limbic cortex.

The stratification of the cytoarchitectonical layers begins at G-20, especially in the deep portions of the cortex. Layers V and VI+VII are distinguished first. At G-32 all layers have already appeared, and the main limbic areas, for example, Brodmann's area 24 and 23 are already established. The development of the anterior and posterior limbic areas is not equal; posterior area 23 develops more rapidly in comparison to anterior area 24. During the second half of prenatal period the limbic *area limitans*, represented by areas 24/32 and area 31, appears and develops intensively. The thickness of the cortex increases, while neuronal density decreases, indicating that dendritic and axonal expansion is in course, as neuronal sizes increase unequally in different layers. This process is better observed first in layer V, then in layer III.

The Development of the Limbic Cortex Continues After Birth and During the Infantile Period

The limbic cortex of a newborn has all limbic areas and subareas: Peritectal areas, propria limbic areas 24 and 23 and limitant areas 24/32 and 31. All cytoarchitectonical layers are very well delimited, but the limbic cortex differs greatly from the same cortex of an adult. For example, the width of the newborn cortex reaches only up to 25 percent of the width of the adult cortex, and has a much

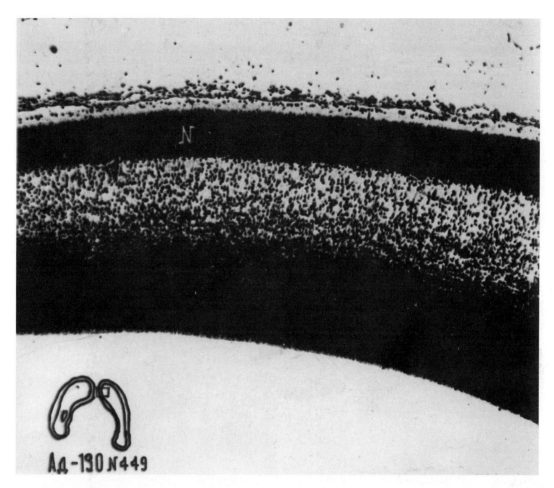

FIGURE 14–1
Cortical cytoarchitecture of the human embryo at the age of
G-10. From the bottom: the ventricular zone, the intermediate
zone, the cortical plate and the marginal zone.

more granular structure (Figures 14–2 and 14–3); layers
II and III in the anterior limbic areas are less developed as
compared to layers V and VI. One remarkable difference
is that the clearly seven-layered, granular structure of the
anterior limbic cortex of the newborn transforms into the
agranular cortex of the adult thanks mostly to changes
involving layer IV. After birth layer III has widened very
much, and layer IV is becoming narrow; as its cells begin
to mix with the cells of layers III and V, it becomes very
difficult to indicate layer IV in the adult brain (Figures
14–3 and 14–4).

The development of the cortex of the cingulate gyrus
continues intensively in the postnatal period: The extension and width of the cortex increase further; cortical cells
grow; the typical shape of pyramidal cells becomes more
evident; the density of neurons decreases. The limbic cortices of the newborn finish their development at different
times: Peritectal area, at the second year after birth; areas
24 and 23, at the fourth year of postnatal period, and
areas 24/32 and 31, at the seventh year of postnatal period.

The Development of Allocortical Cytoarchitectonics in the Hippocampus

The development of another structure of the limbic system – the hippocampus – has attracted the attention of
scientists. Similarly to the cortices of the cingulate gyrus,
which display four cellular zones at the age of G-10, the
telencephalic wall in the parahippocampal region is composed by the ventricular zone, the intermediate zone, the
cortical plate and the marginal zone. The first difference
appears as the telencephalic wall approximates the region
of the hippocampus proper: The cortical plate vanishes,
and the hippocampal region is left with three main zones
only – the ventricular zone, the intermediate zone, and
the marginal zone (Figure 14–5). The hippocampus proper
and its adjoining region, the subiculum, become a protrusion of the lower cortical main layer, originating mainly
from the ventricular zone, which is the widest layer. This
zone has a compact assembly of cells separated from the
intermediate migrational zone. The intermediate zone is
approximately two times narrower than the ventricular

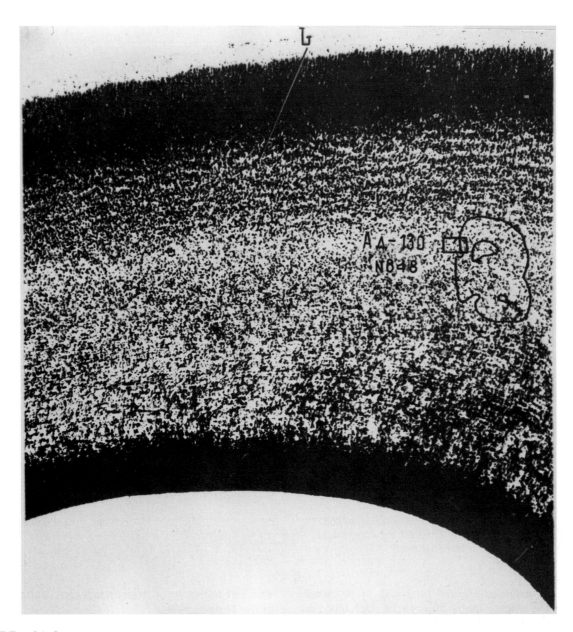

FIGURE 14–2

Cytoarchitecture of the human limbic posterior cortex at G-16: The ventricular zone narrows, the intermediate zone and the cortical plate widen, and the latter starts to divide into two parts, the superior and the inferior, deeper one. Whereas the structure of the superior part is an homogeneous one, that of the inferior part is more laminar.

zone. Neurons migrating from the ventricular zone are placed in the intermediate zone, giving origin to a 'primary hippocampus' and a 'primary fascia dentata'. The cells located in the region corresponding to the primary hippocampus form clusters of three- to five cells, whereas the cells in the primary fascia dentata are more sparsely located (Braitenberg and Schüz, 1983).

Remarkable changes take place between embryonal weeks G-22 and G-25: Cell differentiation begins for the first time in hippocampal ontogeny; the pyramidal layer of the hippocampus is formed in the intermediate zone and separated from the internal sublayer by a cell-free zone; the fascia dentata can be identified and the hippocampus can be already divided into fields, each one bearing its own construction (Figure 14–6). At G-27 the folding of hippocampus over itself has practically completed, the fascia dentata is clearly identified, as well as all hippocampal fields. They acquire the typical bended form, with the borders represented by hippocampal fields h1-h2 (Figure 14–7). Cell differentiation continues, with the development of distinctive sizes and forms of the cellular components in each of the different fields. Between G-32 and G-35 some changes in the disposition of the hippocampus are observed, notably an increase in length and

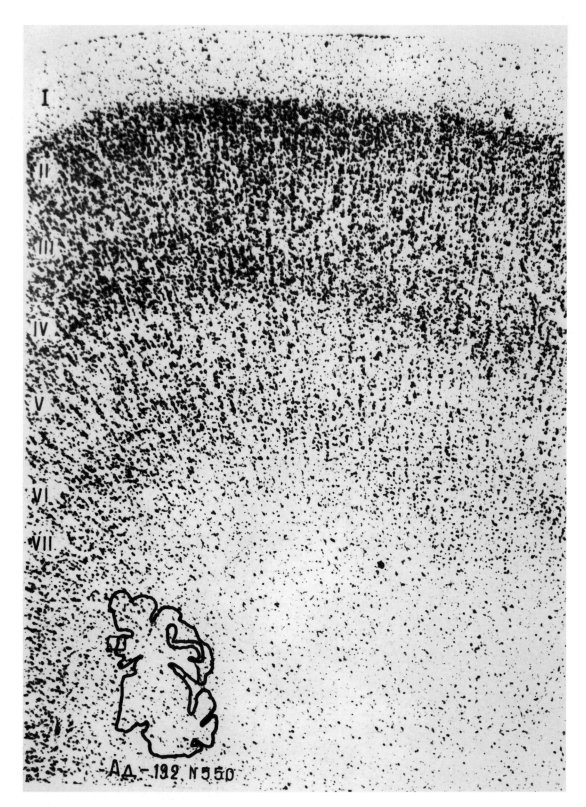

FIGURE   14–3
Cytoarchitecture of the limbic posterior cortex of the newborn:
all cytoarchitectonical layers are very well delimited.

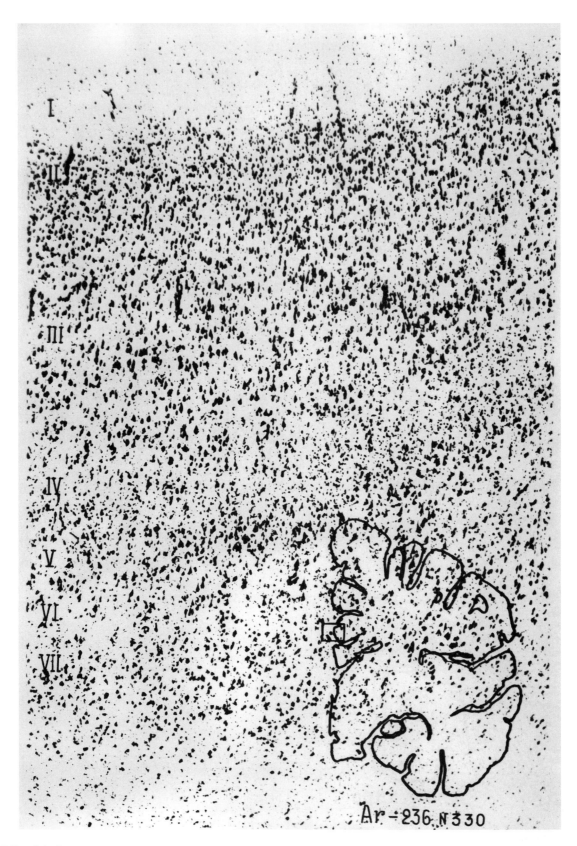

FIGURE   14–4

Cytoarchitecture of the limbic posterior cortex of the adult.
The clearly seven-layered, granular structure of the limbic cortex
of the newborn (compare with Figure 14–2) has transformed
into an agranular cortex in which the indentification of layer
IV is very difficult.

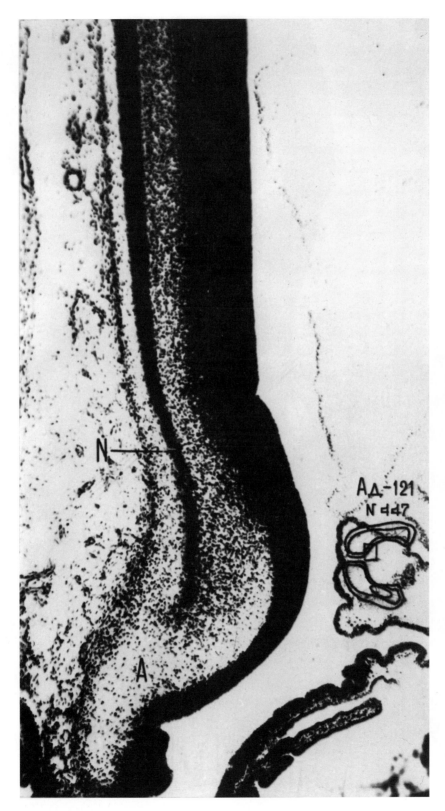

FIGURE   14–5

Cytoarchitecture of the human hippocampus at the age of G-10. As the telencephalic wall approximates the region of the hippocampus proper (A), the cortical plate (N) vanishes, resulting in that the hippocampal region consists of three main zones – the ventricular zone, the intermediate zone, and the marginal zone.

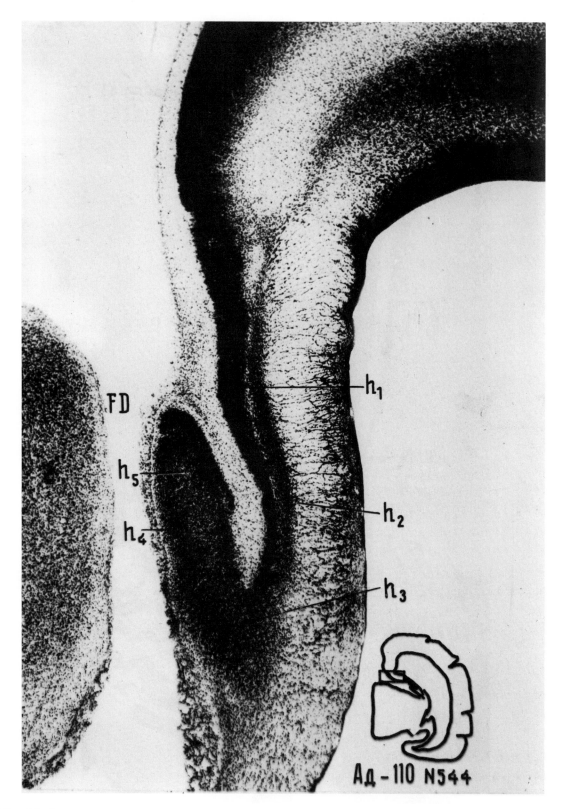

FIGURE   14–6

Cytoarchitecture of the human hippocampus at G-16: Cell differentiation begins for the first time in ontogeny; the pyramidal layer of the hippocampus is formed in the intermediate zone and separated from the internal sublayer by a cell-free zone; the fascia dentata (FD) can be identified and the hippocampus can be already divided into fields (h1-h5), each one bearing on its own construction.

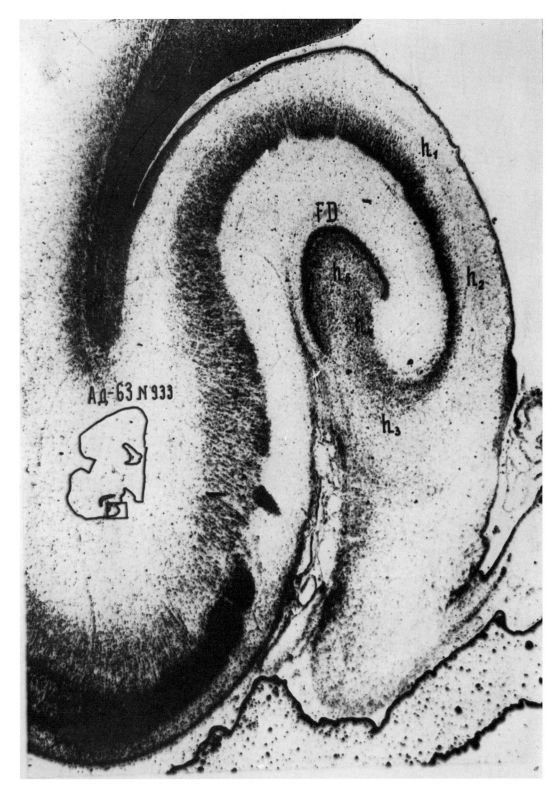

FIGURE   14–7

Cytoarchitecture of the human hippocampus at G-20. The bending of the hippocampus over itself has practically completed, the fascia dentata (FD) is clearly identified, as well as all hippocampal fields (h1-h5). They acquire the typical bended form, with the borders represented by hippocampal fields h1-h2.

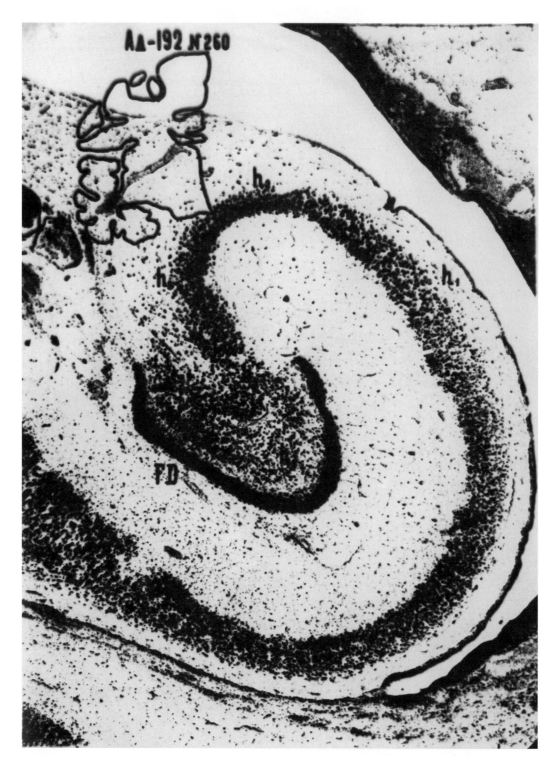

FIGURE   14–8

Cytoarchitecture of the hippocampus of a newborn. The general structure and topography of the hippocampus are similar to those in the adult, except some morphological changes of pyramidal neurons described in the text. The size of the hippocampus of a newborn is only 32–34 percent that of an adult.

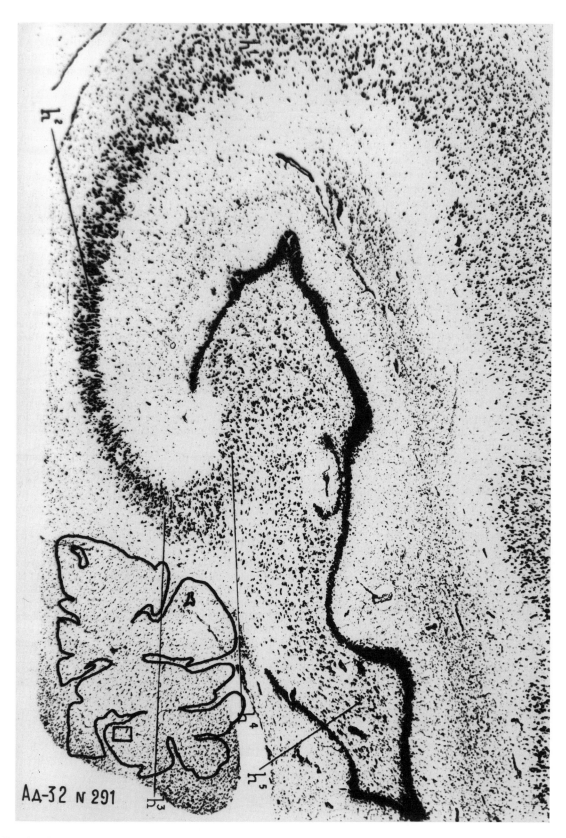

FIGURE   14–9

Cytoarchitecture the adult human hippocampus. From the 4th year of postnatal period on, the vertical orientation of cells is more accentuated than in the newborn; neurons have acquired pyramidal and multiangled form; the width of the pyramidal layer has increased significantly in the different fields, as well as the sizes of the cells and the hippocampal square surface; a cell-free zone surrounds and separates the fascia dentata from field h5.

width of hippocampus and a clear orientation of the cells, perpendicular to the surface of the cortex in each different field. In addition, during this period the differences in cell structure become more clear; field h1 cells are mostly small and the largest cells are those located in fields h2 and h3.

At the moment of birth the general structure and topography of the child's hippocampus are similar to those in the adult (Figures 14–8 and 14–9). However, the child's hippocampus differs considerably in respect to cell structures, sizes and densities. The size of the hippocampus of a newborn is only 32–34 percent that of an adult. In addition, important cytoarchitectonical changes take place in postnatal ontogeny: The vertical orientation of cells accentuates; neurons acquire pyramidal and multiangled form; the width of the pyramidal layer increases significantly in the different fields, as well as the sizes of the cells and the hippocampal square surface; a cell-free zone surrounds and separates the fascia dentata from field h5. Only around the age of 4 years does the cytoarchitectonics of the young hippocampus become similar in all respects to that of the adult (Figure 14–9).

An Overall View

Structures of the limbic system such as the cingulate gyrus and the hippocampus continue their development for years after birth. Cell differentiation seems to begin and terminate earlier in the hippocampus as compared to the cingulate cortex. This is in accord with phylogeny: Hippocampus developed early in the evolution of species; the reptiles already had it. However, the hippocampus has achieved a higher size and a most complicated cytoarchitectonics in man, as compared to reptiles and other taxa. The main neural population in the human hippocampus, the hippocampal pyramidal cells, are very homogeneous in size. Their large cell bodies are concentrated in a narrow band, in striking contrast with the staggering of neural cell bodies in other parts of the cortex, in which the vast majority of neurons are interneurons of invariably smaller sizes. In addition, the number of synapses per neuron is higher in the hippocampus than in the rest of the cortex; comparing the density of synapses with that of neurons, Braitenberg and Schüz (1991) obtained 18,000 synapses per neuron, more than twice the figure for the isocortex. All these features are important not only for determining the role of the hippocampus in learn-

ing and memory, but also for determining, in an as yet poorly understood manner, the rates of neuronal aging and degeneration as observed in this structure.

Selected Readings

Altman, J., and Das, G. 1965. Autoradiographic and histological study of postnatal hippocampal neurogenesis in rats. J. Comp. Neurol. 124:319–336.

Angevine, J. 1965. Time of neuron origin in the hippocampal region. An autoradiographic study in the mouse. Exp. Neurol. Suppl. 2:1–70.

Bogolepova, I. N. 1970. Structure and development of hippocampus of human brain in the prenatal ontogeny. J. Neurol. Psychiatry 70:657–863.

Cajal, S. R. 1955. Studies of the Cerebral Cortex. London.

Chinda, N. 1958. Some results about the structure and development of cells of limbic cortex of human brain after birth. In: Some Questions about Physiology and Pathology of the Human Brain in development, pp. 57–58. Moscow.

Duvernoy, H. M. 1988. The Human Hippocampus. An Atlas of Applied Anatomy. J. F. Bergmann Verlag, München.

Economo, C. F. 1929. The Cytoarchitecture of the Human Cerebral Cortex. Oxford University Press.

Finlay, B. L. 1991. Control of cell number and type in the developing and evolving neocortex. In B. L. Finlay et al. (eds.) The Neocortex, pp. 33–41. Plenum Press, New York.

Rose, M. 1926. Über das histogenische Prinzip der Einteilung der Grosshirnrinde. Zeitschr. Psychol. und Neurol. 32:97–160.

Soriano, E., Del Rio J. A., et al. 1990. Nonpyramidal neurons in the mammalian hippocampus: Principles of organization and development. In B. L. Finlay et al. (eds.) The Neocortex, pp. 185–192. Plenum Press, New York.

References

Braitenberg, V., and Schüz, A. 1983. Some anatomical comments on the hippocampus. In W. Seifert (ed.) Neurobiology of the Hippocampus, pp 21–37. Academic Press, London.

Braitenberg, V., and Schüz, A. 1991. Anatomy of the Cortex. Statistics and Geometry, p. 185. Springer, Heidelberg.

Rakic, P. 1982. Early developmental events: Cell lineages, acquisition of neuronal positions, and areal and laminar development. Neurosci. Res. Prog. Bull. 20:439–451.

Rakic, P. 1990. Radial unit hypothesis of cerebral cortical evolution. In J. C. Eccles, and O. Creutzfeldt (eds.) The Principles of Design and Operation of the Brain, pp. 25–48. Springer-Verlag, Città del Vaticano.

15

Sergio U. Dani

The Metabolic Basis of Encephalization, Prolonged Life Span, and the Evolution of Longevity

'When the concepts concerned with the relation of body size and metabolic rate are clarified,...then comparative physiology of metabolism will be of great help in solving one of the most intricate and interesting problems in biology, namely the regulation of the rate of cell metabolism' (M. Kleiber, 1961)

Because the word 'metabolism' might seem ambiguous, let us define it at the outset. Metabolism is always metabolism of something: carbohydrate metabolism, metabolism of fat, protein metabolism, metabolism of nucleic acids, etc. However, we shall take the word metabolism in its widest sense, namely the integration of different metabolic pathways in the whole body. More specifically, it helps to understand metabolism as enzymatic metabolism, because enzymes are the laborers that bring the concept 'metabolism' to life. Most enzymes are proteins but some are ribonucleic acids (thus called ribozymes). Since the products of the enzymatic function are biological useful molecules of many different classes, it is practical to consider metabolism as a general molecular function, the *basal metabolic rate* (BMR), which is a measure of the rate of molecular synthesis and degradation in the whole animal's body.

In the whole animal's body, molecular synthesis and degradation are both energy-consuming and energy-producing reactions, whereas in the brain these are mainly energy-consuming reactions. In the brain, glycogen is not stored (it constitutes less than 0.2 percent of brain weight) and gluconeogenesis does not occur (the key enzyme involved in gluconeogenesis, *phosphoenolpyruvate carboxykinase*-PEPCK, is not expressed at significant levels in the brain). Nevertheless, neural cells have a highly active metabolism. Some neurons are the largest cells in the body, and require much energy to maintain the transmembrane electrochemical potential, features that accentuate the risk of metabolic failure that these cells run. Neurons are so sensitive to disturbances in the energy supply by the body that they cannot survive in culture even in the presence of adequate oxygen if glucose is not supplied, immediately after the cells are isolated from brains.

This vulnerability of the brain and its parts has been the object of many 'metabolic hypotheses' to account for encephalization. R. D. Martin (1981) linked relative brain size at birth with maternal BMR during development. He pointed out that in placental mammals, brain size may be constrained by the resources channeled to the embryo from the mother. This assumption seems to be partly true: If we consider the higher encephalization of newborn primates as compared to adults, we are led to conclude that the availability of nutrients is likely to be less of a constraint to brain size than it is to the rest of the newborn's body. It is instructive to think of newborn primates as being more encephalized than their mothers, because this realization leads us to conclude that factors such as maternal BMR may not hinder the development of a highly encephalized child. For one thing, although cerebral metabolism is markedly decreased in newborns as compared to adults (neonatal metabolic rates are approximately 30 percent that of adults), the developing brain is a fierce competitor for nutrients, leaving as few as 50 percent of the available glucose for the rest of the developing body. Another very important aspect to be taken into account is that the human brain at birth is only 25 percent of its adult size: The period of maximum growth is in the first three years thereafter, at the end of which period the brain is 75 percent of its adult size, and the brain metabolic values typically surpass the adult values. Thereafter the infantile brain spurt subsides and further growth occurs at a lower rate, with the growth of the body. Whereas the efficiency of the brain to take up oxygen and glucose from the bloodstream drops from the 50 percent of total oxygen and glucose in the newborn to the 20 percent–25 percent in the adult, the adult brain weight is considered insensitive to the factors that may easily change the weight of other organs or of the whole body.

In a refinement of Martin's hypothesis, Armstrong (1983) proposed that the size of the brain will be constrained not only by the size of the system delivering oxygen and glucose but also by the rate at which energy can be expended on supporting the brain's constantly high metabolic demands. She concluded that a major primate adaptation appears to have been the allocation of a larger proportion of the body's energy supply to the brain. This conclusion, like Martin's, seems to be faulty, because it takes a consequence for a cause: The allocation of a larger proportion of the body's energy supply to the brain appears to be a consequence, rather than a cause, of encephalization. Although seizures and developmental delay in the brain have been observed in children with

defective glucose transport across the blood-brain barrier (De Vivo et al., 1991), evidence that less encephalized primates have less efficient delivery-systems is lacking. Comparative studies on the differences in the permeability of the blood-brain-barrier to oxygen and glucose and the rate at which energy is expended on supporting the brain's metabolic demands in different anthropoids could help further to clarify this issue.

In one thing, however, one has to be in accord with Martin and with Armstrong: In the importance of the study of metabolic regulation as a key to understand not only the mechanisms underlying encephalization, but also the development of longevity. The importance of metabolism for the brain can never be overemphasized. Brain and liver are the organs that express the highest number of distinct genes per tissue, one fifth of which are devoted to metabolic functions (Adams et al., 1995). Since brain metabolism is highly dependent on liver metabolism, it is useful to view these two organs as composing a brain-liver metabolic unit. This helps to understand the intricate relationship between the brain and the bodily providers of metabolic resources.

For the present suffice it to say that a primary adaptation achieved with encephalization was a genetic change, or a set of genetic changes which might have been sufficient to alter metabolism in such a way as to affect the rates of tissue and cell growth, differentiation, and maturation. That the regulation of growth rates is an ontogenetic mechanism has been recognized by Napier and Napier (1967:40):

'Accelerations, retardations, retentions and reductions are some of the mechanisms by which innovations in the genotype are reflected in the specificity of the phenotype; these processes act by modifying the differential growth velocities and new phenotypes – new species – may then evolve.'

Brain Size and Complexity Predict Longevity

The specific adaptation of mammals in general and primates in particular was encephalization, or the increase of brain weight relative to body weight (Figure 15–1). The trend in mammalian evolution towards larger brains appears to go hand in hand with a trend towards longer-lived animals. Sacher (1978) found the following explanation for this phenomenon:

'The reproductive success of iteroparous organisms (organisms that reproduce several times along their lives) is dependent on the maintenance of successful reproduction for a time period sufficient for replacement of individuals died from age-independent factors (predation, accident, starvation, and other environmental contingencies) and an adequate rate of population increase. The increase in brain size, which is a trend in the mammalian evolution, would lead to an increase of the replacement time, through decreased random death from environmental contingencies. However, the additional requirement for

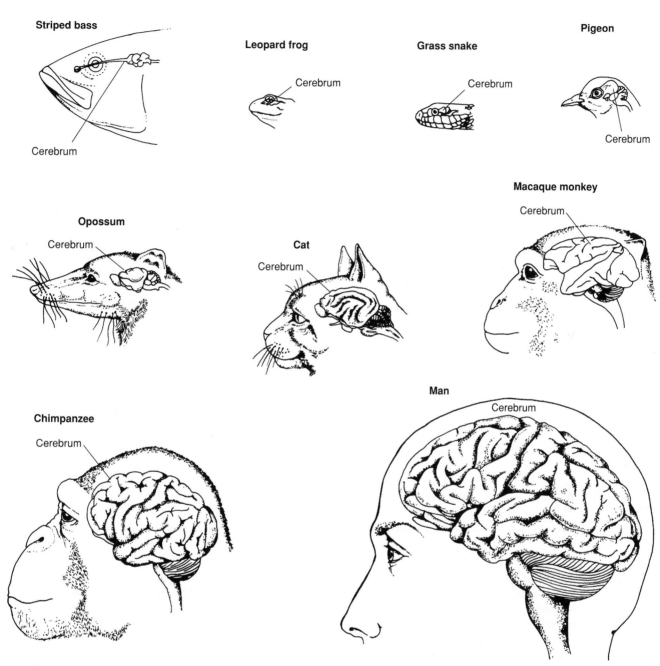

FIGURE 15–1
The brain enlarges progressively in a series of vertebrates drawn to the same scale. The face decreases in size relative to the brain. (Redrawn from Hubel, 1979.)

the maintenance of a very high degree of physiological performance over the full duration of the replacement time gives rise to independent selection for increased physiological stability and resistance to failure, and this selection is reflected in a change of survival parameters.'

The increase in brain size among the primates is a dramatic example of the relationship between brain size,

body size and longevity. Table 15–1 summarizes the data of 30 living primates including man. The maximum life span records in captivity for these animals indicate that life span has been prolonged by a factor of 20 from *Tupaia*, considered by some authors to be the most simple forms, to the most sophisticated *Homo*. In the hominid lineage, too, in 3.5 million years of evolution brain size has increased about threefold from *Australopithecus* (aver-

TABLE **15–1.**   Maximum life span (MLS) record in captivity (male and female average), gestational period and body weight for 30 living primates, including man (*)

Genus or species	MLS record (years)	Gestational period (days)	Body weight (kg, average; male/fem.)
Tupaia glis[a]	5	41–50	0.18/0.16
Urogale[b]	7	54–56	0.35/–
Leontideus	10	132–134	0.6/0.5
Saguinus	7	~140	0.35/0.35
Callithrix	12	~140	0.3/0.2
Loris	7	160–174	0.3/0.2
Tarsius	12	~180	0.13/0.12
Microcebus	15	59–62	0.06
Lemur	27	120–135	2/2
Galago crassicaudatus	14	130–135	1.2/1
Ateles	20	~130	7/6
Galago senegalensis	14	144–146	0.3/0.2
Cynopithecus	7	155–175	10/6
Presbytis entellus	21	~168	12/10
Macaca	29	146–186	11/9
Papio cynocephalus	31	154–183	25/13
Saimiri	21	169–182	0.8/0.6
Erythrocebus	20	170 (estim.)	10/6
Cebus	40	~180	3/2
Nycticebus	13	193	1.3/1.2
Miopithecus	22	196	1.3/0.8
Cercopithecus	31	~180–213	4.8/2.8
Hylobates lar	32	~210	6/5.5
Lagothrix	12	~225	7/6
Symphalangus	16	230–236	11/10
Mandrillus sphinx	28	~245	20/–
Gorilla gorilla	40	251–289	160/140
Pongo pygmaeus	46	275	69/37
Pan troglodytes	45	225	49/41
Homo sapiens	100	250	64/48

(*) data from various sources, compiled in Napier and Napier (1967) and updated for some species in Cutler (1975). Most values are rounded off to avoid appearance of high accuracy. Note the trend to simultaneous increase in longevity, gestational period and body weight, which also corresponds to a trend towards the increase of brain weight and encephalization (not shown).

[a, b] by some authors not allocated to the order Primates (cf. Martin, 1993) but included here because these are extant species that resemble the putative earliest ancestor of primates.

age brain weight 480 g), to *Homo sapiens* (average brain weight 1,350 g), and maximum life span has similarly increased two- to threefold in the same period (Chapter 12). In light of this evidence, two fundamental questions in the biology of neural aging are raised: (i) How do brains grow larger and more complex and, (ii) what has a larger brain to do with life span and longevity of its possessor?

Cell Number Predicts Brain Size and Complexity

Brain size and complexity is determined by different factors including the total number of cells (neurons, glia and other cell types), the size of individual cells, the dendritic arborization, the density of neurons, the amount of white matter (well-myelinated tracts occupy a larger volume than lightly or unmyelinated pathways), and the size of internal cavities or ventricles. Environmental factors (such as diet) as well as the species' genetic blueprint may influence each of these factors.

Of the above factors, the number of nerve cells offer the most plausible explanation to the fact that, within

the class Mammalia, some neural structures – notably the neocortex – differ in size by a factor of more than 200, after adjusting for differences in body size (Stephan, Baron and Frahm, 1988). The remarkable growth of the primate brain during rather short periods was accounted for by the prolongation of cytogenesis and the creation of 'surplus' cells in the brain (Chapters 11 and 12).

Cell Number and Encephalization are Genetically Determined

Although the sequence of genetic changes accounting for evolutive steps in brain morphology and physiology remains largely unknown, comparative cell biology has disclosed some of the basic principles which may be involved. One of such principles is the general trend in evolution towards a positive increase in complexity with increasing minimum (haploid) genome size. The total amount of DNA in the haploid genome is a characteristic of each living species known as its *C value*. The simplest explanation for variation in cell number is the variation in the C value, thus in the genome size, which is also known to correlate positively with cell size. This correlation is extraordinary in amphibians such as frogs and salamanders, which show nearly an order of magnitude variation in genome size within each group: The smaller the genome size, the more numerous the cells, the smaller the cell size, and the more complex the brains (Figure 15–2). This remarkable relationship shows clearly that cell number, cell size and brain complexity are genetically determined. The consequences of this conclusion are breathtaking: Encephalization can be explained in genetic terms.

A straightforward attempt to look for a possible genetic clue of human encephalization is to look for major genetic changes or major genetic accidents that could have rendered the hominid genome markedly differentiated from that of the anthropoid apes. It would appear that a dramatic and life-threatening change, as encephalization probably was for the early hominids, is likely to have been caused by a remarkable genomic change as early as in the late australopithecine stage, when the pronounced trend towards hominid encephalization started (Chapter 12). Being dramatic enough, we may admit that such a change had to occur at higher levels of genome organization. Whereas a change at the lower level of single genes leading to untimely encephalization would easily have disappeared by selection in a fierce environment, a change of the kind affecting the structure and number of chromosomes would have been much more difficult to

get rid of. This initial event driven by chance would then elicit more directed selection.

An unequivocal proof for this hypothesis is difficult to provide because there is no such thing as fossilized chromosomes of early hominids that could be compared between the different ancestor species and modern man. However, we have access to genetic material of extant anthropoid apes, which can provide us with an insight into what kind of changes might have occurred in an early hominid genome which could have been related to the evolution of the human species and its features that help distinguish modern humans from anthropoid apes. The reader should be cautioned that, when we compare the chromosomes of extant apes and humans, we would have no way of knowing which of the changes revealed by cytogenetic analysis were related, phenotypically, to encephalization. However, such changes are instructive as clues for further experimental approaches, in a way similar to employing linkage analysis to find out associations between genes and phenotypes.

Whereas the anthropoid apes *Pongo, Pan and Gorilla* have the same chromosome number (2n = 48), and the same length of chromosome (Chiarelli, 1973:183), the karyotype of the human differs from that of the anthropoid apes in the morphology of some chromosomes. However, the karyotype comparison shows clearly that some chromosomes of the chimpanzee are morphologically and dimensionally very similar or almost identical to corre-

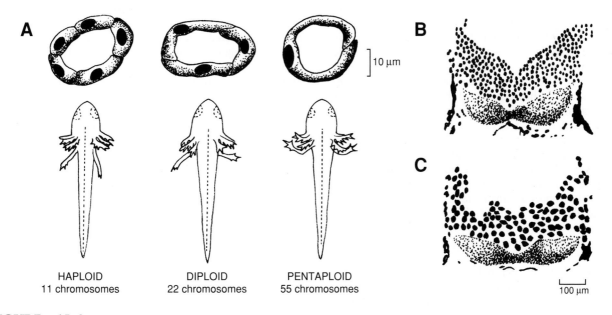

HAPLOID
11 chromosomes

DIPLOID
22 chromosomes

PENTAPLOID
55 chromosomes

10 µm

100 µm

FIGURE   15–2

Genome size determines cell size and brain morphological complexity in frogs and salamanders.

A. Drawings of representative sections of kidney tubules from salamander larvae of different ploidy. Pentaploid salamanders have cells that are bigger than those of haploid salamanders, but the animals and their individual organs are the same size

because each tissue in the pentaploid animal contains fewer cells. From Frankhauser, 1955.

B and **C.** Cross sections of the hindbrain of haploid (**B**) and tetraploid (**C**) salamanders, showing how reduced cell numbers compensate for increased cell size. Simpler brain morphology of salamanders is associated with increases in genome and cell size. Adapted from Frankhauser, 1952.

sponding chromosomes in man (Chiarelli, *op. cit.*: 178). Other chimpanzee chromosomes do not show any real correspondence with the human ones, but they have been aligned with certain human chromosomes because of a general similarity in size. There is, however, a metacentric chromosome in the human karyotype, chromosome no. 2, which does not seem to show any counterpart in the karyotype of chimpanzee. On the other hand, the chimpanzee karyotype has two acrocentric chromosome pairs (numbers 12 and 13) which do not show similarities to any human chromosome. As hypothesized by Chiarelli and coworkers early in 1961 and recently confirmed by DNA hybridization assays, chromosome no. 2 of man resulted from a centric fusion between two acrocentric chromosomes in an early ancestor of man who was closely related to the chimpanzee. This centric fusion might well account for a reduction of the chromosome number from 48 to 46 in one of man's ancestors, creating an important divergence between the karyotypes of anthropoid apes and man (op. cit.:178–180). As a consequence of the diminution of the genome size, the number of cells would increase and the average cell size would decrease, in a manner similar to that described for salamanders. Since the australopithecines did not differ substantially from the modern chimpanzee in many respects, we are tempted to attribute the above described changes not to any ancestor of the australopithecines but to an immediate ancestor of *Homo habilis* of some 2.3 Mya or to *H. habilis* proper, in an effort to provide a possible genetic clue to the burst of encephalization observed in *H. habilis* (Chapter 12).

This hypothesis is attractive, though the evidence is far from complete and certain. The centric fusion of chromosomes 12 and 13 of an early hominid ancestor to make the human chromosome 2 may not have been sufficient to bring about differences in encephalization. In addition, all three extant anthropoid apes differ in encephalization without having gross differences in their karyotypes. This is a feature of the *C value paradox*, namely that there may be large variations in complexity between certain species whose C values apparently does not vary much. We clearly need more evidence from physical mapping of genes, gene homology and gene regulation studies, which are currently underway (for reviews see Goodman *et al.*, 1994; Ruvolo, 1994; Ayala *et al.*, 1994). One such study using chromosomal *in situ* suppression (CISS) hybridization with human chromosome-specific DNA libraries (Jauch *et al.*, 1992) confirmed the high homology between the chromosomes of man and anthropoid apes, and also revealed a reduced hybridization on the heterochromatic short arms of chimpanzee chromosomes 12 and 13, suggesting loss of some genetic material during the formation of human chromosome 2. Whether the lack of this material has been of any importance to human encephalization in a way analogous to what occurs in salamanders and frogs, is a matter of speculation.

Contrary to what could have been expected as an explanation for the extremely rapid evolution of traits such as encephalization and life span prolongation in homi-

nids, it has been inferred (Sacher, 1975; Cutler, 1975) that the genetic changes may have been accomplished by allelic substitution or point mutational changes at a comparatively small number of loci. It has been predicted that about 160–250 genes or 0.4 percent–0.6 percent of the total functional genes have received base substitutions leading to one or more adaptive amino-acid changes in 10,000 generations of hominid evolution (Cutler, 1975). However, if we consider also the highly repetitive, non-coding DNA sequences which spread between the coding regions, the changes in the genome are likely to be more extensive than previously suspected. This is another feature of the *C value paradox*, namely that there is an apparent absolute excess of DNA compared with the amount that could be expected to code for proteins. However, these non-coding regions which are dubbed 'junk DNA' because of their apparent lack of functional meaning, are a main source of variation. What sort of regulatory function, if any, could these stretches of non-coding DNA have? We know that they are not translated into proteins, but they are indeed transcribed and their mRNAs apparently remain in the nucleus, where they may play some role in the regulation of gene expression, cell growth etc.

The molecular genetics of the evolution of encephalization and longevity is in its infancy, and it is widely open for major contributions. While we still do not have any evidence for the genetic blueprint of encephalization and life span prolongation, at least we might argue that these adaptations are likely to have derived from a few changes with a widespread general effect at the cellular level. Because traits such as cell size and organ and body weights are thought to vary on a continuous scale, and this variation is expected to have a polygenic basis (Falconer, 1981), we might rely on classic additive polygenic models of quantitative phenotypic variation to estimate the heritabilities for encephalization and longevity. The question poses itself: Are organ-specific changes necessary and sufficient to account for encephalization, or is there a more general change such as the regulation of cell metabolism involved?

Nerve Cell Size Can Scale Conservatively

In addition to the creation of excess or surplus nerve cells, evolution makes larger brains by increasing the size of the nerve cells (Bekkers and Stevens, 1990) – a phenomenon called 'conservative scaling' – and a combination thereof. However, conservative scaling is not, as indicated by the term, a mechanism of encephalization or the relative increase of brain size. In a 1987 study, Herbert Haug compared different mammals, including whales, primates, ancient species such as the tupaioids and lemur, and modern humans, and found that the average perikaryon projection area of neurons in the brain cortex of humans is smaller than that of large mammals such as whales, or small ancient primates such as the tupaioids and lemur. Notwithstanding, the average perikaryon projection area was slightly larger in humans as compared to that of 11 Old and New World monkeys. This evidence supports the idea that, while the basic mechanism of encephalization in man was largely the creation of a surplus, mainly small-sized nerve cells in the early stages of hominization, a relatively minor degree of conservative scaling could also be observed in the late stages of hominization.

Brain Longevity and Specialization Depend on Cellular Adaptations to Metabolic Constraints

We have been taught to believe that excess nerve cells are important for encephalization and the evolution of intelligence. There is reason to believe that excess cells is important for the evolution of longevity, too. One simple reason is that different cells, or similar cells in different locations, have different thresholds to age related degeneration. Thus a tissue may be viewed as a mosaic of cells with different life spans and longevities. The larger the tissue, the greater the probability that the tissue reserve of healthy cells will compensate for the unhealthy cells for a longer period. While this surely constitutes a strategy of longevity enhancement, the actual mechanism is likely to be found at the level of metabolic regulation in single cells.

Cell Growth is Metabolically Constrained

In the cell, the amount of metabolizing material is proportional to the cell volume, and so is the amount of oxygen required by the cell (Figure 15–3). The *cell viability factor* is defined as the ratio between the maximal amount of oxygen that can be obtained by diffusion through the cell membranes, and the amount of oxygen which is actually demanded for the survival of the cell.

If the cell viability factor is greater than 1 (e.g., small cells with a good oxygen supply or relatively small amounts of metabolizing material), viability equally increases, and the cell may increase its growth rate or start cell division. In general, decreased cell sizes lead to increases in rates of cell metabolism and proliferation. Salamanders with smaller genomes and smaller cells have more cells, including nerve cells, owing to increased cell-proliferation rates. Increased cell proliferation rates is also a feature of immature embryonal nerve cells which are typically smaller than the mature cells.

On the reverse side of the coin, if the cell viability factor is smaller than 1 (e.g. low oxygen supply or a relatively increased amount of metabolizing material), viability equally lowers, metabolic rates are decreased, and cell growth and cell proliferation are retarded. This situation occurs, for example, as cells differentiate and acquire their mature size. Salamanders with larger genomes have decreased cell-proliferation rates owing presumably to a relatively increased amount of intracellular metabolizing material.

The Metabolic Basis of Cortical Specialization and Enhanced Brain Longevity

Owing to metabolic constraints imposed to cell growth, important adaptations had to be met in order to enhance longevity during the course of human encephalization. The explanation has been hinted at previously: Nerve cells are not only the largest cells in the body; they are metabolically the most active cells. As a matter of fact, not only does the size of the nerve cell soma, but also the length, thickness and complexity of dendrites increase as a function of the organism's size (Barasa, 1960; Purves and Lichtman, 1985; Snider, 1987). Since postmitotic cells such as neurons cannot divide, they have to increase their surface area if they are to survive. After a precursor cell becomes irreversibly committed to be a postmitotic neuron, dendritic branching is left as the main strategy to increase its surface area [an other adaptation is the formation of perikaryal projections (Pannese *et al.*, 1983, 1985)]. Owing to their highly irregular shape, characterized by extensive branching, neurons usually have very large surface areas which compensate for the loss of viability accompanying the volume growth of such cells. The considerable extent of the cell surface area is surely one of the most significant neuronal features. It not only facilitates exchange between the neuron and its environment; it also allows the establishment of numerous connections between nerve cells.

Metabolic constraints to cell size may also account for increased specialization of cortical areas seen in highly encephalized animals. J. L. Ringo pointed out that increased specialization of cortical areas may be a necessity as brain size increases. If fixed percentage connectivity was maintained then the volume of connections would rise exponentially which he showed to be unproductive due to the rise in conduction times. Previously J. L. Eilbert had identified three levels of micro-anatomical-functional hierarchy. They are mediated by three populations of neurons: Short-range, long-range directional and long-range diffuse. The short range level is mediated by interneurons and pyramidal-pyramidal connections within a single region. The long-range directional level is mediated by pyramidal cells, the axons of which form the white matter. The long-range diffuse class are the monoamine transmitters. The distinction can be understood as scaling sizes and impulse transmission times: Interneurons with a few hundred microns in size, 10 msec transmission time; pyramidal cells with a few cm, 100 msec; monoamine transmitters with several cm, seconds or longer. Consistent with Ringo's view, it has been postulated that the proportion of pyramidal cells which project cortico-cortically, as opposed to cortico-thalamically, has increased during evolution, to reach the modern limit of 69 out of 71 pyramidal cells in humans (Hofman, 1985).

In view of the metabolic risks that even highly branched neurons run, one is led to accept Herron and Johnson's account of the origin of gyrification and the formation of sulci in the brain: They suggested that during evolution sulci were formed because the length of intracortical axons did not increase at the same rate as the expansion of the brain. Therefore, intracortical-connected cortex had to be pulled inward in order to maintain intracortical connections. Experimental work has shown that cortical folding appears to originate within the cortical

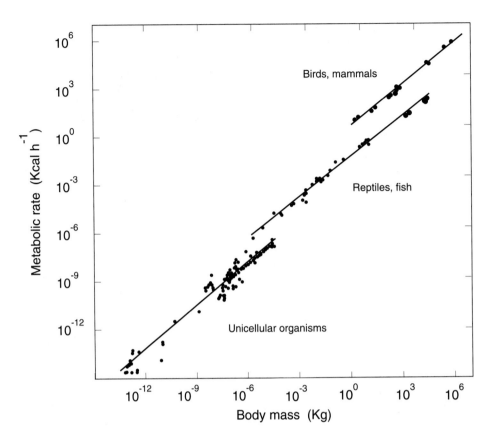

FIGURE   15–3

A log-log graphic to show the relationship between metabolic rate (Kcal h^{-1}) and cell volume/body mass in a wide range of organisms. The amount of metabolizing material is proportional to the cell volume or body mass, and so is the amount of oxygen necessary for the cell or the organism to remain alive. From Hemmingsen, 1960.

sheet and is not caused by external factors such as the pressure of the calvaria. In other words, the cerebral cortex appears to have its own intrinsic geometry (Griffin, 1994) (Figure 15–4).

The Human Brain, Being a Nutrient Sink, Regulates Body Growth Rates and Longevity

The metabolic burden accompanying encephalization is understandable since the brain, highly metabolically active as it is, relies strongly on an efficient nutrient delivery, including, above all, the constant supply of glucose and oxygen. The brain's demand for glucose can be as high as 50 percent to 60 percent of the whole body's demand for glucose in newborn and infantile humans, whereas in adults this figure drops to about 20 percent to 25 percent. Neural cells not only do not store glycogen; they also do not execute gluconeogenesis. Thus blood glucose is the immediate source of brain energy. Glucose is supplied by food intake, glycogen storage and gluconeogenesis in peripheral organs, mainly the liver and, to a lesser extent, the kidneys. When glucose supply is impaired, e.g. in starvation, ketones (2–4 carbon units made from acetate following fatty acid oxidation) can still be used to

supply up to 70 percent of the adult human brain's energy requirements without functional impairment. In comparison to the adult, the infant brain readily accepts ketones for 30–50 percent of its energy requirements under conditions of normal glucose availability (Cremer, 1982). This capacity to utilize ketones is never lost but gradually diminishes after weaning, coincident with the change from a diet in which fat (mainly from breast milk) is the main source of energy and building blocks, to a diet in which carbohydrate is the main energy source (Cunnane et al., 1993).

The liver and the kidneys, the major providers of bodily resources of nutrients to the brain, are likely to exhibit correlated responses to selection for increased relative brain size (Mahaney et al., 1993) such as that observed in the hominid fossil record. However, marked encephalization, by increasing brain-size relative to the rest of the body, leads to the diminution of bodily resources (including carbohydrate, fat, cofactors and vitamins; bodily proteins have a 'carbohydrate value' through gluconeogenesis). Therefore it is assumed that the brain's demands will be met during encephalization, at the expense of the nutrients available to the rest of the body. In other words, the human brain is thought to be an effective 'nutrient sink' causing a nutrient restriction to the rest of the body. This has important repercussions to our understanding of body growth and longevity; it becomes easy to understand why retardation of growth is the hallmark of human development (Box 15–1).

Encephalization may Enhance Human Longevity by Increasing the Nutrient Restriction to the Body

The development of brain structures correlates with increases in cerebral metabolism. The metabolic values increase until the third year when they surpass adult values. The glucose metabolic rate reaches a plateau near the age of four which continues until approximately age nine. The metabolic rate then declines to adult values by the end of the second decade (Chugani, 1987). The retardation and prolongation of the brain-growth period in the infantile, juvenile and young adult stages in humans is by no means supplanted after development. It persists in adults which retain, for example, the cranial proportions that characterize juvenile or even fetal stages of other large primates. This remarkable altricial development in a highly encephalized species speaks for a major role of the brain in the regulation of body growth and life span. It leads to the hypothesis that encephalization, by creating a nutrient sink, may increase human life span and enhance longevity. It is a happy circumstance that rats become obese when the activity of neurons involved in the regulation of energy metabolism is experimentally lowered. In a similar fashion, the increase in body weight in humans after the age of 40 years (Chapter 19) may partly be due to an age-related decrease in neuronal activity.

Nutrient restriction is presently the only reliable experimental model for delaying growth and prolonging life span in a wide range of invertebrates and vertebrates, including mammals (McCay *et al.*, 1935; Masoro *et al.*, 1992). The works of Rubner (1908), Pearl (1928) and Sacher (1977) have led to the hypothesis that dietary restriction increases longevity by decreasing metabolic rate. There is evidence that if an organism is repeatedly subjected to weight loss (as in human dieting patterns), long-term changes may occur; fewer calories will be needed to maintain a given weight. Besides, it is well known that animals with a higher metabolic rate per unit body mass (i.e., a higher utilization of energy per hour per unit of body mass) have smaller bodies and tend to have shorter life spans. However, studies of diet-restricted rats have shown that they have the same metabolic rate as rats fed *ad libitum* yet differ greatly in longevity. This finding led to the idea that the reduction of energy intake per animal apparently modulates aging by altering characteristics of fuel use rather than the rate of use (Masoro *et al.*, 1992).

Whatever mechanism is involved, the nutrition-restriction model calls our attention to the importance of the brain-metabolic adaptation represented by the regulation of body growth rates, life span and longevity.

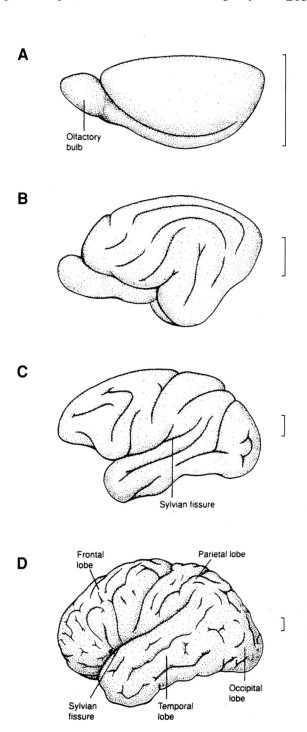

FIGURE 15–4

Progressive folding and gyrification of cerebral hemispheres in a series of increasing body- and brain size and altriciality.

A. In the rat the cerebral hemisphere is not folded, and no gyri are formed.

B. In the cat folding and gyrification are evident; the caudal end of the cerebral hemisphere extends slightly downward.

In the monkey (**C**) and man (**D**) folding (the cerebral hemispheres curves from the frontal lobe into the temporal lobe, which reaches forward), gyrification and deepening of fissures are pronounced. From Nauta and Feirtag, 1986. Scale bars: 1 cm.

Precocious Versus Altricial Development   Box 15–1

The pattern of rapid development and differentiation is referred to as *precocious* (Latin *praecox*, meaning 'precooked'). In precocious animals great amounts of energy per unit body weight and time are required from readily available sources such as carbohydrate and fat, and great amounts of aminoacids are demanded mainly from exogenous proteins to build up the structure of rapidly growing cells and bodies. Respiration and intracellular protein synthesis and degradation are increased. In a word, general metabolism is increased. As a consequence, rapid growth, cell differentiation, and reproductive maturation are attained early in development, and life span is short. Owing to the short developmental period, brain and body size in extremely precocial organisms are typically small. *Altricial* organisms on the contrary are characterized by reduced use of metabolic energy per unit body mass and time; as a consequence they have relatively lowered growth rates.

Since small bodies demand high metabolic rates per unit body mass in precocial animals, the high rates of fuel utilization may decrease the longevity of these animals by increasing macromolecular damage. The use of fuel is essential for life but may have long-term negative consequences. Glucose, for example, undergoes a nonenzymatic reducing reaction called the glycation reaction with the amino groups of proteins, and with nucleic acids (Cerami, 1985). Selection for efficient molecular repair systems is relaxed in precocious animals because such animals complete their life cycles within short periods. It is noteworthy that short life spans correlate with less efficient DNA repair in a wide range of animal species (Hart and Setlow, 1974). Thus, not only early reproduction and short life spans, but also small bodies and brains and decreased longevity are features of precocial animals with high metabolic rates per unit body weight. What we may conclude about such animals is that they are neither capable of creat-

ing a cell surplus to build large bodies and brains, nor are they 'thrifty' enough to live longer. Even when these animals develop behavioral adaptations to reduce nutrient intake, such as hibernation and the reduction of the heart rate, they are invariably short-lived organisms. Of course these considerations are not meant to imply that such animals are less adapted to their ecological niches.

Among all living things, the human species produces the most altricial newborns. Human newborns can be said to be underdeveloped as compared to other mammals or even to other primates. Humans produce absolutely and relatively the largest infant at birth of all primates, but the ossification of the bones of the hand lags far behind that of macaques, and somewhat behind that of chimpanzees (Napier and Napier, 1967:40). At birth the human infant's brain is 25 percent of its adult size compared with the 70 percent of the brains of macaques and gibbons. Thereafter the brain continues to grow in man, the maximum growth period being in the first three years. However, from the time of birth to early adult life, man's development continues slower but for longer, as compared with other primates: Myelination of many nerve tracts is completed, new synapses are formed, the body increases in size relative to the brain, some regions of the brain continue development into the postnatal period, the hippocampus presents differential increase in size and complexity (Chapter 14), total sleep time and percent REM sleep decrease, as reproductive maturity is attained. The retardation and prolongation of the brain-growth period in the infantile, juvenile and young adult stages in humans certainly reflect the complexity of the organization and neuronal connections in the adult. This continued trajectory of early postnatal human growth relative to that in other primates is an example of *neoteny* or 'secondary altricial development'.

An Overall View

Nerve cell metabolic adaptations predict not only the size and complexity of brain substructures that determine the increased complexity of function and 'intelligence' that characterize the brain-behavioral relationships in a given species, but also the longevity or resistance to failure of the species. Encephalization and longevity in the human species are largely determined by the creation of an excess neural cells during embryonal development, followed by a conservative growth of neurons after birth. Since nerve cells are highly metabolically active, the developing brain functions as a nutrient sink to the rest of the body. As a consequence, development is retarded and life span is prolonged. Prolongation of life span would then elicit more directed selection for enhanced longevity.

Selected Readings

Holloway, R. L. 1968. The evolution of the Primate brain: some aspects of quantitative relations. Brain Res. 7:121–172

Jerison, H. J. 1991. Brain Size and the Evolution of Mind. The 59th James Arthur Lecture on the evolution of the human brain, American Museum of Natural History, New York.

Jerison, H. J. 1973. Evolution of the Brain and Intelligence, Academic Press, New York.

Kleiber, M. 1961. The Fire of Life, Wiley, New York.

Peters, A., Harriman, K. M., and West, C. D. 1987. The effect of increase longevity, produced by dietary restriction on the neuronal population and area 17 in rat cerebral cortex. Neurobiol. Aging 8:7–20.

Shimazu, T., and Takahashi, A. 1980. Stimulation of hypothalamic nuclei has differential effects on lipid synthesis in brown and white adipose tissue. Nature 284:62.

Teixeira, V. L., Antunes-Rodrigues, J., and Migliorini, R. H. 1973. Evidence for centers in the central nervous system that selectively regulate fat mobilization in the rat. J. Lipid Res. 14:672.

References

Adams, M. D. *et al.* 1995. Initial assessment of human gene diversity and expression patterns based upon 83 million nucleotides of cDNA sequence. Nature 377, suppl., Genome Directory: 3–17.

Armstrong, E. 1983. Relative brain size and metabolism in mammals. Science 220:1302–1304.

Ayala, F. J., Escalante, A., and O'Huigin, K. J. 1994. Molecular genetics of speciation and human origins. Proc. Natl. Acad. Sci. USA 91:6787–6794.

Barasa, A. 1960. Forma, grandezza e densit dei neuroni della corteccia cerebrale in mammiferi die grandezza corporea differente. Zeitsch. Zellforsch. mikroskop. Anat. 53:69–89.

Bekkers, J. M., and Stevens, C. F. 1990. Two different ways evolution makes neurons larger. Progr. Brain Res. 83:37–45.

Cerami, A. 1985. Hypothesis. Glucose as a mediator of aging. J. Am. Geriat. Soc. 33:626–634.

Chiarelli, A. B. 1973. Evolution of the Primates. An Introduction to the Biology of Man. London and New York: Academic Press.

Chugani, H. T., Phelps, M. E., and Mazziotta, J. C. 1987. Positron emission tomography study of human brain functional development. Ann. Neurol. 22:487.

Cremer, J. 1982. Substrate utilization and brain development. J. Cereb. Blood Flow Metab. 2:394–407.

Cunnane, S. C., Harbige, L. S., and Crawford, M. A. 1993. The importance of energy and nutrient supply in human brain evolution. Nutr. Health 9:219–235.

Cutler, R. G. 1975. Evolution of human longevity and the genetic complexity governing aging rate. Proc. Natl. Acad. Sci. USA 72:4664–4668.

De Vivo, D. C., Trifiletti, R. R., Jacobson, R. I., *et al.* 1991. Defective glucose transport across the blood-brain barrier as a cause of persistent hypoglycorrhachia, seizures, and developmental delay. N. Engl. J. Med. 325:703–709.

Eilbert, J. L. 1988. Axon shape as a basis for multinode functional units in a hierarchical neural model. J. Theor. Biol. 130:95–122.

Falconer, D. S. 1981. Introduction to Quantitative Genetics, 2nd ed., New York: Willey.

Frankhauser, G. 1952. Int. Rev. Cytol. 1:165–193.

Frankhauser, G. 1955. In B. H. Willier, P. A. Weiss, and V. Hamburger (eds.) Analysis of Development, pp. 126–150. Philadelphia: Saunders.

Goodman, M., Bailey, W. J., Hayasaka, K., *et al.* 1994. Molecular evidence on primate phylogeny from DNA sequences. Am. J. Physic. Anthropol. 94:3–24.

Griffin, L. D. 1994. The intrinsic geometry of the cerebral cortex. J. Theor. Biol. 166:261–273.

Hart, R. W., and Setlow, R. B. 1974. Correlation between deoxyribonucleic acid excision-repair and life-span in a number of mammalian species. Proc. Natl. Acad. Sci. USA 71:2169–73.

Haug, H. 1987. Brain sizes, surfaces, and neuronal sizes of the cortex cerebri: A stereological investigation of man and his variability and a comparison with some mammals (primates, whales, marsupials, insectivores, and one elephant). Am. J. Anat. 180:126–142.

Hemmingsen, A. M. 1960. Report of the Steno Memorial Hospital and the Nordisk Insulin Laboratorium 9:1.

Herron, P., and Johnson, J. I. 1987. Organization of intracortical and commissural connections in somatosensory cortical areas I and II in the raccoon. J. Comp. Neurol. 257:359–371.

Hofman, M. A. 1985. Neuronal correlates of corticalization in mammals: a theory. J. Theor. Biol. 112:77–95.

Hubel, D. H. 1979. The brain. Scient. American 241: 45–53.

Jauch, A. Wienberg, J. Stanyon, R., *et al.* 1992. Reconstruction of genomic rearrangements in great apes and gibbons by chromosome painting. Proc. Natl. Acad. Sci. USA 89:8611–8615.

Jerison, H. J. 1970. Gross brain indices and the analysis of fossil endocasts. Primate Brain 1:225–244.

Mahaney, M. C., Williams-Blangero, S., Blangero, J., and Leland, M. M. 1993. Quantitative genetics of relative organ weight variation in captive baboons. Hum. Biol. 65:991–1003.

Martin, R. D. 1981. Relative brain size and basal metabolic rate in terrestrial vertebrates. Nature 293:57–60.

Martin, R. D. 1993. Primate origins: plugging the gaps. Nature 363:223–234.

Masoro, E. J., McCarter, R. J. M, Katz, M. S., and McMahan, C. A. 1992. Dietary restriction alters characteristics of glucose fuel use. J. Gerontol. 47:B202-B208.

McCay, C., Crowell, M., and Maynard, L. 1935. The effect of retarded growth upon the length of the life span and upon ultimate size. J. Nutr. 10:63–79.

Morgane, P. J. *et al.* 1992. In R. L. Isaacson, and K. F. Jensen (eds.) The Vulnerable Brain and Environmental Risks. Vol. 1, chap. 1. New York: Plenum.

Napier and Napier. 1967. A Handbook of Living Primates.

Nauta, W. J. H., and Feirtag, M. 1986. Fundamental Neuroanatomy. New York: Freeman.

Pannese, E., Bianchi, R., Gioia, M., and Ventura, R. 1985. A quantitative electron microscope study of the perykarial projections of sensory ganglion neurons. II. Gecko and lizard. J. Comp. Neurol. 240: 212–218.

Pannese, E., Gioia, M., Carandente, O., and Ventura, R. 1983. A quantitative electron microscope study of the perykarial projections of sensory ganglion neurons. I. Cat and rabbit. J. Comp. Neurol. 214: 239–250.

Pearl, R. 1928. The Rate of Living. Alfred Knopf, New York.

Purves, D., Lichtman, J. W. 1985. Geometrical differences among homologous neurons in mammals. Science 228:298–302.

Ringo, J. L. 1991. Neuronal interconnection as a function of brain size. Brain Behav. Evol. 38:1–6.

Roth, G., Blanke, J., and Wake, D. B. 1994. Cell size predicts morphological complexity in the brains of frogs and salamanders. Proc. Natl. Acad. Sci. USA 91:4796–4800.

Rubner, M. 1908. Das Problem der Lebensdauer und seine Beziehungen zum Wachstum und Ernährung. Oldenburg, Munich.

Ruvolo, M. 1994. Molecular evolutionary processes and conflicting gene trees: The hominoid case. Am. J. Physic. Anthropol. 94:89–113.

Sacher, G. A. 1977. Life table modifications and life prolongation. In C. E. Finch, and L. Hayflick (eds.) Handbook of the Biology of Aging, pp. 582–638. Van Nostrand Reinhold, New York.

Sacher, G. A. 1975. Maturation and longevity in relation to cranial capacity in hominid evolution. In R. Tuttle (ed.), Antecedents of Man and After, Vol. I, Primates: Functional Morphology and Evolution, pp. 417–441. The Hague: Mouton and Co..

Sacher, G. A. 1978. Evolution of longevity and survival characteristics in mammals. In E. L. Schneider, (ed.) The Genetics of Aging, pp.151–168. Plenum Press, New York and London.

Sarnat, H. B. 1985. Histochemical mapping of vertebrate brains for study of evolution. in A. A. Boulton, and G. B. Baker, (eds.) Neuromethods, Vol. 1, General Neurochemical Techniques, chap. 14, pp. 497–535. Humana Press, Clifton.

Snider, W. D. 1987. The dendritic complexity and innervation of submandibular neurons in five species of mammals. J. Neurosci. 7:1760–1768.

Stephan, H., Baron, G., and Frahm, H. D. 1988. Comparative Primate Biology, Vol. 4, pp. 1–38. Liss.

Sergio U. Dani

16

Evolution, Secular Changes and Aging: How Old is Our Brain?

E volution and aging represent a sequence of genetic events in the history of single organisms and species. John Hughlings Jackson in 1884 first clearly articulated a possible relationship between evolution and human neurologic disease. Since then the concept of *phylogenetic diseases* has been developed in relation to other systems. Arthur Keith for example was writing about the ills of uprightness in human evolution 80 years ago, and Phillip Tobias developed the idea in relation to posture and locomotion.

Because aging does not appear to depend on its own unique genetic or biochemical pathways, but rather is an outcome of generally important evolutive mechanisms (Rose and Finch, 1993), it is likely that further progress in knowledge on the cellular and molecular correlates of increased life span, longevity and encephalization will change the present understanding of many age-related neurodegenerative conditions such as the dementias of the Alzheimer type (Alzheimer disease, AD) so that we should come to decide whether we should include them, too, among the phylogenetic diseases, or, eventually, among the so-called *secular diseases* ('mal-du-siècle'). This may give us insights into the present and future evolution of the longevity of our brain, which has important implications for the future of our societies.

The Force of Natural Selection Weakens With Increasing Age and Progressive Evolutive Steps

Put in single-organism terms biological aging is a persistent decline in the age-specific fitness of an organism due to internal physiological deterioration. This progressive loss of vitality has been called *abiotrophy* (*a* = negative + Greek *bios* = life + *trophe* = nutrition), a term which apparently had its origins in the writings of a turn-of-the-century London neurologist, William Richard Gowers (Martin, 1993). Gowers clearly appreciated the possibility that unusual inheritance could explain some late-onset types of neurodegenerative conditions, including what is now known to be X-linked forms of *muscular dystrophy* and *Friedreich disease*.

For George M. Martin, *abiotrophic mutations* are defined as those 'which have relatively delayed expression (and certainly without apparent phenotypes at birth), in which the gene action results in either degenerative types of pathology (the affected cell tissues having previously been functioning well to preclude a clinical diagnosis) or proliferative types of pathology, or both.' (*op. cit.*, p. 267). The very existence of abiotrophy is accounted for by population genetics, based on the declining force of natural selection with age. A quotation from Medawar (1952) helps to make our point:

'The force of natural selection weakens with increasing age – even in a theoretically immortal population, provided only that it is exposed to real hazards of mortality. If a genetical disaster (...) happens late enough in individual life, its consequences may be completely unimportant. Even in such a crude and unqualified form, this dispensation may have a real bearing on the origin of innate deterioration with increasing age'.

Thus, dramatic neurogenetic diseases such as *Huntington disease* (Chapter 32), which has an average age of onset of 35 years, support the idea that early men and women seldom lived much beyond thirty, so postponement of disease onset beyond this age had no selective advantage or disadvantage, and the gene responsible for the condition passed unselected to the next generations. Population genetic interpretations of diseases such as Huntington disease, Friedreich disease, and many other age-related dysfunctions (reviewed by Martin, 1993), show how fundamental the processes of evolution are to our understanding of aging, and neural aging in particular.

Gene loci fall into either of two broad classes of constitutional mutations or *polymorphisms*: (i) Variant genes with little effect of reproductive fitness, and (ii) variants characterized by obvious *pleiotropic effects* (Greek *pleion* = more + *tropos* = tendency, meaning the tendency of an inherited disposition to influence or affect several parts or functions of the organism). Pleiotropic genes are generally selected because of enhanced reproductive fitness, but may have ultimate deleterious effects during the postreproductive life span; this type of gene action has been referred to as negative or *antagonistic pleiotropy*. Since some phylogenetic diseases can be seen as a special case of *antagonistic pleiotropy* of phylogenetic magnitude, a modification of Medawar's assertion to allow for the inclusion of phylogenetic diseases would sound somewhat like this: 'The force of natural selection weakens with increasing age and progressive evolutionary steps – even in

a theoretically immortal population, provided only that it is exposed to real hazards of mortality. If a genetical disaster... happens late enough in individual life *or affects phylogenetically recent structures or adaptations*, its consequences may be completely unimportant, *as opposed to genetical disasters occurring early in life or affecting phylogenetically old structures or adaptations, without which death occurs in early stages of development*. Even in such a crude and unqualified form, these dispensations may have a real bearing on the origin of innate deterioration *with both increasing age and progressive evolutive steps.'*

Some Human Neurodegenerative Diseases Reflect the Relative Vulnerability of Recently Evolved Neural Structures

Examples of human degenerative diseases selectively affecting recently evolved structures have been reviewed by Sarnat (1985): '... *Krabbe leukodystrophy*, a progressive disease of white matter of the brain and peripheral nerves related to deficiencies of *galactocerebroside-beta-galactosidase* and *psychosine galactosidase*, with resulting accumulations of galactolipids in myelin-forming cells followed by death of those cells. The distribution of lesions in the brain and spinal cord suggests an evolutionary pattern because the tracts involved are almost exclusively mammalian structures, while the phylogenetically old and constant pathways found in all classes of vertebrates are spared. Uninvolved structures include the olfactory tracts, fornix, mamillothalamic fasciculus, stria medullaris, and medial longitudinal fasciculus. By contrast, the corticospinal tracts, subcortical white matter of the *centrum semiovale*, and dorsal columns of the spinal cord are severely affected. Mammals have more galactolipids in cerebral myelin, but less phospholipids, than do nonmammalian vertebrates, even though structural differences between white matter in various species cannot be demonstrated. By contrast with Krabbe's disease, *Niemann-Pick disease* results from a deficiency of *sphingomyelinase* and impaired phospholipid metabolism; no selective involvement of new or old structures of the brain is evident.

Other examples of selective vulnerability of phylogenetically recent structures of the CNS in human disease include *olivo-ponto-cerebellar atrophy* and (as above cited) Friedreich ataxia, the original examples cited by Jackson. *Leber optic atrophy* may be yet another example. The optic nerve is fundamentally different in mammals than in other vertebrates because more than 90 percent of its fibers project to the midbrain in nonmammalian species and more than 95 percent of mammalian optic nerve fibers terminate in the thalamus.' (pp. 506–508).

Sarnat goes further to cite other examples of pathologic conditions in humans reminiscent of normal anatomy in other animals, including 'agenesis of the corpus callosum in marsupials such as the opossum and kangaroo, congenital muscle fiber-type disproportion in rodents, and the abnormal pyramidal cells with loss of basal dendritic spines in human *Pick disease*, which resemble large cortical 'candelabra' neurons normally found in reptiles.' (*op. cit.*, pp. 507–508).

Encephalization and Alzheimer Disease May be Viewed as Effects of Pleiotropic Genes

The proposition that neurodegenerative diseases such as AD should be included in the group of phylogenetic diseases, is based on the assumption that AD represents a dramatic outcome of the very metabolic changes that led to encephalization and altricial development in early hominids. Since major evolutionary changes are generally assumed to have a meaning for survivorship, we may wonder how the postponement of development and maturation could have represented an advantage for the survival of early hominids and a disadvantage for modern humans.

Encephalization in primates was mainly due to the evolution of the mammals-specific neocortex which accounts for about 40 percent of the brain weight. This enormous increase in neocortex – an associative cortex – occurred in response to the need to increase the capacity and complexity of the processing of information coming from the external world through the organs of sense. Harry Jerison linked the origins of consciousness in primates with the solution of the problem represented by the necessity to analyze and integrate information from different sources. The adaptive value of a consciousness is based on its endowing the ability to convey new information to a brain's own image of the external world, allowing the animal to change its patterns of behavior accordingly. Before this improvement, most animals survived by using more or less elaborated reflexive responses to their environment.

Although we are generally taught to believe that the increase in brain size relative to body size was advantageous in many respects, encephalization and the evolution of consciousness were an actual trade-off, as almost every evolutionary change is. While consciousness increases the fitness value of other species-specific adaptations, a large brain represents a metabolic burden for the rest of the body. Therefore, from an evolutionary perspective, there are good reasons to suppose that encephalization was in many regards up to a mischief whenever it obtruded during hominid evolution (Chapter 12). Especially children carrying a genetic information for larger brains were at higher risk to die early in their lives. These individuals experienced the hazards of a tremendous selection force that costed many lives. As pointed out by Acsadi and Nemeskeri (1970):

'(...) the child mortality was so high that only few of them could reach adolescent age. But those of them who attained it had probably sufficient resistance to environmental influences, and acquired all the knowledge that was needed to maintain life up to old age' (p:181).

Surprisingly, dramatic bursts of encephalization were tolerated inasmuch as they represented a somewhat successful attempt to conform to exacting conditions. Those children who managed to survive were adapted to make the best use of limited resources over a prolonged developmental period. They were probably endowed with a *thrifty phenotype* (i.e., a highly efficient metabolic phenotype) that allowed their large brains to develop slowly but fully and safely, at the expenses of the bodily resources. Now there is reason to believe that this, too, was a makeshift development, for adult life and old age were not devoid of the threatens of age-related pathological changes including neurodegenerative diseases. Such age-related changes have a direct bearing on the evolution of longevity.

A Highly Efficient Metabolic Phenotype, Selected For in a Nutrient-poor Environment, Leads to Decreased Longevity in a Nutrient-rich Environment

The antagonistic pleiotropy theory of senescence, based on the idea advanced by Medawar, posits that some individual loci/alleles have different effects on fitness at different ages, and at different phylogenetic steps in the case of phylogenetic diseases as well. The possibility that an increase in neurodegeneration would be largely an outcome of the very metabolic adaptations which led to encephalization and altricial development early in life can be viewed under this general scope. If the metabolic adaptations had a positive effect on fitness at a relatively early age and a deleterious effect in older individuals, the positive effect on fitness would outweigh the negative effect because of their relative positioning in life history. This was probably the case during hominid encephalization, and we shall come to the amazing hypothesis that prolonged development and encephalization constitute actual challenges for the evolution of longevity at advanced ages.

While a thrifty phenotype may be the most convenient to cope with a scarce resource basis that is further limited by the resource requirements of growth and maturation, this very phenotype may become deleterious in adult life, especially if the resource basis is expanded beyond the actual bodily needs. In the thrifty phenotype, the effect of nutrient restriction on plasma glucose results in the efficient use of an important but potentially toxic fuel (glucose). Encephalization itself may be viewed as the fundamental mechanism in the thrifty phenotype, since an enlarged brain, being a nutrient sink (Chapter 15), cares for the maintenance of plasma glucose at sustained lower concentrations, and presumably at concentrations that are less damaging over the long run. There are numerous instances in which a highly efficient metabolic phenotype, selected for in a nutrient-poor environment, leads to decreased longevity in a nutrient-rich environment. The classical example is the development of diabetes in human populations exposed to high-calorie diets to which they had not previously become adapted (Neel, 1962; Zimmet *et al.*, 1990; Diamond, 1992; Mobbs, 1993).

It happens that expansion of the resource basis is consistent with the late stages of encephalization, since more encephalized hominids including humans are able to adopt brain-behavioral adaptations to get more food more efficiently. The human brain being a fierce nutrient sink is assumed to cause a nutrient surplus to this organ, if the nutrient intake is higher than the actual nutrient demand. This condition has an important repercussion on brain metabolism and longevity, namely the fact that the brain is rendered more vulnerable to phenotypic ill-adaptations during development, and macromolecular damage in the long run. In the human brain the metabolic constraint represented by encephalization has been circumvented partly by a decrease in average cell size, an increase in the cell surface of neurons, and partly by folding and specialization of cortical areas (Chapter 15). All these adaptations are attained in great part during intrauterine development. However, many neocortical areas do continue their development in the postnatal stage. One example is the limbic system which continues its development after birth up to the 7th year of the infantile period or longer (Chapter 14). Nutrient surplus during this period is assumed to cause phenotypic ill-adaptations which may have repercussions on the rate of neurodegeneration (Chapter 19).

Secular Changes, Life Span Prolongation, and Alzheimer Disease

We have seen that the increased metabolic burden of a larger brain led many hominids to die earlier relative to what could be expected from the size of their brains (Chapter 12). Since the demographic trend of high infantile mortality continued across species boundaries from *H. habilis* to *H. erectus* and *H. sapiens*, one may speculate that the proposed genetic change(s) (Chapter 15) underlying the coupled processes of postponement of development and maturation, and the increase in encephalization, persisted firmly until natural selection forced anew a further improvement in the resistance to failure. In other words, further increases in brain weight and life span might have demanded further developments in longevity (the resistance to age-specific metabolic failure). Unless the latter adaptation had been attained, further spurts of encephalization were likely to have met unbearable evolutionary costs reflected in increased death and extinction probabilities.

From the demographic data reviewed (Chapter 12), one is led to conclude that early hominid children under the age of 20 were especially vulnerable to the miscarriages of encephalization. While it might be easy to accept that those children or young adults died as a result of infections or of malnutrition when the resource basis was reduced, for many of us it might be difficult to concede that many of these children died from neoplasia, or as a consequence of senescent or *progeroid phenotypes* (Chapter 30), especially when the resource basis was expanded. Here we admit this possibility and hypothesize that degenerative diseases such as AD claimed its first victims among the early hominids, possibly when they were as young as 40 years. This is the very age of exponential onset of AD-like degenerative changes (Chapter 19) in some extant species of monkeys and apes including man, and in the Down syndrome brain.

To support further these hypotheses, it might help to review some recent evidence on the aging brain, not from fossil specimens, of course – because brains do not fossilize – but from real modern human brains. It would be most relevant to the discussion if these data could be presented in the context of changing rates of encephalization, for this would enable us to test the bearing of encephalization on the longevity of the brain. Unfortunately, no further encephalization than that already achieved in the late Pleistocene can be detected in modern human brain series to our knowledge. Some authors even believe that the selective pressures towards encephalization seem to have relaxed somewhat, a few thousand years ago (Chapter 12). However, changes of life style in a number of modern societies have caused and are still causing important secular changes in body mass and brain weight (Haug, 1984; Jolicoeur *et al.*, 1988; Lynn, 1990), and have also allowed a larger proportion of people to survive to ages closer to the species *maximum life span* (MLS) (Figure 16–1). These two facts of modern life, the secular changes of body- and brain size and the prolongation of life expectancy nearing the MLS, may provide us with a suitable model to be explored in our argument. Another less evident model that we shall refer to *en passant* is that of animal domestication causing a decrease in relative brain size (Kruska, 1988).

Changes in Life Style Have Important Repercussions on Body Metabolism, Body- and Brain Size, Average Life Span, and Neural Aging

Variations in body size, brain size and neuronal size distribution in the brain can be due to differences in genotype, diet and/or environment, since each factor influences rates of change at the molecular, cellular and organ levels (Finch, 1993). Notwithstanding, it is well known that brain size correlates with body size and nutritional status (Dekaban and Sadowsky, 1978; Morgane *et al.*, 1992) and that human populations all over the world are experiencing secular changes in body size (Sidhu *et al.*, 1982; Chamla, 1983; Kapoor *et al.*, 1984; Ohyama *et al.*, 1987; Matsumoto, 1982; Malina, 1990; Ling and King, 1987; Seth *et al.*, 1989). These changes are referred to as positive, if they involve increase in body dimensions, or negative, in case contrary. Herbert Haug (1984) showed how regularly positive secular changes are observed in distinct populations, a secular increase of 10 cm in body length corresponding to an increase of about 60 g in brain weight, although, as Tobias and others have shown, negative secular trends (towards decreased stature) are evident in mainly Third World populations.

The positive secular changes evident in First World populations have been attributed mainly to environmental changes (including socio-economic, cultural, nutritional, hygienic and health fields), but also to the effect of assortative selection and mating. However, above all causes of

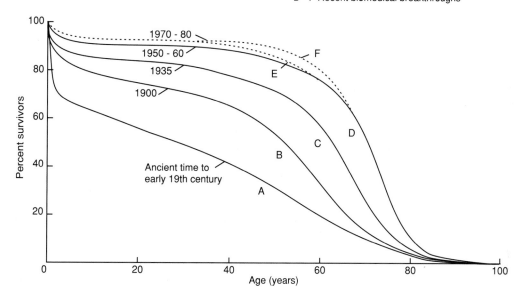

FIGURE   16–1

Impact of technical and cultural developments on human life span trends, from ancient times to present. Curves A-E represent male or female survivalship. The major technological achieve- ments which presumably account for the shifts from a lower- to a higher survivalship curve are indicated. Redrawn from Gold- man and Côté (1991), after Strehler (1975).

secular changes, the quality and the quantity of nutrition are decidedly most important. Positive secular trends in human brain size since the mid-nineteenth century have shown a gradual and consistent increase in 'Western' so- cieties, in line with an improvement in the general nutri- tion (Lynn, 1990). This trend has led to what appears to be great progress in certain human societies, yet, remark- ably, neither encephalization, nor MLS or longevity have increased. Secular trends are, by definition, not evolution- ary trends. In the best situations, what appears to have happened is a decrease in infantile mortality and a general increase in life expectancy reflected by an increase in the average life span.

The rapid changes in human body dimensions accom- panying industrialization are only one example of how man-made environmental factors are likely to regulate body metabolism. Figure 16–2 shows the dramatic changes in the *per capita* energy consumption in different stages of human evolution, from the heyday of *Homo erectus* to the present. The daily bodily energy intake has increased fivefold during this period, to reach as many as 6,000 Kcal daily:

'In America and in Europe there are, at present, unlim- ited supplies of food available. At little cost we are able to feed ourselves to satiation, ingesting daily as many as 6,000 Kcal, while our average daily requirements are about 3,000 to 3,500 Kcal. Overeating is one of the most *frequent causes of death, in some of these regions. In other parts of the world, on the other hand, 1,500 Kcal per day constitute an exceptional diet; for much of the population of southern Asia 800 Kcal represent the nor- mal condition'* (Chiarelli, 1973, p.32).

The situation is even more provocative if we consider the other categories of energy utilization, including do- mestic use, and use in industry, agriculture and transpor- tation. Energy consumption in these sectors of human ac- tivity has jumped dramatically from the modest 2,000 Kcal/day in the early days of *Homo sapiens* to more than 200,000 Kcal/day in some modern industrial societies (Figure 16–2). Although these types of energy are not di- rectly absorbed by the human body, their use has direct and important repercussions on the energetic balance of the body. For example, central heating decreases the dissi- pation of body heat, and automobiles offer people an al- ternative to walking as a means of transportation. The re- sult is that not only has food intake increased, but energy dissipation by the human body has decreased.

While these changes in life style do have an important repercussion on the metabolism of the whole body, as suggested by the secular increases in body size referred to above, it is almost impossible that they do not have a ma- jor impact on the most metabolically active organ and its parts, the brain and its neurons. This suspicion has been documented in recent geographic, cross-cultural, transna-

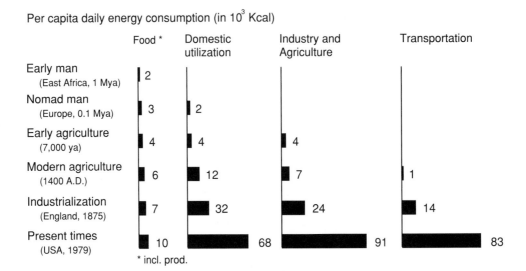

FIGURE   16–2
Per capita daily energy consumption in different stages of
human history. (From Goldemberg, 1979.)

tional, comparative epidemiologic studies of risk factors
for AD (for a review see Osuntokun *et al.*, 1992). It has
been suggested that AD is the consequence of exposure
to some environmental factors to which humans are not
adapted, and which are ubiquitous in Western societies
but not present in nonindustrialized countries (Henderson, 1986, 1988). In the United States, an estimated 4
million people suffer from degenerative dementias of the
Alzheimer type (DDAT), more than 100 thousand of
whom die every year from this irreversible condition affecting old people (Wurtman, 1985; AFAR, 1995). If the
number of annually newly diagnosed cases of DDAT in
USA is multiplied by the average duration of the condition after diagnosis (4–5 years) and by the average cost of
specialized care for these persons (US$ 7 thousand per
year is a modest estimate), the staggering annual cost of
US$ 3.15 billion is obtained. Actually, the total cost of in-
stitutional care for patients with dementia was estimated
in 1985 to exceed US$ 25 billion annually (Katzman,
1986), or more than 5 percent of the total cost of national
health care, and US$ 100 billion in 1995 (AFAR, 1995).
In addition to the economic distress, one must consider
the emotional and psychological problems that occur in a
family with a DDAT relative. The degenerative dementia
is now being dubbed 'the epidemic of the 21st century',
'the disease of industrialized societies'; it is already the
third leading cause of death in the United States. An intriguing feature of this condition is that it affects almost exclusively the recently evolved neocortex and an old structure – the limbic system – which has increased in size
and complexity during the evolution of the human brain.
It may turn out in the near future that the factors underlying secular increases in the human body and brain, an
ongoing phenomenon in many industrialized societies, do
play a part in triggering a previously not manifested vul-

nerability of the brain to this and other neurodegenerative
conditions.

The hypothesis that degeneration of the Alzheimer
type might be linked with changes in life style is indeed
tantalizing. On the one hand we have the paleontological
evidence suggesting that environmental conditions leading to undernourishment were fierce enough to select for
a thrifty phenotype in the human lineage. Encephalization and increased life span were the outcome of this phenotype, and increased longevity was largely the outcome
of this phenotype being constantly challenged by the
environment. Now the thrifty phenotype is being challenged again, though by an 'overconsumption phenotype'
and we are filled with dismay because the incidence of
abnormal protein precipitation in the brain (mainly in the
form of amyloid deposits, see Chapter 19) and the clinical
manifestations of this condition (degenerative dementias)
are increasing in industrialized regions of the world. What
is the mechanism by which a highly efficient metabolic
phenotype, selected for in a nutrient-poor environment,
leads to decreased longevity in a nutrient-rich environment?

*Under Conditions of High Nutrient Intake, the
Thrifty Phenotype may be Selected Against or Not,
Depending on the Age of Onset of the Deleterious
Effects and the Kind of Inheritance*

In humans, studies on genetic susceptibilities to diet-induced impairments of protein metabolism and neuronal
function with aging are in their infancy. However, there
is no reason to believe that protein neurotoxicity is not as
common as high-calorie, diet-induced glucose toxicity,
which is extremely common in many indigenous populations, possibly due to the selection for the thrifty pheno-

type (Neel, 1962; Zimmet *et al.*, 1990; Diamond, 1992; Mobbs, 1993). It has been hypothesized that in human populations which were subject to periods of low food availability or famine, genotypes are selected which utilize nutrients very efficiently (Neel, 1962). However, when these genotypes are exposed to a high-nutrient diet for extended periods of time, this very efficiency leads to obesity and conceivably other complications as well, and thus becomes deleterious. Under conditions of high nutrient intake, the thrifty phenotype may be selected against or not, depending on the age of onset of the deleterious effects and the kind of inheritance. Efficient utilization of glucose for example, may lead to juvenile diabetes, and is likely to be selected against because juvenile diabetes is manifested early enough in life to affect reproductive life span. AD, however, like late-onset diabetes, is mainly a late-onset phenotype, thus it is likely that efficient utilization of glucose and protein or its building blocks, amino-acids, will remain unselected for a longer time. But we cannot be sure, because our knowledge about the early manifestations of AD is still far from complete. As far as the genetics of AD is concerned, there is no such thing as one single Alzheimer gene, and there is no good reason to doubt that a great many genes are at work (Chapters 6 and 7). Nor is there any reason not to believe that the genes so far associated with the condition interact in a way we can describe as additive or co-operative. In this kind of genetics, higher levels of metabolic regulation are likely to be much more decisive than regulation by specific loci.

The Future Evolution of the Human Brain and Longevity

Any discussion about the future of biological processes is an invitation to error. The notion of the man of the future, formerly invariably conceived as possessing a large brain and a relatively small body, is an example of such prognostication, which has not found a correlate in reality, as pointed out in these witty remarks by Loren Eiseley:

'There's just one thing we haven't quite dared to mention. It's this, and you won't believe it. It's all happened already. Back there in the past, ten thousand years ago. The man of the future, with the big brain, the small teeth. Where did it get him? Nowhere. Maybe there isn't any future. Or, if there is, maybe it's only what you find in a little heap of bones on a certain South African beach. Many of you who read this belong to the White race. We like to think about this man of the future as being White. It flatters our ego. But the man of the future in the past I'm talking about was not White. He lived in Africa. His brain was bigger than your brain. His face was straight and small, almost a child's face. He was the end evolutionary product in a direction quite similar to the one anthropologists tell us is the road down which we are traveling' (pp.129–130).

When one takes a long-term evolutionary look at the problem as did Phillip Tobias (Chapter 12), it seems that a larger brain-size may once have been vitally important in aiding survival, though, beyond a certain stage in the increase of brain size, we have no evidence that further increase in any way improved man's adaptive abilities. On the contrary, we have discussed evidence that increases in brain size, coupled with prolonged life expectancy in modern societies, may even constitute a risk factor for degeneration in the long run. However, we have also discussed the basic mechanism by which longevity emerges as an aftermath of encephalization, provided that environmental conditions are favorable for this kind of development. But no further encephalization has been observed. Maybe the man-made environment as we know it today is incompatible with further encephalization. In modern human societies, when we talk about favorable environmental conditions, we may imply not only improved nutrition and life ways, but also – and markedly – progress in education and science, in Medawar's words 'incomparably the most successful activity human beings have ever engaged upon'. Thus, if we decide that increasing longevity, or the age-specific resistance to failure, is likely to be much more important now and in the future than simply increasing the size of our brains or the average life span in our societies, it may be time to engage more decisively in research on longevity and aging.

We are led to accept that our genetic make-up is currently in the process of being tried out by factors that cause secular increases in body- and brain size and gradual increases in average life expectancy (though not necessarily an increase in longevity). These poorly understood factors have disclosed how vulnerable our brain can be to devastating conditions such as the degenerative dementias of the Alzheimer type. The mechanism of trial-and-error, adaptation-and-blunder is not new in the evolution of hominid brain size and longevity. What is new is our brain and the scientific achievements that it has made possible. Thus it is in our hands to understand better the metabolism and genetics of its longevity and to act accordingly to promote it.

An Overall View

Organ systems and their portions have evolved and senesce at different times. Of all specialized organ systems, the brain has changed the most in phylogenesis; this fact accounts not only for the evolution of higher intellectual abilities in our species; it also helps explain why our brain or portions of it may be selectively vulnerable to age-related *phylogenetic diseases*.

There is evidence that encephalization directs the evolution of longevity through metabolic adaptations. The adaptation represented by a thrifty phenotype might have been a necessary condition for the postponement of development and maturation in early hominids, thus increasing the early age-specific fitness of large-brained individuals. In the late stages of hominid evolution, increases in brain size and longevity appear to go hand in hand, but reminders of the miscarriages of encephalization still persist in the modern human brain. In spite of its surprising longevity, the modern human brain still shows a pattern of selective vulnerability to age-related degeneration which seems to recapitulate phylogeny: Phylogenetically older structures such as the hindbrain are more resistant, whereas recent structures, such as the neocortex, or recently changed structures in the limbic system, are more vulnerable. The variability that characterizes the self-maintenance capacity of these structures is greatly a result of evolution failing to 'pay attention' to the problem of becoming old in the human species, but is also partly a result of environmental, non-evolutionary contingencies.

Changes in life style in modern human societies have disclosed how imperfect our genome can be or how inadequate the man-made environment is for many of us. The importance of this realization to our natural history, our societies, medical care systems and environment is far-reaching and fills us with dismay: Prolonged life span has disclosed characteristics of our brain that endows it with unique susceptibilities to pathological changes in a resource-rich environment. Genes or combinations of genes that presumably play a part in the regulation of longevity may be in the process of being tried out. The incidences of degenerative diseases and cancer have increased, as well as the time and resources needed to provide an ever aging, commonly dependent population, with long-term care and integration in society.

There is thus enough reason to believe that, to become old with a well-maintained nervous system, is very important to our species and our societies, that is, longevity and the means of promoting it have significance for our evolutionary fitness. There is no reason to believe that the adoption of any measures to promote longevity would have biologically malign effects, or that this would be any different from other measures aimed at improving the welfare of humankind. To this extent, a continued effort directed to research on aging and evolution of the brain is likely to yield important changes in our understanding of these biological phenomena, in the ability of medicine to further extend life span with better life quality and at supportable costs, and in our ability to change adverse – including man-made – environmental and biological conditions. In the words of Peter Medawar:

'The brain makes it possible for organisms to evolve in a much more efficient way than by natural selection... It is a profound truth that Nature does not know best; that a genetical evolution, if we choose to look at it liverishly instead of with fatuous good humour, is a story of waste, makeshift, compromise, and blunder... We can then improve upon nature; but the possibility of our doing so depends, very obviously, upon our continuing to explore into Nature and to enlarge our knowledge and understanding of what is going on...'

And he concludes:

'The inference we can draw from an analytical study of the differences between ourselves and other animals is surely this: that the bells which toll for mankind are – most of them, anyway – like the bells on Alpine cattle; they are attached to our own necks, and it must be our fault if they do not make a cheerful and harmonious sound.' (1991:174–177)

Selected Readings

Holloway, R. L. 1968. The evolution of the Primate brain: some aspects of quantitative relations. Brain Res. 7:121–172

Jackson, J. H. 1984. Croonian lectures. Br. Med. J. 1:501,660,703.

Jerison, H. J. 1991. Brain Size and the Evolution of Mind. The 59th James Arthur Lecture on the evolution of the human brain. American Museum of Natural History, New York.

Sarnat, H. B., and Netsky, M. G. 1984. Hypothesis: Phylogenetic diseases of the nervous system. Can. J. Neurol. Sci. 11: 29–33.

Martin, G. M. 1993. Abiotrophic gene action in Homo sapiens: potential mechanisms and significance for the pathobiology of aging. Genetica 91:265–277.

References

Acsadi, G., and Nemeskeri, J. 1970. History of Human Life Span and Mortality. Budapest.

AFAR-American Federation for Aging Research. 1995. Putting Aging on Hold: Delaying the Diseases of Old Age. An Official Report to the White House Conference on Aging.

Chamla, M. C. 1983. L'évolution récente de la stature en Europe occidentale (Période 1960–1980). Bull. Mém. Soc. d'Anthrop. Paris, t.10, sér. XIII, 2, 195–224.

Chiarelli, A. B. 1973. Evolution of the Primates. An Introduction to the Biology of Man. London and New York: Academic Press.

Dekaban, A. S., and Sadowsky, D. 1978. Changes in brain weights during the span of human life: Relation of brain weights to body heights and body weights. Ann. Neurol. 4:345–356.

Diamond, J. M. 1992. Diabetes running wild. Nature 357:362–363.

Eiseley, L. 1956. The Immense Journey. New York, Random House, Inc.

Finch, C. E. 1993. Neuron atrophy during aging: Programmed or sporadic? Trends Neurosci. 16:104–110.

Goldemberg, J. 1979. Energia no Brasil. São Paulo, Livros Técnicos e Científicos.

Goldmann, J., and Côté, L. 1991. Aging of the brain: dementia of the Alzheimer's type. In E. R. Kandel, J. H. Schwartz, and T. M. Jessel (eds.) Principles of Neural Science, 3rd Ed., Chapter 62, p. 974–983. New York, Elsevier.

Haug, H. 1984. Der Einfluss der sekularen Acceleration auf das Hirngewicht des Menschen und dessen Änderung während der Alterung. Gegenbaurs Morphol. Jahrb. 130:481–500.

Henderson, A. S. 1986. The epidemiology of Alzheimer's disease. Br. Med. Bull. 42:3–10.

Henderson, A. S. 1988. The risk factors for Alzheimer's disease:

a review and a hypothesis. Acta Psychiatr. Scand. 78: 257–275.

Jerison, H. J. 1970. Gross brain indices and the analysis of fossil endocasts. The Primate Brain 1:225–244.

Jerison, H. J. 1973. Evolution of the Brain and Intelligence, Academic Press, New York.

Jolicoeur, P., Baron, G., and Cabana, T. 1988. Cross-sectional growth and decline of human stature and brain weight in 19th-century Germany. Growth. Dev. Aging 52:201–206.

Kapoor, S., Kapoor, A. S., Kumbnani, H. K., and Bhalla, R. 1984. Anthropometry of newborns: change over a decade. Acta Med. Auxol. 16: 223–226.

Katzman, R. 1986. Alzheimer's disease. N. Engl. J. Med. 314: 946–973.

Kruska, D. 1988. Mammalian domestication and its effect on brain structure and behavior. In H. J. Jerison and I. Jerison (eds.) Intelligence and Evolutionary Biology. NATO ASI Series, Vol. G17, pp. 211–250. Springer, Berlin.

Ling, J. Y. K., and King, N. M. 1987. Secular trends in stature and weight in southern Chinese children in Hong Kong. Ann. Hum. Biol. 14:187–190.

Lynn, R. 1990. The role of nutrition in secular increases in intelligence. Person. Indiv. Diff. 11:273–285.

Malina, R. M. 1990. Research on secular trend in auxology. Anthrop. Anz. 48:209–227.

Matsumoto, K. 1982. Secular acceleration of growth in height in Japanese and its social background. Ann. Hum. Biol. 9:399–410.

Medawar, P. B. 1952. An Unsolved Problem of Biology. H. K. Lewis, London.

Medawar, P. B. 1991. The Threat and the Glory. Reflections on Science and Scientists. Oxford University Press.

Mobbs, C. V. 1993. Genetic influences on glucose neurotoxicity, aging, and diabetes: a possible role for glucose hysteresis. Genetica 91:239–253.

Morgane, P. J. et al. 1992. In R. L. Isaacson and K. F. Jensen (eds.) The Vulnerable Brain and Environmental Risks. Vol. 1, chap. 1. New York: Plenum.

Neel, J. V. 1962. Diabetes mellitus: a thrifty genotype rendered detrimental by 'progress'? American J. Hum. Genet. 14:353–362.

Ohyama, S., Hisanga, A., Inamasu, T., Yamamoto, A., Hirata, M., and Ishinishi, N. 1987. Some secular changes in body height and proportion of Japanese medical students. Am. J. Phys. Anthrop. 73: 179–183.

Osuntokun, B. O., Hendrie, H. C., Ogunniyi, A. O., et al. 1992. Cross-cultural studies in Alzheimer's disease. Ethnicity Dis. 2: 352–357.

Rose, M. R., and Finch, C. E. 1993. The janiform genetics of aging. Genetica 91:3–10.

Sarnat, H. B. 1985. Histochemical mapping of vertebrate brains for study of evolution. in A. A. Boulton, and G. B. Baker (eds.) Neuromethods, Vol. 1, General Neurochemical Techniques, chapt 14, pp. 497–535. Humana Press, Clifton..

Seth, V., Patnaik, K. K., Rai, A., Gupta, M., and Sundram, K. R. 1989. Secular trend in height and weight of pre-school children in urban slums of Delhi (India). Acta Med. Auxol. 21:79–84.

Sidhu, L. S., Bhatnagar, D. P., and Dubey, A. P. 1982. Secular trends in heights and weights of Punjabi boys. Anthrop. Anz. 40:187–192.

Wurtman, R. J. 1985. Alzheimer's disease. Scient. Am. 252:62–74.

Zimmet, P. Z., Dowse, G. K., and Finch, C. F. 1990. The epidemiology and natural history of NIDDM – lessons from the South Pacific. Diabetes Metab. Rev. 6:91–124.

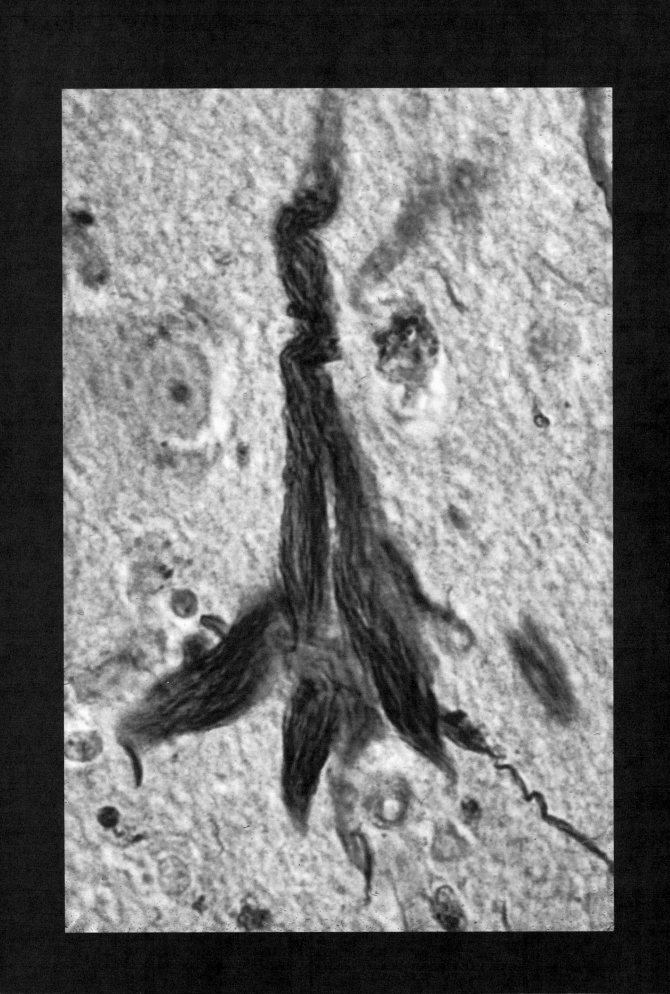

III

Tissue and Cellular Changes

A pyramidal neuron in the human parahippocampal gyrus. The soma of the neuron is completely filled with neurofibrillary tangles, stained by colloidal silver impregnation. Preparation and photograph by S.U. Dani.

III

Financial and Policy Changes

17

Rafael Linden

Neuron Death: A Developmental Perspective

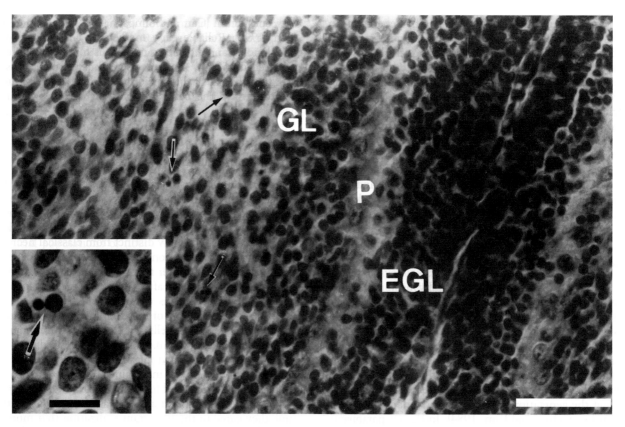

FIGURE   17–1

Section through the cerebellum of a 7-day-old rat, stained by hematoxylin-eosin. Arrows point to pyknotic nuclei. The inset shows a degenerating cell at higher magnification. Notice the presence of dying postmigratory cells at the time of granule cell migration. Calibration bars: 50 μm, and 10 μm (inset). Abbreviations: EGL, external granular layer; P, Purkinje cells layer; GL, granular layer. From E. Lopes and R. Linden, unpublished results.

tion of the size and cellular composition of tissues in physiological conditions.

Wyllie and colleagues in the 1980's showed that cell death by apoptosis was accompanied by *internucleosomal cleavage* of DNA, caused by the activation of *endonucleases* (Cohen and Duke, 1984; Arends *et al.*, 1990; McCabe *et al.*, 1992; Fernandes and Cotter, 1993; Matsubara *et al.*, 1994). This type of DNA degradation is revealed by electrophoresis as a 'ladder' of DNA bands at multiples of 180–200 base pairs. The pattern of DNA cleavage is distinct from the seemingly random degradation that occurs during necrosis, and the *DNA ladder* eventually became recognized as a biochemical hallmark of apoptosis (Kerr and Harmon, 1991).

Apoptotic nuclei can be easily recognized in cell cultures using the morphological method of identification alone, or in combination with other techniques such as DNA electrophoresis and flow cytometry (Darzynkiewicz *et al.*, 1992). However it is much more difficult to recognize apoptotic nuclei *in vivo* on a morphological basis alone, since apoptotic nuclei may be indistinguishable from necrotic nuclei, lymphocytes or telophases (Wijsman *et al.*, 1993). An alternative technique is the *in situ* labeling of fragmented DNA by DNA polymerase (Gold *et al.*,

1993; Wood *et al.*, 1993; Wijsman *et al.*, 1993) and terminal deoxynucleotidyl transferase (TdT) (Gavrieli *et al.*, 1992), in order to incorporate labeled nucleotides in the 3'-hydroxyl-recessed termini of DNA breaks produced by endonuclease. Although this technique is not specific for apoptosis, it has been applied to many tissues of nervous origin (Migheli *et al.*, 1994) appearing to be of great help.

Apoptosis is the Most Common Mechanism of Programmed Cell Death in the Developing CNS

Likewise the concept of apoptosis, the concept of *programmed cell death* appeared also in the sixties, based on observations by Lockshin and Williams of the metamorphosis of insects and the morphogenesis of avian limbs by Saunders. A series of experimental studies led to the concept that certain cells of the embryo engaged in a program of intracellular events controlled by the genome, that finally led to cell death (Lockshin and Zakeri, 1991). This operational concept was initially distinct from that of apoptosis. Nonetheless, the finding that inhibition of RNA or protein synthesis abrogate apoptosis led to the indiscriminate usage of the terms apoptosis or programmed cell death to designate several instances of cell attrition, especially the selective degeneration of immune cells.

The impropriety of intermixing the concepts of apoptosis and of programmed cell death has been pointed out (Lockshin and Zakeri, 1991; Martin *et al.*, 1994, see also Box 17–1). There is now abundant evidence that certain instances of programmed cell death do not conform to either the morphological or the biochemical criteria of apoptosis. This distinction, far from being trivial, suggests that the molecular mechanisms that lead to classical apop-

tosis in some cells may be distinct from other instances of programmed cell death. Even in canonical cases, evidence is available that the degradation of DNA may be dissociated from the morphological changes in chromatin (Sun *et al.*, 1994), thus casting doubt on the unity of the apoptotic process and on the common belief that the internucleosomal cleavage of DNA is the initial event of apoptosis. Many examples of apoptosis published in the literature may have to be reviewed as to the criteria em-

---

Programmed Cell Death, Apoptosis, Necrosis, and Oncosis   **Box 17–1**

Cell death as a physiological event was discussed almost as soon as stains became available. It was born with a bang in 1885 in a paper by the same Walther Flemming who created the terms chromatin and mitosis. Flemming studied ovarian follicles in mammals and noticed that the epithelial lining of regressing follicles was littered with cells the nuclei of which were breaking up. His careful *camera lucida* drawings illustrate the half-moons of pyknotic chromatin typical of apoptosis as well as apoptotic bodies loose in the cavity of the follicle. Flemming gave a name to the process, chromatolysis, referring to the fact that the broken up nucleus ultimately disappears. The term chromatolysis was later adopted by neuropathologists to mean something entirely different, namely the apparent breakdown of Nissl substance after transection of the axon.

The phenomenon properly called *programmed cell death* received its name before apoptosis; it referred to situations in which cells are programmed to die at a fixed time. Dramatic examples are the absorption of the tadpole's tail during metamorphosis, and the death of a group of cells in the chick embryonic plate to help create the outline of a wing. This form of cell death is programmed in the sense that a genetic clock selects a given time for the death of certain cells. However, when the time has come, a different program must dictate to these cells how to engineer suicide (e.g., apoptosis).

In recent years there has been an unfortunate tendency to use programmed cell death and apoptosis interchangeably, because in both cases genetic programs are involved. This is confusing. The genetic program of programmed cell death is a clock specifying the time of suicide, whereas the genetic program of apoptosis specifies the weapons (the means) to produce instant suicide. Apoptosis is thus not a program to carry out suicide, but a program to trigger the suicidal program.

Apoptosis is characterized by cell shrinkage, as implied in the original name shrinkage necrosis given by Kerr in 1971. The chromatin becomes pyknotic and

packed into smooth masses applied against the nuclear membrane, creating curved profiles that have inspired the descriptive terms for over a century, such as half-moon-, horse-shoe-, sickle-, lancet-, and ship-like (navicular). The nucleus may also break up (karyorhexis), and the cell emits processes (the budding phenomenon) that often contain pyknotic nuclear fragments. These processes tend to break off and become apoptotic bodies, which may be phagocytized by macrophages or neighboring cells or remain free; however, the cell may also shrink into a dense, rounded mass, as a single apoptotic body. There is little or no swelling of mitochondria or other organelles.

Biochemically, the DNA is broken down into segments that are multiples of approximately 185 bp, due to specific cleavage between nucleosomes. The process is under genetic control and can be initiated by an internal clock, or by extracellular agents such as hormones, cytokines, killer cells, and a variety of chemical, physical, and viral agents. Apoptosis can run its course very fast, even in minutes (e.g. 34 minutes from the onset of budding to complete breakup). For this reason apoptosis is remarkably unobtrusive in tissue sections. In routine sections the best cytological marker of apoptosis is karyorhexis, especially in an isolated cell. Fortunately, recent technical advances by Gavrieli and colleagues and Gold and coworkers make the identification of apoptosis a matter of simple histochemistry, a method that takes advantage of the fact the DNA breaking points (nicks) expose molecular endings that are chemically specific. Random DNA cleavages occur as a late event in necrosis, but these are preferentially detected by nick translation methods which label single strand breaks. It remains to be solved whether early genome digestion is a universal feature of apoptosis *in vivo* and whether it can be regarded as a specific marker for apoptosis.

A strong argument for a final common pathway of apoptosis can be made, from the ability of anti-apoptotic genes such as *bcl-2* to protect against apoptotic deaths triggered by a variety of stimuli. However, the rapidly developing tale of apoptosis warns us that generalizations are dangerous because, first, cell suicide does not always take the form of apoptosis; second, cell murder by cytotoxic lymphocytes leads to apoptosis; third, there seem to be several varieties of apoptosis and fourth, different cell types may follow different rules.

Necrosis is commonly used to designate cell death not by apoptosis but it is not appropriate, because it does not indicate a form of cell death but refers to changes secondary to cell death by any mechanism, including apoptosis. Cell death and necrosis are two very different things. Cell death is a process that leads to the point of no return, which, for liver cells submitted to total ischemia, lies at approximately 150 minutes, at which time scarcely any changes can be seen in histological sections. Necrosis is full-blown only after 12 to 24 hours. In other words, cells die long before any necrotic changes can be seen by light microscopy. Necrosis is signaled by irreversible changes in the nucleus (karyolysis, pyknosis, and karyorhexis) and in the cytoplasm (condensation and intense eosinophilia, loss of structure, and fragmentation). We can safely assume that these are the features of a cell's cadaver, whatever the mechanism of the cell's death, be it ischemia, heat, toxins, mechanical trauma, or even apoptosis. Accordingly, the second phase of apoptosis should be called apoptotic necrosis, as opposed to ischemic, toxic, or massive necrosis.

It is true that apoptotic cells do not seem to attract neutrophils or lymphocytes characteristic of inflammation. This could reflect a qualitative difference of apoptotic cell death, but it could also mean that cells dying singly (as apoptotic cells usually do) release such small quantities of chemoattractants that not all the molecular species reach the vascular endothelium in effective concentrations (the endothelial cells are responsible for initiating the sequence of leukocyte emigration). The Greek name apoptosis is most felicitous, suggesting as it does the discrete image of leaves dropping off here and there from a tree (*apó*, meaning from, and *ptósis*, meaning fall) as opposed to the massive cell death of an infarct. When apoptosis occurs in a large scale, however, as in certain phases of embryonic development, hordes of phagocytes appear in the scene. One inflammatory feature of apoptosis does seem unusual, namely, the fact that the cell debris (*apoptotic bodies*) are often phagocytized by neighboring cells as epithelial cells, which are not professional phagocytes. This does appear to be cellular cannibalism, but it is not clear whether it is specific to apoptosis, or it represents a general tendency of cells to devour their disabled neighbors, however they may have died.

The term *oncosis* (derived from the Greek *ónkos*, meaning swelling) was proposed in 1910 by the German pathologist von Recklinghausen precisely to mean cell death with swelling. Oncosis leads to necrosis with karyolysis and stands in contrast to apoptosis, which leads to necrosis with karyorhexis and cell shrinkage. An example of oncosis is seen in ischemic cell death, which can be considered an entity of its own, caused by failure of the ionic pumps of the plasma membrane by lack of ATP, followed by swelling, and accompanied by intense blebbing. Ischemic liver cells swell for 6 to 7 hours, then lose water and shrink. Early in the swelling process they die. Protein denaturation begins while the cell is still alive, being detectable at 30 minutes. During ischemic cell death and the subsequent coagulation necrosis, large amounts of calcium are taken up by the affected cells.

Adapted from G. Majno and I. Joris. 1995. Apoptosis, oncosis, and necrosis. An overview of cell death. American Journal of Pathology, 146 (1):3–15

---

ployed for diagnosis and, especially, as to their pertinence to a single mode of cell death.

It is likely, however, that apoptosis is at least one, and possibly the most common type of programmed cell death (Bowen, 1993; Evans, 1993). Still, the mechanisms of apoptosis seem to vary in distinct cell types, or in various conditions. Blockade of RNA or protein synthesis for example prevents the apoptosis of thymocytes induced by glucocorticoids (Wyllie *et al.*, 1984), supporting the idea that apoptosis results from the induction of specific genes. Nevertheless, blockade of protein synthesis also produces apoptosis, defined both by morphological and by biochemical criteria, in the HL-60 leukemia cell lineage and in CD4+ human T lymphocytes (Martin *et al.*, 1990; Martin, 1993). Apoptosis can be triggered also by mild harmful stimuli, which induce necrosis when in higher doses or intensities (Bursch *et al.*, 1992). The latter cases do not qualify as strictly programmed as implied by the original concept.

Morphological Diversity Indicates Multiple Mechanisms of Neuronal Degeneration

Ultrastructural studies led to the identification of various forms of developmental neuronal death. Some cell types show the early chromatin condensation typical of classical apoptosis, whereas other cells show distinct forms of degeneration (Clarke, 1990). The data accumulated for various types of neurons demonstrate that programmed cell death in the nervous system does not always coincide with the criteria of apoptosis (Server and Mobley, 1991). Rather, the morphological diversity of degenerating neurons suggests multiple mechanisms of programmed cell death (Clarke, 1990).

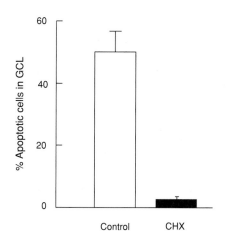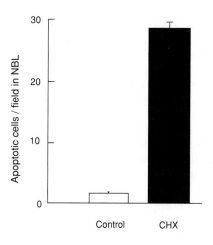

FIGURE   17–2

Apoptosis in the retina *in vitro*. The graphics show the paradoxical effects of cycloheximide (CHX) upon the incidence of apoptosis among the populations of cells in the ganglion cell layer (GCL, left) or in the neuroblastic layer (NBL, right) of both the control and the experimental explants: Blockade of protein synthesis by CHX prevents apoptosis in the GCL but causes apoptosis in the NBL. Both effects were prevented by inhibitors of endogenous endonuclease.

Experimental procedure: Explants of the retina of neonatal rats were kept for 24 hours in an orbital shaker in culture medium supplemented with 5% fetal calf serum. Some explants were supplemented with 1 μg/ml of cycloheximide which produces approximately 90% blockade in the incorporation of S35-methionine into acid-precipitable protein. From Rehen and Linden, 1994.

We have shown that the rate of cell death inferred by nuclear pyknosis effectively predicts the changes in neuron loss following either axon damage or deafferentation of neurons of the mesencephalic parabigeminal nucleus (Linden and Pinon, 1987). However, following simultaneous deafferentation and axon damage, the rate of encounter of pyknotic nuclei ceased to be an effective predictor of cell loss, suggesting that alternative modes of cell death may occur among the developing neurons, depending on interactive trophic support by both targets and afferents (Pinon and Linden, 1996).

Experimental studies have been directed at the mechanisms of apoptosis in some types of developing neurons. The apoptosis of sympathetic neurons deprived of NGF *in vitro* depends on RNA and protein synthesis, but the cells did not respond to zinc, a blocker of endogenous endonuclease activity (Martin *et al.*, 1988; Martin and Johnson, 1991; Deckwerth and Johnson, 1993). Both the natural and experimentally induced degeneration of lumbar motoneurons in the chick embryo show the classical apoptotic morphology (Chu-Wang and Oppenheim, 1978) and depend on protein synthesis (Oppenheim *et al.*, 1990), although the cleavage of DNA has yet to be examined in these cells.

Distinct Modes of Apoptosis Coexist in the Retina

The retina has been often used as a model for studies of development in the central nervous system. The long-axon ganglion cells are typical projection neurons, while other retinal cell types serve as representative cases of intrinsic neurons. Naturally occurring ganglion cell death in the rat retina is accompanied by chromatin condensation and phagocytosis by retinal macrophages, both typical of classical apoptosis (Perry *et al.*, 1983; Linden *et al.*, 1986). A later wave of natural degeneration, identified by the presence of pyknotic nuclei, sweeps across the remaining retinal layers (Beazley *et al.*, 1988).

The death of ganglion cells following axon damage is also accompanied by nuclear pyknosis both *in vivo* and *in vitro*. We showed that blockade of protein synthesis prevents the apoptosis of the axotomized ganglion cells in either retinal explants or cultures of dissociated retinal cells maintained *in vitro*. On the other hand, the blockade of protein synthesis caused apoptosis of other retinal cell types located in the neuroblastic layer (Rehen and Linden, 1994) (Figure 17–2). Both instances of cell death are accompanied by internucleosomal cleavage of DNA, and the degeneration induced by protein synthesis blockade is prevented by inhibitors of endogenous endonuclease (Rehen *et al.*, 1996). Thus, it appears that two distinct modes of apoptosis coexist in the retina. One mode is triggered by axotomy and depends on the synthesis of killer proteins. In addition, there seems to be a latent mechanism of apoptosis that is continually blocked by repressor proteins.

Cell Death or Cell Survival May be Determined by the Balance Between the Expression of Killer and Protective Genes

Studies of the molecular genetics of programmed cell death in the nematode *C. elegans* have shown that cell death is controlled by antagonist genes. The genes *ced-3* and *ced-4* are required for cell death to occur, whereas the gene *ced-9* protects cells from degeneration (Ellis and Horvitz, 1986). In vertebrates, the *bcl-2* gene was shown to protect cells from various types of degeneration including classic apoptosis (Hockenbery *et al.*, 1990; Sentman *et al.*, 1991; Veis *et al.*, 1993), while the counteracting gene *bax* has the opposite effect. The two gene products are neutralized by heterodimerization, indicating that the balance between the expression of *bcl-2* and *bax* may determine either cell death or cell survival (Oltvai *et al.*, 1993; Korsmeyer *et al.*, 1993). Recent work seems to implicate the gene ICE as a mammalian homologue of the gene *ced-3*, with a similar role in the induction of cell death (Miura *et al.*, 1993).

In the retina *in vitro*, the ganglion cells are axotomized, and therefore prevented from receiving retrogradely transported neurotrophic factors from their targets. These cells are also at a more advanced stage of development than the other cell types located in the neuroblastic layer. It is possible that the dominance of either mechanism of apoptosis relates to the type of cell, to effects of direct damage, or the state of neurotrophic support of each cell. Each of these conditions may alter the balance between the expression of killer and protective genes, and therefore determine the response to protein synthesis blockade. In addition, cell proliferation is still under way in the neuroblastic layer in postnatal rats, and may be linked with a distinct mechanism of apoptosis. These possibilities remain to be investigated, as well as their implications for the control of cell death *in vivo*. Nonetheless, the data indicate that multiple mechanisms may lead to apoptosis in the developing retinal tissue.

Competitive Interactions and the Neurotrophic Theory: Target Availability Controls Neuronal Survival in Normal Development

The competition hypothesis has long served as a useful conceptual framework for the interpretation of developmental neuron death and other events of neurogenesis. A series of remarkable experiments started in the forties provided the initial impulse for studies of trophic interactions of neurons with their peripheral targets, and established the foundations of the pervasive *neurotrophic theory* that followed the examination of cellular and molecular mechanisms of peripheral competition.

Developing neurons appear to compete for space within their targets to accomodate their growing axons, and cells denied the appropriate target space degenerate during the period of naturally occurring neuronal death. Early evidence of neuronal competition for survival stemmed from the work of Victor Hamburger and Rita Levi-Montalcini showing increased degeneration of dorsal root ganglion cells after the early removal of their peripheral targets (Figure 17–3, A, B). Enhancement of the rate of developmental neuronal death after target removal has since been confirmed by many authors in various populations of neurons from both the peripheral and the central nervous system (reviewed in Oppenheim, 1991; Linden, 1994).

The fact that cell loss following early target ablation is cotemporal with naturally occurring neuronal death sup-

ports the idea that target availability controls neuronal survival in normal development. This idea was strengthened by the converse experiment, in which enlargement of the peripheral target field led to the rescue of increased numbers of innervating neurons (Hollyday and Hamburger, 1976; Boydston and Sohal, 1979) (Figure 17–3, C).

Neurons Compete for a Limited Amount of Resources Needed for Survival

Quantitative matching of neurons with their targets was tested in various cell populations. Surgical manipulation

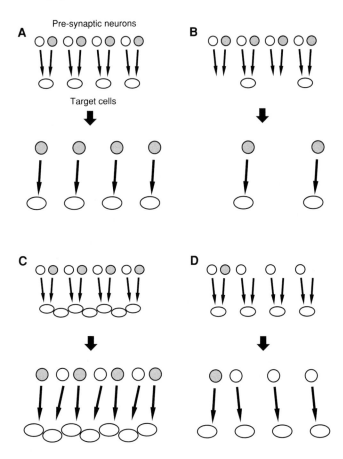

FIGURE   17–3

Major experiments related to the target control of developmental neuron death. In each diagram, the top drawing represents the situation early in development, and the bottom drawing below the thick arrow shows the outcome in the adult animals. Thin arrows represent axonal projections. Filled and open circles represent distinct neurons.

A. During normal development, the number of neurons (circles) adjusts to the available target cells (ellipses).

B. Early removal of axonal targets leads to reduced numbers of surviving neurons.

C. Augmented target fields support an increased number of neurons.

D. Early removal of some neurons increases the chances of survival of the remaining neurons.

of individual muscles or whole limbs suggested a linear relationship between the final number of surviving motoneurons and the number of target cells available at a critical stage of development (McLennan, 1982; Habgood *et al.*, 1984; Tanaka and Landmesser, 1986). In the central nervous system, experiments with chimeric mice with various degrees of Purkinje cell degeneration also showed a linear relationship between the numbers of granule cells and the numbers of their target Purkinje cells available at critical stages of cerebellar development (Wetts and Herrup, 1983; Herrup and Sunter, 1987). Further work showed that the removal of part of the neurons that project to an area of the developing brain enhances the survival of other populations that innervate the same targets (Figure 17–3, D). The axons of the remaining neurons spread across the partially denervated area (Pilar *et al.*, 1980; Sengelaub and Finlay, 1981; Jeffery and Perry, 1981; Linden and Serfaty, 1985). These data support the hypothesis that the neurons compete for a limited amount of resources needed for survival, and offered to the ingrowing axons by their target cells.

The outcome of target removal depends on the formation of anomalous pathways. We have shown that neonatal ablations of the superior colliculus in the rat, a procedure that removes the target of the contralateral parabigeminal nucleus of the mesencephalon, failed to produce a net cell loss in the latter (Linden and Perry, 1983; Linden and Pinon, 1987; Linden and Renteria, 1988). The parabigeminal nucleus forms an aberrant projection to the thalamus, within an area that is denervated by the removal of projections from the ablated superior colliculus. The anomalous target sustains a normal number of parabigeminal neurons, despite the lack of the specific projection field. There is a linear relationship between the number of neurons in the anomalous thalamic target and the number of surviving neurons in the parabigeminal nucleus (Linden, 1990). The quantitative matching of neurons with their targets may therefore hold even for abnormal projections.

Dendritic Competition

The complementary concept of dendritic competition emerged from a series of experimental studies of the mammalian retina (Linden and Perry, 1982; Perry and Linden, 1982) (Figure 17–4). We and others showed that the early degeneration of part of the ganglion cells in the neonatal rat retina resulted in increased survival of neighboring ganglion cells whose targets in the brain were intact (Linden and Perry, 1982; Leventhal *et al.*, 1988b). Further, the dendrites of the surviving ganglion cells oriented down the experimentally induced gradient of cell density, towards the depleted territory (Perry and Linden, 1982; Linden and Perry, 1982; Eysel *et al.*, 1985; Leventhal *et al.*, 1988a; Linden, 1993a). To account for these results, we proposed that during development immature neurons compete for locally-derived trophic support available to their growing dendrites, and cells that fail in the competi-

tion degenerate during the period of naturally-occurring neuron death (Linden, 1992, for a review).

It has been pointed out that plastic responses to damage in the immature brain may sometimes result from the expression of abnormal mechanisms that do not operate in the normal brain (Guillery, 1988). Yet, the results obtained for various cell populations subject to multiple experimental approaches are consistent with the current usage of the term competition, according to which the chances of survival of any neuron are reduced in the presence of other similar elements. In addition, observations of normal development offer further support to the competition hypothesis. Schall and Leventhal have shown in 1987 that the dendritic trees of most retinal ganglion cells in normal cats are laterally displaced away from the area centralis down the centro-peripheral gradient of cell density. These data support the contention that dendritic competition occurs among normal neurons, and is not an artifact induced by severe experimental conditions.

Neurons Depend Directly on Neurotrophins and Indirectly on Electrical Activity for Survival

The competition hypothesis was strengthened by the demonstration that developing neurons do in fact depend on specific neurotrophic factors present in minute quantities in their target cells (Barde, 1989; Thoenen, 1991; Barbacid, 1995). Current data indicate that during normal development the growing neurons pass through several stages of neurotrophic dependence. At early stages, before the formation of contacts between the immature cells and their targets, precursor cells capable of mitotic activity depend on specific neurotrophins for their survival (Bloom *et al.*, 1993; Birren *et al.*, 1993). Later, the trophic dependence shifts toward one or more distinct *neurotrophins* (Birren *et al.*, 1993; Davies, 1994), of which at least some are produced by the peripheral targets of the developing axons at the time of innervation (Davies *et al.*, 1987). At this stage, the survival of the maturing neurons depends on electrical activity (Oppenheim, 1987), which appears to affect primarily the uptake of the target-derived *neurotrophic factors* (Tanaka, 1987).

With regard to the mechanisms of dendritic competition, various hypotheses have been tested in recent experimental studies of the rat retina. It has been shown that the blockade of electrical activity with *tetrodotoxin* (TTX) results in increased degeneration of ganglion cells in cultures of dissociated retinal cells from postnatal rats (Lipton, 1986). The chances of survival of ganglion cells thus appeared to be enhanced by functional contacts, and the dendrites might be competing for synapses formed with the ingrowing afferents. It should be noted that morphologically identifiable synapses are found in the inner plexiform layer of the rat retina only after the period of naturally occurring ganglion cell death (Weidman and Kuwabara, 1968; Horsburgh and Sefton, 1987). Notwithstanding, early junctions can be shown in the same layer well within the cell death period (Fernandes *et al.*, 1989),

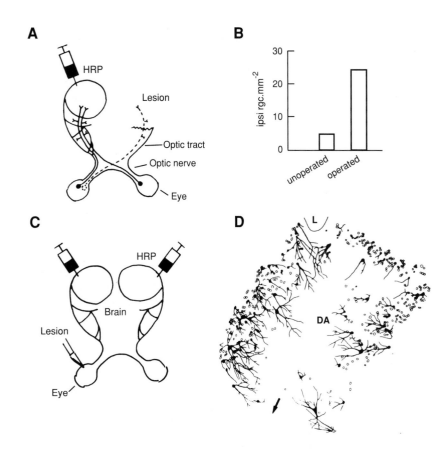

FIGURE   17–4

Evidence for dendritic competition in the developing retina.

A. Ganglion cells with uncrossed axons were retrogradely labeled with horseradish peroxidase (HRP) in adult rats, following a lesion to the optic tract at birth, that causes retrograde degeneration of ganglion cells with crossed axons (interrupted line).

B. The density of ganglion cells with ipsilateral projections found in the retina (left retina in A) was increased in operated rats when compared with unoperated controls.

C. Following localized retinal lesions at birth, massive injections of HRP were made in the adult rats to label the dendrites of ganglion cells.

D. The cells located at the borders of a depleted area (DA) peripheral to the lesion (L) directed their dendrites towards the depleted area. The arrow indicates the direction away from the optic nerve head. After Linden, 1992.

and these might possibly mediate an early form of synaptic transmission.

The electrical activity, however, appeared to be needed for either the production or the release of soluble trophic molecules rather than for the survival of the active ganglion cells themselves. Further work showed that the *vasoactive intestinal peptide* (VIP), that is found in some amacrine cells of the rat retina, can compensate for electrical activity through an increase in cyclic AMP (Kaiser and Lipton, 1990). The data suggested that the release of VIP by active amacrine cells helps sustain ganglion cells that become dependent on activity for survival. However, VIP seemed to act exclusively upon the degeneration experimentally induced by TTX, and not on the spontaneous degeneration that occurred among ganglion cells maintained in control conditions *in vitro* (Kaiser and Lipton, 1990). Thus, it is unlikely that VIP is the actual endogenous factor that controls ganglion cell death *in vivo*.

We approached the mechanisms of local control of cell death by studying the release of neurotrophic factors by retinal cells. Ganglion cell survival *in vitro* was enhanced by culture media previously conditioned by aggregates or explants of either rat or chick retina (Araujo and Linden, 1990, 1993; Ary-Pires *et al.*, 1992; Rehen *et al.*, 1993). The trophic activity is non-dialyzable and is sensitive to temperature. Explants of rat retinae kept *in vitro* for various periods of time secreted the trophic activity as long as the ganglion cell and inner plexiform layers were reasonably well preserved, while medium conditioned by ex-

plants of cerebral hemispheres had no effect (Araujo and Linden, 1993). The data indicate that retinal cells located in either the ganglion cell layer or the inner nuclear layer, or both, release neurotrophic factors capable of preventing ganglion cell degeneration *in vitro*. These factors may be similar to those implied in the target control of naturally-occurring neuron death. An active protein fraction was recovered from media conditioned by chick retina, by precipitation with 25–75 percent ammonium sulphate, and NGF was unable to reproduce the effect of the conditioned medium (R. Ary-Pires, S. K. Rehen and R. Linden, unpublished results). Other neurotrophins had been tested in preparations of retinal cells, and both BDNF (Johnson *et al.*, 1986) and NT-3 (Rodriguez-Tebar *et al.*, 1989) were found to increase the survival of ganglion cells *in vitro*. It is not clear at present whether or when these molecules are active *in vivo*, although evidence has been reported for the production of both the neurotrophins and their receptors (Carmignoto *et al.*, 1991; Zanellato *et al.*, 1993; Carri *et al.*, 1993).

Further characterization and ultimately the study of the localization and expression of the trophic molecules will be needed to evaluate their possible role in the control of developmental neuronal death *in vivo*, as well as their relationship with neurotransmitters and neuropeptides, and with the degeneration induced by activity blockade.

Reorganization of Nerve Connections Following Brain Damage May be Impaired by the Mismatch Between Cell Populations

Elucidation of the basis of the neurotrophic theory and of the mechanisms of competition is far from complete. Several questions remain open, some of which are particularly relevant to the reorganization of nerve connections following brain damage (Linden, 1993b).

Although the replacement of normal targets with an abnormal projection within the central nervous system may be able to maintain a normal number of neurons (Linden, 1990), the mismatch of two cell populations may prevent trophic support from heterologous targets. Partial deletions of the limb in developing *Xenopus* produce total loss of the innervating motoneuron pool, although the motor axons transiently innervate a distinct part of the limb (Lamb, 1979, 1981). Thus, competition for trophic factors is clearly modulated by other requirements of neurogenesis. In addition, competitive interactions among either axons or dendrites may have distinct requirements during development. In the retina, almost all ganglion cells rescued by increased target availability had small somas, whereas large cells were relatively favored following diminished dendritic competition (Linden and Serfaty, 1985). It is unknown whether these differences are intrinsic to the various cell classes or result from asynchronous development of distinct populations of ganglion cells in the retina (Linden, 1987; Perry, 1989).

The Afferent Control of Developmental Neuron Death: Neuronal Populations are Matched With Their Afferents

Evidence for *afferent control of neuronal death* is similar to that for target dependence (Figure 17–5). Deafferentation increased neuronal degeneration within the period of naturally occurring cell death in various areas of the developing brain (reviewed in Linden, 1994) (Figure 17–5, A, B), while hyperinnervation by an experimentally enlarged supply of retinofugal axons was reported to increase neuronal survival in subcortical optic targets in the rat (Cunningham *et al.*, 1979) (Figure 17–5, C). Experimental data are also consistent with a model of quantitative matching based on the availability of afferents. We assessed neuron numbers in the parabigeminal nucleus after various degrees of partial deafferentation, and a linear relationship was found between the numbers of surviving parabigeminal neurons and their major afferents (Linden and Renteria, 1988). In addition, the experiments reviewed in the previous section suggest that developing dendrites compete for afferents within the developing retina (Figure 17–5, D).

The data therefore strongly support the idea that neuronal populations are quantitatively matched with their afferents, as well as with their targets. Targets and afferents appear to act in concert upon the same cells. For example, in the ciliary ganglion of the chick a minority of neurons survive either target removal or deafferentation, but the

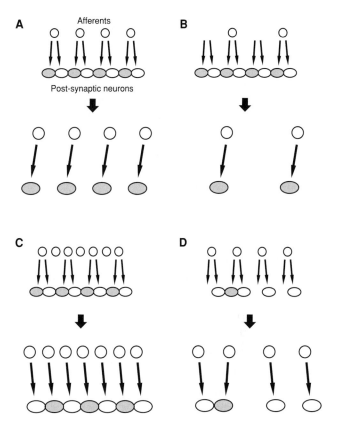

FIGURE   17–5

Afferent control of developmental neuron death. The conventions are the same as for Figure 17–4.

A. Normal quantitative adjustment of developing neurons to their afferents.

B. Deafferentation increases neuronal death.

C. Enlargement of the afferent supply increases neuronal survival.

D. Removal of some neurons increases the chance of survival of other neurons with intact axonal targets.

simultaneous removal of both sets of connections leads to complete neuron loss in the ganglion (Furber *et al.*, 1987). In the parabigeminal nucleus of the rat, a normal number of neurons may be supported by an anomalous target in the thalamus (Linden, 1990, see above). This, however, depends on the integrity of the tectal afferents. Bilateral tectal lesions, that remove simultaneously the targets and the afferents of the parabigeminal nucleus, lead to complete neuron loss in the latter (Linden and Perry, 1983). Developmental studies showed that the effects of target removal/axon damage and of deafferentation are interactive. Thus, the rate of cell death detected by nuclear pyknosis immediately after combined deafferentation and target ablation, was higher than the sum of the rates of cell death induced by the isolated ablation of each set of connections (Pinon and Linden, 1990), indicating a synergistic effect. The mode of cell death may also depend on an interaction of target- and afferent-derived trophic influences. Data from experimental studies of the isthmo-optic nucleus of the chick showed that afferents and targets differentially affect the mode of developmental neuron death in individual cells (Clarke and Egloff, 1988).

The demonstration that the afferents control the amount of neuronal death during development warrants re-evaluation of earlier data on the quantitative matching of neurons with peripheral targets (Habgood et al., 1984; Tanaka and Landmesser, 1986). For example, dorsal root ganglion cells are also affected by deletions of the limb (Hamburger and Levi-Montalcini, 1949) and this might in turn affect the final number of motoneurons (Okado and Oppenheim, 1984). On the other hand, the afferent control of neuron numbers is relevant to experiments that failed to provide evidence of quantitative matching of neurons with their target cells (Lamb, 1980; Sohal et al., 1985). For example, support from the afferent supply may explain why the total number of motoneurons from both sides of the spinal cord forced to innervate a single hindlimb in Xenopus exceeds the number that normally projects to each limb (Lamb, 1980).

Mechanisms Involved in The Afferent Control of Neuronal Survival

Various mechanisms may be involved in the afferent control of neuronal survival. Most data support the involvement of activity-dependent processes, which can be mediated by *neurotransmitters* and *neuromodulators*, and by *neurotrophic factors*.

Electrical Activity and Axoplasmic Transport

Evidence for the role of electrical activity in the anterograde control of neuronal survival was gathered both *in vitro* and *in vivo*. Depolarization enhances neuronal survival *in vitro* (Scott, 1977; Bennet and White, 1981), an effect mediated by calcium influx through L-type voltage-dependent calcium channels (Gallo et al., 1987; Collins and Lile, 1989; Koike et al., 1989; Collins et al., 1991; Larmet et al., 1992). In turn, blockade of voltage-sensitive sodium channels with tetrodotoxin increased the degeneration of neurons in dorsal root-spinal cord dissociated cell cultures and of ganglion cells in dissociated retinal cultures (Brenneman et al., 1983; Lipton, 1986). These data were taken as evidence that the survival of developing neurons depends on post-synaptic electrical activity. Notwithstanding, spike activity mediated by voltage-dependent sodium channels was not required for the trophic effects of potassium-induced depolarization on various cell types (Gallo et al., 1987; Collins and Lile, 1989; Koike et al., 1989; Larmet et al., 1992).

Studies of the auditory system *in vivo* also provided evidence for a role of electrical activity on the control of neuronal survival. Blockade of afferent activity in the auditory nerve led to degeneration in target brainstem neurons, an effect that could not be compensated by antidromic stimulation of those neurons in brainstem slices maintained *in vitro* (Rubel et al., 1990). These results sug-

gest that the pre-synaptic, rather than the post-synaptic, activity is crucial for the trophic effects of afferents on developing neurons.

In the visual system, blockade of electrical activity in the optic nerve leads, both in the optic tectum of the chick and in the superior colliculus of the rat, to an increase in cell death above the rates of naturally-occurring cell degeneration. This is followed by decreased cell death accompanying the return of the optic nerve activity (Catsicas et al., 1992; Galli-Resta et al., 1993). In contrast, neuron death in a subset of tectal neurons in the chick was independent of pre-synaptic activity, while blockade of axoplasmic transport in the afferent retinotectal axons resulted in increased cell death among this subset of tectal cells (Catsicas et al., 1992). Both electrical activity and axoplasmic transport are likely to affect the release of neuroactive molecules with an effect upon the post-synaptic neurons.

Neurotransmitters

The anterograde trophic effects may be mediated by *neurotransmitters*. In autonomic ganglia *in vivo*, the blockade of post-synaptic receptors with specific antagonists increased neuron loss during the period of naturally-occurring cell death (Wright, 1981; Meriney et al., 1987; Maderdrut et al., 1988). However, the effects of the neurotransmitters may be independent of electrical activity in post-synaptic cells. For example, NGF-deprived sympathetic neurons were rescued by activation of nicotinic cholinergic receptors, without requiring either the activation of L-type calcium channels or extracellular calcium (Koike et al., 1989). Instead, the effect was prevented by chelation of intracellular calcium. This suggests that the trophic effect may be due to voltage-independent release of intracellular calcium stores via the inositol triphosphate pathway (Giovanelli et al., 1991). In addition, depletion of intracellular calcium stores induces neuron death prior to the expression of L-type calcium channels in nodose ganglion neurons *in vitro* (Larmet et al., 1992).

Therefore, the data favor the interpretation that pre-synaptic activity results in the release of molecules with neurotrophic activity upon post-synaptic cells. It is possible that the effects of either activity blockade or depolarization described in mixed cell cultures (see above) reflect changes in the release of trophic agents by the afferent neurons. In addition, the direct entry of calcium induced by high potassium concentrations *in vitro* may compensate for distinct events normally mediated by metabotropic receptors due to modified levels of free calcium. These possibilities remain to be explored with suitable preparations.

Neurotrophins

Neurotrophic factors are likely to be involved in the afferent control of neuronal survival. It was shown that depolarizing stimuli and impulse activity specifically increase NGF gene expression in hippocampal cells *in vitro* (Lu et

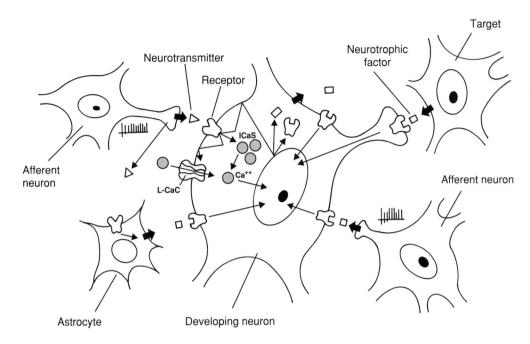

FIGURE 17–6

A summary diagram of various possible mechanisms of anterograde neurotrophic control. Release of molecules is indicated with thick arrows, intracellular events are represented by thin arrows.

Top right: Target-derived neurotrophic factors combine with neurotrophin receptors and act upon the nucleus of developing neurons, preventing the action of death genes. This mechanism of control of neuron death by the axonal targets interacts with several possible actions of the afferent supply.

Top left: Active afferent neurons release neurotransmitters and/or neuromodulators. Neurotransmitter receptors on the membrane mediate various effects (clockwise): Depolarization of the membrane activates L-type calcium channels (L-CaC),

allowing the influx of calcium into the cytoplasm; Voltage-independent mobilization of intracellular calcium stores (ICaS) results in the release of calcium. The modified calcium concentration ([Ca]) affects the activity of death genes; Depolarization produced by the action of neurotransmitters increases the expression of neurotrophic factors and autocrine effects; Depolarization also increases the expression of neurotrophin receptors.

Bottom left: Astrocytes activated by neuromodulators release neurotrophic factors that combine with receptors at the surface of the membrane and therefore affect neuronal survival.

Bottom right: Active afferents release neurotrophic factors that affect neuronal survival following combination with membrane receptors. Redrawn from Linden, 1994.

al., 1991). These data are relevant for afferent control because of recent evidence for the coexpression of neurotrophic factors and their receptors in some populations of neurons (Wetmore *et al.,* 1991; Schecterson and Bothwell, 1992; Wright *et al.,* 1992). Thus, the increased expression of neurotrophins following depolarization might help the survival of developing neurons by an autocrine or paracrine mechanism. In addition, depolarization increased the expression of messenger RNA for the high-affinity subunit of the NGF receptor, and induced functional responsiveness to NGF in a sympathoadrenal cell line (Birren *et al.,* 1992). Therefore, the afferent supply may control the responsiveness of developing neurons to target-derived growth factors, as well as affect autocrine mechanisms.

The hypothesis that neurotrophic factors may be released by the afferent supply or intervening non-neuronal cells is under investigation. Recently, Brenneman and co-workers purified an 'activity-dependent neurotrophic factor' from medium conditioned by astrocytes, which appears to mediate a rescuing effect of the neuropeptide VIP (vasoactive intestinal peptide) on degeneration induced by blockade of electrical activity (Brenneman *et al.,* 1991). It

is unclear, however, whether this protein relates to the afferent control of neuronal survival within the spinal cord or to other local neurotrophic interactions.

Anterograde release of neurotrophic factors by active afferents may also apply to the local control of ganglion cell death in the rat retina. It is, however, still not known whether the neurotrophic proteins released by retinal cells in vitro (see above) are produced by neurons or glial cells.

Various events that affect calcium fluxes or other second messenger systems may cooperate with the action of neurotrophic factors in the afferent control of neural development and survival, as well as interact with target-derived factors (Figure 17–6). For example, it has been shown that depolarizing stimuli and trophic factors interact in the control of Purkinje cell survival *in vitro* (Cohen-Cory *et al.,* 1991). In addition, the levels of cytoplasmic free calcium modulate the sensitivity of developing neurons to neurotrophic factors *in vitro* (Koike and Tanaka, 1991), although the survival effects of neurotrophic factors are not mediated by calcium (Larmet *et al.,* 1992).

An Overall View

Compelling evidence gathered in a variety of systems show that naturally occurring neuron death is a major event in vertebrate neurogenesis, controlled by the mutual exchange of neurotrophic molecules between contacting immature cells, and dependent on competitive interactions modulated by neural activity. Programmed cell death may either conform to the classical criteria of apoptosis or occur according to various forms suggestive of distinct mechanisms, and multiple pathways of trophic support may operate concurrently *in vivo*.

Neural pathways retain in the adult a potential for growth and reorganization that can be elicited, albeit in limited ways, by various perturbations. In several instances, the reorganizing nervous system seems to replay the basic mechanisms of growth of the immature brain. It is likely that the mature neurons retain the principles of neurotrophic support outlined above, long after the period of developmental neuron death. Cell demise in the senescent brain may thus be qualitatively similar to that in the developing nervous system, and the data discussed above may be useful to interpret the changes of neuronal populations associated with aging, both in normal and in pathological conditions.

Selected Readings

Barbacid, M. 1995. Neurotrophic factors and their receptors. Curr. Opin. Cell Biol. 7, 148–155.

Clarke, P. G. H. 1990. Developmental cell death: Morphological aspects and multiple mechanisms. Anat. Embryol. 181:195–213.

Guillery, R. W. 1988. Competition in the development of visual pathways. In J. G. Parnavelas, C. D. Stern, and R. V. Stirling (eds.) The Making of The Nervous System. pp. 356–380. Oxford: Oxford University Press.

Linden, R. 1994. The survival of developing neurones: A review of afferent control. Neuroscience 58:671–682.

Majno, G., and Joris, I. 1995. Apoptosis, oncosis, and necrosis. An overview of cell death. Am. J. Pathol. 146:3–15.

Martin, S. J., Green D. R., and Cotter, T. G. 1994. Dicing with Death – Dissecting the Components of the Apoptosis Machinery. Trends Biochem. Sci. 19:26–30.

Oppenheim, R. W. 1991. Cell death during development of the nervous system. Ann. Rev. Neurosci. 14:453–501.

References

Araujo, E. G., and Linden R. 1990. Survival of retinal ganglion cells: The effect of conditioned medium from retinal cell aggregates. Brazilian J. Med. Biol. Res. 23:743–746.

Araujo, E. G., and Linden, R. 1993. Trophic factors produced by retinal cells increase the survival of retinal ganglion cells in vitro. Eur. J. Neurosci. 5:1181–1188.

Arends, M. J., Morris, R. G., and Wyllie, A. H. 1990. Apoptosis: The role of the endonuclease. Am. J. Pathol. 136:593.

Ary-Pires, R., Rehen, S. K., and Linden, R. 1992. Evidence for a developmentally regulated neurotrophic activity from chick retina affecting the survival of retinal ganglion cells from newborn rats. Brazilian J. Med. Biol. Res. 25:845–848.

Barde, Y. A. 1989. Trophic factors and neuronal survival. Neuron 2:1525–1534.

Beazley, L. D., Perry, V. H., Baker, B., and Darby, J. E. 1987. An investigation into the role of ganglion cells in the regulation of division and death of other retinal cells. Dev. Brain Res. 33:169–184.

Bennett, M. R., and White, W. 1981. The survival and development of cholinergic neurons in potassium-enriched media. Brain Res. 173:549–553.

Birren, S. J., Lo, L. C., and Anderson, D. J. 1993. Sympathetic Neuroblasts Undergo a Developmental Switch in Trophic Dependence. Development 119:597–610.

Birren, S. J., Verdi, J. M., and Anderson, D. J. 1992. Membrane depolarization induces p140trk and NGF responsiveness, but not p75LNGFR, in MAH cells. Science 257:395–397.

Bloom, E. D. C., Friedman, W., and Black, I. B. 1993. NT-3 stimulates sympathetic neuroblast proliferation by promoting precursor survival. Neuron 11:1101–1111.

Bowen, I. D. 1993. Apoptosis or programmed cell death? Cell Biol. Intern. 17:365–380.

Boydston, W. R., and Sohal, G. S. 1979. Grafting of additional periphery reduces embryonic loss of neurons. Brain Res. 178:403–410.

Brenneman, D. E., Barth R., Warren, D., Davidson, A., and Gozes, I. 1991. Purification of activity dependent neurotrophic factor (ADNF). Soc. Neurosci. Abstr. 17:754.

Brenneman, D. E., Neale, E. A., Habig, W. H., et al. 1983. Developmental and neurochemical specificity of neuronal deficits produced by electrical impulse blockade in dissociated spinal cord cultures. Dev. Brain Res. 9:13–27.

Carmignoto, G., Comelli, M.C., Candeo, P., et al. 1991. Expression of NGF receptor and NGF receptor messenger RNA in the developing and adult rat retina. Exp. Neurol. 111:302–311.

Carr, V. M., and Farbman, A. I. 1993. The Dynamics of Cell Death in the Olfactory Epithelium. Exp. Neurol. 124:308–314.

Carr, V. M., and Simpson, S. B. 1982. Rapid appearance of labeled degenerating cells in the dorsal root ganglia after exposure of chick embryos to tritiated thymidine. Dev. Brain Res. 2:157–162.

Carri, N. G., Williams, R., Backstrom, A., et al. 1993. Neurotrophin receptors during development of the chick and rat retina. Soc. Neurosci. Abstr. 19:1298.

Catsicas, M., Pequignot, Y., and Clarke, P. G. H. 1992. Rapid onset of neuronal death induced by blockade of either axoplasmic transport or action potentials in afferent fibers during brain development. J. Neurosci. 12:4642–4650.

Chu-Wang, I., and Oppenheim, R. W. 1978. Cell death of motoneurons in the chick embryo spinal cord. I. A light and electron microscopis study of naturally occurring and induced cell loss during development. J. Comp. Neurol. 177:33–58.

Clarke, P. G. H., and Egloff, M. 1988. Combined effects of deafferentation and de-efferentation on isthmo-optic neurons during the period of their naturally occurring cell death. Anat. Embryol. 179:103–108.

Clarke, P. G. H. 1990. Developmental cell death: Morphological aspects and multiple mechanisms. Anat. Embryol. 181:195–213.

Cohen, J. J., and Duke, R. C. 1984. Glucocorticoid activation of a calcium-dependent endonuclease in thymocyte nuclei leads to cell death. J. Immunol. 132:38–42.

Cohen-Cory, S., Dreyfus, C. F., and Black, I. B. 1991. NGF and excitatory neurotransmitters regulate survival and morphogenesis of cultured cerebellar Purkinje cells. J. Neurosci. 11:462–471.

Collins, F., and Lile, J. D. 1989. The role of dihydropiridine voltage-gated calcium channels in potassium-mediated neuronal survival. Brain Res. 502:99–108.

Collins, F., Schmidt, M. F., Guthrie, P. B., and Kater, S. B. 1991. Sustained increase in intracellular calcium promotes neuronal survival. J. Neurosci. 11:2582–2587.

Cowan, W. M., Fawcett, J. W., O'Leary, D. D. M., and Stanfield, B. B. 1984. Regressive events in Neurogenesis. Science 225:1258–1265.

Cunningham, T. J., Huddleston, C., and Murray, M. 1979. Modification of neuron numbers in the visual system of the rat. J. Comp. Neurol. 184:423–434.

Dani, S. U., Pitella, J. E. H., Hori, A., et al. 1994. Different rates of neuronal degeneration: An exquisite variation of the 'cascade' hypothesis. Dementia 5:110–118.

Davies, A. M. 1994. Neurotrophic Factors – Switching Neurotrophin Dependence. Curr. Biol. 4:273–276.

Davies, A. M., Bandtlow, C., Heumann, R., et al. 1987. Timing and site of nerve growth factor synthesis iin developing skin in relation to innervation and expression of the receptor. Nature 326:353–358.

Darzynkiewicz, Z., Bruno, S., Del Bino, G., et al. 1992. Features of apoptotic cells measured by flow cytometry. Cytometry 13:795–808.

Deckwerth, T. L., and Johnson, E. M. 1993 Temporal analysis of events associated with programmed cell death (apoptosis) of sympathetic neurons deprived of nerve growth factor. J. Cell Biol. 123:1207–1222.

Ellis, R. E., and Horvitz, H. R. 1986. Genetic control of programmed cell death in the nematode C. elegans. Cell 44:817–829.

Evans, V. G. 1993. Multiple pathways to apoptosis. Cell Biol. Intern. 17:461–476.

Eysel, U. T., Peichl, L., and Wassle, H. 1985. Dendritic plasticity in the early postnatal feline retina: Quantitative characteristics and sensitive period. J. Comp. Neurol. 242:134–145.

Fernandes, A. J., Martinez, A. M. B., and Linden, R. 1989. Estruturas juncionais precoces na camada plexiforme interna da retina do rato em desenvolvimento. Resumos do XII Colóquio da Sociedade Brasileira de Microscopia Eletrônica, pp. 225–226. SBME, Caxambu.

Fernandes, R. S., and Cotter, T. G. 1993. Activation of a calcium/magnesium independent endonuclease in human leukemic cell apoptosis. Anticancer Res. 13:1253–1259.

Flemming, W. 1885. Über die Bildung von Richtungsfiguren in Säugetiereiern beim Untergang Graaf'scher Follikel. Arch. Anat. Entwicklungsgesch. 1885:221–244.

Furber, S., Oppenheim, R. W., and Prevette, D. 1987. Naturally-occurring neuron death in the cilliary ganglion of the chick embryo following removal of preganglionic input: Evidence for the role of afferents in ganglion cell survival. J. Neurosci. 7:1816–1832.

Galli-Resta, L., Ensini, M., Fusco, E., Gravina, A., and Margheritti, B. 1993. Afferent spontaneous electrical activity promotes the survival of target cells in the developing retinotectal system of the rat. J. Neurosci. 13:243–250.

Gallo, V., Kingsbury, A., Balasz, R., and Jorgensen, O. S. 1987. The role of depolarization in the survival and differentiation of cerebellar granule cells in culture. J. Neurosci. 7:2203–2213.

Gavrieli, Y., Sherman, Y., and Ben-Sasson, S. A. 1992. Identification of programmed cell death in situ via specific labeling of of nuclear DNA fragmentation. J. Cell Biol. 119:493–501.

Giovanelli, A., Grassi, F., Mattei, E., et al. 1991. Acetylcholine induces voltage-independent increase of cytosolic calcium in mouse myotubes. Proc. Natl. Acad. Sci. USA 88:10069–10073.

Gold, R., Schmied, M., Rothe, G., et al. 1993. Detection of DNA fragmentation in apoptosis: application of in situ nick translation to cell culture systems and tissue sections. J. Histochem. Cytochem. 41:1023–1030.

Gold, R., Schmied, M., Giegerich, G., et al. 1994. Differentiation between cellular apoptosis and necrosis by the combined use of in situ tailing and nick translation techniques. Lab. Investig. 71:219–225.

Guillery, R. W. 1988. Competition in the development of visual pathways. In J. G. Parnavelas, C. D. Stern, and R. V. Stirling (ed.) The Making of the Nervous System, pp. 356–380. Oxford: Oxford University Press.

Habgood, M. D., Hopkins, W. G., and Slack, J. R. 1984. Muscle size and motor unit survival in mice. J. Physiol. 356:303–314.

Hamburger, V., and Levi-Montalcini, R. 1949. Proliferation, differentiation and degeneration in the spinal ganglia of the chick embryo under normal and experimental conditions. J. Exp. Zool. 111:457–501.

Herrup, K., and Sunter, K. 1987. Numerical matching during development: Quantitative analysis of granule cell death in staggerer mouse chimeras. J. Neurosci. 7:829–836.

Hockenbery, D. M., Nunez, G., Millman, C., et al. 1990. Bcl-2 is an inner mitochondrial membrane protein that blocks programmed cell death. Nature 348:334.

Hollyday, M., and Hamburger, V. 1976. Reduction of the naturally occurring motor neuron loss by enlargement of the periphery. J. Comp. Neurol. 170:311–320.

Jacobson, M. 1991. Developmental Neurobiology. pp. 1–776. New York: Plenum Press, 3 Ed.

Jeffery, G., and Perry, V. H. 1981. Evidence for ganglion cell death during development of the ipsilateral retinal projection in the rat. Develop. Brain Res. 2:176–180.

Johnson, J. E., Barde, Y. A., Schwab, M., and Thoenen, H. 1986. Brain derived neurotrophic factor supports the survival of cultured rat retinal ganglion cells. J. Neurosci. 6:3031–3038.

Kaiser, P. K., and Lipton, S. A. 1990. VIP-mediated increase in cAMP prevents tetrodotoxin-induced retinal gangolion cell death 'in vitro'. Neuron 5:373–381.

Kerr, J. F. R. 1965. A histochemical study of hypertrophy and ischaemic injury of rat liver with special reference to changes in lysosomes. J. Pathol. Bacteriol. 90:419.

Kerr, J. F. R., and Harmon, B. V. 1991. Definition and incidence of apoptosis: An historical perspective. In L. D. Tomei, and F. D. Cope (eds.) Apoptosis: The Molecular Basis of Cell Death, pp. 5–29. Plainville, NY: Cold Spring Harbor Laboratory Press.

Kerr, J. F. R., Wyllie, A. H., and Currie, A. H. 1972. Apoptosis: A basic biological phenomenon with wide-ranging implications in tissue kinetics. Br. J. Cancer 26:239–257.

Koike, T., and Tanaka, S. 1991. Evidence that nerve growth factor dependence of sympathetic neurons for survival in vitro may be determined by the levels of cytoplasmic free Ca^{2+}. Proc. Natl. Acad. Sci. USA 88:3892–3896.

Koike, T., Martin, D. P., and Johnson, E. M., Jr. 1989. Role of Ca^{2+} channels in the ability of membrane depolarization to prevent neuronal death induced by trophic-factor deprivation: Evidence that levels of internal Ca^{2+} determine nerve growth factor dependence of sympathetic ganglion cells. Proc. Natl. Acad. Sci. USA 86:6421–6425.

Korsmeyer, S. J., Shutter, J. R., Veis, D. J., et al. 1993. Bcl-2/Bax – A Rheostat That Regulates an Anti-Oxidant Pathway and Cell Death. Semin. Cancer Biol. 4:327–332.

Krinke, G. J., and Eisenbrandt, D. L. 1994. Nonneoplastic changes in the brain. In U. Mohr, D. L. Dungworth, and C. C. Capen (eds.) Pathobiology of the Aging Rat. Vol. 2, pp. 3–19. Washington, D.C.: ILSI Press.

Lamb, A. H. 1979. Evidence that some developing limb motoneurons die for reasons other than peripheral competition. Dev. Biol. 71:8–21.

Lamb, A. H. 1980. Motoneurone counts in Xenopus frogs reared with one bilaterally-innervated hindlimb. Nature 284:347–350.

Lamb, A. H. 1981. Target dependency of developing motoneurons in Xenopus laevis. J. Comp. Neurol. 203:157–171.

Larmet, Y., Dolphin, A. C., and Davies, A. M. 1992. Intracellular calcium regulates the survival of early sensory neurons before they become dependent on neurotrophic factors. Neuron 9:563–574.

Leventhal, A. G., Schall, J. D., and Ault, S. J. 1988. Extrinsic determinants of retinal ganglion cell structure in the cat. J. Neurosci. 8:2028–2038.

Linden, R. 1992. Dendritic competition: A principle of retinal development. In R. Lent (ed.) The Visual System: From Genesis to Maturity. pp. 86–103. Boston: Birkhauser.

Linden, R. 1993b. Neuron death and the neurotrophic theory – some open issues. IBRO News 21:5.

Linden, R. 1987. Competitive interactions and regulation of developmental neuronal death in the retina. In C. Chagas, and R. Linden (eds.) Developmental Neurobiology of Mammals, pp. 109–140. The Vatican: Pontifical Academy of Sciences.

Linden, R. 1990. Control of neuronal survival by anomalous targets in the developing brain. J. Comp. Neurol. 294:594–606.

Linden, R. 1993a. Dendritic competition in the developing retina: Ganglion cell density gradients and laterally displaced dendrites. Vis. Neurosci. 10:313–324.

Linden, R., Araujo, E. G., and Pires, R. A. 1991. Intraretinal neurotrophic factors prevent ganglion cell death in vitro. Soc. Neurosci. Abstr. 17:228.

Linden, R., Cavalcante, L. A., and Barradas, P. C. 1986. Mononuclear phagocytes in the retina of developing rats. Histochemistry 85:335–340.

Linden, R., and Perry, V. H. 1983. Retrograde and anterograde-transneuronal degeneration in the parabigeminal nucleus following tectal lesions in developing rats. J. Comp.Neurol. 218:270–281.

Linden, R., and Pinon, L. G. P. 1987. Dual control by targets and afferents of developmental neuronal death in the mammalian central nervous system: a study in the parabigeminal nucleus of the rat. J. Comp. Neurol. 266:141–149.

Linden, R., and Renteria, A. S. 1988. Afferent control of neuron numbers in the developing brain. Dev. Brain Res. 44:291–295.

Linden, R., and Serfaty, C. A. 1985. Evidence for differential effects of terminal and dendritic competition upon developmental neuronal death in the retina. Neuroscience 15:853–868.

Linden, R., and Perry, V. H. 1982. Ganglion cell death within the developing retina: a regulatory role for retinal dendrites? Neuroscience 7:2813–2827.

Lipton, S. A. 1986. Blockade of electrical activity promotes the death of mammalian retinal ganglion cells in culture. Proc. Natl. Acad. Sci. USA 83:9774–9778.

Lockshin, R. A., and Williams, C. M. 1964. Programmed cell death. II: Endocrine potentiation of the breakdown of the intersegmental muscles of silkmoths. J. Insect Physiol. 10:643.

Lockshin, R. A., and Zakeri, Z. F. 1991. Programmed cell death and apoptosis. In L. D. Tomei, and F. D. Cope (eds.) Apoptosis: The Molecular Basis of Cell Death, pp. 47–60. Plainville, NY: Cold Spring Harbor Laboratory Press.

Lu, B., Yokoyama, M., Dreyfus, C., and Black, I. B. 1991. Depolarizing stimuli regulate nerve growth factor gene expression in cultured hippocampal neurons. Proc. Natl. Acad. Sci. USA 88:6289–6292.

Maderdrut, J. L., Oppenheim, R. W., and Prevette, D. 1988. Enhancement of naturally occurring cell death in the sympathetic and parasympathetic ganglia of the chicken embryo following blockade of ganglionic transmission. Brain Res. 444:189–194.

Martin, D. P., and Johnson, E. M., Jr. 1991. Programmed cell death in the peripheral nervous system. In L. D. Tomei, and F. D. Cope (eds.) Apoptosis: The Molecular Basis of Cell Death, pp. 247–261. Plainville, NY: Cold Spring Harbor Laboratory Press.

Martin, D. P., Schmidt, R. E., DiStefano, P. S., et al. 1988. Inhibitors of protein synthesis and RNA synthesis prevent neuronal death caused by nerve growth factor deprivation. J. Cell Biol. 106:829–844.

Martin, S. J. 1993. Protein or RNA synthesis inhibition induces apoptosis of mature human CD4+ T cell blasts. Immunol. Lett. 35:125–134.

Martin, S. J., Lennon, S. V., Bonham, A. M., and Cotter, T. G. 1990. Induction of apoptosis (programmed cell death) in human leukemic HL-60 cells by inhibition of RNA or protein synthesis. J. Immunol. 145:1859–1867.

Matsubara, K., Kubota, M., Adachi, S., et al. 1994. Different mode of cell death induced by calcium ionophore in human leukemia cell lines – Possible role of constitutive endonuclease. Exp. Cell Res. 210:19–25.

McCabe, M. J., Jr., Nicotera, P., and Orrenius, S. 1992. Calcium-dependent cell death: Role of the endonuclease, protein kinase C and chromatin conformation. Ann. N.Y. Acad. Sci. 663:269–278.

McLennan, I. S. 1982. Size of motoneuron pool may be related to number of myotubes in developing muscle. Dev. Biol. 92:263–265.

Meriney, S. D., Pilar, G., Ogawa, M., and Nunez, R. 1987. Differential neuronal survival in the avian ciliary ganglion after chronic acetylcholine receptor blockade. J. Neurosci. 7:3840–3849.

Migheli, A., Cavalla, P., Marino S., and Schiffer D. 1994. A study of apoptosis in normal and pathologic nervous tissue after in situ end-labeling of DNA strands breaks. J. Neuropathol. Exper. Neurol. 53:606–616.

Miura, M., Zhu, H., Rotello, R., Hartwieg, E. A., and Yuan, J. Y. 1993. Induction of apoptosis in fibroblasts by IL-1 beta-converting enzyme, a mammalian homolog of the C. elegans cell death gene ced-3. Cell 75:653–660.

Okado, N., and Oppenheim, R. W. 1984. Cell death of motoneurons in the chick embryo spinal cord. IX: The loss of motoneurons following removal of afferent inputs. J. Neurosci. 4:1639–1652.

Oltvai, Z. N., Milliman, C. L., and Korsmeyer, S. J. 1993. Bcl-2 heterodimerizes in vivo with a conserved homolog, Bax, that accelerates programmed cell death. Cell 74:609–619.

Oppenheim, R. W. 1987. Muscle activity and motoneuron death in the spinal cord of the chick embryo. In G. Bock, and M. O'Connor (eds.) Selective Neuronal Death, pp. 96–112. New York: Wiley.

Oppenheim, R. W., Prevette, D., Tytell, M., and Homma, S. 1990. Naturally occurring and induced neuronal death in the chick embryo in vivo requires protein and RNA synthesis: Evidence for the role of cell death genes. Dev. Biol. 138: 104–113.

Pearson, H. E., Payne, B. R., and Cunningham, T. J. 1993. Microglial invasion and activation in response to naturally occurring neuronal degeneration in the ganglion cell layer of the postnatal cat retina. Dev. Brain Res. 76:249–255.

Perry, V. H. 1989. Dendritic interactions between cell populations in the developing retina. In B. L. Finlay, and D. R. Sengelaub (eds.) Development of the vertebrate retina, pp. 149–172. New York: Plenum Press.

Perry, V. H., Henderson, Z., and Linden, R. 1983. Postnatal changes in retinal ganglion cell and optic axon populations in the pigmented rat. J. Comp. Neurol. 219, 356–370.

Perry, V. H., and Linden, R. 1982. Evidence for dendritic competition in the developing retina. Nature 297:683–685.

Pilar, G., Landmesser, L., and Burstein, L. 1980. Competition for survival among developing ciliary ganglion cells. J. Neurophysiol. 43:233–254.

Pinon, L. G. P., and Linden, R. 1990. Interactive effects of deafferentation and target removal on cell death in the parabigeminal nucleus of developing rats. Braz. J. Med. Biol. Res. 23:659–662.

Pinon, L. G. P., and Linden, R. 1996. Target and afferents interact to control developmental neuronal death in the parabigeminal nucleus of the rat. J. Neurosci. Res. 45:174–182.

Prestige, M. C. 1970. Differentiation, degeneration and the role of the periphery: Quantitative considerations. In F. O. Schmitt (ed.) The Neurosciences, 2nd study program, pp. 73–82. New York: Rockefeller University Press.

Raff, M. C., Barres, B. A., Burne, J. F., et al. 1993. Programmed cell death and the control of cell survival: Lessons from the nervous system. Science 262:695–700.

Recklinghausen, F. von. 1910. Untersuchungen über Rachitis und Osteomalacie. Jena: Verlag Gustav Fischer.

Rehen, S. K., and Linden, R. 1994. Apoptosis in the developing retina: Paradoxical effects of protein synthesis inhibition. Brazilian J. Med. Biol. Res. 27:1647–1651.

Rehen, S. K., Ary-Pires, R., and Linden, R. 1993a. Intraretinal neurotrophic activity prevents the degeneration of ganglion cells in retinal explants. Brazilian J. Med. Biol. Res. 26:955–959.

Rehen, S. K., Varella, M. H., Freitas, F. G., Moraes, M. O., and Linden, R. 1996. Contrasting effects of protein synthesis inhibition and of cyclic AMP on apoptosis in the developing retina. Development 122:1439–1448.

Rubel, E. W., Hyson, R. L., and Durham, D. 1990. Afferent regulation of neurons in the brain stem auditory system. J. Neurobiol. 21:169–196.

Saunders, J. W. 1966. Death in embryonic systems. Science 154:604–612.

Schall, J. D., and Leventhal, A. G. 1987. Relationships between ganglion cell dendritic structure and retinal topography in the cat. J. Comp. Neurol. 257:149–15.

Schecterson, L. C., and Bothwell, M. 1992. Novel roles for neurotrophins are suggested by BDNF and NT-3 mRNA expression in developing neurons. Neuron 9:449–463.

Scott, B. S. 1977. The effect of elevated potassium on the time course of neuron survival in cultures of dissociated dorsal root ganglia. J. Cell Physiol. 91:305–316.

Seeburger, J. L., and Springer, J. E. 1993. Experimental rationale for the therapeutic use of neurotrophins in amyotrophic lateral sclerosis. Exp. Neurol. 124:64–72.

Sengelaub, D. R., and Finlay, B. L. 1981. Early removal of one eye reduces normally occurring cell death in the remaining eye. Science 213:573–574.

Sentman, C. L., Shutter, J. R., Hockenbery, D. M., et al. 1991. Bcl-2 inhibits multiple forms of apoptosis but not negative selection in thymocytes. Cell 67:879–888.

Server, A. C., and Mobley, W. C. 1991. Neuronal cell death and the role of apoptosis. In L. D. Tomei, and F. D. Cope (eds.) Apoptosis: The Molecular Basis of Cell Death, pp. 263–278. Plainville, NY: Cold Spring Harbor Laboratory Press.

Sohal, G. S., Stoney, S. D., Arumugan, T., et al. 1985. Influence of reduced neuron pool on the magnitude of naturally occurring motor neuron death. J. Comp. Neurol. 247:516–528.

Sun, D. Y., Jiang, S., Zheng, L. M., et al. E. 1994. Separate metabolic pathways leading to DNA fragmentation and apoptotic chromatin condensation. J. Exp. Med. 179:559–568.

Swaab, D. F. 1991. Brain aging and Alzheimer's disease: 'Wear and tear' versus 'use or lose it'. Neurobiol. Aging 12:317–324.

Tanaka, H., and Landmesser, L. 1986. Cell death of lumbosacral motoneurons in chick, quail and chick-quail chimera embryos: A test of the quantitative matching hypothesis of neuronal cell death. J. Neurosci. 6:2889–2900.

Terry, R. D., DeTeresa, R., and Hansen, L. A. 1987. Neocortical cell counts in normal human adult aging. Ann. Neurol. 21:530–539.

Thoenen, H. 1991. The changing scene of neurotrophic factors. Trends Neurosci. 14:165–170.

Tomei, L. D., and Cope, F. D. 1991. Apoptosis: The molecular basis of cell death. Plainville, NY: Cold Spring Harbor Laboratory Press.

Tomlinson, B. E. 1992. Ageing and the dementias. In: J. H. Adams, and L. W. Duchen (eds.) Greenfield's Neuropathology, p. 1284. London: Edward Arnold.

Veis, D. J., Sorenson, C. M., Shutter, J. R., and Korsmeyer, S. J. 1993. Bcl-2 deficient mice demonstrate fulminant lymphoid apoptosis, polycystic kidneys and hypopigmented hair. Cell 75:229–240.

Weidman, S., and Kuwabara, T. 1968. Postnatal development of the rat retina: an electron microscopic study. Arch. Ophtalmol. 79: 470–484.

Wetmore, C., Cao, Y. H., Pettersson, R. F., and Olson, L. 1991. Brain-derived neurotrophic factor – Subcellular compartmentalization and interneuronal transfer as visualized with anti-peptide antibodies. Proc. Natl. Acad. Sci. USA 88:9843–9847.

Wetts, R., and Herrup, K. 1983. Direct correlation between Purkinje and granular cell number in the cerebella of lurcher chimeras and wild-type mice. Dev. Brain Res. 10:41–47.

Wijsman, J. H., Jonker, R. R., Keijzer, R., et al. 1993. A new method to detect apoptosis in paraffin sections: in situ endlabeling of fragmented DNA. J. Histochem. Cytochem. 41:7–12.

The brain consists of many parts. The functionally most important structure is the gray matter, containing numerous nerve cells and a network of neuronal processes. This network of long extensions like axons and dendrites interfaces through the synapses. One nerve cell, depending on its size, can have between hundreds and many thousands of such connections (Haug, 1981). The other substance is the white matter; it contains the myelinated fibers that make up the connections between the different grays (Chapter 21).

An important neuronal feature is the fact that the neurons had their last mitosis before birth. This can be easily understood by function. The neuron and their functional connections do not allow mitosis; each mitosis would only be possible if all processes were retracted. However, this would cause a loss of synaptic connections and thus loss of memory. Therefore, the life time of a human neuron has the same span as the whole life time of the individual.

Different gray matters have different levels of function. Some operate without the individual being aware of them. Others with higher capacities are located in the cortex cerebri. The latter has overtaken various functions of the higher nervous activities, like sensory analysis, higher analysis of sensory input, speech, and motor output. It takes the responsibility for motivation as well as to inhibitory behavior, connected with consciousness and mind. One distinguishes between about 40 cortical areas having specific cytoarchitectonic structures (Brodmann, 1909; v. Economo and Koskinas, 1925; Vogt and Vogt, 1926).

An important question is whether the brain ages similarly in all parts or differently in the various parts. The Vogts introduced in 1929 the term *pathoklise* meaning that every part of the human brain has its own susceptibility and response to pathological events. The Vogts' definition has been rarely used, but the fact is well known. Our group investigated consequently different areas with various functions. The aim was to explore whether the biological aging of the various grays has a different character in time and shape (Haug *et al.*, 1983, 1984).

Stereological Procedures are Used to Study the Complex 3D Structure of the Brain

Why is aging in the brain and its cortex insufficiently understood? This has two main reasons. The first is the inherent complexity of the substrate, with neurons of the various grays arranged in highly different cytoarchitectonics like globuli or layers. The second reason has to do with the distortive influence of our preparative and morphometric techniques on the brain tissue. An interdependence connects both reasons and influences therefore the results (Haug, 1986).

Fixation and the histological treatment of the brain tissue cause a volume change, mostly a shrinkage. The expression shrinkage is due to the postmortem volume changes during preparative procedures, and diminution or decrease regard the premortem, thus vital loss of volume of the brain and its parts. In morphometry, the ratio of thickness of section to the size of the estimated structure is important. The technical error grows with decreasing section thickness and increasing structure size (Haug, 1967). However, the distorted data can be transformed into three-dimensional magnitudes by *stereology*, which was unknown 50 years ago (Box 18–1). Stereology in connection with sensitive morphometric equipment is an invaluable technique to estimate three-dimensional sizes at all levels, from macroscopy to electron microscopy. The shrinkage during preparation has to be accurately determined in order to correct all evaluated morphometric data and to achieve precise results for neuron density and size, synapses and microvessels, according to the situation in the living brain. In addition, the evaluation procedures have to observe the layering of cortical cytoarchitectonics.

A further aspect to be considered is the choice of the animal models. Results gained through animal research can be transferred to human aging with caution. The aging of rats is in some respects different from that of human beings (Haug, 1990). This can easily be understood in evolutionary terms. Rodents and primates were separated at the end of the Earth's middle age long before the Tertiary. Furthermore, the life span of rats is about 20 times shorter than that of humans. Therefore, some results of experimental aging research in rats cannot be transferred directly to humans. On the other hand, experimental aging research ideally uses a species with a relatively short life span. The problem with the study of human material is thus not only to find procedures where the postmortem changes are kept minimal; in order to compensate for the high individual variability of the structures and progress of age-related changes, a large amount of specimens and objects have to be examined. We have evaluated the brain macroscopically, the size and number of neurons microscopically and the synapses and microvessels by electron microscopy. All pathological changes, including presenile dementia (Alzheimer disease), have been omitted from our investigation.

Studies of Human Brain Aging Require Extensive Evaluations

The modern procedures of stereology allow not only to estimate the total brain size but also the volume fractions of the various parts of the brain. It is now possible to determine whether the various parts of the brain undergo changes at the same rate or if they are aging in different manners and at different speeds.

Physiological investigations have opened new vistas on human brain aging that relate to morphological results. All efforts to enlarge our knowledge on aging require sensitive techniques and large quantities of material. This means that future investigation of aging in the human brain will lead to increasing expense. Both the high variability of human brain and the changes of tissue during preparation affect the results of studies on the aging process.

To give an idea about figures, the macroscopic reports in this chapter are from individuals 20 to 100 years old. The age-related changes are based on 1,130 brain weights

Stereological Procedures in the Morphometry of the Brain   BOX 18–1

Morphometric problems arise from the ratio of section thickness to structural size (Figure 18–1). In addition, nearly all preparative procedures are influenced by the histological shrinkage, by the treatment during staining, and by the variability of section thickness or physical focus depth. The latter depends on the optical aperature used. This leads always to a procedural bias in the results. A certain degree of shrinkage is found during plastic embedding also (Dethlefsen, 1988).

With stereology it is possible to minimize the error of estimation. The term *stereology* was introduced by Elias, Haug *et al.* in the 70's, but some stereological procedures had been introduced much earlier, by Floderus, in 1944. Further procedures were developed by Weibel in 1979 and in the last years by Gundersen *et al.* In the last years *dissector procedures* were introduced which are 'bias free' at least in regard to the correct mathematical basis (Gundersen *et al.*, 1988). However Pover and Coggeshall (1991) found that even the dissector procedures show unexpected variabilities of the results; some technical procedures have been developed further to circumvent the morphometrical bias (Clarke, 1993; Duyckaerts *et al.*, 1994; Witelson *et al.*, 1992, and others). I am astonished that in most 'bias free' papers nothing is said about the preparative influences. However, one can easily understand why the various authors who measured correctly found different sizes

in their samples. Today these differences are relatively small within a size range of about 20 percent. This range overlaps with the variation due to preparative shrinkage in our own investigation (Eggers *et al.*, 1981; Sass, 1982). We consequently regard the differences within the above range as similar.

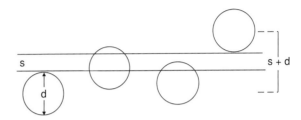

FIGURE 18–1

Particles of size *d* which are partly contained in a slice of thickness *s* have centers lying inside an outside of the slice. The visual aspect of 2-D profiles do not reflect 3-D size whether in number or in size. Therefore these particles can not simply be sampled without bias. A stereological correction of the morphometrical histological data is inherent. Arbitrary-shaped neurons, or spherical nuclei, all of variable size, hit by a 2-D section plane (knife blade) are seen in different appearance to their actual number and size present in the 3-D reference space. The sampling of taller structures in a slide leads to larger bias as of smaller ones.

---

and 22 human brains for the morphometry of the various parts. Morphometric analysis of neurons was performed on more than 150 human brains, 18 to 111 years old. We excluded all brains with signs of neuropathological changes. Nearly 300 evaluations in four cortical areas and the striatum were performed. In each area, 1,500–2,000 neurons were estimated in all layers. Each cell was measured semi-automatically over the drawing mirror of a microscope with a computerized digitizer (Haug, 1976). The following data were stored on computer diskettes: Number and type of neurons and glial cells, size of perikaryon of both cells and the gravity coordinates of each cell. The latter values allow the construction of artificial cytoarchitectonic figures by the computer (Haug, 1979; Schmitt *et al.*, 1995).

We examined neuron densities and sizes in cortical parts with different functions in both genders. A total of four areas (Brodmann, 1909) and one subcortical griseum were measured. Their functional meaning is as follows (Haug *et al.*, 1984): Area 6 in the convexity of the frontal lobe has according to Eccles (1982) an extrapyramidal function; area 11 in the orbital section of the frontal lobe is a typical human area and linked with psychosocial functions; area 7 in the convexity of the parietal lobe operates in the sensory and especially speech analysis; area 17 or visual cortex in the occipital lobe performs analysis

of visual input; the *corpus striatum* is important for the performance of movements within the extrapyramidal system (Eggers and Haug, 1989).

The influence of procedures on the results is important. We found that the shrinkage of brain tissue depends on the individual age. The difference between the fresh, unfixed brain volume and the morphometrically evaluated section is called residual volume (Haug, 1984; Eggers *et al.*, 1981; Sass, 1982). The residual volume of the histological section is expressed in percent fresh volume of the brain tissue (after brain removal and before fixation). Figure 18–2 shows the size of the volume changes during embedding using methyl-benzoate as an intermedium. The shrinkage in the younger individuals is high, and low in the older individuals. This is probably caused by a decreasing water content of the brain tissue (Desbordes and Cohadon, 1987).

The magnitude of shrinkage affects the density of measured neurons. The higher shrinkage of the younger individuals leads to a higher density of neurons because the microscopic distances between the neurons are smaller. The difference in shrinkage during embedding amounts to about 15 percent, when we compare 20 and 75 year old brain material. If we do not observe this fact, we have consequently a 15 percent lower neuron density in the aged individuals as compared to younger ones. The age

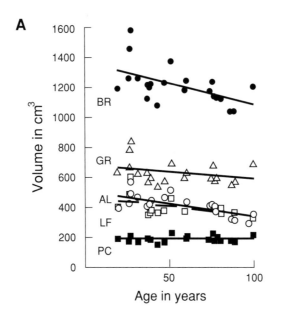
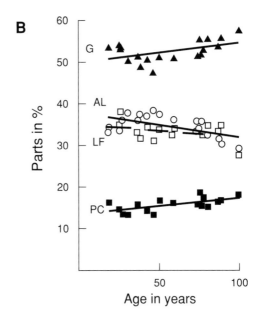

FIGURE 18–4

The absolute (A) and relative (B) volume changes of the brain parts. The latter are expressed in percentage of the individual human brains. Abbreviations: BR = entire brain (equals 100%);

GR or G = griseum; AL = Album, LF = Frontal lobe (including the white matter); PC = postcentral convexity from parietal and temporal cerebral cortex.

occipital lobe (CO) do not change its proportional volume.

The brain stem (mesencephalon and myelencephalon) (BS) ages similarly as the entire brain. The ventricles increase in weight by 150 to 200 percent. This fact is well known. It is necessary to mention that the volume parts of the ventricles are not contained in the 100 percent of the brain. Sullivan and colleagues (1995) have examined with magnetic resonance imaging (MRI) the volumina of the hippocampus and the temporal lobe. However, because they measured after their fig. 1 only a restricted region of the brain, it is questionable if they have examined the entire temporal lobe. After their fig. 1 they have estimated the hippocampus correctly and did not find any volume decline for the hippocampus. They found a slight significant right-left difference. Otherwise, the temporal lobe shows a certain diminution in volume, which is in contrast to our own results. I think this difference in results is due to the restricted evaluation of the brain and the difficulty to determine the border between temporal and occipital lobe.

In summary, the various regions of the brain undergo different macroscopic alterations during aging. This also applies to the cerebral cortex, where the frontal cortex has the tendency to decline. In contrast in the parieto-occipital cortex the changes are only minute. These results are probably connected with the functional use of the cortical grays: While the sensory input still connects the social surrounding with the life of the elderly, the motor activity decreases mostly in the higher age. The macroscopic decrease of the white matter (AL) is about twice to three-fold that of the gray matter (GR); after Meier-Ruge and col-

leagues (1992) this is probably caused by the diminution of the diameters of myelinated fibers (Chapter 21).

Microscopic Changes Vary Greatly Depending on Areal Cytoarchitectonics and Functional Specialization

This chapter will concentrate on the isocortical part of the human cortex cerebri. The aging of dendrites and neurotransmitters will only be discussed. All pathological changes, are omitted from our investigation. A set of observations made by using stereological procedures have shed new light on the problem, indicating that diminution of neuron size, rather than neuron loss, is the main change in normal human brain aging.

A pure random selection of samples for microscopic evaluation is only useful for tissues with an uniform function such as lung and liver. However, the cytoarchitectonic and functional specialization of the different brain parts creates the need for the morphometric evaluation in selected locations. Within such locations, samples may be also evaluated in a randomized way. In the cortex cerebri we perform randomized measurements in parallel strips or ribbons arranged perpendicularly to the cortical surface (Haug, 1979). The advantage of this procedure is the possibility to evolve artificial cytoarchitectonic charts (Haug, 1986) and calculate neuron distances, examine neighborhood questions, and collect further information on the internal structural composition (Schmitt et al., 1995a, 1995b). Another very important aspect must be taken into account in the morphometric evaluation of the brain cortex, namely the fact that the number and size of neu-

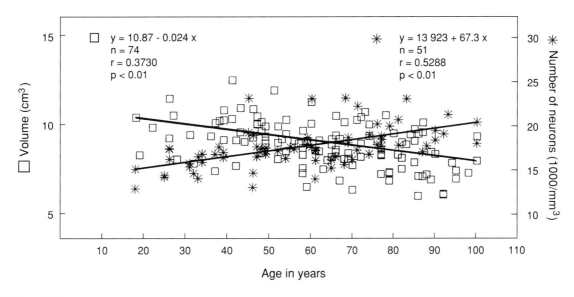

FIGURE   18–5

The connection between volume changes of the neostriatum (open squares) and neuronal density (asterisks) in the aging striatum. Both regressions are with $p < 0.01$ highly significant. (Eggers and Haug, 1989).

rons vary greatly within a population. Therefore, our estimates are based on measurements of at least 50 brains for
each area. Because the shrinkage of the tissue during histological treatment are a major source of bias (Eggers *et
al.*, 1981; Sass, 1982), all results of microscopy must be
corrected for fresh or unfixed brain as well.

Eggers [personal communication and Eggers and Haug
(1989)] describes in Figure 18–5 the connection between
neuronal density and the changes in volume of the *neostriatum* during aging. The volume was estimated by the
Cavalieri principle (Gundersen *et al.*, 1988), and the density of neurons, counted as usual in the same neostriatum, was expressed in $1,000/mm^3$. The lines of linear regression have the same, though inverse steepness. The
absolute volume was found to decrease by 12 percent between 40 and 90 years. The entire brain volume diminishes by 10 percent. The volume decrease is followed
by a density increase because the neurons move together.
The neuronal size decreases inverse to the density increase. Eggers calculated the total number of neurons in
the neostriatum from the density and volume figures of
this nucleus. The total number of nerve cells with the

usual variance is constant during the life: 120 million
(Eggers and Haug, 1989).

*Increased Neuronal Density Reflects the Diminution
of Gray and Cell Volume with Aging*

The volume of a cortical area itself cannot be estimated
directly, because the borders of an area are unrecognizable
in the macroscopic level. The density of neurons increases in all areas (Figure 18–6A) and their perikaryal size
decreases (Figure 18–6B) with aging. This behavior is
found in different degrees in most grays (Haug and Eggers,
1991). Area 6 shows the striking result that the increase
of neuron density per mm^3 is very high (Haug *et al.*,
1984, 1984). The sensory area 7 has an increasing pattern
similar to that of the psychosocial area 11. Area 17 (visual
cortex) presents an increase as well. The changes of the
neuronal size, estimated by the microscopic projection
area, are seen in Figure 18–6, B. The supplementary motor cortex, area 6, exhibits a striking degree of diminution
of neuron size during aging, with a remarkable decrease
of the neuronal perikaryal size. The visual area 17 shows

TABLE **18–2**   Mean values (MV) and statistics of the results regarding neuronal densities and sizes
in four human cortical areas during aging. DEN, density in 1,000 per mm^3. SIZE, size of
perikaryon in μm^2. Significant changes ($p < 0,05$) printed in bold.

AREA		6			7			11			17	
	n	DEN	SIZE	n	DEN	SIZE	n	DEN	SIZE	n	DEN	SIZE
MV	67	15,0	211,5	51	23,1	133,2	60	22,1	139,2	50	41,3	91,6
MV<65	43	**14,6**	**225,7**	32	22,6	136,0	39	21,6	**146,9**	33	40,1	93,9
MV>64	24	**15,8**	**186,1**	19	23,8	128,4	21	23,0	**126,9**	17	43,6	87,0
female	19	**17,4**	**192,8**	6	**27,8**	117,7	23	**24,7**	134,8	3	**48,7**	79,5
male	48	**14,1**	**218,9**	45	**22,4**	135,2	37	**20,8**	141,6	47	**40,8**	92,4

thin section were equal in the areas 6, 7 and 11 (Haug et al., 1989).

Figure 18–8 shows the changes in number of synapses in an arbitrary area, in three different areas. The linear regression has in area 6 an insignificant progress with p = 0,87. The other areas have a highly significant decrease with p < 0,0001. The amount in area 6 is highly variable, but the synapses do not diminish. Nevertheless, this result indicates an actual decrease in number of synapses per neuron, because in this area 6 the neuron density (Figure 18–6, A) increases by over 18 percent. This means that a loss of synapses per neuron is possible in the magnitude of about 20 percent. In contrast to the small changes in the macroscopic and microscopic levels, area 7 exhibits a distinct numerical decrease of synapses in the magnitude of 10 to 15 percent. However, the neuron density increases only a little, so that the number of synapses per neuron diminishes similarly to area 6. In Area 11 the decrease of synapses with age is a bit stronger than that observed in area 7. A loss of about 20 percent per neuron results from the analysis of the density increase in both areae. Similar observations were published by Adams and Jones (1987), Masliah and colleagues (1993), and Saito and colleagues (1994).

The electron microscopic results show that in the synaptic level the aging process is independent from the stability of neuron number. This fact provides a possible explanation why the functional use of cortical structures inhibits the involution usually associated with aging. The synapses are dynamic structures with a certain plasticity (Eccles, 1979). Our own investigation as well as those of Huttenlocher (1979), Uemura (1985), Bertoni-Freddari and colleagues (1993), and Jones and Calverley (1992) demonstrate that the density of synapses decreases with higher age. However, in many cases elderly people live in an impoverished situation before their death. This might lead to a loss of synapses, in combination with restrictions imposed by bad health. In our material we did no get information on the situation of the elderly before death. It is unknown, for example, if the material includes individuals who were a longer time in a restricted surrounding, like in a nursing home for elderly. Probably the high variability of numbers is due to the great differences in the *premortem* living situation.

Cerebral Capillaries Undergo Minor Changes During Normal Aging

The capillaries of the brain are also relatively well preserved if the fixation is performed within about 48 hours after the death. This is especially due to the stability of the basal lamina. We have estimated the capillaries in 515 electron microscopes of 45 cortical samples (19 from area 7 and 26 from area 11). Only in 4 individuals both areas were evaluated. A total of 43 individuals aged between 19 and 96 years were studied. 23 estimations came from females and 24 from males. We selected a few structures (out of 50 measured details) for the sake of the present discussion (for details see Haug et al., 1991; Weis et

al., 1990; Weis and Haug, 1989). The capillary including the pericytes are surrounded by the basal lamina. In the entire capillary we evaluated the total area, the diameter of the capillary and of the lumen, as well as the areal fraction of lipofuscin in the capillaries. In the endothelial cells we measured the area and thickness. In the pericytes we reported on the area and number per capillary. We also observed the thickness of the basal lamina and counted the number of the different vacuoles within the basal lamina (Weis and Haug, 1989). In the beginning we have differentiated between 4 types of empty and filled vacuoles. However, since they have a similar behavior, we combined them under one general type. The results of our analyses did not show any statistical differences in the various sizes, neither for age nor for gender nor for area 7 and 11. Only the number of vacuoles increased in the older age group above 65 years, with a high statistical significance (Figure 18–9). This possibly influences the stability of the basal lamina that decreases with age. It is unknown if this change can influence the function of the blood-brain-barrier (Rapoport, 1994).

The results of our measurements demonstrate that the cerebral capillaries have only minor changes during aging. This fact was unexpected. Later on, Heinsen and Heinsen (1983), Hennerici (1995), Kalaria (1994), Peters and colleagues (1991), and Burns and colleagues (1983) reported relatively similar results both in humans and monkeys. Probably the rats show more important changes (Atkinson et al., 1992). We conclude that the most changes within the cerebral vessels do not regard the capillaries. Rather, vascular changes are often observed in the smaller and thicker parts of the arterioles and venules, in addition to the changes frequently observed in large vessels (Chapter 27). We did not investigate individuals with diabetes or neurological diseases like Alzheimer or cerebro-vascular dementia.

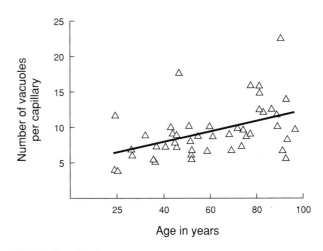

FIGURE   18–9

Age and brain capillaries. The number of vacuoles in the capillary basement membrane of the human cortex (area 7 and 11) tend to increase with aging.

The Functional Meaning of Areal Differences

The results of Haug (1990, 1991), Chui and colleagues (1984), Leuba and Kraftsik (1994), and Terry (1992), in the human brain; and Curcio and Coleman (1982), Pakkenberg and colleagues (1995), Peters and colleagues (1994), and Voytko and colleagues (1995), in monkeys and rats led to dedicated insights into the morphological and functional changes of the aging brain. Our measurements were made only in brains without signs of psychological or pathological illness. The different localization of our samples allow a first statement. The various locations within the brain age very differently. However, the aging behavior of neurons shows some similarities in locations with similar function. This can be observed in the major brain systems such as the motor, the sensory and the association cortices.

Aging does not Invariably Lead to Neuron Loss

Even today, some scientists still believe that increasing numbers of neurons will be invariably lost throughout the life span of an individual. This belief is founded on research published about 50 years ago. The basis was the work of Brody (1955). At this time the preparative shrinkage and the influence of the section's thickness on counting neurons were unknown. Scientists did not observe both facts. Brody expressed his view in vague terms because his statistical basis was too small for a definite statement. However, subsequent interpretations by other scientists and in the press have created the conviction that neurons are lost throughout life. About 20 to 30 years ago, this interpretation led to the opinion that the dementia of aging people begins at about 40 years. In some American companies, managers above 40 years were dismissed. However, the lack of experience of the younger managers caused problems within the companies. After only a few years this nonsense was totally stopped. Wickelgren (1996) gives a critical statement on the present dispute regarding the neuron loss in human brain during aging. She reports on an increasing number of papers which neglect a loss of neurons in the human cortex cerebri beginning with Haug and colleagues (1984) and Terry and colleagues (1987). Wickelgren reports as well on results with magnetic resonance imaging (MRI). Some scientists think that the decrease of gray volume leads to a loss of neurons. But, our results demonstrates clearly that the neuron density increases in order to compensate for the volume decrease of the grays. MRI shows as well that the volume decrease in aging is in the white matter higher than in the gray matter.

Reports on centenarians (Hauw *et al.*, 1986; Mizutani, 1992) have shown that nearly 50 percent of the centenarians have relatively high brain weights and that the incidence of Alzheimer disease is unexpectedly low in this group of patients. Possibly this is a kind of selection, since individuals with illnesses are likely to depart before their 100th year of age (Riggs, 1992). It is probable that the time and speed of aging are dependent on a genetic program.

However, it is evident that the generally determined timetable of age changes occurring in the various parts of the cerebral cortex may be slowed or accelerated. This depends on the degree of functional use, and the use is connected with the psychosocial environment. From this viewpoint we can understand why individuals who work beyond the normal retirement age retain their mental ability.

Changes in Motor Cortices and Neostriatum Begin Relatively Early

Aging differs in time, extent, and rate for the gray matter of different regions. However, we see in any localization a certain conformity of the results. The human cerebral cortex show in all examined levels only small changes before the age of 60–65 years. The motor cortex is an exception. Changes in the human supplementary motor cortex and the neostriatum begin relatively early, possibly at about 40 years (Eggers and Haug, 1989; Haug and Eggers, 1991). Everybody knows that sport records are limited by the age. Both grays are part of the extrapyramidal motor function that acts upon the course of the movement (Eccles, 1982). This concerns the macroscopic decrease of the frontal lobe (LF, in Figure 18–4,) and the neurons in area 6 (Figure 18–6); and neostriatum (Figure 18–5). Both have a high neuronal density increase and a distinct decrease of size (Table 18–2).

Higher Sensory Processes are Preserved up to Advanced Ages in the Parietal Cortex

Area 7 (PC, in Figure 18–4 and Table 18–1) is very different from area 6. Age changes of this area in the convexity of the parietal lobe begin late in life. This area plays an important function in higher sensory processes. During aging the convexity of the parietal lobe does not diminish in volume and has an increase of its percentage in the brain. A lifelong high sensibility is important for the daily life and this is probably the reason of the few age-changes up to high ages.

Area 17 or the visual cortex is located in the occipital cortex. The decrease in size is insignificant because the variability is high. The increase of neuronal density is highly significant, but the diminution of neuron sizes is relatively minute.

Psychosocial Functions of the Basal Prefrontal Cortex are Maintained Until Retirement Age

Psychosocial functions are regulated in the basal prefrontal cortex. In the area 11, located within the *sulcus rectus,* a special neuronal behavior is found. The neurons have no significant changes until retirement age. After the age of 65 the perikaryon size diminishes and a density increase is noticed (Table 18–2).

The 'Use It or Lose It' Paradigm Applies for the Aging Brain

Cortical dendrites generally diminish in their length, and each neuron loses about 15 to 20 percent of its synapses in an age-dependent fashion. However, neurons sprout sometimes in late adulthood as well as during exercises in higher age (Coleman and Flood, 1992; Flood, 1993). After Ehrenberg and Pöhl (1954), and Rance and colleagues (1993), a size increase of larger neurons is observed in the 60's. After this age these neurons diminish in size. Pyapali and Turner (1996) measured the extent of the dendrites in rat CA1 hippocampal neurons. The total dendritic length of the apical and basal dendrites is in the aged animal longer as in the younger ones. This is probably due to a functional plasticity of the system. Brizzee and colleagues (1983) and Schlote and Boellaard (1983) published equivalent results on lipofuscin. These observations have led to an increasing amount of papers dealing with plasticity.

For the neuronal plasticity in advanced ages including the changes in number and size of neurons and synapses speak mainly the experiments with aged rats. Such experiments were originally performed by a Californian group, being then followed by others (Diamond and Connor, 1982; Gool et al., 1987; Black et al., 1987; Saito et al., 1994; Lowenthal, 1994; Pyapali and Turner, 1996). They demonstrated that environment exerts a strong influence on the aging process. Older rats were housed in narrow cages comparable to the restricted environment of some nursing homes for the elderly. After a certain time they had a considerable loss of synapses and synaptic spines in the cerebral cortex. However, rats identical in age and breeding, though living in large cages with an enriched environment together with rats of every age, revealed no loss of synapses after the same period of observation. The results of experiments with enriched environments demonstrate that neuronal structures can regenerate also up to high age. The presupposition is that the neuron itself is intact.

These findings suggest the following. The use of cortical connections permits the conservation of the structure and their functions. According to present knowledge, the dynamic features of synapses are important, because these structures can degenerate in the case of reduced use. They are able to rebuild themselves in case of increasing demand for use. This is not a new phenomenon as it is known that muscles that are not used undergo hypotrophy and will regenerate after exercise.

The evidence as well as the long conservation of the sensory cerebral cortex speaks for the fact, that the 'use it or lose it' paradigm is a profound truth (Haug and Eggers, 1991; Swaab, 1991a, b). It is well known in human psychology that work and activity helps to conserve mental ability (Baltes, 1989). We can now understand that some active older men had influenced the political decisions in a consequent and positive way. On the other hand, the sensory cortical areas are usually preserved in the elderly, even if used in an environment of poor quality.

An Overall View

The morphometric investigation of the brain is difficult. This situation is created by the complicated brain structures, which developed during phylogenesis, and the increasing functional complexity. The complexity is faced in all levels of investigations, from macroscopy to electron microscopy. Furthermore, the various locations participate in different degrees in the specific functions. Consequently each efficient examination must be performed in a location of functional significance. The functional neurobiological aspect is important for any scientific investigation including the aging changes. A random selection within the entire brain is less valuable for qualitative and quantitative results. The presented results show a high difference in the aging behavior and underline the necessity of examinations in different functional locations.

Every morphometric investigator intends to obtain results as accurate as possible. But this is difficult, because various factors influence the results. These are the pre- and postmortem changes often unknown or neglected. Furthermore, the preparative influences are seldom examined, presumably because scientists are usually eager to obtain results to the main question. They do not like long examinations of the preparative changes in the tissues. Consequently, the different results in the literature arise often from preparation and measurement procedures. We have demonstrated the importance of preparative changes by the age dependent shrinkage of the brain tissue (Haug et al., 1984).

The results of our investigation indicate that the aging processes are different in the various parts of the brain. The different cortical lobes show a diminution beginning in the 60's that is very small in the parietal lobe and distinct in the frontal lobe. During normal aging no neurons in the cerebral cortex are lost, but a diminution of neuron size can be observed with different degrees in the various areas. The numbers of synapses per neuron decrease with age, too. The frontal lobe cortex with the specific human function for activity and behavior is more affected by aging than the parieto-occipto-temporal lobe. These parts of the brain are responsible for the connection of the individual with its environment. Our findings have implications for the debate on retirement age. The long stability of this brain part speaks for 'Use It or Lose It' and not for 'Wear and Tear'.

Selected Readings

Desbordes, P., and Cohadon, F. 1987. Brain water and aging. J. Gerontol. 42:655–659.

Flood, D. G. 1993. Critical issues in the analysis of dendritic extent in aging humans, primates, and rodents. Neurobiol. Aging 14:649–654.

Gundersen, H. J. G., Bagger, P., Bendtsen, T. F., et al. 1988. The new stereological tools: Dissector, fractionator, nucleator and point sampled intercepts and their use in pathological research and diagnosis. APMIS 96:857–881.

Haug, H. 1986. History of neuromorphometry. J. Neurosci. Meth. 18:1–17.

Haug, H., and Eggers, R. 1994. Das menschliche Gehirn – Gewicht, Alterung und säkulare Akzeleration. Ann. Anat. 176, Suppl. 171.

Haug, H., Kühl, S., Mecke, E., Sass, N.-L., and Wasner, K. 1984. The significance of morphometric procedures in the investigation of age changes in the cytoarchitectonic structures of human brain. J. Hirnforsch. 25:353–374.

Haug, H., and Eggers, R. 1991. Morphometry of the human cortex cerebri and corpus striatum during aging: Neurobiol. Aging 12:336–338.

Huttenlocher, P. R. 1979. Synaptic density in human frontal cortex – developmental changes and effects of aging. Brain Res. 163:195–205.

Leuba, G., and Kraftsik, R. 1994. Changes in volume, surface estimate, three-dimensional shape and total number of neurons of the human primary visual cortex from midgestation until old age: Anat. Embryol. 190:351–366.

Saito, S., Kobayashi, S., Ohashi, Y., Igarashi, M., Komiya, Y., and Ando, S. 1994. Decreased synaptic density in aged brains and its prevention by rearing under enriched environment as revealed by synaptophysin contents. J. Neurosci. Res. 39:57–62.

Swaab, D. F. 1991a. Brain aging and Alzheimer's disease, 'wear and tear' versus 'use it or lose it'. Neurobiol. Aging 12:317–324.

Swaab, D. F. 1991b. Author's response to commentaries. Neurobiol. Aging 12:352–355.

Wickelgren I. (1996). The aging brain. For the cortex, neuron loss may be less than thought. Science 273, 48–50.

Witelson, S. F., Kigar, D. L., and McKanna, J. A. 1992. A computer-assisted direct-imaging system to obtain numerical densities of neurons in human cortex. Brain Res. Bull. 29:441–447.

References

Adams, I., and Jones, D. G. 1987. Effects of normal and pathological aging on brain morphology: Neurons and synapses: 1–84. Current topics in research on synapses,Vol.4. Alan R. Liss.

Atkinson, J., Lartaud, I., and Capdeville-Atkinson, C. 1992. Age-related changes in regulation of cerebral blood flow: Presse Med., 21:1227–1230.

Baltes, P. B. 1989. Erfolgreiches Altern: Mehr Jahre und mehr Leben. In P. B. Baltes, Jahrestagung der Deutschen Gesellschaft für Gerontologie (Sektion 3: Psychologie und Sozialwissenschaften). Berlin.

Bertoni-Freddari, C., Fattoretti, P., Casoli, T., et al. 1993. Morphological plasticity of synaptic mitochondria during aging. Brain Res. 628:193–200.

Black, J. E., Greenough, W. T., Anderson, B. J., and Isaacs, K. R. 1987. Environment and the aging brain. Can. J. Psychol., 41:111–130.

Bloom, F. E., and Aghajanian, G. K. 1968, Fine structural and cytochemical analysis of the staining of synaptic junctions with phosphotungist acid. J. Ultrastruct. Res., 22:361–375.

Brizzee, K. R., Samorajski, T., Brizzee, D. L., et al. 1983. Age pigments and cell loss in the mammalian nervous system: Functional implications. Aging 21:211–229.

Brodmann, K. 1909. Vergleichende Lokalisationslehre der Grohirnrinde. Leipzig, J. A. Barth.

Brody, H. 1955. Organization of the cerbral cortex. III. A study of aging in the human cerbral cortex. J. Comp. Neurol., 102:511–556.

Burns, E. M., Kruckeberg, T. W., Gaetano, P. K., and Shulman, L. M. 1983. Morphological changes in cerebral capillaries with age. Aging 21:115–132.

Chui, H. C., Bondareff, W., Zarow, C., and Slager, U. 1984. Stability of neuronal number in the human nucleus basalis of Meynert with age. Neurobiol. Aging 5:83–88.

Clarke, P. G. H. 1993. An unbiased correction factor for cell counts in histological sections. J. Neurosci. Meth. 49:133–140.

Coleman, P. D., and Flood, D. G. 1992. Proliferation and involution of dendrites in normal aging and Alzheimer's disease. In K. Fujisawa, and Y. Morimatsu (eds.) Development and Involution of Neurones, pp. 235–247. Japan Scientific Societies Press: Tokyo.

Curcio, C. A., and Coleman, P. D. 1982. Stability of neuron number in cortical barrels of aging mice. J. Comp. Neurol. 212:158–172.

Dani, S. U. 1994. Larger neuronal size overwhelms maintenance capacity with aging. Med. Hypotheses 42:208–210.

Dani, S. U., Pittella, J. E. H., Hori, A., et al. 1994. Different rates of neuronal degeneration: An exquisite variation of the 'cascade' hypothesis. Dementia 5:110–118.

Dani, S. U., Pittella, J. E. H., Boehme, A., Hori, A., Schneider, B. 1997. Progressive formation of neuritic plaques and neurofibrillary tangles in exponentially related to age and neuronal size: A morphometric study of three geographically distinct series of aging people. Dementia and Geriatric Cognitive Disorders 8:217–227.

Desbordes, P., and Cohadon, F. 1987. Brain water and aging. J. Gerontol. 42:655–659.

Dethlefsen, J. F. 1988. Mikroskopisch-morphometrische Untersuchung des Einflusses verschiedener Einbettverfahren auf die Groesse von Nervenzellen der Hirnrinde sowie eine Analyse der Perikarion-Kern-Volumenverhältnisse für verschieden grosse Nervenzellen. Diss., Medical University, Lübeck.

Diamond, M. C., and Connor, J. R. J. 1982. Plasticity of the aging cerebral cortex. In S. Hoyer (ed.) Physiological and Pathophysiological Aspects, pp. 36–44. Springer Verlag, Berlin, Heidelberg, New York.

Duyckaerts, C., Godefroy, G., and Hauw, J.-J. 1994. Evaluation of neuronal numerical density by Dirichlet tessellation. J. Neurosci. Meth. 51:47–69.

Eccles, J. C. 1982. The initation of voluntary movements by supplementary motor area. Arch. Psychiatr. Nervenkr. 231:423–441.

Eccles, J. C. 1979. Synaptic plasticity. Naturwissenschaften 66:147–153.

Eggers, R., and Haug, H. 1989. Morphometry of aging human neostriatum. Bulletin de Association des Anatomistes, pp. 33–34.

Eggers, R., Haug, H., and Kunkel, M. 1987. Altersveränderungen des Volumens des menschlichen Corpus striatum und seiner Nervenzelldichte. Anat. Anz. (Jena) 163:149.

Eggers, R., Haug, H., and Manfeldt, H. 1981. Ueber die Grösse der Einbettungsschrumpfung und ihren Einfluss auf die Ergebnisse morphometrischer Untersuchungen. Acta Anat. 111:37–38.

Ehrenberg, R. and Pöhl, M. 1954. Altersgänge in der Grosshirnrinde des Menschen. Z. Naturforsch., v. 9b:796–798.

Elias, H., Hennig, A., and Schwartz, D. E. 1971. Stereology: Application to biomedical research. Physiol. Rev. 51:158–200.

Elias, H., and Hyde, D. M. 1983. A guide to practical stereology. Basel-New York, Karger.

Floderus, S. 1944. Untersuchungen über den Bau der menschlichen Hypophyse mit besonderer Berücksichtigung der quantitativen mikromorphologischen Verhältnisse. Acta Pathol. Microbiol. Scand., Suppl, 53.

Flood, D. G. 1993. Critical issues in the analysis of dendritic extent in aging humans, primates, and rodents. Neurobiol. Aging 14:649–654.

Göser, G. 1997. Postmortale Veränderungen im Lobus parietalis der Ratte. Eine elektronenmikroskopische Untersuchung mit morphometrischer Bestimmung der Synapsendichte und deren Grössenverteilung bei unterschiedlicher Präparation. Diss., Medical University, Lübeck.

Gool, W. A. v., Pronker, H. F., Mirmiran, M., and Uylings, H. B. M. 1987. Effect of housing in an enriched environment of the size of the cerebral cortex in young and old rats. Exp. Neurol. 96:225–232.

Gundersen, H. J. G., Bagger, P., Bendtsen, T. F., et al. 1988. The new stereological tools: Disector, fractionator, nucleator and point sampled intercepts and their use in pathological research and diagnosis. APMIS 96:857–881.

Haug, H. 1967. Number of particles per unit volume. In H. P. Elias (ed.) Stereology. Proceedings of the Second International Congress for Stereology, pp. 199–210. Springer INC: New York.

Haug, H. 1976. Experiences with optomanual automated evaluation-systems in biological research, especially in neuromorphometry. In E. E. Underwood, R. de Wit, and G. A. Moore (eds.) Proceedings of the Fourth International Congress for Stereology, Gaitherburg, pp. 167–172. U.S. Gouvernment Printing Office: Washington D.C.

Haug, H. 1979. Nervous tissue. In E. R. Weibel (ed.) Stererological methods – Practical methods for biological morphometry, v.1 (8):311–322. Academic Press: New York, London.

Haug, H. 1981. Die Evolution der Interneurone in der Hirnrinde von Affen und Delphinen sowie ihre Bedeutung für komplexe Funktionen einschliesslich der Sprache. Nova Acta Leopoldina N. F. 54:245,763–777.

Haug, H. 1984a. Der Einfluss der säkularen Acceleration auf das Hirngewicht des Menschen und dessen Änderung während der Alterung. Morph. J. B. (Leipz.) 130:481–500.

Haug, H. 1984b. Macroscopic and microscopic morphometry of the human brain and cortex: A survey in the light of new results. Brain Pathol. 1:123–149.

Haug, H. 1985. Are neurons of the human cerebral cortex really lost during aging? A morphometric examination. In J. Traber, and W. H. Gispen (eds.) Senile dementia of the Alzheimer type, pp. 150–163. Springer, Berlin Heidelberg.

Haug, H. 1986. History of neuromorphometry. J. Neurosci. Meth. 18:1–17.

Haug, H. 1989. The aging human cerebral cortex: Morphometry of areal differences and their functional meaning. In D. Platt (ed.) Gerontology, pp. 139–158. Springer, Berlin-Heidelberg.

Haug, H. 1990. Morphometric evaluation of the aged human brain. Changes in volume of various grays, in the neuronal composition and ultrastructure. 74 XIth International Congress of Neuropathology W-13-4. International Society of Neuropathology: Kyoto, Japan.

Haug, H. 1991. Aging of the brain. In F. C. Ludwig (ed.) Life Span Extension. Consequencies and Open Questions. pp. 55–67. Springer Publishing Company: New York.

Haug, H., Barmwater, U., Eggers, R., et al. 1983. Anatomical changes in aging brain: Morphometric analysis of the human prosencephalon. Aging 21:1–12.

Haug, H., and Eggers, R. 1991. Morphometry of the human cortex cerebri and corpus striatum during aging. Neurobiol. Aging 12:336–338.

Haug, H., and Eggers, R. 1994. Das menschliche Gehirn – Gewicht, Alterung und säkulare Akzeleration. Ann. Anat. 176, Suppl. 171.

Haug, H., Knebel, G., and Lodd, M. 1989. Die Dichte der Synapsen im menschlichen Cortex. Eine Untersuchung zur Alterung der Areae 6 und 7. Ver. Anat. Ges. 82:895–897.

Haug, H., Kühl, S., Mecke, E., Sass, N.-L., and Wasner, K. 1984. The significance of morphometric procedures in the investigation of age changes in the cytoarchitectonic structures of human brain. J. Hirnforsch. 25:353–374.

Haug, H., Weis, S., Eller, S., and Knebel, G. 1991. Die Alterung der Kapillaren der menschlichen Hirnrinde. Immunhistochemische, elektronenmikroskopische und morphometrische Untersuchungen. Ver. Anat. Ges. 84:643–645.

Hauw, J.-J., Vignolo, P., Duyckaerts, C., et al. 1986. Étude neuropathologique de 12 centenaires: La fréquence de la démence sénile de type Alzheimer n'est pas particulièrement élevée dans ce groupe de personnes trés âgées. Rev. Neurol. (Paris) 142:107–115.

Heinsen, H., and Heinsen, Y. L. 1983. Cerebral capillaries. Qualitative and quantitative observations in young and senile rats. Anat. Embryol. 168:101–116.

Hennerici, M. 1995. Vascular dementia: A changing concept: Arzneimittelforschung 45:366–370.

Ho, K.-C., Roessmann, U., Straumfjord, J. V., and Monroe, G. 1980. Analysis of brain weight. I. Adult brain weight in relation to sex, race, and age. (pp. 635–639) II. Adult brain weight in relation to body height, weight, and suface area. (pp. 640–645). Arch. Pathol. Lab. Med. 104:635–645.

Holubek, B. 1994. Makroskopisch-stereologische Untersuchungen am menschlichen Gehirn mit einem Verfahren der semiautomatischen Bildanalyse unter Berücksichtigung von Altersveränderungen und Seitendifferenzen. Diss.: Medical University Lübeck.

Huttenlocher, P. R. 1979. Synaptic density in human frontal cortex – developmental changes and effects of aging. Brain Res. 163:195–205.

Inoue, T., and Otsu, S. 1987. Statistical analysis of the organ weights in 1,000 autopsy cases of japanese aged over 60 years. Acta Pathol. Jpn. 37:343–359.

Jones, D. G., and Calverley, R. K. S. 1992. Changes of synapses with age: The respective contributions of non-perforated and perforated synapses in neocortex. In K. Fujisawa, and Y. Morimatsu (eds.). Development and involution of neurones. pp. 249–262. Japan Scientific Societies Press: Tokyo.

Kalaria, R. N. 1994. Brain microvasculature in aging. Neurobiol. Aging 15:765–766.

Leuba, G., and Kraftsik, R. 1994. Changes in volume, surface estimate, three-dimensional shape and total number of neurons of the human primary visual cortex from midgestation until old age. Anat. Embryol. 190:351–366.

Lowenthal, D. T. 1994. Effects of exercise on age and disease. South. Med. J. 87:S42-S46.

Madeira, M. D., Sousa, N., Santer, R. M., Paula-Barbosa, M. M., and Gundersen, H. J. G. (1995). Age and sex do not affect the volume, cell number, or cell size of the suprachiasmatic nucleus: An unbiased stereological study. J. Comp. Neurol 361: 585–601.

Masliah, E., Mallory, M., Hansen, L., Deteresa, R., and Terry, R. D. 1993. Quantitative synaptic alterations in the human neocortex during normal aging. Neurology 43:192–197.

Medvedev, Z. A. 1991. The structural basis of aging. In F. C. Ludwig (ed.) Life span extension, pp. 9–17. Springer Puiblishing Company: New York.

Meier-Ruge, W., Ulrich, J., Brühlmann, M., and Meier, E. 1992. Age-related white matter atrophy in the human brain. Ann. N. Y. Acad. Sci. 673:260–269.

Mizutani, T. 1992. Neuropathology of the centenarian brains. In K. Fujisawa, and Y. Morimatsu (eds.) Development and involution of neurones. pp. 187–202. Japan Scientific societies Press: Tokyo.

Pakkenberg, B. 1993. Total nerve cell number in neocortex in chronic schizophrenics and controls estimated using optical disectors. Biol. Psychiatry 34:768–772.

Pakkenberg, H., Andersen, B.B., Burns, R.S. and Pakkenberg, B. (1995). A stereological study of substantia nigra in young and old rhesus monkeys. Brain Res. 693, 201–206.

Peters, A., Josephson, K., and Vincent, S. L. 1991. Effects of aging on the neuroglial cells and pericytes within area 17 of the rhesus monkey cerebral cortex. Anat. Rec. 229:384–398.

Peters, A., Leahu, D., Moss, M. B., and McNally, K. J. 1994. The effects of aging on area 46 of the frontal cortex of the rhesus monkey. Cereb. Cortex, 4:621–635.

Pover, C. M., and Coggeshall, R. E. 1991. Verification of the disector method for counting neurons, with comments on the empirical method. Anat. Rec. 231:573–578.

Pyapali, G.K. and Turner, D.A. 1996. Increased dendritic extend in hippocampal CA1 neurons from aged F344 rats. Neurobiol. Aging 17: 601–611.

Rance, N. E., Uswandi, S. V., and McMullen, N. T. 1993. Neuronal hypertrophy in the hypothalamus of older men. Neurobiol. Aging 14:337–342.

Rapoport, S. I. 1994. Aging and the blood-brain barrier. Neurobiol. Aging 15:759–760.

Regeur, L., Badsberg Jensen, G., Pakkenberg, H., et al. 1994. No global neocortical nerve cell loss in brains from patients with senile dementia of Alzheimer's type. Neurobiol. Aging 15:347–352.

Riggs, J. E. 1992. Aging and mortality: Manifestations of natural 'non-selection'. Mech. Ageing Dev. 62:127–135.

Saito, S., Kobayashi, S., Ohashi, Y., et al. 1994. Decreased synaptic density in aged brains and its prevention by rearing under enriched environment as revealed by synaptophysin contents. J. Neurosci. Res. 39:57–62.

Sass, N.-L. 1982. The age-dependent variation of the embedding-shrinkage of neurohistological sections. Mikroskopie (Wien) 39:278–281.

Schlenska, G. 1969. Messungen der Oberfläche und der Volumenanteile des Gehirnes menschlicher Erwachsener mit neuen Methoden. Z. Anat. Entwicklungsgesch. 128:47–59.

Schlote, W., and Boellaard, J. W. 1983. Role of lipopigment during aging of nerve and glial cells in the human nervous system. In J. Cervós-Navarro, and H. I. Sarkander (eds.) Brain Aging: Neuropathology and Neuropharmacology, pp. 27–74. Aging, 21. Raven Press: New York.

Schmitt, O., Eggers, R., and Haug, H. 1995a. Quantitative investigations into the histostructural nature of the human putamen. I. Staining, cell classification and morphometry. Ann. Anat. 177:243–250.

Schmitt, O., Eggers, R., and Haug, H. 1995b. Quantitative investigations into the histostructural nature of the human putamen. II. The differentiated topological distribution of certain neuron type arrangements. Ann. Anat. 177:455–465.

Sturrock, R. R. 1991, Stability of neuron number in the subthalamic and entopeduncular nuclei of the ageing mouse brain. J. Anat. 179:67–73.

Sturrock, R. R., and Rao, K. A. 1985. A quantitative histological study of neuronal loss from the locus coeruleus of ageing mice. Neuropathol. Appl. Neurobiol. 11:55–60.

Sullivan, E.V., Marsh L., Mathalon D.H., Lim K.O., and Pfefferbaum A. (1996). Age-related decline in MRI volumes of temporal lobe gray matter but not hippocampus. Neurobiol. Aging 16. 591–606.

Swaab, D. F. 1991a. Brain aging and Alzheimer's disease, 'wear and tear' versus 'use it or lose it'. Neurobiol. Aging 12:317–324.

Swaab, D. F. 1991b. Author's response to commentaries. Neurobiol. Aging 12:352–355.

Terry, R. D. 1992. Neuronal and synaptic loss in aging and in Alzheimer disease. In K. Fujisawa, and Y. Morimatsu (eds.) Development and involution of Neurones, pp. 219–226. Japan Scientific Societies Press, Tokyo.

Terry, R. D., Deteresa, R., and Hansen, L. A. 1987. Neocortical cell counts in normal human adult aging. Ann. Neurol. 21:530–539.

Uemura, E. 1985. Age-related changes in the subiculum of Macaca mulatta: 1. Synaptic density (403–411); 2. Dendritic branching pattern (412–427). Exp. Neurol. 87:403–427.

Uemura, E., and Hartmann, H. A. 1978. RNA content and volume of nerve cell bodies in human brain. I. Prefrontal cortex in aging normal and demented patient. Neuropathol. Exp. Neurol. 34:487–496.

v. Economo, C., and Koskinas, G. N. 1925. Die Cytoarchitektonik im Hirnrinde des Menschen. Eine makroskopisch-morphometrische Untersuchung. Wien und Berlin, Springer.

Vijayashankar, N., and Brody, H. 1977. A study of aging in the human Abducens nucleus. J. Comp. Neurol. 173:433–438.

Vijayashankar, N. and Brody, H. 1979, A quantitative study of the pigmented neurons in the nuclei Locus coeruleus and subcoeruleus in man as related to aging: J. Neuropath. Exp. Neurol. 38, 490–497.

Vogt, C., and Vogt, O. 1926. Die vergleichende architektonische und vergleichende reizphysiologische Felderung der Großhirnrinde mit besonderer Berücksichtigung der menschlichen. Naturwissenschaften 14:1190–1194.

Vogt, C., and Vogt, O. 1929. Über die Neuheit und den Wert des Pathoklisenbegriffes. J. Psychol. Neurol. 38:147–154.

Voytko, M. L., Sukhov, R. R., Walker, L. C., Breckler, S. J., Price, D. L., and Koliatsos, V. E. 1995. Neuronal number and size are preserved in the nucleus basalis of aged rhesus monkeys. Dementia 6:131–141.

Weibel, E. R. 1979. Stereological Methods: Vol. 1, Practical methods for biological morphometry. London, Academic Press.

Weis, S., and Haug, H. 1989. Capillaries of the human cerebral cortex: A quantitative electronmicroscopical study. Acta Stereol. 8:139–144.

Weis, S., Haug, H., Mittwede, T., et al. 1990. Stereologische Untersuchungen zur Mikrovaskularisation der Hirnrinde. Ein Vergleich zwischen Norm und AIDS-Demenz. Zentralbl. allg. Pathol. Anat. 136:637.

Witelson, S. F., Glezer, I. I., and Kigar, D. L. 1995. Women have greater density of neurons in posterior temporal cortex. J. Neurosci. 15:3418–3428.

Witelson, S. F., Kigar, D. L., and McKanna, J. A. 1992. A computer-assisted direct-imaging system to obtain numerical densities of neurons in human cortex. Brain Res. Bull. 29:441–447.

Sergio U. Dani

Histological Markers of Neuronal Aging and Their Meaning

Neuron Shrinkage with Age is Compatible with Neuron Survival

> Neuron Loss Varies According to the Different Parts of the Brain

Accumulation of Lipofuscin is the Most Regular Finding During Aging

Neuritic Plaques and Neurofibrillary Tangles Increase Exponentially with Age and Neuronal Size

> The Age of Onset of NP and NFT may be Tightly Determined, but the Progression of the Changes Vary Greatly, According to Neuronal Size
>
> Interaction with Glial Cells may Influence the Onset and Progression of NP and NFT
>
> The Ability to Process NP and NFT in the Brain may be Linked with Maintenance of Mental Functions
>
> Progressive Reduction of RNA within Neurons Precedes and Aggravates the Formation of NP and NFT

***Corpora Amylacea* are Related to Neuronal Dysfunction**

An Overall View

S ome neurons are among the largest cells in the human body and have the largest amounts of distinct macromolecules per cell. Although there is general agreement that these superlative features are necessary for the accomplishment of neuronal functions, little is known about their consequences for neuronal aging. The relationships between the impairment of neuronal molecular turnover with age and the accumulation of abnormal cytoskeletal proteins have been intensely investigated. The cytoskeleton controls both the shape and size of cells and the distribution of membrane proteins.

Since a great proportion of the genes of the human genome are believed to direct the synthesis of macromolecules that are present in significant quantities only in the central nervous system, it is likely that metabolic adaptations have evolved to cope with the burden represented by such large macromolecular pools. However, as neurons become old, altered rates of molecular turnover may rapidly produce long lasting modifications in the anatomy and surface chemistry of cells and their processes; those very metabolic adaptations are gradually surmounted and the maintenance capacity is exceeded, giving rise to senescent phenotypes.

In this chapter we shall examine some of the most common histological markers of neuronal aging, including neuron shrinkage, neuron loss, and precipitation of macromolecules in the form of lipofuscin, neuritic plaques (NP) and neurofibrillary tangles (NFT), and Lafora bodies or *corpora amylacea*.

Neuron Shrinkage with Age is Compatible with Neuron Survival

A relatively well understood way by which large molecular pools are reduced during aging is neuron shrinkage. This can occur through an imbalance between the rates of protein synthesis and degradation favoring a net reduction in the accumulation of molecules. Reductions in neuronal protein synthesis and degradation do occur with aging (Chapter 7), but neuron shrinkage or atrophy is not restricted to senescence and is not necessarily detrimental to cell function, being compatible with neuron survival (Finch, 1993).

In the brain, considerable age-related shrinkage of large neurons occurs with a consequent increase in the number of small neurons. Morphological changes of pyramidal cells due to aging comprise loss of dendritic spines, swellings, varicosities and distortions of the horizontal branches, followed by progressive swelling of the cell body, loss of basilar dendrites and of branches of the apical shaft and terminal arches (Scheibel 1978, 1979a,b). These changes may result in either shrinkage alone, or shrinkage with accumulation of abnormal macromolecules within the cytoplasm and in the karyoplasm. The decision between shrinkage alone or shrinkage with accumulation of abnormal macromolecules is presumably dependent upon neuronal size (Dani, 1994a), among other poorly understood factors. Thus, it is likely that a limit to neuronal size has been set during brain evolution, beyond which the ability of a neuron to dispose of excess macromolecules is exceeded, giving rise to toxic precipitations as the cell becomes old.

Although the majority of neurons undergo atrophy, showing reduced perikaryal RNA content and reduction in the rates of protein synthesis with age, some pyramidal cells can undergo considerable dendritic growth in normal old age, possibly as a response to loss of adjacent neurons (Mehraein et al., 1975; Buel and Coleman, 1979, 1981). In addition, decrease in the number of synapses found during aging can be compensated for by means of increase in the length of the postsynaptic contact zone (Cragg, 1975; Adams, 1987). The repercussions of these reactive enlargements to the maintenance ability of neurons during aging are poorly understood.

Neuron Loss Varies According to the Different Parts of the Brain

In the view of Herbert Haug, neuronal shrinkage and not neuronal loss is the one significant change which occurs in the human cerebral cortex in old age. He considered that tissue shrinkage during processing produces such large differences between young and old age groups that correction for this factor largely eliminates significant evidence of loss of neurons in the cortex (Chapter 18). Nonetheless, there is evidence that at greater ages and in neurodegenerative conditions neuron loss may occur at variable degree. By age 80 the human brain normally has decreased in weight by less than 15 percent, but in some demented patients the decrease may be much greater (Tomlinson et al., 1968, 1970), the gyri are thin and the sulci prominent. The constant neuronal density associated with diminished cortical volume clearly indicates that some loss of neurons occurs with age.

Neuron loss and change in dendritic extent vary according to the different parts of the brain in normal aging and neurodegenerative conditions. Whereas in some parts of the brain the numbers of neurons apparently remain unchanged or slightly reduced (Chapter 18), the number of nerve cells in the nucleus basalis of Meynert, the main source of cholinergic fibers to the brain, and in locus caeruleus, the main source of noradrenergic fibers to the brain, decays with age, so that around the tenth decade up to 35–40 percent of the original cell complement has been lost, and the capacity to synthesize proteins for physiological integrity is reduced in the remaining cells (Mann et al., 1984). In AD there is excess neuron loss and dendritic regression in some, but not all, brain regions (Figure 19–1). Measures of morphologic substrates of brain function in autopsied people may show appreciable overlap between AD and control groups. However the static, post mortem status of brain morphology may not adequately reflect the functional capabilities of the dynamic morphology of the living brain.

Corresponding brain regions do not always change with age in similar ways in rodents and primates. Coleman and Flood (1987) suggested that such differences may, in part, be due to inconsistent definitions of 'aged' among species, and that neuron numbers and sizes may show similar age-related changes in human and animal brains only for sharply defined brain subdivisions, such as CA1 of cornu ammonis.

Accumulation of Lipofuscin is the Most Regular Finding During Aging

The accumulation of lipoprotein pigment in nerve cells is the most regular finding during the aging process. In normal neurons, membranes are continuously repaired and recycled with the help of lysosomes. In mammalian cells lysosomal degradation of intracellular proteins occurs mostly under stressed conditions like starvation. Lipofuscin originates from secondary lysosomes which transform into lipopigment granules. These pigments may be formed as a result of the interaction between the products of polyunsaturated fatty acid peroxidation and several biologically useful molecules or by nonenzymatic glycosylation, mainly of long-lived proteins and nucleic acids, resulting in sugar groups that can be oxidized to form massive cross-links between proteins, lipids, and nucleic acids. Some of these conjugates are fluorescent, and the crosspolymers are hydrolytically indigestible or difficult to digest, accumulating as residual bodies within the cytoplasm (Figure 19–2). The fact that all biological molecules may become constituents of lipopigments is in accordance with the ultrastructural heterogeneity of neuronal lipofuscin as observed by J. W. Boellaard and W. Schlote (1986).

A

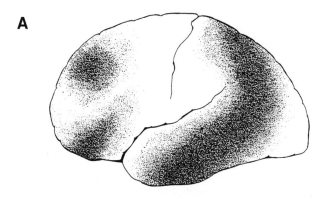

B

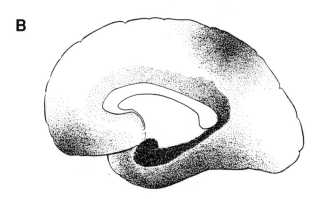

FIGURE 19–1

Distribution of histological markers of neurodegeneration in Alzheimer disease. The dark zones represent the cortex regions where the markers are most frequently observed and in remarkable densities. (From Allard *et al.*, 1988.)

A. Lateral view of the left hemisphere showing the involvement of frontal and temporal parietal regions.

B. Medial view of the right hemisphere showing the involvement of frontal medial, temporal medial, and parietal regions. Observe the remarkable involvement of the hippocampus and cingulate cortex, which are component structures of the limbic system.

Lipofuscin accumulation is apparently a function of total metabolic activity, rather than of chronological age alone (Lippmann, 1983). Comparison of rodent, canine, and human lipofuscin accumulation patterns indicates an inverse relationship between rate of accumulation and species longevity (Rose, 1991). The rate of absolute (cytosolic) RNA decrease is concomitant with that of mean lipofuscin increase during aging (Mann and Yates, 1974). H. Barden (1970) linked a reduction in Golgi enzyme activity with the extent to which lipofuscin accumulates within the nerve cell body in the brain of the aging rhesus monkey. Similarly, decreased synthesis and abnormal activity of lysosomal enzymes such as proteases have been maintained as the major pathogenetic factors in the group of diseases known as neuronal ceroidlipofuscinosis, lyso-

somal enzymopathies or lysosomal storage diseases, even though some enzymatic activity may still be displayed by lipofuscin throughout life (Maslinska *et al.*, 1984).

Neuritic Plaques and Neurofibrillary Tangles Increase Exponentially with Age and Neuronal Size

Neuritic plaques (NP) and neurofibrillary tangles (NFT) are the two hallmarks of structural protein precipitation in neuronal aging and Alzheimer disease (AD). Their morphological and biochemical features strongly suggest a common neuronal pathology. NP consist of loosely arranged aggregates of glial and neuronal processes containing intracytoplasmic deposits of structural neuronal proteins such as microtubule-associated tau-protein and membrane-associated β-amyloid protein (βA) and varying degrees of extracellular deposits which are considered to be byproducts of neurodegeneration (Hyman *et al.*, 1993a, 1993b). Any hypothesis of neurotoxic agents es-

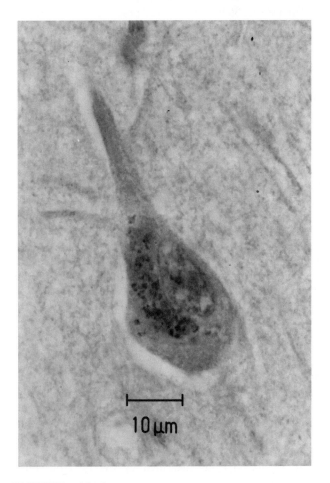

FIGURE 19–2

Lipofuscin is the most regular finding in the aging neuron. This picture shows a pyramidal neuron in the human entorhinal cortex (parahippocampal gyrus). The paranuclear dark structures are granules of lipofuscin. Howell-Black/Reusche silver impregnation.

caping from blood vessels as the initiators of NP is questionable, since there are cortical areas in which persistent absence of NP has been reported (Pearson *et al.*, 1985; Esiri *et al.*, 1986). NFT also consist of deposits of structural proteins, mainly bundles of abnormal filaments typically found within neuronal cell bodies, but also within many small neuronal processes, dendrites and terminal arborizations of axons. The principal component of these bundles is a paired helical filament (PHF) containing abnormal tau-protein, with varying degrees of involvement of other proteins, including βA (Box 19–1, Figures 19–3 and 19–4).

The typical pathology of NP and NFT is difficult to reproduce in any known animal model, and our present knowledge of NP and NFT pathophysiology has been almost entirely derived from *post mortem* human specimens. Quantitative morphometry has disclosed that an increased tendency to develop NP and NFT is a feature of certain groups of neurons that have in common a large cell size. These include pyramidal neurons in layers III and V of the neocortex, subiculum, and layer II of the entorhinal cortex. One of the best procedures to stain NP and NFT in brain sections, found incidentally by E. Reusche in 1991, is a silver impregnation procedure originally developed by W. Howell and D. Black in 1980, for staining nucleolus organizer regions (Box 19–2). Using the Reusche method in extensive quantitative analyses of the incidence of NP and NFT in the entorhinal cortex of geographically and ethnically different people, we have shown that NP and NFT incidences increase exponentially with age and increasing mean neuronal size (Figure 19–5). The spatial distribution in the cortex and the timing pattern show a clear, though nonlinear, relationship between these two markers. A significant correlation can be found in severely affected brain regions such as the entorhinal cortex, in which formation of NP precedes that of NFT. The evidence suggests further that NP and NFT are different phases of the same degenerative process, in that NP signalize a primary neuronal change affecting neurites which, with time, can progress to the onset of NFT in the perikaryon (Box 19–3, Figures 19–6 and 19–7).

The Age of Onset of NP and NFT may be Tightly Determined, but the Progression of the Changes Vary Greatly, According to Neuronal Size

The mean age of onset of NP and NFT in the entorhinal cortex does not seem to vary greatly either between geographically and ethnically distinct people, nor between sexes. This remarkable finding suggests that neurodegeneration is tightly programmed in our species. The incidence of NP and NFT, however, and the progression from NP to NFT, as measured by the NFT:NP ratio (Dani, 1994c; Dani and Weis, 1994) can be significantly increased in brains with great proportions of larger neurons. We had a clear picture of this problem when we compared series of aging people with different patterns of neuronal size distribution in the entorhinal cortex. Compared to the series with small proportions of large neu-

rons, the series with higher proportions of large neurons had heavier brains with about twice as many medium and large neurons in the entorhinal cortex, with almost half the figures for small neurons, along with a twofold increase in the incidence of NP and NFT, and an almost twofold increase in the NFT:NP ratio (Figure 19–8).

The evidence that heavier brains tend to have a higher proportion of medium and large neurons can be viewed under the scope of the phenomenon of conservative scaling. This very phenomenon seems to account for the fact that the proportion of large neurons is usually greater in men as compared to women, as males tend to have higher brain weights than women, but with the same total number of neurons in the cerebral cortex (Haug *et al.*, 1984). In studies of aging people, however, the relationship between brain size and neuronal size distribution is not clear-cut: Significant positive correlation between brain weight and neuronal size is typically found before 65 years of age, when brain shrinkage is less important. Thereafter, there is a negative correlation between brain weight, neuronal size and the incidence of NP and NFT, which peaks at the eighth decade of life when brain atrophy is already important. This is understandable in the sense that increased brain atrophy correlates with increased NP and NFT. Neary and colleagues (1986) found a correlation between increase in NP and increase in the degree to which some perikaryal measures are reduced, and also between increase in NFT frequency and cell loss. Since larger neurons tend to undergo a more intense degeneration with age, it is likely that larger brains containing a great proportion of large neurons are more susceptible to undergo higher degrees of macroscopic atrophy, thereby masking the positive correlation between brain size, neuronal size distribution, and susceptibility to neurodegeneration.

These findings raise the possibility that increased proportions of large neurons may be a risk factor for AD, as the degree of brain shrinkage, the incidence of NP and NFT, the rate of progression from NP to NFT, and neuron loss are typically much greater in AD than in normal aging. A variety of human and animal degenerative neurological diseases result from dysfunction and death of specific groups of neurons, the so called 'system degenerations', instances of which are *amyotrophic lateral sclerosis* and Parkinson disease. According to Price and colleagues (1987), AD should also be regarded as a system degeneration. Consequently, increased formation of NP and NFT in AD might be viewed as a feature of neural systems with great proportions of large neurons.

Interaction with Glial Cells may Influence the Onset and Progression of NP and NFT

A tendency to reduction in size and numbers of NP with age has been noticed (Figure 19–4), and propositions have been made that factors inherent to the nervous tissue may contribute to reduce NP size or even to eliminate it. NP size reduction can be imputed to degeneration of the terminals of affected neurons which contribute to the

Neuritic Plaques (NP) and Neurofibrillary Tangles (NFT)   Box 19–1

Neuritic plaques (NP) were originally described by Blocq and Marinesco more than 100 years ago. NP are focal degenerative alterations observed in the neuropil, with irregular outline, tending to circular shape in histological preparations (Figure 19–3, A). The denomination 'senile plaque', as proposed by Simchowicz, will not be used in this chapter, because there are types of senile plaques such as those seen in amyloid angiopathy (Chapter 27) which may not be signs of neuronal or neuritic degeneration. A morphological classification of senile plaques has been proposed by Wisniewski and Terry, following from the study of von Braunmühl, which recognizes the existence of 'primitive', 'classic' and 'compact' forms of senile plaques. This classification, in the author's view, is not helpful in biological studies, nor does it take into account the potential evolution indicators of the histological marker.

In histological sections, NP size ranges from 30 μm^2 (one single neuron involved) to 30,000 μm^2 or more (NP become confluent owing to the involvement of many neurons), which corresponds to a spheric volume range of 125 μm^3 to 3,500,000 μm^3. The average size of NP in the human entorhinal cortex varies between 250 μm^2 and 720 μm^2, depending on factors such as age, brain size, and neuronal size distribution in the brain cortex (Dani et al., 1993a). NP diameter may also be constrained by interfascicular distances between bundles of axons where the NP are located (Kosik et al., 1987). Their microscopic aspect is that of a lattice of altered neurites, containing variable levels of amyloid material, usually deposited at the central portions of the lesions (Figure 19–4, C). Large NP with diffuse neurites and poorly defined shape (Figure 19–4, A) are most frequently observed in younger subjects. NP with a more regular circular shape (Figure 19–4, B) are observed preferentially in middle-aged subjects, and NP with increasing amounts of amyloid (Figure

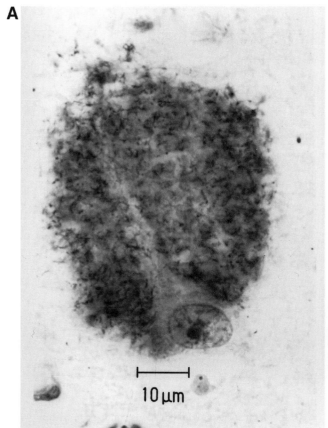

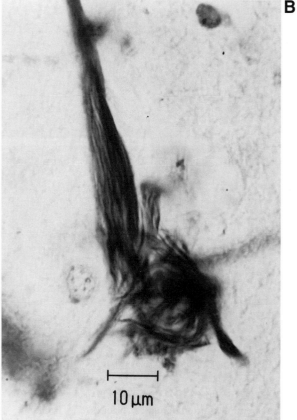

FIGURE   19–3

Histological aspects of a neuritic plaque (**A**) and neurofibrillary tangles (**B**) in two human pyramidal neurons in the parahippocampal gyrus, as stained by the Howell-Black/Reusche silver staining (see Box 19–2). Neuritic plaques (NP) and neurofibrillary tangles (NFT) are considered to be different phases of the same cytoskeletal degeneration in neurons, with the formation of NP usually preceding that of NFT. NP and NFT vary dynamically in size and may vanish completely, depending upon as yet poorly understood recycling ability of the components of the brain cortex.

19–4, C) and cellular debris (Figure 19–4, D) are most frequently observed in elderly patients. Contrarily to the poor association of 'young' NP with NFT in the same cortex region, association of 'old' NP with NFT is most evident. β-amyloid protein (βA), which is derived from a large precursor (APP) (Chapters 8 and 9), is the major constituent of NP amyloid. This protein is composed of 4–8 nm fibrils, whose β-pleated sheet molecular conformation provides amyloid with birefringence after *Congo red* staining, and fluorescence after thioflavine S treatment. In the typical NP, amyloid fibrils appear intermingled with and surrounded by large numbers of neuronal processes. In addition to βA, there is evidence that other protein species and a number of different substances such as carbohydrate and lipids take part in NP and NFT.

Neurofibrillary tangles (NFT) were identified as 'fibrillary changes' by Alois Alzheimer in 1907. At light microscopy, NFT present as bundles of fibrillary material, characteristically observed within perikarya, which may be partially or fully filled with NFTs (Figure 19–3, B). Electron microscopy has revealed morphologic heterogeneity of these lesions which contain, among other elements, straight filaments and paired helical filaments (PHF). Staining methods used for the detection of NP proved also most adequate for the demonstration of NFT.

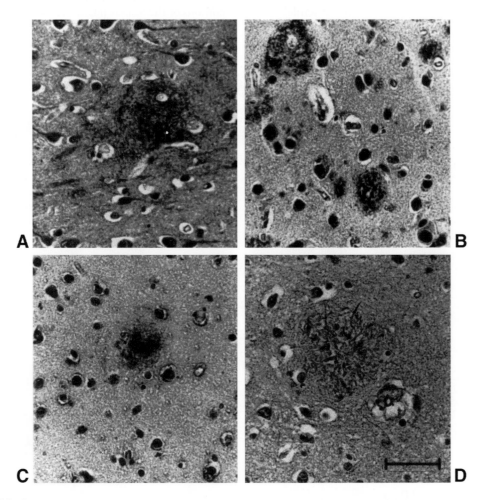

FIGURE 19–4

Morphological evolution of neuritic plaques (NP), from 'young' plaques (**A, B**) to 'old' plaques (**C, D**). (From Dani, 1993c.) Scale bar = 50 μm.

A. Large, diffuse plaques consisting of altered neurites are formed in the neuropil by confluent smaller plaques, indicating the involvement of more than one neuron.

B. Neuritic plaques such as in (A) become more circumscribed as they are gradually processed by glial cells.

C. In a later stage, amyloid deposits condensate within plaques to form the classic 'amyloid core' type of plaque.

D. Neuritic plaques, neurofibrillary tangles and remaining cell debris may vanish completely. Structures called *neuropil threads* can be seen which are sometimes difficult to differentiate from NP or NFT.

PHF are the major constituents of NFT. These paired helical filaments are thought to be composed mostly by the microtubule-associated protein tau (Goedert *et al.*, 1988). Tau exists in four or five isoforms (MW 55,000–62,000) derived from alternative splicing of a single tau gene. PHF have an alternated width between 8 nm and 20 nm, with an apparent period of about 80 nm. By treating PHF with acid or alkali it is possible to untwist them completely into uniform flat ribbons about 20 nm wide (Goedert *et al.*, 1991).

Straight filaments, which also contain tau, represent a minority species in NFT preparations. Quite rarely, hybrid filaments showing a sharp transition from a segment of PHF into a segment of SF can be seen (Goedert *et al.*, 1991). Likewise the tendency to variation in size observed in NP, variation in size and aspect of NFT has been also observed, in that NFT located outside the cytoplasm look enlarged and less compact. Sometimes they look diffuse, making it difficult to differentiate them from a NP (Figure 19–4, D).

Histochemistry for Neuritic Plaques (NP) and Neurofibrillary Tangles (NFT): The Howell-Black/Reusche Method   Box 19–2

The Howell-Black silver impregnation method was incidentally found by E. Reusche to be an effective method to stain both NP and NFT in brain sections. This valuable method was originally developed by W. M. Howell and D. A. Black for demonstration of nucleolus organizer regions. Recently, it has proved to be as sensible as immunostaining for demonstration of intracellular and extracellular accumulation of βA and tau-protein (Abe *et al.*, 1994), the main components of respectively NP and NFT, among other protein deposits:

1. Stock solutions: (i) 2 g gelatin in 100 ml 1 percent aqueous formic acid; (ii) 50 g $AgNO_3$ in 100 ml distilled water; (iii) 3 percent Na-thiosulfate, stored in dark bottles.

2. Using latex gloves, solutions (i) and (ii) are mixed respectively 1:2 just before use.

3. Deparaffinized brain slides previously washed in distilled water are brought into humid dark-chamber, dropped each with 200 μl of the fresh mixture, coverslipped and let stain for 60 minutes. The slides are then washed in distilled water, treated with solution (iii) for 2 minutes, rinsed in distilled water, dehydrated in ascending aqueous concentrations of ethanol, cleared in an organic solvent, mounted, and examined under the microscope. There are variations of the method designed by E. Reusche and colleagues for electron-microscopic examination of NP and NFT.

A

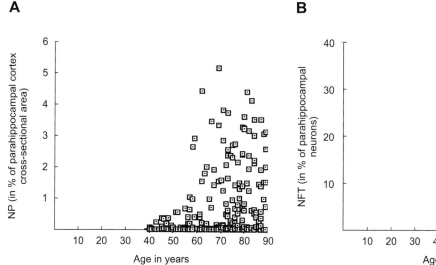

B

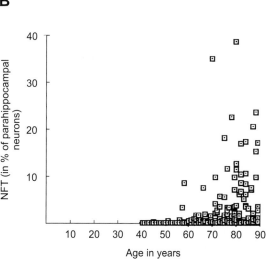

FIGURE 19–5

Incidence of neuritic plaques (**A**) and neurofibrillary tangles (**B**) in the entorhinal cortex of 351 autopsied patients, including 321 non-demented and 30 Alzheimer disease patients. NP and NFT increase exponentially with age and neuronal size. While most patients in the base line had small proportions of large neurons, the majority of patients over the base line had great proportions of large neurons. Notice that NFT increase is somewhat elapsed in relation to NP increase, indicating that the formation of NP precedes that of NFT. (From Dani *et al.*, 1997.)

formation of NP. There is evidence that degradation of cytoskeletal proteins initiates at nerve terminals (Sandberg et al., 1980; Glass and Griffin, 1991), and that proteolytic activity is very intense in neuronal perikarya and proximal axons (Hamakubo et al., 1986), especially during the assembly of cytoskeletal structures (Lazarides et al., 1984). The conclusion may be that age-related failure of proteolysis is most likely to occur first at neuronal terminals (NP) and only then within perikarya (NFT). Thus, NP might be viewed as an earlier, milder, neuronal change.

In another vein, there is evidence that NP and, to a lesser extent, also NFT are dynamically processed by glial cells outside the affected neurons, either when neurons are disrupted and their constituents are released into the neuropil, or through a direct interplay of glial cells in delaying the onset of NP and NFT. This latter possibility cannot be discarded in view of the report by Cavanagh and colleagues (1990) that glial cells actively remove detritus from within nerve cells. The putative role of interstitial processing of NP and NFT in the neuropil deserve further studies. NP and NFT sometimes become confluent with glial processes, thus foreshadowing the observation of complex modifications in size, composition, and frequency with age. Cataldo and Nixon (1990) have demonstrated anti-cathepsin D immunoreactivity in both lysosomes and lipofuscin released in the neuropil, and Défossez and Delacourte (1987) reported on the transformation of degenerating neurofibrils into amyloid substance within the NP. Such chemical modifications may be mediated either by spontaneous chemical modifications of nerve cell debris released in the neuropil, or by active participation of glial cells, which apparently maintain protein synthetic capabilities, even in the presence of important RNA loss in neurons (Doebler et al., 1988).

Whatever the mechanism involved, it seems that NP and NFT as demonstrated in histological sections are a lesser proportion of the actual quantities of NP and NFT formed and vanished (turned over) in vivo, before the time of histological observation.

The Ability to Process NP and NFT in the Brain may be Linked with Maintenance of Mental Functions

Attempts to correlate psychological measures to measures of NP frequency have yielded conflicting results. A significant correlation between NP and dementia has been reported, but a much higher significant correlation has been found between presence and severity of dementia and the number of NFT in the cerebral cortex. Similarly, changes in nerve cell function have been found to correlate less with NP than with NFT (Mann and Yates, 1981; Wilcock et al., 1982). This evidence agrees well with the notion than NP are a milder, earlier sign of neurodegeneration, as compared to NFT.

Gibson found that in non-demented patients the majority of plaques are of 'discrete form' (old, processed plaques), indicating that the ability to organize and/or to vanish NP could be somehow linked to maintenance of nervous tissue normal function. In AD, however, the 'amorphous form' (young, non-processed plaques) dominate. Since the most remarkable feature of the neocortex is its role in cognitive processes, it might be interesting to test further whether reduction in size or elimination of NP result in a compensation for impairments in cognitive abilities due to NP themselves or due to progression of the degeneration to NFT. The occurrence of NP in deeper or 'inner' cortical layers as compared to NFT-bearing neurons brings about some suppositions concerning the relation of NP to the clusters of apical dendrites and their influences upon cognitive processes. A worth testing approach is the hypothesis that NP could disturb the putative mind-brain interactions based on clusters of apical dendrites that John Eccles once called 'dendrons'.

Progressive Reduction of RNA within Neurons Precedes and Aggravates the Formation of NP and NFT

In spite of the fact that studies on ribosomal changes during cellular aging have so far been very limited, an age-related decline in the number of ribosomes, thermal stability, levels of ribosomal proteins and rRNA, and the efficiency of ribosomal binding to aminoacyl-tRNAs have been observed in various organisms or on isolated organs from rats, mice and birds (Reff, 1985). Much has been said about these quantitative aspects of RNA depletion during aging, but little has been studied concerning the meaning of RNA reduction to the pathogenesis of NP and NFT.

Depletion of RNA in sites in which there is little or no NP or NFT formation has been alleged as a challenge to the notion that the latter are consequence of the former. However, this view underscores a wealth of evidence pointing to a dysregulation in neuronal RNA/protein metabolism during aging and AD, such as: (i) The accumulation of β-amyloid-protein (βA) and the microtubule-associated protein tau within NP and NFT; (ii) the fact that the cellular localization of βA-precursor and tau transcripts in the central nervous system is neuronal (Goedert and Spillantini, 1990); (iii) the lack of evidence that overproduction of amyloid βA-precursor or tau-protein alone is the reason for NP and NFT formation rather than being by-products of neuronal dysfunction and death; (iv) the evidence suggesting that RNA loss in AD may be limited to the neuronal compartment (where NP and NFT start to accumulate), with astrocytes maintaining protein synthetic capability; and (v) the evidence that reduction of transcriptionally active euchromatin fraction of neuronal chromatin (Crapper et al., 1979), as well as RNA depletion (Sajdel-Sulkolwska et al., 1983) is more intense in brains of AD patients as compared to age-matched controls.

The problem of determining the relationship between total RNA depletion and the formation of NP and NFT has been addressed by multivariate analysis of variance – MANOVA in a study (Dani et al., 1993). The amount of

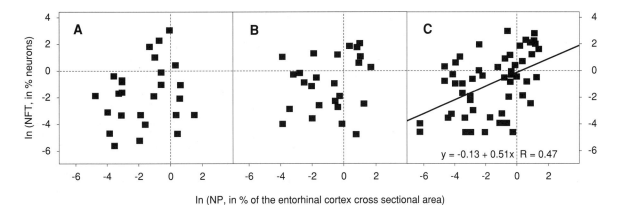

In (NP, in % of the entorhinal cortex cross sectional area)

FIGURE 19–8

The incidence of NP and NFT and the average NFT:NP ratio increase in three series of entorhinal cortices of each 100 autopsied people with increasing proportions of large neurons (A = B < C). In the plots, the ordinate is given as y = ln [NFT] and the abscissa as x = ln [NP], with ln [NFT] = natural logarithm of [(NFT counts)/(absolute number of neurons) x 100], and ln [NP] = natural logarithm of [(ΣNP-cross sectional area)/(gray matter-cross sectional area) x 100]. The NFT:NP ratio can be calculated as a measure of the rates of progression of neurodegenerative changes. In accord with the definition of the NFT:NP ratio, namely a ratio expressing the progression from an early stage of neurodegeneration (NP) to a later stage (NFT), only cases bearing both NP and NFT were plotted, i.e., cases with only NP, only NFT, or none of these, were excluded from this analysis. Linear regression was performed to obtain the estimate of the average NFT:NP ratio, expressed by the regression coefficient (r) to the linear equation: ln [NFT] = (b) + (a) ln [NP], where (a) = slope, and (b) is the value of ln [NFT] when ln [NP] = 0 (i.e.,

the intercept of the linear equation at the ordinate). A high NFT:NP ratio is ascertained when r > 0.45, a > 0, and b approaching zero. (From Dani *et al.*, 1997.)

A. Out of a series of 100 non-demented patients with low proportions of large neurons in the entorhinal cortex and aged 40–90 years, only 26 patients showed a combined incidence of NP and NFT.

B. Out of the second series of another 100 non-demented patients with low proportions of large neurons in the entorhinal cortex, and aged 40–90 years, only 25 patients showed a combined incidence of NP and NFT.

C. Out of the third series of another 100 non-demented patients with great proportions of large neurons in the entorhinal cortex, and aged 40–90 years, 55 patients showed a combined incidence of NP and NFT, and the highest NFT:NP ratio of the three series. Linear regression is shown.

neuronal ab-RNA decreased regularly with age in the entorhinal cortex, though significant covariance of ab-RNA loss by age was found only within the interval between the 5th and 7th decades, corresponding to the age of exponential onset of NP and NFT (compare with Figure 19–5). MANOVA indicated not only isolated effects of age and ab-RNA but also interactive effects of these two parameters upon the frequency of NP and NFT. In the same study it was assumed that most of these ab-RNA loss reflects rRNA loss, since the greater part of tissue RNA is ribosomal. The results of the study stress a qualitative aspect of RNA depletion, namely the fact that the variation in the otherwise constant RNA depletion rates is concomitant to the onset of neurohistological changes. It has been put forward that the rate at which RNA is depleted, rather than the depletion alone, may be important in the etiology of the process leading to NP and NFT formation. Thus, progressive total RNA depletion may be involved in the pathophysiology of the neurodegeneration as featured by the formation of NP and NFT.

Corpora Amylacea are Related to Neuronal Dysfunction

Corpora amylacea have been observed in astrocytes, in increasing frequencies starting as early as within the third

life decade in humans (Scholz, 1957). Similar inclusion bodies, the *Lafora bodies*, are frequently found intra-axonally, more commonly in neurodegenerative diseases (Anzil *et al.*, 1974; Takahashi *et al.*, 1977). The fine structure of these inclusion bodies has been described by R. J. Ramsey in 1965 as an aggregate of randomly oriented, ramified fibrils of 6 to 10 nm in width with amorphous densities, identified as polymers of carbohydrate. *Corpora amylacea* measure ca. 10 to 20 μm in diameter, sometimes contain an eosinophilic or argentophilic core suggesting the presence of proteins (Figure 19–9). The favorable spherical form and the localization patterns of *corpora amylacea* give some clues about possible transport mechanisms from the site of production to the site of accumulation: *Corpora amylacea* are frequently found clustered under the *pia mater*, the ependyma or along the margins of blood vessels (all regions of loose neuropil), in relation to astrocytic processes, or located between nerve fibers (that may provide orientation for migration of these spheric bodies, as often observed in the fimbria of the hippocampus), but rarely seen within the gray matter. The exception is CA4 of hippocampus, which often contains appreciable numbers of *corpora amylacea*. The conclusion may be that the granular layer of the dentate gyrus represents a natural barrier for the migration of *corpora amylacea* through the neuropil in the CA4 region.

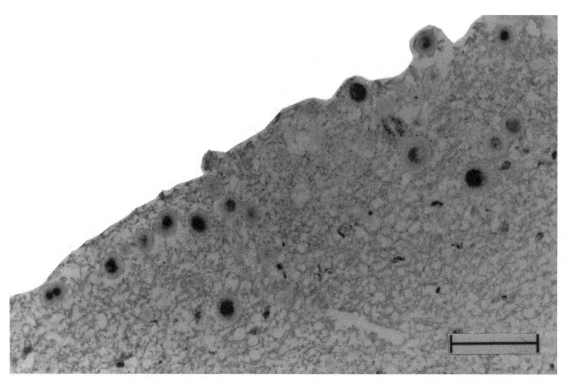

FIGURE   19–9

Corpora amylacea are commonly observed in subpial aspects of the brain during aging. This picture shows a subpial portion of a human parahippocampal gyrus with various *corpora amylacea* stained by the Howell-Black/Reusche method. Note the argento-philic cores of *corpora amylacea* indicating the presence of polypeptide species, surrounded by a halo of carbohydrate polymers. Scale bar = 50 μm.

There is work showing that the formation of *corpora amylacea* is related to neuronal dysfunction. Schwalbe and Quadbeck (1975) held that *corpora amylacea* of the brain may be caused by the glucose requirement of the organ being reduced, while the supply of glucose is normal. Neuronal loss with increasing age has been associated with an exquisite topographical replacement by *corpora amylacea* in the Purkinje layer of the cerebellum (Mittal and Olszewski, 1985). Singhrao and collaborators insisted that *corpora amylacea* occurring in Alzheimer disease differ from those in other conditions, in that they appear in much larger numbers than in normal aged brain, and presumably show more variable immunoreactivity. In our experience, however, they often show non-specific positive reactions with various antibodies. In addition, analysis of their protein fraction revealed several polypeptides suggesting the involvement of distinct protein species, of which ubiquitin (Chapter 7) has been already identified (Cissé *et al.*, 1991; Martin *et al.*, 1991). A MANOVA study revealed isolated and interactive effects of age and *corpora amylacea* on the frequency of lipofuscin, NP, NFT, and percent of gray matter cross-sectional area occupied with NP in the hippocampal formation and entorhinal cortex in a series of aging people (Dani, 1994c). A significant increase in the rate of total neuronal RNA depletion correlated with significant onset of lipofuscin, NP, NFT and *corpora amylacea*. The results suggest that decreased levels of RNA are associated with severity of the markers, leading to the conclusion that RNA depletion and consequently decreased macromolecular turnover might play an important role in the etiology of neuronal aging and dysfunction.

An Overall View

Age-related reductions in macromolecular turnover appear to account for neuron shrinkage, intracellular accumulation of macromolecules, and neuron death. While neuron shrinkage is compatible with neuron survival, accumulation of macromolecules is usually a sign of more severe neuronal dysfunction. It is likely that neuronal size and the rate at which total RNA is reduced with age play important roles in deciding whether neurons shrink or progressively accumulate macromolecules up to a point of no return, when cell death occurs. In normal aging, changes are mild and limited in time, as opposed to neurodegenerative diseases, in which a loss of homeostatic capacity is associated with rapid dysfunction and death. Higher proportions of large neurons in the brain may increase the severity or extent of the neurodegeneration.

Selected Readings

Barden, H. 1970. Relationship of Golgi thiaminepyrophosphatase and lysosomal acid phosphatase to neuromelanin and lipofuscin in cerebral neurons of the aging rhesus monkey. J. Neuropathol. Exp. Neurol. 29:225–240.

Boellaard, J. W., and Schlote, W. 1986. Ultrastructural heterogeneity of neuronal lipofuscin in the normal human cerebral cortex. Acta Neuropathol. 71:285–294.

Cataldo, A. M., Paskevich, P. A., Kominami, E., and Nixon, R. A. 1991. Lysosomal hydrolases of different classes are abnormally distributed in brains of patients with Alzheimer disease. Proc. Natl. Acad. Sci. USA 88:10998–11002.

Cavanagh, J. B., Nolar, C. C., and Brown, A. W. 1990. Glial cell intrusions actively remove detritus due to toxic chemicals from within nerve cells. Neurotoxicology 11:1–12.

Coleman, P. D., and Flood, D. G. 1987. Neuron numbers and dendritic extent in normal aging and Alzheimer's disease. Neurobiol. Aging 8:521–545.

Curcio, C. A., McNelly, and Hinds, J. W. 1984. Intranuclear inclusions in rat piriform cortex: increase with age and preferential location within superficial layer II. Anat. Rec. 210:657–662.

Doebler, J. A., Markesbery, W. R., Anthony, A., et al. 1988. Astrocyte RNA in relation to neuronal RNA depletion in Alzheimer's disease. Acta Neuropathol. 75:272–276.

Gibson, P. H. 1983. Form and distribution of senile plaques seen in silver-impregnated sections in the brains of intellectually normal elderly people and people with Alzheimer-type dementia. Neuropathol. Appl. Neurobiol. 9:379–389.

Gibson, P. H., Stones, M., and Tomlinson, B. E. 1976. Senile changes in the human neocortex and hippocampus compared by the use of the electron and light microscopes. J. Neurol. Sci. 27:389–405.

van Hoesen, G. W., Hyman, B. T., and Damasio, A. R. 1986. Cell-specific pathology in neural systems of the temporal lobe in Alzheimer's disease. Prog. Brain Pathol. 70:321–335.

Hyman, B. T., Marzloff, K., and Arriagada, P. V. 1993. The lack of accumulation of senile plaques or amyloid burden in Alzheimer's disease suggests a dynamic balance between amyloid deposition and resolution. J. Neuropathol. Exp. Neurol. 52:594–600.

Ivy, G. O., Schottler, F., Wenzel, J., Baudry, M., and Lynch, G. 1984. Inhibitors of lysosomal enzymes: accumulation of lipofuscin-like dense bodies in the brain. Science 226:985–987.

Kidd, M. 1964. Alzheimer's disease: an electron microscopical study. Brain 87:307–321.

Kosik, K. S. 1992. Alzheimer's disease: A cell biological perspective. Science 256:780–783.

Mann, D. M. A., and Sinclair, K. G. A. 1978. The quantitative assessment of lipofuscin pigment, cytoplasmic RNA and nucleolar volume in senile dementia. Neuropathol. Appl. Neurobiol. 4:129–135.

Mann, D. M. A., Yates, P. O., and Marcyniuk, B. 1984. Alzheimer's presenile dementia, senile dementia of Alzheimer type and Down's syndrome in middle age form an age related continuum of pathological changes. Neuropathol. Appl. Neurobiol. 10:185–207.

Masters, C. L., et al. 1985. Neuronal origin of a cerebral amyloid: neurofibrillary tangles of Alzheimer's disease contain the same protein as the amyloid of plaque cores and blood vessels. Eur. Mol. Biol. Organ. J. 4:2757–2763.

Price, D. L., et al. 1987. Dysfunction and death of neurons in human degenerative neurological diseases and in animal models. Selective neuronal death. Wiley, Chichester Ciba Foundation Symposium 126:30–48.

Probst, A., Langui, D., and Ulrich, J. 1991. Alzheimer's disease: a description of the structural lesions. Brain Pathol. 1:229–239

Raes, M. 1991. Involvement of microtubules in modifications associated with cellular aging. Mutat. Res. 256:149–168.

Ringborg, U. 1966. Composition and content of RNA in neurons of rat hippocampus at different ages. Brain Res. 2:296–298.

Rogers, J., and Morrison, J. H. 1985. Quantitative morphology and regional and laminar distributions of senile plaques in Alzheimer's disease. J. Neurosci. 5:2801–2808.

Roses, A. D. 1993. Molecular genetics of neurodegenerative diseases. Curr. Opin. Neurol. Neurosurg. 6:34–39.

Schmidt, M. L., Murray, J. M., and Trojaknowski, J. Q. 1993. Continuity of neuropil threads with tangle-bearing and tangle-free neurons in Alzheimer disease cortex. A confocal laser scanning microscopy study. Mol. Chem. Neuropathol. 18:299–312.

Snow, A. D., et al. 1990. Early accumulation of heparan sulfate in neurons and in the beta-amyloid protein-containing lesions of Alzheimer's disease and Down's Syndrome. Am. J. Pathol. 137:1253–1270.

Sparkmann, D. R., Goux, W. J., Jones, C. M., et al. 1991. Alzheimer disease paired helical filament core structures contain glycolipid. Biochem. Biophys. Res. Commun. 181:771–779.

Tabaton, M., Mandybur, T. I., Perry, G., et al. 1989 The widespread alteration of neurites in Alzheimer's disease may be unrelated to amyloid deposition. Ann. Neurol. 26:771–778.

Terry, R. D., Gonatas, N. K., and Weiss, M. 1964. Ultrastructural studies in Alzheimer's presenile dementia. Am. J. Pathol. 44:269–297.

Trojanowski, J. Q., Schmidt, M. L., Otvos Jr., L., Arai, H., Hill, W. D., and Lee, V. M.-Y. 1990. Vulnerability of the neuronal cytoskeleton in Alzheimer's disease: Widespread involvement of all the three major filament systems. Ann. Rev. Gerontol. Geriat. 10:167–182.

Zeman, W. 1971. The neuronal ceroid lipofuscinoses-Batten-Vogt syndrome: a model for human aging? Adv. Gerontol. Res. 3:147–170.

References

Abe, H., Mehraein, P., and Weis, S. 1994. Modified NOR silver impregnation technique for amyloid plaques and neurofibrillary tangles: Comparative assessment. Neuropathol. Appl. Neurobiol. 20:478–486.

Adams, I. 1987. Plasticity of the synaptic contact zone following loss of synapses in the cerebral cortex of aging humans. Brain Res. 424:343–351.

Allard, M., Signoret, J.-L., and Stalleicken. 1988. Alzheimer Demenz. Springer-Verlag, Berlin, Heidelberg.

Alzheimer, A. 1907. Über eine eigenartige Erkrankung der Hirnrinde. Zentralbl. Nervenheilk. 18:177–179

Anzil, A. P., Herlinger, H., Blinzenger, K., and Kronski, D. 1974. Intraneuritic corpora amylacea: Demonstration in orbital cortex of elderly subjects by means of early postmortem brain sampling and electron microscopy. Virchows Arch. A 364:297–301.

Ball, M. J. 1977. Neuronal loss, neurofibrillary tangles and granulovacuolar degeneration in the hippocampus with ageing and dementia – a quantitative study. Acta Neuropathol. 37:111–118.

Bekkers, J. M., and Stevens, C. F. 1990. Two different ways evolution makes neurons larger. Progr. Brain Res. 83:37–45.

Blocq, P., and Marinesco, G. 1892. Sur les lésions et la pathogénie de l'épilepsie dite essentielle. Semaine Médicale 12:445–446

Boellaard, J. W., and Schlote, W. 1986. Ultrastructural heterogeneity of neuronal lipofuscin in the normal human cerebral cortex. Acta Neuropathol. 71:285–294.

Braak, H. 1984. Architectonics as seen by lipofuscin stains. In A. Peter, and E. G. Jones (eds.) Cerebral Cortex, Vol. 1, Cellular Components of the Cerebral Cortex. Plenum, New York, pp. 1–32.

Braak, H., Braak, E., and Bohl, J. 1993. Staging of Alzheimer-related cortical destruction. Eur. Neurol. 33:403–408.

Braak, H., and Braak, E. 1991. Neuropathological staging of Alzheimer-related changes. Acta Neuropathol. 82:4,239–259.

Blessed, G., Tomlinson, B. E., and Roth, M. 1968. The association between quantitative measurements of dementia and of senile changes in the cerebral grey matter of elderly subjects. Br. J. Psychiatry 114:797–811.

Brun, A., and Englund, E. 1981. Regional pattern of degeneration in Alzheimer's disease: neuronal loss and histopathological grading. Histopathology 5:549–564.

Buel, S. J., and Coleman, P. D. 1979. Dendritic growth in the aged brain and failure of growth in senile dementia. Science 206:854–856.

Buel, S. J., and Coleman, P. D. 1981. Quantitative evidence for selective dendritic growth in normal human aging but not in senile dementia. Brain Res. 214:23–41.

Cataldo, A. M., and Nixon, R. A. 1990. Enzymatically active lysosomal proteases are associated with amyloid deposits in Alzheimer brain. Proc. Natl. Acad. Sci. USA 87:3861–3865.

Cavanagh, J. B., Nolar, C. C., and Brown, A. W. 1990. Glial cell intrusions actively remove detritus due to toxic chemicals from within nerve cells. Neurotoxicology 11:1–12.

Cissé, S., Lacoste-Royal, G., Laperriäre, J., et al. 1991. Ubiquitin is a component of polypeptides purified from corpora amylacea of aged human brain. Neurochem. Res. 16:429–433.

Coleman, P. D., and Flood, D. G. 1987. Neuron numbers and dendritic extent in normal aging and Alzheimer's disease. Neurobiol. Aging 8:521–545.

Cragg, B. G. 1975. The density of synapses in neurons in normal, mentally defective and aging human brains. Brain 98:81–90.

Crapper, D. R., Quittkat, S., and De Boni, U. 1979. Altered chromatin conformation in Alzheimer's disease. Brain 102:483–495.

Dani, S. U. 1994a. Larger neuronal size overwhelms maintenance capacity with aging. Med. Hypotheses 42:208–210.

Dani, S. U. 1994b. Spatial patterns of plaques and tangles in Alzheimer's disease. Dementia 5:53.

Dani, S. U. 1994c. Neuronal Aging and Degeneration: A Multivariate Histopathological Study on the Incidence of Neuritic Plaques and Neurofibrillary Tangles in the Human Hippocampal Formation. Thesis, Medizinischen Hochschule Hannover, Germany.

Dani, S. U., Bergmann, B., Walter, G. F., et al. 1993. A multivariate approach to the relationship between aging, RNA depletion and the incidence of plaques and tangles. Neuropathology (Kyoto) 13:243–249.

Dani, S. U., Pittella, J. E. H., Hori, A., et al. 1994. Different rates of neuronal degeneration: An exquisite variation of the cascade hypothesis. Dementia 5:110–118.

Dani, S. U., Pittella, J. E. H., Boehme, A., Hori, A., Schneider, B. 1997. Progressive formation of neuritic plaques and neurofibrillary tangles is exponentially related to age and neuronal size: A morphometric study of three geographically distinct series of aging people. Dementia and Geriatric Cognitive Disorders (July issue, in press).

Dani, S. U., and Weis, S. 1994. Looking for histological correlates of dementia: The neurodegeneration progression rate (NDPR). Clin. Neuropathol. 5:240–241.

Défossez, A., and Delacourte, A. 1987. Transformation of degenerating neurofibrils into amyloid substance in Alzheimer's disease: Histochemical and immunohistochemical studies. J. Neurol. Sci. 81:1–10.

Doebler, J. A., Markesbery, W. R., Anthony, A., and Rhoads, R. E. 1987. Neuronal RNA in relation to neuron loss and neurofibrillary pathology in the hippocampus in Alzheimer's disease. J. Neuropathol. Exp. Neurol. 46:28–39.

Doebler, J. A., Markesbery, W. R., Anthony, A., Scheff, S. W., and Rhoads, R. E. 1988. Astrocyte RNA in relation to neuronal RNA depletion in Alzheimer's disease. Acta Neuropathol. 75:272–276.

Doebler, J. A., Rhoads, R. E., Anthony, A., and Markesbery, W. R. 1989. Neuronal RNA in Pick's and Alzheimer's disease. Comparison of disease susceptible and disease resistant cortical areas. Arch. Neurol. 46:134–137.

Eccles, J. 1990. A unitary hypothesis of mind-brain interaction in the cerebral cortex. Proc. Royal Soc. London, Series B 240:433–451.

Esiri, M. M., Pearson, R. C. A., and Powell, T. P. S. 1986. The cortex of the primary auditory area in Alzheimer's disease. Brain Res. 366:385–387.

Finch, C. E. 1993. Neuron atrophy during aging: Programmed or sporadic? Trends Neurosci. 16:104–110.

Gibson, P. H. 1983. Form and distribution of senile plaques seen in silver-impregnated sections in the brains of intellectually normal elderly people and people with Alzheimer-type dementia. Neuropathol. Appl. Neurobiol. 9:379–389.

Glass, J. D., and Griffin, J. W. 1991. Neurofilament redistribution in transected nerves: Evidence for bidirecional transport of neurofilaments. J. Neurosci. 11:3146–3154.

Goedert, M., and Spillantini, M. G. 1990. Molecular neuropathology of Alzheimer's disease: In situ hybridization studies. Cell. Mol. Neurobiol 10:159–174.

Goedert, M., Spillantini, M. G., and Crowther, R. A. 1991. Tau proteins and neurofibrillary degeneration. Brain Pathol. 1:279–286.

Hamakubo, T., Kannagi, R., Murachi, T., and Matus, A. 1986. Distribution of calpains I and II in rat brain. J. Neurosci. 6:3103–3111.

Hardy, J. A., and Higgins, G. A. 1992. Alzheimer's disease: The amyloid cascade hypothesis. Science 256:184–185.

Haug, H., Kuhl, S., Mecke, E., Sass, N. L., and Wasner, K. 1984. The significance of morphometric procedures in the investigation of age changes in cytoarchitectonic structures of human brain. J. Hirnforsch. 25:353–374.

Hyman, B. T., Marzloff, K., and Arriagada, P. V. 1993. The lack of accumulation of senile plaques or amyloid burden in Alzheimer's disease suggests a dynamic balance between amyloid deposition and resolution. J. Neuropathol. Exp. Neurol. 52:594–600.

Hyman, B. T., Weniger, J. J., and Tanzi, R. E. 1993. Nonisotopic in situ hybridization of amyloid beta protein precursor in Alzheimer's disease: Expression in neurofibrillary tangle bearing neurons and in the microenvironment surrounding senile plaques. Mol. Brain. Res. 18:253–258.

Howell, W. M., and Black, D. A. 1980. Controlled silver-staining of nucleolus organizer regions with a protective colloidal developer: a 1-step method. Experientia 36:1014–1015.

Jamada, M., and Mehraein, P. 1968. Verteilungsmuster der senilen Veränderungen im Gehirn. Die Beteiligung des limbischen Systems bei hirnatrophischen Prozessen des Seniums und bei Morbus Alzheimer. Arch. Psychiatr. und Nervenkrankh. 211:308–324.

Kosik, K. S., Rogers, J., and Kowall, N. W. 1987. Senile plaques are located between apical dendritic clusters. J. Neuropathol. Exp. Neurol. 46:1–11.

Lazarides, E., Nelson, W. J., and Kasamatsu, T. 1984. Segregation of two spectrin forms in the chicken optic system: A mechanism for establishing restricted membrane-cytoskeletal domains in neurons. Cell 36:267–278.

Lippmann, R. D. 1983. Lipid peroxidation and metabolism in aging: A biological, chemical, and medical approach. Rev. Biol. Res. Aging 1:315–342

Mandybur, T. I., and Chuirazzi, B. A. 1990. Astrocytes and the plaques of Alzheimer's disease. Neurology 40:635–639.

Mann, D. M. A., and Yates, P. O. 1974. Lipoprotein pigments - their relationship to ageing in the human nervous system. Brain 97:481–488.

Mann, D. M. A., and Yates, P. O. 1981. The relationship between formation of senile plaques and neurofibrillary tangles and changes in nerve cell metabolism in Alzheimer type dementia. Mech. Aging Dev. 17:395–401.

Mann, D. M. A., Yates, P. O., and Marcyniuk, B. 1984. Alzheimer's presenile dementia, senile dementia of Alzheimer type and Down's syndrome in middle age form an age related continuum of pathological changes. Neuropathol. Appl. Neurobiol. 10:185–207.

Mann, D. M. A., Yates, P. O., and Marciniuk, B. 1985. Some morphometric observations on the cerebral cortex and hippocampus in presenile Alzheimer's disease, senile dementia of the Alzheimer's type and Down's syndrome in middle age. J. Neurol. Sci. 69:139–159

Martin, J. E., Mather, K., Swash, M., et al. 1991. Heat shock protein expression in corpora amylacea in the central nervous system: clues to their origin. Neuropathol. Appl. Neurobiol. 17:113–119.

Maslinska, D., Boellard, J. W., and Schlote, W. 1984. Acid phosphatase activity in human neuronal and glial lipofuscin. Acta Neuropathol. 64:222–228.

Mehraein, P., Yamada, M., and Tarnowska-Dziduszko, E. 1975. Quantitation studies on dendrites in Alzheimer's disease and senile dementia. In G. W. Kreutzberg (ed.) Physiology and Pathology of Dendrites. Raven Press, New York, pp 453–458.

Mittal, K. R., and Olszewski, W. A. 1985. Widening of inter-Purkinje cell distances in association with corpora amylacea. J. Gerontol. 40:700–702.

Motte, J., and Williams, R. S. 1989. Age-related changes in the density and morphology of plaques and neurofibrillary tangles in Down syndrome brain. Acta Neuropathol. 77:535–546.

Neary, D., et al. 1986. Alzheimer's disease: a correlative study. J. Neurol. Neurosurg. Psychiatry 49:229–237.

Pearson, R. C. A., Esiri, M. M., Hiorns, R. W., et al. 1985. Anatomical correlates of the distribution of the pathological changes in the neocortex in Alzheimer's disease. Proc. Natl. Acad. Sci. USA 82:4531–4534.

Price, D. L., et al. 1987. Dysfunction and death of neurons in human degenerative neurological diseases and in animal models. Selective neuronal death. Wiley, Chichester Ciba Foundation Symposium 126:30–48.

Probst, A., Ulrich, J., and Heitz, P. U. 1982. Senile dementia of Alzheimer type: Astroglial reaction to extracellular neurofibrillary tangles in the hippocampus. An immunocytochemical and electron-microscopic study. Acta Neuropathol. 57:75–79.

Rafalowska, J., Barcikowska, M., Wen, G. Y., and Wisniewski, H. M. 1988. Laminar distribution of neuritic plaques in normal aging, Alzheimer's disease and Down's syndrome. Acta Neuropathol. 77:21–25.

Ramsey, H. J. 1965. Ultrastructure of corpora amylacea. J. Neuropathol. Exp. Neurol. 24:29–39.

Reff, M. E. 1985. In C. E. Finch and E. L. Schneider (eds.) Handbook of the Biology of Aging. New York: Van Nostrand Reinhold, 2nd edition, pp. 225–249.

Reusche, E. 1991. Silver staining of senile plaques and neurofibrillary tangles in paraffin sections. A simple and effective method. Pathol. Res. Practice 187:1045–1049.

Rose, M. R. 1991. Evolutionary Biology of Aging. Oxford University Press, New York.

Sajdel-Sulkolwska, E. M., Coughlin, J. F., Staton, D. M., and Marotta, C. A. 1983. In vitro protein synthesis by messenger RNA from the Alzheimer disease brain. In R. Katzman (ed.) Biological Aspects of Alzheimer's Disease, Banbury Report 15. Cold Spring Harbor Laboratory, Cold Spring Harbor, NY, pp. 193–200.

Sandberg, M., Hamberger, A., Jacobson, I., and Karlsson, J.-O. 1980. Role of calcium ions in the formation and release of low molecular weigth substances from optic nerve terminals. Neurochem. Res. 5:1185–1198.

Scheibel, A. B. 1978. Structural aspects of the aging brain: spine systems and the dendritic arbor. In R. Katzman, R. D. Terry, and K. L. Bick (eds.) Aging, vol. 7., pp. 353–373. Alzheimer's Disease, Senile Dementia and Related Disorders. Raven Press, New York.

Scheibel, A. B. 1979a. Aging in human motor control systems. In J. M. Ordy and K. Brizzee (eds.) Aging, vol. 10. Sensory Systems and Communication in the Elderly, pp. 297–310. Raven Press, New York.

Scheibel, A. B. 1979b. The hippocampus organisational patterns in health and senescence. Mech. Ageing Dev. 9:89–102.

Scholz, W. 1957. Allgemeine Daten zu Degenerationsprozessen; in W. Scholz (ed.) Handbuch der speziellen Pathologischen Anatomie und Histologie, 13. Band; 1. Teil; Teil A: Erkrankungen des zentralen Nervensystems I, pp. 227–229. Springer-Verlag, Berlin.

Schwalbe, H.-P., and Quadbeck, G. 1975. Die Corpora amylacea im menschlichen Gehirn. Virchows Arch. A 366:305–311.

Singhrao, S. K., Neal, J. W., and Neuman, G. R. 1993. Corpora amylacea could be an indicator of neurodegeneration. Neuropathol. Appl. Neurobiol. 19:269–272.

Takahashi, K., Iwata, K., and Nakamura, H. 1977. Intra-axonal corpora amylacea in the CNS. Acta Neuropathol. 37:165–167.

Tomlinson, B. E., Blessed, S., and Roth, M. 1968. Observations on the brains of non-demented old people. J. Neurol. Sci 7:331–356.

Tomlinson, B. E., Blessed, S., and Roth, M. 1970. Observations on the brains of demented old people. J. Neurol. Sci. 11:205–242.

Vaughan, D. W., and Peters, A. 1981. The structure of neuritic

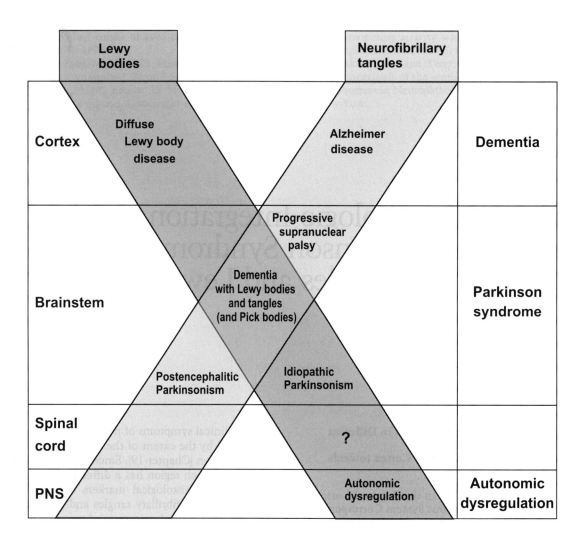

FIGURE 20–1

The topographical distribution of neurofibrillary tangles and Lewy bodies correlates with the clinical symptoms. There are various schemes of overlapping and transition of the distribution patterns of the degeneration as well as of clinical manifestations. Diffuse Lewy body disease is also called 'Lewy body variant of Alzheimer disease' (Hansen *et al.*, 1990)

distribution of neurofibrillary tangles in the brain. Furthermore PSP patients may also manifest organic psychic symptoms including dementia. The ultrastructure of neurofibrillary tangles of PSP (straight tubules) generally differs from that of neurofibrillary tangles in Alzheimer disease (paired helical filaments or twisted ribbons) (Pollanen *et al.*, 1994, 1995).

In contrast to Alzheimer disease, the distribution of neurofibrillary tangles in postencephalitic parkinsonism is stressed in the *substantia nigra* and other brainstem areas. This disorder, a parkinsonian state with personality changes, was described in patients long after the *von Economo encephalitis (encephalitis lethargica)*. Despite the fact that the von Economo encephalitis was well observed and documented several decades ago, the von Economo virus has not been identified and the disease is now believed to be deceased. The distribution of morphological changes in postencephalitic parkinsonism is similar to that in the *'Parkinsonism-dementia complex on Guam'* (PDC on Guam), which was described by Hirano and coworkers in the early 60's. Before their reports, PDC on Guam was indeed thought to be a postencephalitic parkinsonism (Kurland and Mulder, 1954). Papers discussing this idea appeared very late (Hori and Iizuka, 1978; Hudson and Rice, 1990). The distribution of neurofibrillary tangles in postencephalitic parkinsonism and/or in PDC on Guam, stressed in the brainstem, correlates very well with the clinical manifestations. This suggests that the shift of the distribution of neurofibrillary tangles from the cortex towards the brainstem makes the difference between dementia and parkinsonism which may overlap to some extent (Figure 20–1.)

The Distribution of Lewy Bodies in the Cerebral Cortex, Brainstem, and Peripheral Nervous System Corresponds to Dementia, Parkinsonism, and Peripheral Autonomic Dysregulatory Disorders, Respectively

Lewy bodies were originally described by Lewy in 1912 in Parkinson disease in the dorsal vagal nucleus and *substantia innominata* (basal ganglia of Meynert), and not in the *substantia nigra*. The name 'Lewy bodies' was proposed in 1919 by Trétiakoff who contributed to the understanding of the morphology of Parkinson disease.

In a disease called *diffuse Lewy body disease* which clinically manifests dementia, the distribution of Lewy bodies is shown diffusely in the neocortex. In contrast, *idiopathic parkinsonism* (synonyms: Parkinson disease; parkinsonism of Lewy body type) displays Lewy body distribution in the *substantia nigra, locus coeruleus*, and further in the hypothalamus and vagal nuclei etc., i.e., in the brainstem. It is not rare that a small amount of Lewy bodies are found also in the cerebral cortex of Parkinson disease patients. In a case of diffuse Lewy body disease, a supranuclear gaze palsy was observed as a brainstem dysfunction (Fearnley et al., 1991). Jackson and colleagues (1995) found Lewy bodies mainly in the dorsal vagal nuclei in two old patients who developed dysphagia without Parkinson disease.

The distribution of Lewy bodies in Parkinson disease can be shifted to the peripheral nervous system. Kupsky and colleagues (1987) observed Lewy bodies in enteric ganglion cells in patients with acquired megacolon in addition to Parkinson disease. Oyanagi and coworkers (1990) found Lewy bodies in the preganglionic parasympathetic neurons innervating the anal sphincter in a patient with clinical constipation, one of the most frequent autonomic dysfunctions in Parkinson disease.

Thus, the distribution of Lewy bodies in several disorders resembles the general scheme already described for neurofibrillary tangles. The distribution of Lewy bodies predominantly in the cortex, in the brainstem, and in the peripheral nervous system corresponds to dementia, parkinsonism, and peripheral autonomic dysregulatory disorders, respectively (Figure 20–1.) Similar to the accumulation of neurofibrillary tangles in the infant brains in different disorders, Lewy bodies have also been described in several disorders in children, such as *subacute sclerosing panencephalitis* (SSPE) (Gibb et al., 1990) (see Chapter 30).

We should consider that the metabolic dispositions which lead to the accumulation of Lewy bodies in different parts of the nervous system may be an *integrated disease entity*. Parkinson disease is not a purely motor disorder but reflects only an aspect of a possibly wider systemic disease of the central and peripheral nervous system, including the autonomic nervous system. Therefore the reportedly favorable short-term prognostics of the autologous transplantation of spinal ganglia or adrenal medullary chromaffin cells into the brain of Parkinson patients does not actually provide a reason for enthusiasm

(Date et al., 1995; Diamond et al., 1994; Itakura et al., 1994). As a matter of fact, eosinophilic inclusion bodies were found by den Hartog Jager in the adrenal medulla (adrenal bodies) of Parkinson disease patients. A comparative study between adrenal bodies and Lewy bodies was performed by Kimula and coworkers (1983); neurofibrillary tangles and paired helical filaments were also recognized in pheochromocytoma cells of the adrenal medulla (Izumiyama et al., 1990) (see below).

Alzheimer Disease and Diffuse Lewy Body Disease may Belong to the Same Spectrum of Neurodegeneration

There are opinions that Alzheimer disease and diffuse Lewy body disease (including Parkinson disease) belong to the same spectral disease process, or that both diseases share some common pathogenic mechanisms. Neurofibrillary tangles and Lewy bodies share some characteristics (Hakim and Mathieson, 1979; Dickson et al., 1989). The amyloid precursor protein observed in Alzheimer disease has been detected in Lewy bodies (Arai et al., 1992), and filamentous subunits are deposited in the Lewy body fibrils (Pollanen et al., 1993) which are antigenically identical with neurofilaments. It is well known that Lewy bodies and neurofibrillary tangles may manifest simultaneously in a patient (see Chapter 30; Figure 30–2). Popovitch and coworkers (1987), for example, found the combination in a clinically demented young adult. Unique was an old demented patient in whom not only neurofibrillary tangles and Lewy bodies but also Pick bodies were observed in the cerebral cortex (Kosaka et al., 1976). Hansen and colleagues (1990) and Förstl and colleagues (1993) described a 'Lewy body variant' of Alzheimer disease clinically showing extrapyramidal signs in addition to Alzheimer type dementia, and pathologically showing both neurofibrillary tangles and Lewy bodies. It should be mentioned that older Down syndrome patients may display Lewy bodies in addition to Alzheimer pathology (Raghavan et al., 1993).

Not only similarities but also differences were pointed out between neurofibrillary tangles and Lewy bodies (Galloway et al., 1988; Harrington et al., 1994): from the point of view of 'tau protein pathology' – a microtubule-binding protein aggregates in form of insoluble paired helical or straight filaments in degenerative diseases – the pathomechanisms of Alzheimer and Parkinson diseases may be different; the Alzheimer pathology is rather related to that of Pick disease and PSP. Ince and colleagues (1991) reported that Alzheimer disease, diffuse Lewy body disease, and Parkinson disease differed from each other on the basis of the intensity and distribution of 'Alzheimer type pathology' (neurofibrillary tangles, neuritic plaques, and granulovacuolar degeneration), and neuronal density in the hippocampus and entorhinal cortex. Dickson and colleagues (1991) insisted on the differences in the type of neuritic degeneration between diffuse Lewy body disease and Alzheimer disease, based on the immunohistochemical reaction for ubiquitin, neurofila-

José Eymard H. Pittella

21

Changes in the White Matter

In the elderly, intense immunoreactivity is also observed in the periventricular region, being more prominent and diffuse when compared to young adults. More conspicuous *periventricular* and *perivascular gliosis* in the elderly suggest that it may depend on circulatory factors, e.g., reduced blood flow into the white matter secondary to the thickening of the wall of medullary small arteries and arterioles and cardiovascular disturbances such as hypertension. Age related cerebral white matter gliosis not accompanied by demyelination has been reported also in other mammal species such as the mouse (Bronson *et al.*, 1993).

The Accumulation of Various Substances in the Aging White Matter May be Related to Enzyme Deficiencies

Age related deposition and/or accumulation of various substances in the white matter has been described by many authors: Proteinase inhibitor region of amyloid precursor proteins (APPI), ubiquitin, transferrin, ferritin and glycogen. Anti-APPI aggregates 20–40 μm in diameter have been observed by the immunohistochemical method, corresponding exclusively to fibrous astrocytes and associated with the presence of lipofuscin. Such association suggests that the APPI may be related to lysosomal proteinases, since the lipofuscin corresponds to a residual body derived from the lysosome resulting chiefly from cell autophagy. Finely granulated ubiquitin deposits have also been identified by the immunohistochemical method. Myelinated neurites laden with dense ubiquitin-positive bodies were observed on electron microscopy. A few neurites had dense amorphous ubiquitin-positive areas. Myelin displayed focal swellings containing large floccular structures diffusely labeled by ubiquitin. Presence of ubiquitin within lysosomal dense bodies is consistent with the notion that the ubiquitin proteolysis system is not independent of the lysosomes (Chapter 7). Accumulation of ubiquitin in the lysosomes might indicate an age-dependent impairment of the lysosomal system of proteolysis and contribute to the formation of dystrophic myelinated neurites.

Changes in regional distribution of transferrin and ferritin, respectively involved in the mobilization and storage of iron, have been reported in the white matter of elderly individuals, although the amount of residual iron remained unchanged. Since such molecules are located predominantly in the oligodendrocytes, changes might occur in the iron homeostasis resulting in some loss of myelin. Another frequent change in the white matter of elderly individuals, which have not been observed in younger individuals, is the accumulation of glycogen in the form of granules making up not-membrane-bound bodies associated with cell processes, sometimes identified as astrocytic. Such finding has been linked with an alteration in carbohydrate metabolism secondary to a latent enzymatic deficiency that is unmasked during the aging process (Gertz *et al.*, 1985).

Neuro-Imaging Helps Identify Age-related White Matter Changes in vivo

The introduction of new and more sophisticated and sensitive imaging techniques have permitted better visualization of brain morphology and provided an increased capacity for differentiating brain diseases (Chapters 28 and 29). The two main advantages of the neuro-imaging studies over those based on autopsy material are the opportunity to conduct anatomic and prospective studies on healthy living individuals. In addition, neuro-imaging studies remove possible sources of error in postmortem investigations, i.e., selection bias, influence of cause of death, and fixation artifacts. Below are described white matter age-related changes as identified by *computerized tomography* (CT) and magnetic resonance imaging (MRI), and the anatomic basis, etiopathogenesis and clinical significance of such changes. Some images appear in Chapter 28, to which the reader is referred.

Age-related white matter changes as visualized by CT consist of diffuse or more circumscribed, bilateral and usually symmetric, hypodensity areas (*lucencies*) of periventricular and deep white matters. The incidence of these changes seems to increase with age, from 7 percent of individuals between 55–69 years, to 24 percent between 70–85 years (Fukuda *et al.*, 1990; Rezek *et al.*, 1987). However, they are not observed in individuals under 50 years.

Since the introduction of MRI it has been possible to get more precise anatomic images than CT alone. MRI increased the sensitivity of CT, offering a better contrast between tissues of different densities, like gray and white matter. This technical progress rendered possible age-related white matter changes to be more effectively assessed and described. On the coronal plane, which enables an optimal visualization of the brain anatomy, MRI images of white matter changes are bilateral and symmetrically located in the periventricular and deep white matters, and characterized by isolated or multiple areas of increased signal intensity. The visualization of the images can be improved by special techniques, such as highlighting T_2 relaxation with a long spin-echo pulse sequence (Chapter 28). The incidence of the findings varies greatly, from 8 to 74 percent of elderly subjects, depending, similarly to what was stated for the CT, on the age range considered. One study found white matter changes at MRI in 100 percent of the individuals examined in the 71–80 year group. As age increases, not only the incidence of affected individuals but also the number and size of the changes increase. Generally, discrete and moderate changes predominate.

Leuko-araiosis Comprises a Group of White Matter Changes Characterized by a Decrease in White Matter Representation in CT and MRI, Caused or Aggravated by Vascular Pathology

Comparative studies have shown a five times greater sensitivity of MRI than CT in identifying white matter changes. For example, *punctiform hyperintensities* visualized by the MRI, including initial confluent changes, are not similarly represented by CT. However, it is possible that the pathology producing hyperintensities at MRI and lucencies at CT are similar and that such changes account for different stages of the same process, the lesions identified by MRI possibly representing the most initial stage. In 1987, Hachinski and coworkers proposed the designation *leuko-araiosis* (Greek *leuko* = white + *araios* = thin) for those white matter changes identified by CT and MRI, and characterized by a decrease in the white matter representation density (Chapter 28).

Few are the studies attempting to correlate the CT and MRI findings with neuropathologic findings. Hypodensity at CT was noted in a few cases of white matter infarct, while lacunes, gliosis, myelin pallor and dilatation of perivascular spaces are the lesions usually associated with high intensity signals observed by MRI. One of such studies demonstrated a correlation between the number of lacunes and the severity of diffuse periventricular hyperintense lesions. On the other hand, cases of neuropathologic changes (e.g., diffuse myelin pallor) have occasionally been described with no corresponding changes being detected by MRI, and *vice-versa*.

Even though some recent studies were not able to show any relation between leuko-araiosis and hypertension, there is a compelling body of evidence that a persistent increase in blood pressure may act as a risk factor for the development and/or worsening of leuko-araiosis. Hypertension is usually associated with arteriolosclerosis of long medullary arteries and hypoperfusion resulting from the narrowing of the vascular lumen, worsened by systemic factors (e.g., arterial hypotension episodes, congestive heart failure). CT-based studies showed that hypertension was present in 57–63 percent of individuals with leuko-araiosis, compared to 25–38 percent of individuals without leuko-araiosis. Neuropathologic findings commonly associated with leuko-araiosis (lacunes, gliosis, myelin pallor, dilatation of perivascular spaces) also suggest that a decreased white matter blood perfusion caused by the mechanisms mentioned above, is likely to be the principal factor for the development and/or worsening of leuko-araiosis.

Another possible cause of decrease in white matter blood flow and, consequently, of leuko-araiosis development is the presence of *artery and arteriole tortuosities* in the white matter, which are more commonly found in the elderly compared to adults (Figures 21–5 and 21–6). The tortuosities reduce the blood flow in affected vessels by increasing local vascular resistance; by increasing the length of affected vessel; or by changing laminar flow into turbulent flow. As a consequence, higher hydrostatic pressures are required to keep tortuous vessels opened.

New methods for measuring regional brain blood flow and cerebral metabolism have confirmed occurrence of hypoperfusion during aging. Decrease in blood flow and O_2 extraction rate was observed, although O_2 utilization rate remained unchanged. Blood pressure decrease was greater in the frontal lobes. In certain cases the contribution of a lesion in the blood-brain barrier to the leuko-araiosis genesis should not be disregarded. During aging

white matter capillaries become thinner owing to loss of pericytes and thinning of endothelial cell cytoplasm. Since the pericyte seems to act as a second line of defense in the *blood-brain barrier* by phagocytizing molecules passing the endothelium, loss of such cells with age would decrease the ability of the blood-brain barrier to compensate for transient leaks. Finally, since a few studies have highlighted the correlation between leuko-araiosis severity and the degree of cerebral hypotrophy, and white matter lesions are always bilateral and symmetric and increase with age, it is possible that the white matter decrease observed during aging may contribute to the genesis and progression of leuko-araiosis.

Since the age related neuroradiological changes observed in the cerebral white matter are characterized by decreased white matter representation density, and have as anatomic basis various lesions whose common denominator is the focal or diffuse loss of white matter components, it should be expected that cognitive and motor deficits occur as a consequence of such changes. When evaluated by psychometric testing, individuals with leuko-araiosis have a poorer performance in many cognitive tasks than individuals without leuko-araiosis. Differences remain significant even when the results are adjusted for age, education and brain infarct effects. More prominent diffuse periventricular changes are particularly associated with decreased cognitive functions. Motor changes (e.g., gait disturbances and presence of pathologic reflexes) are also more prominent in individuals with leuko-araiosis. However, some studies have failed to find any correlation between presence of leuko-araiosis and cognitive deficit. Such discrepancies may be explained by selection bias, conflicting definition of changes viewed by MRI, and type of psychometric test used. Even when not associated with cognitive and/or psychomotor decline, leuko-araiosis should contribute to reducing the white matter and, as a result, rendering individuals prone to subsequent functional impairments.

Biochemical Changes

Few are the studies dealing with biochemical changes in cerebral white matter during aging. Decrease by about 25 percent in myelin has been observed in individuals between 30–90 years, resulting from partial loss of lipids and myelin proteins. Decrease in cholesterol by 17–27 percent has been noted in individuals above 70 years. Phospholipid content seems to be significantly reduced (by around 20 percent) in higher age ranges, especially from 70 years. However, no qualitative difference has been observed in the composition of phospholipids (phosphatidyletanolamine, phosphatidylcholine, sphingomyelin). Reduction in total white matter protein by 20–50 percent was reported between 30–90 years, the rate of loss of myelin protein being slightly higher than the loss of total protein. Here again, no qualitative change was noted in the composition of the two main myelin proteins: Proteolipid and myelin basic protein. *Racemization* (i.e., non-enzymatic change of L-amino acids into D-enan-

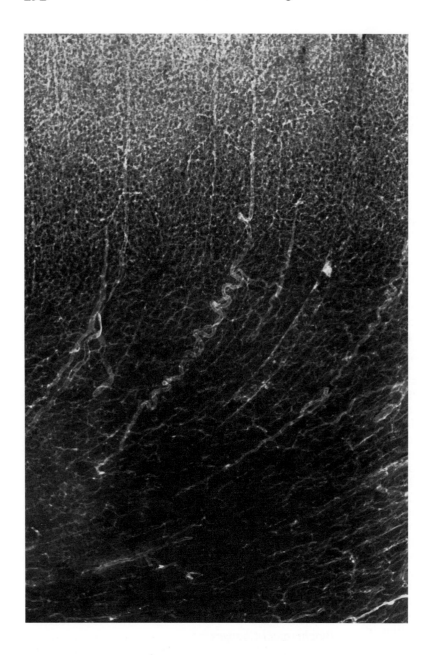

FIGURE   21–5
Typical tortuous medullary arteriole in older and hypertensive patients. After a straight course without branching through the cortex (dense capillary bed at top of illustration), there is extreme tortuosity in the subcortical region. This vessel is 60 μm in diameter. Reproduced, with permission, from Moody *et al.*, 1991.

tiomers) of aspartic acid of myelin protein was found in individuals above 20 years, increasing with age (Matsubara *et al.*, 1994). Another age related biochemical change refers to the water content in the white matter, which was reported to increase from 67 percent at 30 years to 72 percent at 90 years of age. The latter finding may represent one exception to the general rule of decreasing water content of tissues with increasing aging.

The functional consequences of such biochemical changes are still unknown. Since cholesterol and phospholipids contribute to the preservation of the various properties of the cell membranes (stability, permeability, enzyme activity), such quantitative changes might affect some of those properties. Likewise, the high content of D-aspartic acid in the myelin proteins might affect the conformation and function of these proteins, thus possibly causing a change in the speed of nerve impulse transmission.

An Overall View

Among all components of the brain tissue, the white matter develops the most slowly. Owing of the large volume it occupies in the brain, the continuity it keeps with the perikarya of the neurons situated in the cortical and subcortical gray matter and the type of arterial supply occurring in it, the white matter undergoes important changes after development and maturation. These changes are partly dependent on neuronal changes and partly related to changes in medullary artery walls and/or in the cerebral blood flow.

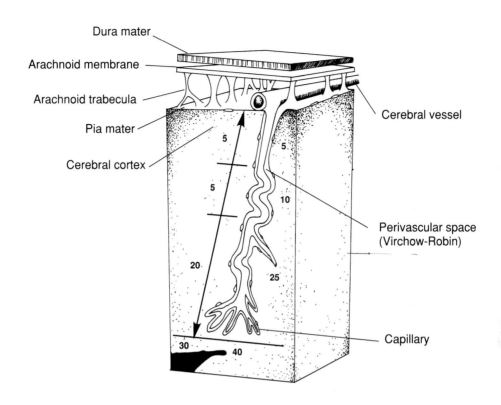

FIGURE   21–6

Scheme of typical cerebral medullary arterioles from older and hypertensive patients. In the subcortical region the vessel traveled 10 mm to gain 5 mm in depth. There is less tortuosity in deep white matter. In addition to the pressure losses caused by the extra length of the tortuosity, there would be further losses if the kinks and loops transformed laminar flow into turbulent flow. Adapted from Moody *et al.*, 1991.

Selected Readings

Braffman, B. H., Zimmerman, R. A., Trojanowski, J. Q., *et al.* 1988. Brain M.R.: pathologic correlation with gross and histopathology. 2. Hyperintense white-matter foci in the elderly. Am. J. Radiol. 151:559–566.

Bronson, R. T., Lipman, R. D., and Harrison, D. E. 1993. Age-related gliosis in the white matter of mice. Brain Res. 609:124–128.

Doraiswamy, P. M., Figiel, G. S., Husain, M. M., *et al.* 1991. Aging of the human corpus callosum: magnetic resonance imaging in normal volunteers. J. Neuropsychiat. Clin. Neurosci. 3:392–397.

Dozono, K., Ishii, N., Nishihara, Y., and Horie, A. 1991. An autopsy study of the incidence of lacunes in relation to age, hypertension, and arteriosclerosis. Stroke 22:993–996.

Fukuda, H., Kobayashi, S., Koide, H., *et al.* 1990. Age-related changes in cerebral white matter measured by computed cranial tomography. Comput. Med. Imaging Graph. 14:79–84.

George, A. E., de Leon, M. J., Gentes, C. I., *et al.* 1986. Leukoencephalopathy in normal and pathologic aging: 1. CT of brain lucencies. Am. J. Radiol. 7:561–566.

George, A. E., de Leon, M. J., Kalnin, A., *et al.* 1986. Leukoencephalopathy in normal and pathologic aging: 2. MRI of brain lucencies. Am. J. Radiol. 7:567–570.

Grafton, S. T., Sumi, S. M., Stimac, G. K., *et al.* 1991. Comparison of postmortem magnetic resonance imaging and neuropathologic findings in the cerebral white matter. Arch. Neurol. 48:293–298.

Hunt, A. L., Orrison, W. W., Yeo, R. A., *et al.* 1989. Clinical significance of MRI white matter lesions in the elderly. Neurology 39:1470–1474.

Kawamura, J., Terayama, Y., Takashima, S., *et al.* 1993. Leuko-araiosis and cerebral perfusion in normal aging. Exp. Aging Res. 19:225–240.

Klekamp, J., Riedel, A., Harper, C., and Kretschmann, H.-J. 1989. Morphometric study on the postnatal growth of noncortical brain regions in Australian Aborigines and Caucasians. Brain Res. 485:79–88.

Kluger, A., Gianutsos, J., de Leon, M. J., and George, A. E. 1988. Significance of age-related white matter lesions. Stroke 19:1054–1055.

Kobari, M., Meyer, J. S., and Ichijo, M. 1990. Leuko-araiosis, cerebral atrophy, and cerebral perfusion in normal aging. Arch. Neurol. 47:161–165.

Leys, D., Soetaert, G., Petit, H., Fauquette, A., Pruvo, J.-P., and Steinling, M. 1990. Periventricular and white matter magnetic resonance imaging hyperintensities do not differ between Alzheimer's disease and normal aging. Arch. Neurol. 47:524–527.

Romeu R. de Souza

22

Nerve Cell Loss in the Myenteric Plexus

The Type and Intensity of Age-related Changes Vary Regionally in the Gut

    Age-related Neuronal Loss in the Myenteric Plexus of the Esophagus Has Been Associated with Disordered Esophageal Motility in the Elderly

    Nerve Cell Loss May be Linked with the Age-related Reduction of Gastric Motility, and Secretory and Morphologic Changes in the Stomach

    Neuron Loss in the Myenteric Plexus may Have Important Repercussions for Motility, Absorption of Nutrients and Release of Hormones in the Small Intestine

    The Decrease in the Myenteric Neuron Density with Age may be Involved in Colon Motility Problems Such as Constipation

An Overall View

The myenteric plexus, also termed *Auerbach plexus* after the German physiologist Leopold Auerbach (1828–1897), is a ganglionated plexus situated between the layers of the muscle coat of the alimentary tract, from the esophagus to the anus. It can be visualized histologically as a mesh-like laminar structure consisting of wide and thin ganglia of multipolar neurons joined to each other by connecting strands. The small nerves emerging from this plexus provide autonomous innervation to the muscle layers of the wall of the gut.

Each myenteric ganglion, likewise the gray matter of the central nervous system, is composed of two cell types: nerve cells and glial cells. In man these cell types and their processes are tightly packed within a meshwork of connective tissue (De Souza *et al.*, 1988), differently from other adult animals, in which the connective tissue does not penetrate the ganglia (Gabella, 1979). The total number of myenteric neurons in the human gut is extremely high – probably in the order of hundreds of millions, thus approximately one tenth of the total neuron complement of the brain. The number of nerve cells in each ganglion varies from 300 to only a few in man (De Souza *et al.*, 1988) and from 5 to 160 nerve cells in other mammalian species (Wilson *et al.*, 1981).

Normal aging usually results in a decrease in the number of myenteric neurons. In humans, the decrease in number of these cells seems to accentuate especially after the age of 70 (Koeberle, 1968). Since myenteric neurons play important direct and indirect roles in physiological processes like the motility of the gut, absorption of nutrients and the immune response, age-related changes in their content and distribution have important consequences to the organism. For example, the reduction in number of myenteric neurons with aging may determine changes in the content and distribution of a number of substances that act as neurotransmitters and hormones in the gut. Among the numerous neurotransmitters synthesized and released by myenteric neurons, acetylcholine is the most common one. Acetylcholine is released by myenteric neurons to intestinal smooth muscle, playing an important role in the regulation of the diffuse, worm-like movement termed *peristalsis* (Greek *peri* = around + *stalsis* = contraction), by which the gastrointestinal tube propels its contents. Many other gastrointestinal peptides seem to serve a hormonal action in the alimentary tract and have a neurotransmitter role in the myenteric plexus, like vasoactive intestinal polypeptide (VIP), somatostatin (SOM), substance P (SP), calcitonin gene-related peptide, enkephalin, neurotensin, gastrin, gastrin- releasing peptide, galanin and gama-aminobutyric acid transaminase (Schultzberg *et al.*, 1980).

The Type and Intensity of Age-related Changes Vary Regionally in the Gut

Several studies have been devoted to examine changes in number of neurons in the different parts of the human gut. There is evidence that regional changes do occur and may be related to the physiological functions of each of the different portions of the gut. For this reason we shall review the changes observed in each of these portions.

Age-related Neuronal Loss in the Myenteric Plexus of the Esophagus Has Been Associated with Disordered Esophageal Motility in the Elderly

Neuron loss in the human esophagus has been reported by a number of authors. In one study we showed that, in the entire esophagus, there was a decrease in the number of neurons of at least 15 percent, with the most pronounced loss being 60 percent in the upper third of the organ (Table 22–1).

The normal motor activity of the esophagus consists of an orderly peristaltic contraction that propagates from the upper sphincter through the striated and smooth muscle parts and terminates in closure of the lower esophageal sphincter. Esophageal peristalsis is under a central control mechanism, but there is also an intrinsic peripheral control mechanism located in the myenteric plexus of the esophageal wall. The control of the function of the lower esophageal sphincter is not well understood but it appears to depend on local neural mechanisms (myenteric plexus) together with the modulating effect of circulating hormones (Diamant and El-Sharkawy, 1977). In support to this idea are some functional studies showing that vasoactive intestinal polypeptide, somatostatin or nitric oxide synthase deficiencies may contribute to the dysfunction of the lower esophageal sphincter, e. g., *achalasia* (a = negation + Greek *kalasis* = relaxation, meaning the failure to relax) (Guelrud *et al.*, 1992; Murray *et al.*, 1991).

TABLE **22–1**   Nerve cell loss in the myenteric plexus of various portions of the alimentary tract in several species with aging.

Species	Region	Neurons/cm^2		Loss (%)	Ref.
		Young	**Aged**		
Human	Esophagus:				(i)
	• upper	887	337	62	
	• middle	1,962	1,746	11	
	• lower	1,267	850	33	
	• lower	2,253	1,685	25	(ii)
Human	Stomach:				(iii)
	• fundus	1,005	643	36	
	• body	2,169	1,489	31	
	• antrum	3,249	1,599	51	
Human	Duodenum	7,506	4,663	38	(iv)
	Jejunum	6,900	4,583	34	
	Ileum	6,907	4,376	37	
Rat	Jejunum	5,477	3,290	40	(v)
	Ileum	8,169	4,692	43	
	Colon	14,214	5,128	64	
	Rectum	9,716	5,612	42	
Guinea-Pig	Small intestine	8,600	2,489	71	(vi)

Data are from: (i) Meciano Filho *et al.*, 1995; (ii) Eckardt and LeCompte, 1978; (iii) Anaruma, 1994; (iv) De Souza *et al.*, 1993; (v) Santer and Baker, 1988; (vi) Gabella, 1989.

Age-related neuronal loss in the myenteric plexus of the esophagus has been associated with disordered esophageal motility in the elderly. Soergel and colleagues described a disturbance of esophageal motility in elderly subjects, consisting of disorganization of the response to deglutition, as a result of a defect in initiating relaxation of the lower esophageal sphincter, and of primary peristalsis. Hollis and Castell found weakening of esophageal smooth muscle with an intact neural pathway. The conflicting data from the preceding reports stress the need for additional studies, both anatomic and functional, regarding the neural control in the aging esophagus.

Nerve Cell Loss May be Linked with the Age-related Reduction of Gastric Motility, and Secretory and Morphologic Changes in the Stomach

Gastric motility, too, decreases with advancing age. This may lead not only to delayed emptying and maldigestion but also affect the rate and extent of absorption of orally administered drugs. Because no detailed knowledge has arisen as yet from either structural or functional studies on the microcircuitry of the myenteric plexus in the stomach, it is still difficult to define the role of this plexus in intrinsic reflexes that control the gastric motility. However, there is evidence that myenteric neurons of the stomach mediate locally the powerful inputs coming from the central nervous system via the *nervus vagus*. These vagal inputs are involved in the receptive relaxation and accommodation to increase in volume of the gastric contents, and they also play an important part in the evocation of antral peristalsis in the distal stomach. Similarly, the dominant role of vagal pathways in controlling the secretion of gastric acid, pepsin, and some hormones, notably gastrin, appears to be mediated by myenteric plexus neurons which innervate the acid-secreting parietal cells and gastrin-secreting cells located within the mucosa of

the stomach. Aging of the stomach is also associated with secretory and morphologic changes characterized by diminished acid and pepsin secretion and mucosal atrophy. In an extensive study of the number of myenteric neurons in the stomach of aged humans, C. A. Anaruma observed reductions of 34 percent-54 percent of the number of neurons in relation to young adult individuals (Table 22–1). However, it is still difficult to establish whether the nerve cell loss in the myenteric plexus alone is responsible for these changes. Thus, there is a need for morphologic and physiologic studies in the elderly to look for the effects of myenteric nerve cell loss in the gastric motility and secretion.

Neuron Loss in the Myenteric Plexus may Have Important Repercussions for Motility, Absorption of Nutrients and Release of Hormones in the Small Intestine

Neuron loss has been reported in the aging myenteric plexus of the human small intestine (Table 22–1). Significant reductions of at least 34 percent in the number of neurons in the ganglia of the myenteric plexus of old subjects were recorded in all regions of the small intestine, especially in the duodenum, where the number of neurons decreased by over 38 percent (Figure 22–1). Age-related changes in neuron content in the small intestine of rodents are as impressive as those seen in humans. Santer and Baker (1988) recorded significant reductions of 40 percent in the number of neurons in the myenteric plexus of the 24-month rat small intestine. Gabella (1989) found similar figures in the small intestine of the aging guinea-pig.

These remarkable reductions may play an important part in the age-related regulation of some physiological activities of the small intestine, namely motility, absorption of nutrients and release of hormones. The neural control of intestinal motility is mediated through motor myen-

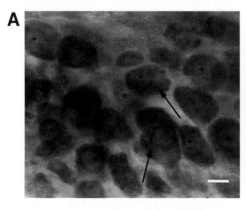
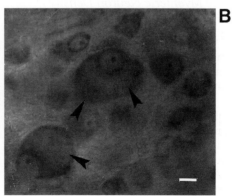

FIGURE   22–1

Whole-mount preparations of the myenteric plexus of the human small intestine (Barbosa, 1978), stained by the Giemsa's method.

A. A group of neurons in a ganglion of young duodenum (arrows). Calibration bar: 5 μm.

B. Two large neurons in a ganglion of the aged ileum (arrowheads). The neuronal staining intensity is weaker than in the young ileum. Calibration bar: 3 μm.

teric neurons. The latter act on the circular and longitudi-nal smooth muscle coats of the external musculature of the small intestine. The motor neurons to the circular muscle are activated via local reflex pathways entirely contained within the wall of the intestine. Distension evokes polarized reflexes – contraction on the oral side and relaxation on the anal side – which together consti-tute the *peristaltic reflex*. Studies of age-associated changes of small intestinal motility have yielded conflict-ing data. One study showed that intestinal transit of bar-ium from the stomach to the cecum was the same in young adults and elderly subjects who had no gastroin-testinal disease (Kim, 1968). The results of another study suggested that there is a reduction of intestinal motility in response to meal in the elderly (Anuras and Sutherland, 1984).

One important age-related change that is well docu-mented in the literature is the reduction in villus height of small intestine mucosa, beginning at approximately age 60 years in most individuals. This reduction of the mucosa surface area is thought to contribute to the age-re-lated reduced absorption of substances such as calcium, iron, fat and carbohydrates. Since the mucosa of the small intestine is richly supplied with nerve endings (Furness *et al.*, 1985) that are involved in the transport of water and electrolytes, the enhancement of blood flow and in the control of the release of some hormones, notably motilin, it is tempting to speculate that the decrease in number of myenteric neurons in the aged might be one of the under-lying mechanisms responsible for the atrophy of the in-testinal mucosa. In support to this hypothesis is an im-munocytochemical study by Fehér and Pénzes (1987) showing that the overall number of substance P-, vasoac-tive intestinal polypeptide- and somatostatin-nerve pro-cesses closely related to epithelial cells, blood vessel base-ment membranes, and smooth muscle cells of the wall of the small intestine was decreased in senile rats in com-parison to young controls.

The Decrease in the Myenteric Neuron Density with Age may be Involved in Colon Motility Problems Such as Constipation

Data concerning changes in the myenteric plexus of the colon with aging have been obtained from studies in lab-oratory animals. Santer and Baker reported a reduction of 60 percent in the number of neurons in the colon of 24-months rats (Table 22–1). Neuron counts have been made on laminar preparations of the colon. Characteristi-cally, in ganglia of aged guinea-pigs the nerve cells are less densely packed (Figure 22–2, B) than in younger adult ani-mals (Figure 22–2, A); moreover, the nerve cells are small-er in the aged and many of them display an irregular pro-file. The same appearance of the myenteric plexus has been observed by Gabella (1989) in the guinea-pig small intestine.

The main function of the colon appears to be the com-pletion of the absorption of water, electrolytes and bile acids, the secretion of potassium and possibly bicarbo-nate, and the production of considerable amounts of mu-cus. Colonic movements include segmentation of the lu-men by stationary narrow *contraction rings* and another type of propulsive activity called *mass movement* or *mass peristalsis*. In the guinea-pig, motor neurons supplying the circular and longitudinal muscles of the large intes-tine have cell bodies located in the myenteric ganglia.

Colonic changes with aging include mucosal atrophy, morphologic abnormalities of mucosal glands, hypertro-phy of the *muscularis mucosae* and atrophy of the muscle layer. The colonic epithelium is rich in mucous cells. Nerve fibers come close to the mucous cells on the sur-face epithelia, so that all have the potential to be in-fluenced by the innervation. T. E. Phillips and coworkers demonstrated a nerve-mediated secretion of mucus in the colon, and Hultén and colleagues showed that there are vasodilator myenteric neurons in the colon.

Common problems in the elderly are *diverticulosis* and *constipation*. The precise mechanism of diverticular formation with aging is uncertain but a large body of lit-erature suggests that diverticulosis is a disorder of muscle function with a pressure gradient developing between the colonic lumen and the serosa, with a second contributory factor being the weakness of the wall of the colon. The mechanism of constipation is poorly understood. It would appear that constipation in the aged is multifactorial, due to a decrease in the muscle tonus and motor function of the colon; a rise of the threshold of pressure for the per-ception of rectal distension and the initiation of the defe-cation reflex; an impaired propulsion in the colon, and nerve cell lesions due to laxative abuse. The decrease in the myenteric neuron density with age is assumed to be involved in all problems cited above.

Novel immunohistochemistry techniques have ad-vanced our understanding of motility disorders that re-sult from myenteric plexus abnormalities. T. R. Koch and colleagues found depleted VIP-containing nerves in pa-tients with slow transit constipation. This evidence not-withstanding, additional studies on the myenteric plexus are required for a better understanding of the influence of nerve cell loss on colonic function in the aged.

An Overall View

The decrease in the number of myenteric neurons with age is probably due to nerve cell death. Since nerve cells are postmitotic, they are not replaced when lost. This leads to the assumption that nerve cell loss represents an irreversible, degenerative process in the myenteric plexus. However, age-related loss of neurons may not always be regarded as a degenerative process; during development, for instance, it simply represents an elimination of redun-dant neurons (Chapter 17), accompanied by a compensa-tory increased efficiency of the surviving cells. Although there is evidence indicating that regional changes in nerve cell numbers do occur with aging which may be related to function abnormalities in each of the different portions of the gut, additional studies are still required in order to clarify further this issue.

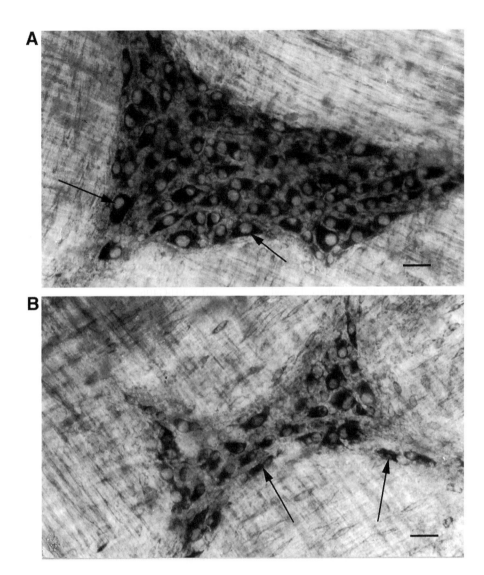

FIGURE   22–2

Whole-mount preparations of the myenteric plexus of the guinea-pig colon stained by the NADH histochemical technique (Gabella, 1987).

A. A myenteric ganglion in the young colon showing a great number of neurons (arrows).

B. A myenteric ganglion in the aged colon showing the dispersed distribution of nerve cells and the relative small size and the irregular profile of most nerve cells (arrows). Calibration bars: 40 µm. Courtesy of E. A. Liberti.

Selected Readings

Armbrecht, H. J., Zenser, T. V., Bruns, M. E., and Davis, B. B. 1979. Effect of age on intestinal calcium absorption and dietary calcium. Am. J. Physiol. 236:E769-E774.

Bird, T., Hall, M. R., and Schade, R. O. 1977. Gastric histology and its relation to anemia in the elderly. Gerontology 23:309–321.

Geokas, M., Conteas, C., and Majundar, A. 1985. The aging gastrointestinal tract, liver and pancreas. Clin. Geriat. Med. 1:177–205.

Greenstein, R. J., Ybanez, M. M., Zhang, R.-L., and Bauman, W. A. 1991. Is aging preprogrammed? Observations from the brain/gut axis. Mech. Ageing Dev. 61:113–121.

James, O. F. W. 1983. Gastrointestinal and liver function in old age. Clin. Gastroenterol. 12:671–691.

Warren, P. M., Pepperman, M. A., and Montgomery, R. D. 1978. Age changes in small intestinal mucosa. Lancet 2:849–850.

Webster, S. G. P., and Leeming, J. T. 1975. The appearance of the small bowel mucosa in old age. Age Ageing 4:168–174.

Yamagata, A. 1965. Histopathological studies of the colon due to age. Jpn. J. Gastroenterol. 62:224–235.

References

Anaruma, C. A. 1994. Morphologic and quantitative study of the myenteric plexus of the human stomach in the elderly. PhD Thesis, Universidade de São Paulo. pp. 39–43.

The peripheral nervous system (PNS) undergoes a variety of changes with age which have been demonstrated by clinical, electrophysiological and pathological studies. These changes may be or may not be considered as 'abnormal', depending on arbitrary criteria such as the degree of functional impairment, the underlying cause of the abnormality, and the population basis on which the concept of 'normality' rests should be applied.

Pathological aging of the PNS is difficult to define, as the 'normality' concept itself depends upon arbitrary criteria. A 'normal conduction velocity' for example, may signify Gaussian, average (or median, modal), habitual, or optimal ('fittest') conduction velocity (Murphy, 1972; Gallen and Gambino, 1975). Ideally, aging as such should be studied longitudinally, and on an individual basis, from which 'normal values' could be obtained for each particular life period, e.g., the measurement of nerve conduction velocity of the same nerve at different ages in the same individual.

In populational studies, however, the concept of normality depends on the methodology adopted to sort and average the individual measurements. Besides, while some age-related changes of the PNS inducing clinical signs and symptoms can be regarded as non-specific, most age-related PNS abnormalities may be accounted for by the increasing prevalence of many age-related diseases such as diabetes mellitus in the population. Therefore the whole population could be examined within given age ranges, or it could be divided into two or more groups of differently aging individuals: The 'normal aging individuals', and the patients affected by one or more diseases.

We focused this chapter on the aging human PNS, some studies on aging animals being quoted at the end of the chapter.

Methodologic Pitfalls in the Study of the Aging PNS can be Circumvented by a Combination of Different Epidemiological Approaches

The main difficulty in the study of PNS neuropathology arises from pathological changes observed in the main *peripheral neuropathies* (PN) being qualitatively similar to some of those seen with increasing prevalence in the so-called normal aging. Thus, the distinction between PN and normal aging of PNS can be difficult, especially in the oldest patients, which make more difficult the diagnosis of the late onset forms of peripheral neuropathies.

Which are the criteria for normality? Seventy-five percent of the population over 70 are affected by at least one significant chronic disease, while half have two or more disorders (Vital and Vital, 1991; Vallat et al., 1992). Could the minority that escaped serious illnesses be considered as normal? As mentioned in the beginning, a 'gold standard' for normality does not exist, and 'normality' has thus to be defined for each study. In some cases, it may be more appropriate to specify the population to be studied in terms of functional ability, or status, or by exclusion of specific diseases or functional impairments. In other cases, a 'normal range' can be used.

Other pitfalls such as cohort effects have been neglected in aging studies for a long time. The comparison between 20-year-old individuals and 80 year-old individuals is biased by secular effects, as individuals were born at a 60 year interval. This kind of methodologic problem could be solved using a combination of cross-sectional and longitudinal studies: Cross-sectional studies tend to overemphasize age differences, while longitudinal studies tend to underemphasize such differences (Metter *et al.*, 1992); longitudinal studies rule out the cohort effects, but are very long and expensive. However this combinatorial approach has not been applied to studies of the peripheral nervous system. The only available data on changes in peripheral motor and sensory systems with aging are cross-sectional.

The Normal Nerve Comprises Many Compactly Ensheathed Layers of Distinct Cells with Different Susceptibilities to Degeneration and Regeneration

The normal nerve comprises myelinated fibers, each of them being made of an axon surrounded by compacted rolled up processes from the membranes of an individual chain of *Schwann cells* (the myelin sheath). Non-myelinated axons lie recessed within a separate cleft in the surface of cords of other Schwann cells. The connective tissue, also named interstitial tissue or interstitium, comprises (Figure 23–1): (i) The *endoneurium*, which surrounds directly the myelinated fibers, unmyelinated axons and Schwann cells, and includes some fibrocytes, rare mastocytes and a few small blood vessels from the microcirculation. (ii) The *perineurium*, that ensheaths each nerve fascicle, and is made of several layers of compactly arranged flattened cells. The perineural cells have basement membranes, and are linked by tight junctions. (iii) The *epineurium* embodies each fascicle, extending to the common connective tissue surrounding the nerve and to adjacent vessels. These comprise the main artery of the nerve, that reaches usually a diameter of 100–200 μm.

Age-related as well as traumatic lesions may affect each of the different structures which comprise the nerve. We shall examine these lesions and the mechanisms of repair in some depth.

Primary Degeneration of Axons and Nerve Cell Bodies

Destruction of axons causes concomitant degeneration of the myelin, but this usually does not destroy the basement membrane that outlines the myelinated fiber, at the external surface of the Schwann cell. Three main mechanisms are involved, namely Wallerian degeneration, dying-back neuropathy or distal axonal degeneration, and neuronopathy.

Wallerian degeneration is the degeneration of axon and myelin sheaths distal to the axonal section (Figure 23–2, C). It is followed by fast proliferation of distal Schwann cells which remain inside the basement membrane of the same nerve fiber, constituting the *Büngner*

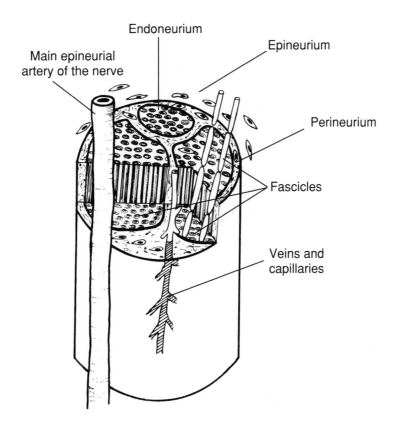

FIGURE 23–1
Diagram of the different compartments, and of the blood supply, of a nerve (Redrawn from J. J. Hauw and B. Eymard, 1995).

bands. Small nerve buds sprout from the injured axon at, and proximal to, the section level. These numerous small regenerating axons grow distally into the Büngner bands and produce clusters of closely-apposed small fibers, some of which become myelinated, the so-called fascicles of regeneration of Nageotte (Figure 23–3).

Dying-back neuropathy is a slow distal axonopathy involving first the longest fibers, which are also the largest ones. Its mechanism is not fully understood. Dysmetabolism of the perikaryon, disturbances of axonal transport, lack of distal growth factors, and action of toxic factors have been suggested. Axonal degeneration occurs concomitantly in the central processes (posterior columns of the spinal cord) and in the peripheral processes of sensory neurons. In this slowly evolving process, axonal degeneration and regeneration (distal and collateral sprouting) are similar to, although milder than, those seen in Wallerian degeneration (Figure 23–2, D).

Neuronopathy is a more rapidly evolving neuronal death, in which the perikaryon and its neurites degenerate simultaneously. There is often a selective vulnerability of the small or of the large neurons of the spinal root ganglia. The mechanisms of neuronopathy, and the cause of the selective involvement of some neuronal populations remain unclear. Other lesions of the axon include axonal atrophy and axonal swelling. Axonal atrophy is

seen mainly in large fibers, and best shown by morphometry. The axon diameter is smaller than it should be in myelinated fibers of the same diameter range. This is often due to abnormalities in neurofilament synthesis. Axonal atrophy may be associated with secondary demyelination, that may be severe. Axonal swelling results from focal accumulation of neurofilaments as a consequence of abnormalities of the slow axonal transport. In proximal axonopathies, axonal swelling is seen initially in proximal axons. Axonal atrophy or degeneration occurs distally.

Two main morphological aspects are associated with primary axonal and neuronal degeneration: (i) *Acute* (or recent) *axonal involvement* is indicated by ovoids and balls of degenerating axons and myelin. They are best seen on teased fibers preparations, but can also be found on longitudinal sections, and even cross-sections, of nerves. Morphometric studies may show a higher density of myelinated fibers than normal, and reveal a shift to the left of the distribution of the diameters of myelinated fibers because of the high number of regenerating axons. Büngner's bands made up by Schwann cell proliferation are usually easy to recognize. (ii) *Chronic axonal involvement* is indicated by rarefaction of nerve fibers, hypertrophy, and sometimes proliferation of Schwann cells and fibrocytes, and increase in their density. Clusters of regeneration may still be seen.

Primary Schwann Cell-Myelin Involvement

Myelin degeneration occurs with relative sparing of axons and of the external basal lamina that outlines the external surface of the Schwann cell.

In *acute segmental demyelination and remyelination,* destruction of myelin involves scattered internodes along the myelinated fiber. It usually begins in the paranodal region (Figure 23–2, B). When this occurs on a few scattered internodes, their remyelination may be performed by their own Schwann cell after phagocytosis of the degenerated myelin by Schwann cells and monocyte-macrophages. This leads to a thin internode of normal length. If proliferated Schwann cells remyelinate longer segments of demyelinated axons, this leads to internodes of irregular lengths and thickness (Figure 23–4). Morphometric study of the so-called *g factor* (internal diameter/external diameter of myelinated fibers) may be helpful to detect milder lesions. Teased nerve fiber preparations provide the best data, however, and allow to quantify easily the proportion of fibers affected by demyelination-remyelination or by axonal degeneration.

Chronic segmental demyelination-remyelination induces Schwann cell proliferation around the intact axon. This leads to a concentric arrangement of Schwann cells and basement membranes called 'onion bulbs' (Figure 23–5). There is also frequently an increase of the non-cellular component in the endoneurium (collagen, proteoglycans).

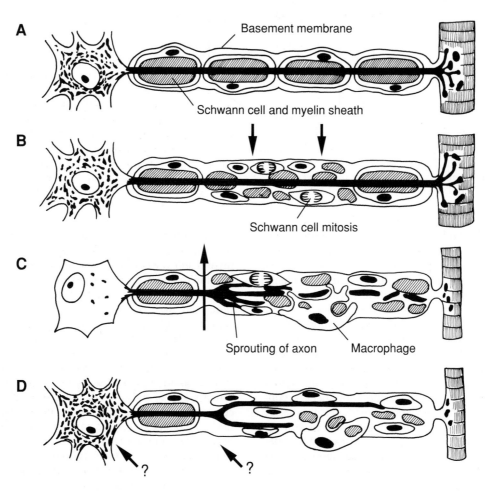

FIGURE 23–2

Diagram of the main degenerative-regenerative processes affecting peripheral nerves.

A. Normal myelinated fiber: Regular internodes of the same length and thickness are seen.

B. In segmental demyelination, there is patchy damage (arrows) of individual Schwann cells and/or myelin sheaths. The neuronal cell body is not affected; there is no denervation atrophy.

C. In Wallerian degeneration, the section (arrow) of the axon causes central chromatolysis of the nerve cell body, and denervation atrophy of the muscle.

D. In dying-back neuropathy, axonal breakdown may be due to a pathologic condition of the nerve cell body or axon (arrows with question marks). There is denervation atrophy of the muscle, and usually no central chromatolysis

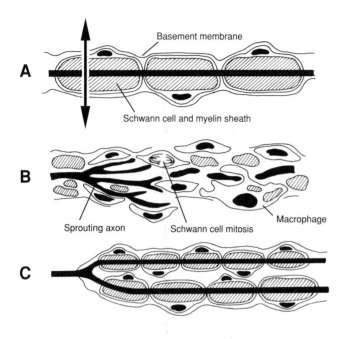

FIGURE 23–3

Diagrammatic representation of the course of Wallerian degeneration and regeneration.

A. Axonal section in a normal myelinated fiber.

B. Distal degeneration of axons and myelin, removal of debris by Schwann cells and macrophages, proliferation of Schwann cells within the basement membrane of the previous myelinated fiber (called Büngner's bands), and sprouting of proximal portion of axon.

C. Regeneration of two small myelinated fibers with short internodes into the basement membrane of the previous myelinated fiber, clusters (or fascicles) of regeneration.

(Redrawn from J. J. Hauw and B. Eymard, 1995).

Nerve Electrophysiological Data Have Been Related to Nerve Morphological Changes

Electrophysiological data have been related to the basic lesions of peripheral nerve. As summarized by Buchthal (1984), slowing of nerve conduction velocity is associated with demyelination. This is the case in the experimental neuropathy and in acute or chronic human disorders with segmental demyelination-remyelination. Mild or moderate slowing in conduction and reduction in amplitude occurs in the absence of marked demyelination and is often by axonal degeneration. In contrast, the conduction velocity is normal in *spinal muscular atrophy*. The slowed conduction found in certain *polyneuropathies* remains more difficult to understand on pure morphological grounds. It may be related to changes in axonal membrane, as we will see later. In addition, marked focal reductions of the amplitude of motor potentials without significant reduction in the conduction velocity (conduction blocks) are not explained by morphological changes.

Neurophysiological Changes With Age

Neurophysiological changes with age include decrease in sensory and motor nerve conduction and denervation-reinnervation changes. The respective roles of aging *per se* versus associated risk factors in determining such changes has never been established.

Sensory and Motor Nerve Conductions are Decreased With Age

In aged individuals, all studies showed a clear decline in velocity and especially in amplitude of potentials with age. Cruz Martinez and colleagues studied the sensory velocity of digital nerves in 47 healthy subjects from 21 to 77 years. It steadily declines from 57 to 48 meters per second, and the amplitude of sensory potentials drops from 43 to 21 microvolts. This is a very early process, since the motor nerve conduction velocity slows at a rate of 1 meter per second per decade from 20 to 55 years of age and 3 m/sec per decade after 55 years of age (Buchthal et al., 1984).

The decrease in nerve conduction velocity and in amplitude of the motor and sensory potentials was often described using linear models. Taylor, however, showed that most changes were better fitted by degree 2 regression, i.e., by a quadratic parabolic model, which shows that changes accelerate with advancing age. Interestingly enough, Taylor's data on terminal motor latency show no age dependence. Buchthal and colleagues observed that

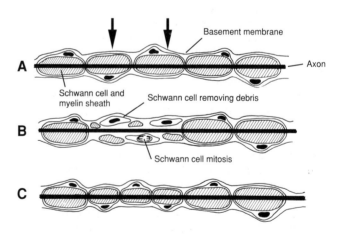

FIGURE 23–4

Diagrammatic representation of the lesions of segmental demyelination and remyelination.

A. Destruction of scattered Schwann cells and/or myelin internodes (arrows) along the myelinated fiber, with axon sparing.

B. Degeneration of myelin, removal of debris by Schwann cells and macrophages, proliferation of Schwann cells within the basement membrane of the previous myelinated fiber.

C. Remyelination of involved internodes leads to myelinated fibers with internodes of irregular lengths and thickness.

(Redrawn from J. J. Hauw and B. Eymard, 1995).

now chaotic form of differentiation, cannot be ascertained in light of the present knowledge of the genetic mechanisms of oncogenesis.

For the following argumentations it must be borne in mind that dedifferentiation may reflect chaotic differentiation, thus a no-way-back. Even if the biological qualities of a tumor in question strongly resemble the qualities of undifferentiated tumors, there is no possibility of redifferentiation, or maturation as seen in primitive undifferentiated tumors.

In pathology, it is common to speak about embryonal tumors, or mature and immature tumors, reflecting the grade of differentiation of a tumor entity, but also more or less unconsciously describing the ontogenetic age of a tumor in question. However, there are few studies which have compared the molecular markers of ontogenetic maturation of the human central nervous system with the expression of these markers in tumors. In an investigation of *primitive neuroectodermal tumors* (PNETs), at least an idea of the grade of maturation – the ontogenetic age – of the individual tumor within this group of PNETs could be given (Kleinert, 1991a, b). An initiated cell can be (i) totally undifferentiated as in germinomas, (ii) almost totally undifferentiated, leading to a usually malignant embryonal tumor; (iii) poorly differentiated, leading to an immature, eventually malignant tumor with a pattern of molecular marker expression as in fetal tissue; or (iv) differentiated, leading to a benign or malignant tumor resembling mature adult tissue. Undifferentiated tumors can further differentiate; differentiated tumors can only dedifferentiate without the possibility of redifferentiation.

Fetal, Adult, or Senile Tumors? Do Tumors Have Ages?

A systematic approach to discuss tumor ages as defined above has to regard not only the grade of cellular differentiation or dedifferentiation but also some histogenetic principles.

The *zygote*, and later the *totipotential blastoderm*, differentiates into three major cell lines, namely the *germ cell line*, the *extraembryonal cell line*, and the *somatic cell line*. And indeed, tumors of all ages can be found within the dysontogenetic tumors derived from germ cells (Walter and Kleinert, 1987). To date, it is generally accepted that all primordial germ cells are produced in the normal fetal yolk sac and migrate along the midline to the gonadal folds (Witschi, 1948; McKay *et al.*, 1953), thereby also passing the later pineal region. Misplaced germ cells may acquire neoplastic properties while keeping their ontogenetic potentiality, explaining the development of the not rare mixed dysontogenetic tumors. *Germinomas* in brain such as all below mentioned dysontogenetic tumors mainly localized in the pineal region, are totally undifferentiated and totipotential, thus corresponding to the preembryonal germ cells. *Embryonal carcinomas* may contain embryoid bodies comparable to normal embryos of the age of 1–2 gestational weeks (Evans, 1957), justifying a tumor subtype called *polyembryoma*. About the same

ontogenetic tumor age have extraembryonal tumors such as *endodermal sinus tumor* deriving from the yolk sac endoderm, and *choriocarcinoma* deriving from trophoblasts of the placenta, as well as the frequent mixed dysontogenetic tumors in which a multipotential initiated cell develops in different cellular directions (Figure 24–1).

The *somatic cell line* further differentiates into three germ layers, i.e. *ectoderm* including *neuroectoderm*, *mesoderm*, and *endoderm*. Tumors of vestigial tissues, e.g. *teratoma*, *dermoid*, *epidermoid*, and *craniopharyngioma*, are clearly of malformative origin. The heterotopic tissue can derive from germ cells as described above, or from heterotopias caused by combined malformations such as in dermoids and epidermoids seen in association with *spina bifida* and other dysraphic malformations. In classical benign mature teratomas, all three germ layers have developed well differentiated tumor tissue comparable to tissue in adult persons. It is readily conceivable that only one or two germ layers may develop as tumor or tumor-like lesion in the brain as it is the case in epidermoids deriving solely from the ectodermal layer or dermoids deriving from both ectoderm and mesoderm. In immature teratomas and teratoid neoplasms, a clear histological recognition of the different germ layers is difficult; the features resemble sometimes fetal tissue, and the histological identity may be unsure (Figure 24–2). These tumors have different grades of dignity depending on the amount of immature tissue (Gonzalez-Crussi, 1982.)

Tumors Deriving from the Neuroectoderm can be Divided in Glial and Neuronal Tumors

Tumors deriving from the *neuroectoderm* can roughly be divided in glial and neuronal tumors. The most instructive example of glial tumors or *gliomas* with respect to ontogenetic ages are the astrocytic tumors. In the international WHO-classification of tumors of the central nervous system (Kleihues *et al.*, 1993), grade I (benign) is reserved for well differentiated and well circumscribed tumors. The histologically well differentiated *fibrillary*, *protoplasmatic*, or *gemistocytic astrocytomas* are characterized by grade II (semibenign) owing to their diffuse intracerebral growth with slightly worse prognosis than grade I tumors. In the most malignant astrocytic tumor, the *glioblastoma*, the very fast tumor growth leads to necroses because the tumor vessels are not growing fast enough to ensure a sufficient blood supply of the tumor tissue (Figure 24–3). Mutations of the *p53* gene play the central role in the initiation of these astrocytic tumors (Louis *et al.*, 1993; Koga *et al.*, 1994). The absence of recurrence and malignant transformation over a considerably long period in many grade II astrocytomas suggests that *p53* mutation may not be sufficient for the progression from grade II to grade III (semimalignant), then called *anaplastic astrocytoma* which is histologically characterized by dedifferentiated focal or diffuse tumor areas (Figure 24–4). Additional genetic alterations may be necessary for the progression to grade IV (malignant) represented by a dedifferentiated astrocytic tumor histologi-

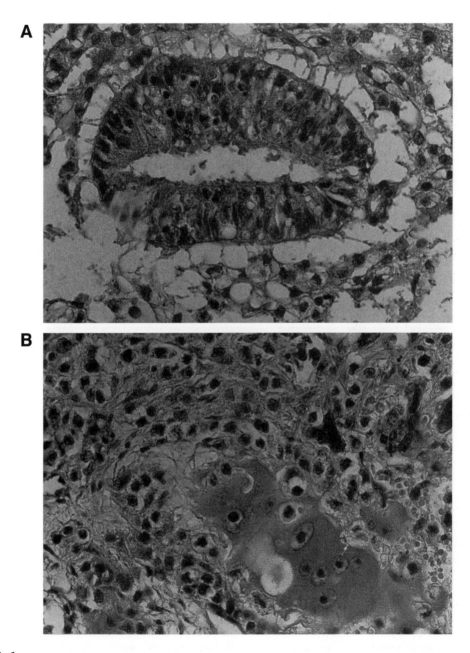

FIGURE   24–1
Examples of embryonal dysontogenetic tumors.

A. Embryonal tumor with polyembryoma body. Hematoxylin-eosin, X 150

B. Extraembryonal tumor from placental tissue (choriocarcinoma) exhibiting syncytiotrophoblastic giant cells. Hematoxylin-eosin, X 150

cally exhibiting features of a seemingly embryonal tumor, the glioblastoma. Consequently, this progression into an anaplastic astrocytoma or a glioblastoma could also be seen as retrogression from an ontogenetic point of view. As already mentioned, *anaplasia* means 'back-formation', or a kind of development bringing the tumor 'backwards' to a younger ontogenetic age. But how can an anaplastic tumor become younger or 'more chaotic' which is also 'younger' in a sense? There is increasing evidence that the progression from grade II astrocytoma to anaplastic as-

trocytoma and glioblastoma is associated with the acquisition of multiple genetic alterations, involving not only chromosome 17p with the *p53* gene, but also other different chromosomes. In glioblastomas, the *loss of heterozygosity* (LOH) for alleles on chromosome 10 and *epidermal growth factor receptor* (EGFR) gene amplification play a crucial role (Bigner and Vogelstein, 1990; von Deimling *et al.*, 1992). However, glioblastomas may eventually occur as primary poorly differentiated tumors, too, deriving from remnants of poorly differentiated glioblasts.

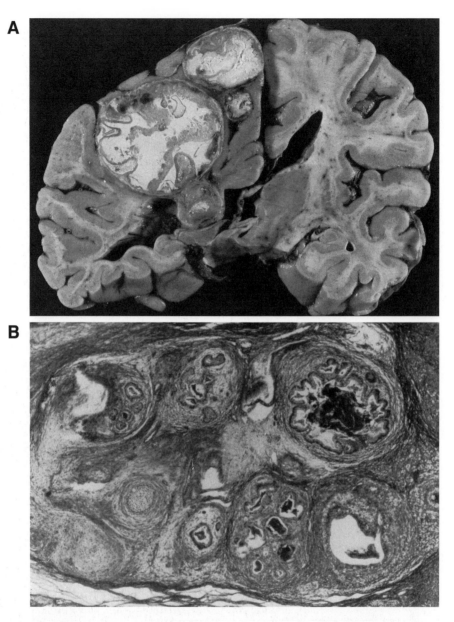

FIGURE 24–2

Examples of mature dysontogenetic tumors

A. Polycystic dermoid as example of an adult-type slow growing tumor with a known course of five decades. The patient refused an operation and actually did not die because of this tumor.

B. Teratoma with a mixture of mature adult-type and immature fetal-type tissues. Masson-trichrome. X 40

One benign grade I astrocytic tumor type has to be mentioned, the *pilocytic astrocytoma*, which usually remains in grade I. Why this difference with other astrocytic tumors? Pilocytic astrocytomas arise in phylogenetically old brain structures along the midline, e.g., the cerebellum, the optic chiasm, and the optic nerve. The pilocytic (hair-like) tumor cells strongly resemble tanycytes (Figure 24–5), the slender glial cells already seen in the brains of chondrichthyes (selachii) such as sharks and rays (Horstmann, 1954). Therefore, it is suggestive that pilocytic as-

trocytomas derive from a phylogenetically older sort of glia (Walter, 1978). Since the pilocytic (tanycytic) astrocytes are localized in phylogenetic and ontogenetic older brain structures, they are presumably more stable from a genetic point of view. Therefore when initiated they cause benign, slowly growing tumors in the above described typical brain locations. Though highly differentiated, they could be regarded as very young tumors reaching back even in our phylogenetic ancestry, thus, being an example of the so called phylogenetic diseases (Chapter 16).

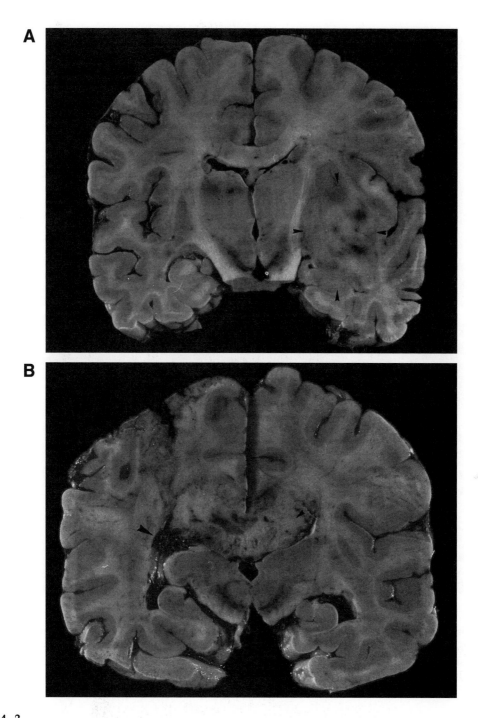

FIGURE 24–3

Examples of glial tumors

A. Astrocytoma WHO-grade II. Note the diffuse growth (arrow heads).

B. Glioblastoma WHO-grade IV ('butterfly glioma' crossing the *corpus callosum*) with necroses (small arrow head) and tumor hemorrhage (large arrow head).

On the reverse side of the coin, an example of a very old tumor would be a tumor with senile features as actually described in a few cases of *ganglioglioma*, a mixed astrocytic and neuronal tumor, in which the ganglionic tumor cells contain neurofibrillary tangles, a feature usually seen in senile brains, Alzheimer disease, or other degenerative conditions (Hori *et al.*, 1988; Soffer *et al.*, 1995). Certainly neurofibrillary tangles are not an exclusive hallmark of senile brains or degenerative brain disease in aging people, nevertheless, their incidence is just too obvious in aging brains.

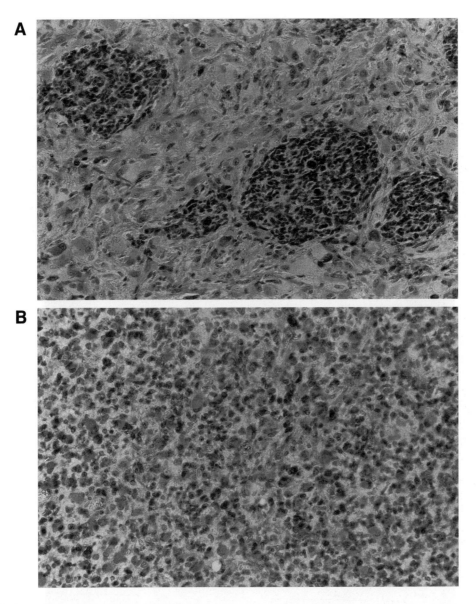

FIGURE   24–4

Examples of dedifferentiation in glial tumors

A. Well differentiated fibrillary astrocytoma with several foci of anaplasia exhibiting clusters of fast growing embryonal-type tumor cells (WHO-grade III). Glial fibrillary acidic protein/hematoxylin, X 80.

B. Anaplastic astrocytoma with diffuse anaplastic transformation of nearly all tumor cells (WHO-grade III). Glial fibrillary acidic protein/hematoxylin, X 80.

Neuronal Tumors Originate From Neuronal Precursor Cells

Also in *neuronal tumors*, the extremes of poorly differentiated embryonal, and well differentiated mature 'adult' tumor entities occur. Since the first attempt of a classification of tumors of the central nervous system by Bailey and Cushing in 1926, poorly differentiated neuronal tumors including *medulloblastoma, pinealoblastoma,* and *neuroblastoma* are familiar to clinicians and neuropathologists (Figure 24–6, A). The obvious relationship between

these entities has lead to the PNET concept uniting all primitive neuroectodermal tumors with embryonal features deriving from neuroblasts (Rorke *et al.*, 1985). Interestingly, the initiated cell may also be a still multipotential stem cell to be sought in an even pre-neuroblast ontogenetic age, then causing a PNET with additional glial or mesenchymal differentiation, e.g. in cases of *medullomyoblastoma* which is a PNET with an additional component of mature striated muscle (Walter and Brucher, 1979). Regarding the PNETs we may talk about an embryonal *dysmaturation*, i.e., the tumors remain in an

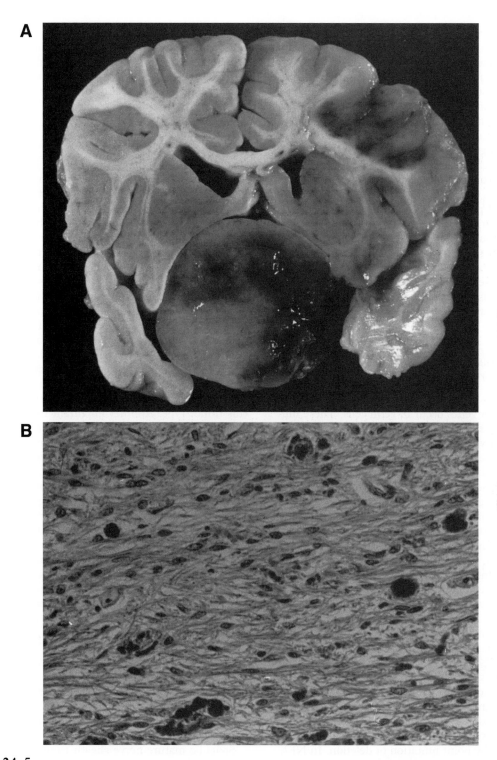

FIGURE   24–5

Pilocytic astrocytoma as model of phylogenetic disease.

A. Pilocytic glioma of the optic nerve in a one year old male patient ('optic glioma').

B. Pilocytic glioma showing hair-like tumor cells with large degenerated Rosenthal-fibers. The tumor cells resemble tanycytes in chondrichthyes. Masson-trichrome, X 80.

embryonal ontogenetic age. However, in some examples of malignant neuroblastoma an impressive further differentiation into *ganglioneuroblastomas* with some mature ganglionic cells, or even into benign mature *gangliocytomas* may occur.

Gangliocytomas are rare and always benign tumors characterized by adult-type ganglionic cells. Since ganglionic cells are postmitotic, a tumorous transformation with growth caused by mitotic division is difficult to understand. It seems not improbable that neuroblasts during their migration from the paraventricular matrix area to their cortical designation have stopped in a heterotopic position. These heterotopias could further differentiate to mature nerve cells giving rise to tumor-like malformations which appear as gangliocytomas, remaining benign because of their postmitotic cells without any capacity to dedifferentiate. On the other hand, though not yet described, one could predict that senile alterations in gangliocytomas, as seen in the few above mentioned cases of ganglioglioma, should occur more often. This would not be unexplicable in the light of the herewith discussed hypothesis. Though mature ganglionic cells are unable to divide, the tumor cells in gangliocytomas often contain multinucleated cells giving evidence that *endomitoses* as expression of incomplete cell divisions have taken place (Figure 24–6, B).

Neurofibromatosis is a Classical Example of Hereditary Tumor Syndromes

The situation is again different when mutations mostly of tumor suppressor genes occur in germ cells. These mutations may provoke hereditary tumor syndromes. The first allele is inactivated in the germ line and the second on a somatic basis. The high likelihood of the second event in at least one susceptible cell explains the apparent dominant inheritance pattern of these syndromes, despite tumor suppressor genes being recessive at the genetic level (Louis and von Deimling, 1995). In contrast to acquired tumors with a mutation in usually only a single somatic cell which initiates tumor growth, in hereditary tumors the genetic defect of germ cells is passed to the next generation and may become phenotypic in entire families of cells. *Recklinghausen disease*, synonymously called *neurofibromatosis type 1* (NF1), is a classical example. An inherited inactivation of the tumor suppressor gene *NF1* on chromosome 17q leads to multiple, often hundreds or thousands of neurofibromas spread over the body (Figure 24–7, A), but also to optic nerve gliomas, and to *hamartomas* of the iris called *Lisch nodules*, next to the typical phakomatous café-au-lait spots of the skin. More common than in NF1, tumors of the central nervous system are observed in *neurofibromatosis 2* (NF2), where the tumor suppressor gene *NF2* on chromosome 22q is inactivated by point mutation or deletion. In NF2, bilateral vestibular schwannomas (acoustic neurinomas), and multiple meningiomas are regular findings (Figures 24–7, B, and 24–8). Usually the tumors of NF1 and NF2 are benign with differentiated adult-type histological features, but malignant transformation is possible.

Among the typical and frequent intracranial tumors, *meningiomas* must not be forgotten. They derive from three meningeal elements, namely arachnoidal cap cells, blood vessels, and fibroblasts. The changing composition of these three histological elements is responsible for the different subtypes of meningiomas (Walter, 1992). Usually meningiomas are benign with well differentiated adult-type tissue, but malignant transformation with anaplasia is possible. The occurrence of multiple meningiomas in NF2 has already been mentioned.

The Age of the Tumor Patient

Primary tumors of the central nervous system and its coverings account for about 1.2 percent of all autopsied deaths and for approximately 9 percent of all primary neoplasms. Eighty-five percent of them are found within the cranial cavity (Rubinstein, 1972). The central nervous system is the second most common site of primary tumor formation in children, who show in this regard a much higher relative incidence than adults. Younger tumors are found in younger patients, adult tissue-type tumors in adults. It can be seen as general rule that undifferentiated embryonal tumors such as germinoma, poorly differentiated dysontogenetic tumors, or PNETs and especially medulloblastoma, occur in childhood or juvenile age. But also mature gangliocytomas are regularly found in children which seems to be in contradiction with the fact that mature tumors should occur in adults, but can easily be understood regarding the malformative pathogenesis of this tumor type. Another important incidental difference between adults and children lies in the localization of intracranial neoplasms. In children 70 percent of all intracranial tumors are infratentorial; in adults 70 percent are supratentorial.

Among the intracranial tumors, those of neuroectodermal origin and here again the glioma group claim priority in number accounting for 40 to 50 percent of all intracranial tumors both primary and metastatic encountered at all ages of life. Differentiated tumors such as astrocytoma grade II typically have a peak in adult middle-aged patients whereas dedifferentiated tumors such as glioblastoma grade IV appear in older adults or in senium. Since the differentiated pilocytic astrocytoma grade I has been suggested to have a special phylogenetic background, its favorite occurrence in children is not astonishing.

Second to gliomas in neurosurgical importance in the adult are the meningiomas. They represent about 15 percent of all primary intracranial tumors. The occurrence of intracranial meningiomas in infancy is extremely rare, in childhood still very rare with about 1.5 percent of all primary intracranial tumors (Mendiratta *et al.*, 1967; Sasaki *et al.*, 1987).

Sporadic mature nerve sheath tumors such as schwannomas and neurofibromas with very rare exceptions are tumors of the adults. This is different in hereditary tumor syndromes where usually already younger patients can be observed. NF1 is the most common hereditary disease predisposing to neoplasia in people (Riccardi and Eichner, 1986). The disease is fully penetrant but highly variable in its expressivity, sometimes producing both mildly affected and severely affected individuals within a single family. Some of the multiple benign tumors can progress and be-

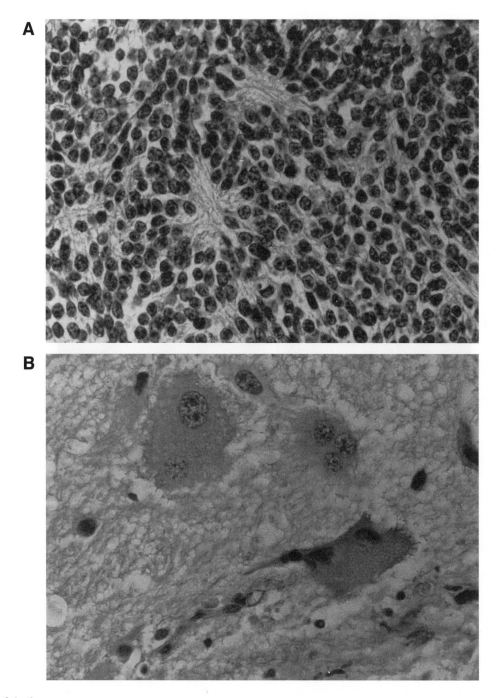

FIGURE   24–6

Examples of neuronal tumors.

A. Primitive neuroectodermal tumor (medulloblastoma) of the cerebellum in a five year old male patient. The tumor is characterized by almost undifferentiated embryonal-type cells, in

places arranging in rosettes. Glial fibrillary acidic protein/hematoxylin, X 150.

B. Gangliocytoma with mature adult-type multinucleated ganglionic cells in a four year old female patient. Hematoxylin-eosin, X 150.

come malignant, other malignant tumors in these patients can arise *de novo*. The mean age of NF1 patients at the time of diagnosis of malignancy was shown to be 38 years, compared to 65 years mean age at diagnosis of malignancy in the general population (Lefkowitz *et al.*, 1990).

Telomeres and Immortalized Cells: Tumor or Eternal Life?

Telomeres are specialized structures found at the ends of eukaryotic chromosomes which protect the chromosome

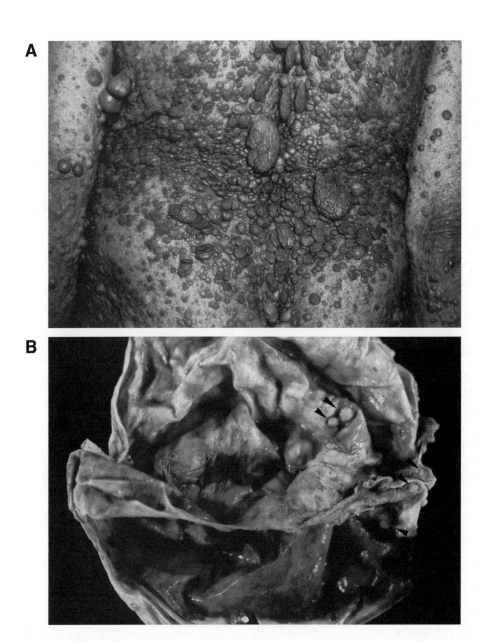

FIGURE   24–7
Examples of hereditary tumor syndromes.

A. Thousands of skin neurofibromas in neurofibromatosis 1 (NF1).

B. Multiple meningiomas adherent to the dura (arrows) in NF2.

ends against degradation and fusion with other ends. Telomeric DNA is highly conserved throughout evolution. The *telomere* hypothesis of cellular senescence (Olovnikov, 1973) postulates that a progressive shortening of the chromosome ends in the somatic cells of multicellular organisms leads to cell cycle exit. For instance, the amount and length of telomeric DNA decreases with continuous passage of normal human fibroblasts *in vitro* (Harley *et al.*, 1990). Telomere length can also predict their replicative capacity; fibroblasts with long telomeres have the greatest proliferation potential (Allsopp *et al.*, 1992). Telomere loss has been associated with aging *in vivo*

(Lindsey *et al.*, 1991). Their loss may also initiate or drive the genomic instability that results in abnormal chromosomes and unchecked cell growth.

It has been proposed that the immortalization of human cells requires the reactivation of the telomere lengthening enzyme *telomerase* (Greider and Blackburn, 1985). Synthesis of DNA at chromosome ends by telomerase may be necessary for indefinite proliferation of human cells – perhaps a key to eternal life? However, there may be still other mechanism of telomere lengthening, at least and probably limited to cells *in vitro* (Bryan *et al.*, 1995). In humans, telomerase activity is present in the germline

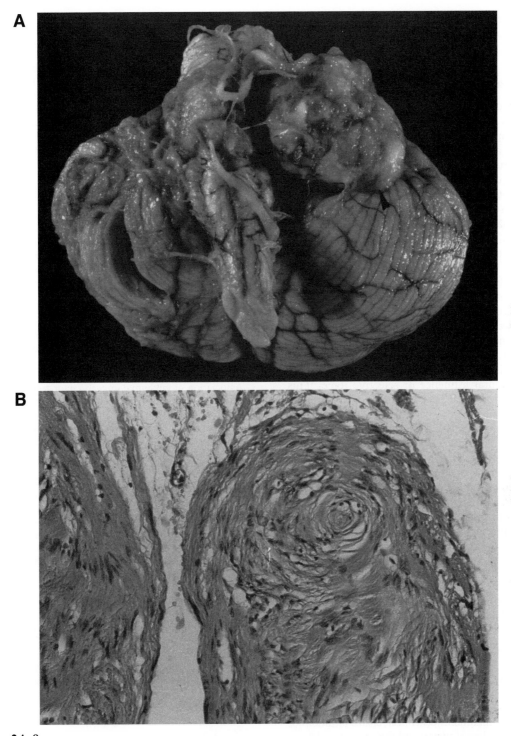

FIGURE   24–8

Examples of hereditary tumor syndromes.

A. Bilateral vestibular schwannomas (acoustic neurinomas) in neurofibromatosis 2 (NF2) with a large tumor of the left cerebel- lopontine angle (arrow head). The tumor of the right cerebello- pontine angle has been operatively removed.

B. Lobular pattern of vestibular schwannoma in NF2. Hematox- ylin-eosin, X 80.

but is not detected in various normal adult tissues. In contrast, telomerase activity has been detected in many human immortal cell lines and in tumor tissues, whereas it is generally absent from primary cell strains and from tumor adjacent tissue samples. Thus, telomerase appears to be stringently repressed in normal human somatic tissues but reactivated in cancer, where immortal cells are likely required to maintain tumor growth (Kim *et al.*, 1994).

An Overall View

All stages of ontogenetic development, from the totipotential zygote to embryonal, fetal, and infantile tissue-types can be recapitulated as tumor tissues. Ongoing differentiation into adult-type tumor tissue can be encountered, and even tumor aging with senile features is possible under certain circumstances. In pilocytic astrocytoma, a retrogression into phylogenetic younger forms seems to occur as otherwise only seen in some malformative syndromes. Teratomas and teratoid tumors are characterized by an important malformative factor, too. But tumors may also exhibit a specific peculiarity which does not appear in any other disease category, namely the possibility for anaplastic dedifferentiation, thus, to become younger from the point of view of tissue differentiation, falling back in embryonal stages with an incessant and explosive exponential growth of cells until the death of the individual patient. So, malignant tumors are as it were restating the possibility of eternal life through evolution (Chapter 3), as long as cells and tissues are not destroyed by any violent environmental influence or selective force. This peculiarity is used in biological research to produce immortalized cell cultures. However, immortalization of cell lines in culture probably has little in common with the 'immortalization' of tumor cells in a complex differentiated individual human being. The selective force is extraordinarily higher in the complex organism, owing to the need for an elaborate interdependence and co-operation of numerous different cell and tissue types. In the last instance, death remains the invincible destiny for individual human life.

Selected Readings

Cox, D., Yuncken, C., and Spriggs, A. I. 1965. Minute chromatin bodies in malignant tumours of childhood. Lancet 11:55–58.

Harris, H., Miller, O.J., Klein, G., Worst, P., and Tachiban, T. 1969. Suppression of malignancy by cell fusion. Nature 223:363–368.

Kim, N. W., Piatyszek, M. A., Prowse, K. R., *et al.* 1994. Specific association of human telomerase activity with immortal cells and cancer. Science 266:2011–2014.

Kleinert, R. 1991. Immunohistochemical characterization of primitive neuroectodermal tumors and their possible relationship to the stepwise ontogenetic development of the central nervous system. 2. Tumor studies. Acta Neuropathol. 82:508–515.

Walter, G. F., and Kleinert, R. 1987. Dysontogenetic brain tumours – proposal for an improved classification. Neuropathol. Appl. Neurobiol. 13:273–287.

Weinberg, R. A. 1991. Tumor suppressor genes. Science 254:1138–1146.

Williams, G. T. 1991. Programmed cell death: apoptosis and oncogenesis. Cell 65:1097–1098.

References

Aaronson, S. A. 1991. Growth factors and cancer. Science 254:1146–1153.

Allsopp, R. C., Vaziri, H., Patterson, C., Goldstein, S., Younglai, E. V., Futcher, A. B., Greider, C. W., and Harley C. B. 1992. Telomere length predicts replicative capacity in human fibroblasts. Proc. Natl. Acad. Sci. USA 89:10114–10118.

Bailey, P., and Cushing, H. 1926. A classification of tumors of the glioma group. Lippincott, Philadelphia.

Bigner, S. H., and Vogelstein, B. 1990. Cytogenetics and molecular genetics of malignant gliomas and medulloblastomas. Brain Pathol. 1: 12–18.

Bishop, J. M. 1983. Cellular oncogenes and retroviruses. Ann. Rev. Biochem. 52:301–354.

Bishop, J. M. 1991. Molecular themes in oncogenesis. Cell 64:235–248.

Brodeur, G. M. 1990. Neuroblastoma – clinical applications of molecular parameters. Brain Pathol. 1:47–54.

Bryan, T. M., Englezou, A., Gupta, J., Bacchetti, S., and Reddel, R. R. 1995. Telomere elongation without detectable telomerase activity. EMBO J. 14:4240–4248.

Cantley, L. C., Auger, K. R., Carpenter, C., *et al.* 1991. Oncogenes and signal transduction. Cell 64:281–302.

Cox, D., Yuncken, C., and Spriggs, A. I. 1965. Minute chromatin bodies in malignant tumours of childhood. Lancet 11:55–58.

Deimling, A. von, Louis, D. N., Ammon, K. von, *et al.* 1992. Association of epidermal growth factor receptor gene amplification with loss of chromosome 10 in human glioblastoma multiforme. J. Neurosurg. 77: 295–301.

Evans, R. W. 1957. Developmental stages of embryo-like bodies in teratoma testis. J. Clin. Pathol. 10:31–39.

Fishel, R., Lescoe, M. K., Rao, M. R. S., *et al.* 1993. The human mutator gene homolog MSH2 and its association with hereditary non polyposis colon cancer. Cell 75:1027–1038.

Friedman, H. S., Burger, P. C., Bigner, S. H., *et al.* 1988. Phenotypic and genotypic analysis of a human medulloblastoma cell line and transplantable xenograft (D-341 Med) demonstrating amplification of c-myc. Am. J. Pathol. 130:472–484.

Gonzalez-Crussi, F. 1982. Extragonadal teratomas. In: Atlas of Tumor Pathology, second series, fascicle 18. Armed Forces Institute of Pathology, Washington, D.C.

Greider, C.W., and Blackburn, E.H. 1985. Identification of a specific telomere terminal transferase activity in *Tetrahymena* extracts. Cell 43:405–413.

Hamilton, S. R., Liu, B., Parsons, R. E., *et al.* 1995. The molecular basis of Turcot's syndrome. N. Engl. J. Med. 332:839–847.

Harley, C.B., Futcher, A.B., and Greider, C.W. 1990 Telomeres shorten during ageing of human fibroblasts. Nature 345:458–460.

Harris, H., Miller, O. J., Klein, G., Worst, P., and Tachibana, T. 1969. Suppression of malignancy by cell fusion. Nature 223: 363–368.

Herskowitz, I. 1987. Functional inactivation of genes by dominant negative mutations. Nature 329:219–222.

Hori, A., Weiss, R., and Schaake, T. 1988. Ganglioglioma containing osseous tissue and neurofibrillary tangles. Arch. Pathol. Lab. Med. 112:653–655.

Horstmann, E. 1954. Die Faserglia des Selachiergehirns. Zeitschr. Zellforsch. 39:588–617.

Jen, J., Harper, W., Bigner, S. H., *et al.* 1994. Deletion of p16 and p15 genes in brain tumors. Cancer Res. 54:6353–6358.

Kim, N. W., Piatyszek, M. A., Prowse, K. R., *et al.* 1994. Specific association of human telomerase activity with immortal cells and cancer. Science 266:2011–2014.

Kleihues, P., Burger, P. C., and Scheithauer, B. W. (eds.) 1993. Histological typing of tumors of the central nervous system. International Histological Classification of Tumours, 2nd ed., Springer, Berlin.

Kleinert, R. 1991a. Immunohistochemical characterization of primitive neuroectodermal tumors and their possible relationship to the stepwise ontogenetic development of the central nervous system. 1. Ontogenetic studies. Acta Neuropathol. 82:502–507.

Kleinert, R. 1991b. Immunohistochemical characterization of primitive neuroectodermal tumors and their possible relationship to the stepwise ontogenetic development of the central nervous system. 2. Tumor studies. Acta Neuropathol, 82:508–515.

Koga, H., Zhang, S., Kumanishi, T., et al. 1994. Analysis of p53 gene mutations in low- and high-grade astrocytomas by polymerase chain reaction-assisted single-strand conformation polymorphism and immunohistochemistry. Acta Neuropathol. 87:225–232.

Lefkowitz, I., Obringer, A., and Meadows, A. 1990. Neurofibromatosis and cancer: incidence and management. In: A. Rubenstein and B. Korf (eds.) Neurofibromatosis: A Handbook for Patients, Families and Health-Care Professionals. pp. 99–110. Thieme, New York.

Lewin, B. 1991. Oncogenic conversion by regulatory changes in transcription factors. Cell 64:303–312.

Lindsey, J., McGill, N. I., Lindsey, L. A., Green, D. K. and Cooke, H. J. 1991. In vivo loss of telomeric repeats with age in humans. Mutat. Res. 256:45–48.

Louis, D. N., Deimling, A. von, Chung, R. Y., et al. 1993. Comparative study of p53 gene and protein alterations in human astrocytic tumors. J. Neuropathol. Exp. Neurol. 52:31–38.

Louis, D. N., and Deimling, A. von. 1995. Hereditary tumor syndromes of the nervous system: overview and rare syndromes. Brain Pathol. 5:145–151.

McKay, D. G., Hertig, A. T., Adams, E. C., and Danziger, S. 1953. Histochemical observations on the germ cells of the human embryos. Anat. Rec. 117:201–219.

Mendiratta, S. S., Rosenblum, J. A., and Strobos, R. J. 1967. Congenital meningioma. Neurology 17:914–918.

Olovnikov, A. M. 1973. A theory of marginotomy. J. Theor. Biol. 41:181–190.

Papadopoulos, N., Nicolaides, N. C., Wei, Y. F., et al. 1994. Mutation of a mutL homologue in hereditary colon cancer. Science 263:1625–1629.

Riccardi, V. M., and Eichner, J. E. 1986 Neurofibromatosis: Phenotype, Natural History, and Pathogenesis. Johns Hopkins University Press, Baltimore.

Rorke, L. B., Gilles, F. H., Davis, R. L., and Becker, L. E. 1985. Revision of the World Health Organization classification of brain tumors for childhood brain tumors. Cancer 56:1869–1886.

Rubinstein, L. J. 1972. Tumors of the Central Nervous System. Atlas of Tumor Pathology, second series, fascicle 6. Armed Forces Institute of Pathology, Washington, D.C.

Ruley, H. E. 1993. Oncogenes. In: Levine, A. J., Schmidek, H. H. (eds) Molecular Genetics of the Nervous System Tumors. Wiley-Liss, New York, pp. 89–100.

Sager, R. 1989. Tumor suppressor genes: the puzzle and the promise. Science 246:1406–1412.

Sasaki, S., Nakagawa, K., Kimura, H., and Ohue, S. 1987. Intracranial meningiomas in infancy. Surg. Neurol. 28:51–57.

Schmidt, E. E., Ichimura, K., Reifenberger, G., and Collins, V. P. 1994. CDKN2 (p16/MTS1) gene deletion or CDK4 amplification occurs in the majority of glioblastomas. Cancer Res. 54:6321–6324.

Soffer, D., Umansky, F., and Goldman, J. E. 1995. Ganglioglioma with neurofibrillary tangles (NFTs): neoplastic NFTs share antigenic determinants with NFTs of Alzheimer's disease. Acta Neuropathol. 89:451–453.

Walter, G. F. 1978. Kleinhirnastrozytome und Opticusgliome – eine vergleichende feinstrukturelle Untersuchung. Virchows Arch. A. 380:59–79.

Walter, G. F. 1992. Pathobiology and neuropathology of meningiomas. In: M. Samii, and M. Ammirati (eds.) Surgery of Skull Base Meningiomas. pp. 123–142. Springer, Berlin.

Walter, G. F. 1994. Gliomas and the p53 gene and protein. Crit. Rev. Neurosurg. 4: 393–400.

Walter, G. F., and Brucher, J. M. 1979. Ultrastructural study of medullomyoblastoma. Acta Neuropathol. 48:211–214.

Walter, G. F., and Kleinert, R. 1987. Dysontogenetic brain tumours – proposal for an improved classification. Neuropathol. App. Neurobiol. 13:273–287.

Weinberg, R. A. 1991. Tumor suppressor genes. Science 254:1138–1146.

Williams, G. T. 1991. Programmed cell death: apoptosis and oncogenesis. Cell 65:1097–1098.

Witschi, E. 1948. Migration of germ cells of human embryos from the yolk sac to the primitive gonadal folds. Contrib. Embryol. 32:67–80.

Davide Schiffer

Dysregulation of Glial Cell Apoptosis in the Basis of Neoplasia

Glial Cell Death by Apoptosis is Part of the General Dynamics of Glial Cell Turnover

    Lethal Stimuli May Prime Glial Cells for Programmed Cell Death

Dysregulation of Apoptosis in the Basis of Carcinogenesis

    Indexes of Apoptosis and Mitosis can be Calculated for Various Tumor Masses

    Large Necroses in Neuroepithelial Tumors may be a Consequence of Inadequate Nourishment of the Increasing Number of Tumor Cells

    Necrosis Alone Does Not Account for the High Cell Loss in Neuroepithelial Tumors

    Restricted Criteria of Apoptosis can Underestimate the Actual Number of Apoptotic Nuclei in Neuroepithelial Tumors

An Overall View

In the beginning of this section we have seen that neurons die during prenatal and postnatal development of the nervous system in order to determine the ultimate size and composition of the neuronal populations (Chapter 17), and that the most common form of neuron death during development is apoptosis, characterized by pyknotic nuclei. Our knowledge about glial cell death during development is less extensive than that of neuron death, but from some contributions it appears clear that developmental glial cell death is as well established as neuron death. Since the staining methods used in most studies to evidence pyknosis cannot make a distinction between neuronal and glial nuclei (Ferrer et al., 1992), it has been considered that, as neurons die during development, there is an intense proliferation and migration of glial cells, which may die as well (Knapp et al., 1986) (Figure 25–1). Although the process is not very well known it probably belongs to programmed cell death occurring in most developing animal tissues in order to keep the cell number in accordance with the development program.

In this chapter we will explore further some mechanisms for the control of glial cells death in development, the failure of which may be in the basis of neoplasia.

Glial Cell Death by Apoptosis is Part of the General Dynamics of Glial Cell Turnover

Glial cells have been shown to proliferate before and during migration and also postnatally (Hubbard and Hopewell, 1979), as opposed to neurons, which do not proliferate any more after differentiation is attained. For the proportions of glial cells to be maintained, a turnover

The ratio between apoptotic nuclei and mitoses has been calculated by Cotter and colleagues (1990). The ratio was 1:1 in untreated tumors, and increased after chemotherapy. Lipponen and Aaltomaa (1994) calculated an *apoptotic index* (AI) for bladder cancer which was found to correlate with mitotic activity. However, this AI was devoid of any prognostic significance. In malignant lymphomas a loose, non-linear correlation, was found between the *mitotic index* (MI) and AI (Del Vecchio et al., 1993). AI and MI were calculated in histologically normal human breasts and in fibrocystic changes as well as in fibroadenomas and carcinomas from breast tissue of the same patients. A reduction of AI and of AI/MI was found in 'normal' breasts with fibrocystic changes and carcinomas. The reduced epithelial cell apoptosis might be causally associated with the development of fibrocystic changes and with an increased risk of carcinoma. Genetically aberrant cells might be preserved favoring neoplastic development (Allan et al., 1992).

In murine tumors it has been demonstrated that in the first few hours following irradiation *in vivo* 10 percent of cells were apoptotic. In responsive tumors there was a longer specific growth delay and a lower TCD50. Not all the tumors were responsive and there was an intra- and inter-tumor heterogeneity (Meyn et al., 1993).

In preneoplastic and neoplastic lesions induced in the rat by N-nitroso-morpholine, an increased [H^3]-*thymidine labeling index* (LI) was found. Also apoptotic nuclei increased, but no statistically significant correlation was found. It means that cell death does not counterbalance cell replication in altered hepatocytes, but rather it occurs more frequently in the course of hepatocarcinogenesis (Zerban et al., 1994).

Apoptosis is an inconspicuous and readily accomplished phenomenon and leaves no residua so that it has been calculated that a small number of apoptotic cells may represent a high cell loss (Kerr et al., 1972; Wyllie et al., 1986). Apoptosis must thus be considered as responsible for at least a proportion of cell loss.

Large Necroses in Neuroepithelial Tumors may be a Consequence of Inadequate Nourishment of the Increasing Number of Tumor Cells

In neuroepithelial tumors, cell death by necrosis and apoptosis is a common, very well known and categorized phenomenon. Three types of necroses can be recognized: (i) Large of coagulative and colliquative aspect, situated at the center of the tumor; (ii) circumscribed with pseudopalisading and (iii) very small necroses (Figure 25–2). The large necroses are usually the consequence of thrombosis or of occlusion of blood vessels or insufficient blood supply to the central part of the tumor. Circumscribed necroses with pseudopalisading are usually found in highly proliferative areas and seem to be due to the imbalance between tumor cell proliferation and angiogenesis, i.e. mitotic imbalance between tumor and endothelial cells.

In our experience, endothelial proliferation produced by mitogenic stimuli originating in tumor cells deforms

the vascular tree of the cortex giving rise to *glomeruloid formations* (Schiffer et al., 1989). The vascular tree, modified by endothelial hyperplasia which gives rise to narrowing of vessels or to blind ended vessels, becomes inadequate to nourish the increasing number of tumor cells, hence the necrosis. Other interpretations have been put forward and the relationship between necrosis and vascular endothelium hyperplasia reversed; necroses have been considered as the source of *fibroblast growth factor* (FGF) which stimulates endothelial cells to proliferate (Paulus et al., 1990). Endothelial proliferations have also been considered as the result of *vascular endothelial growth factor* (VEGF) on its receptors localized in endothelial cells themselves (Schweiki et al., 1992; Plate et al., 1994).

Very small necroses can be found in almost every tumor, but they are especially frequent in *medulloblastoma* and *ependymoma*. Sometimes they are so small that they are limited to a single cell. This occurrence is today considered typical of apoptosis.

Necrosis Alone Does Not Account for the High Cell Loss in Neuroepithelial Tumors

Necrosis can be found in malignant tumors and in the malignant variant of neuroepithelial tumors. Usually it represents a prognostic factor of primary importance. In astrocytic tumors necrosis is considered a hallmark of malignancy and, according to many authors, its occurrence would mark the transition from *anaplastic astrocytoma* to *glioblastoma* (Burger et al., 1985; Kleihues et al., 1993).

Necrosis represents the main source of cell loss in tumors which could be one of the factors responsible for the poor reliability of proliferation markers, as independent prognostic factors (Schiffer et al., 1995). Cell loss is not easy to define or to quantitate in tumors. One approach is to calculate the *cell loss factor* (CLF), i.e. the difference between the expected growth of a tumor based on its proliferation rate and the actual growth rate (Steel, 1977). CLF is calculated to vary from 0.65 and 0.96 (Steel, 1977; Moore, 1983–1987; Kerz and Lamb, 1984). In spite of the frequent appearance of necroses in tumors, necrosis alone does not seem to account for the high cell loss factor in tumors. CLF can be better explained if apoptosis is taken into account.

In medulloblastoma, lymphocyte-like nuclei have been long recognized (Ringertz and Tola, 1954; Zülch, 1956). They stained with *Feulgen reaction* (a method developed by German physiologic chemist Robert Feulgen, to stain nucleic acid after hydrolysis with HCl followed by red staining with decolorized rosaniline), but behaved after fluorochroming with *acridine orange* as denatured DNA. They appeared as compact, round DNA masses, sometimes with satellite smaller masses and were considered as arrested mitoses from which nuclei do not recover. Their aspect could be traced back to atypical mitoses, not infrequent in medulloblastoma (Schiffer et al., 1966). Recently, it has been demonstrated that these nuclei are positive with the *in situ* end labeling (ISEL) technique (see Box 25–1) and show at the electron microscope typical

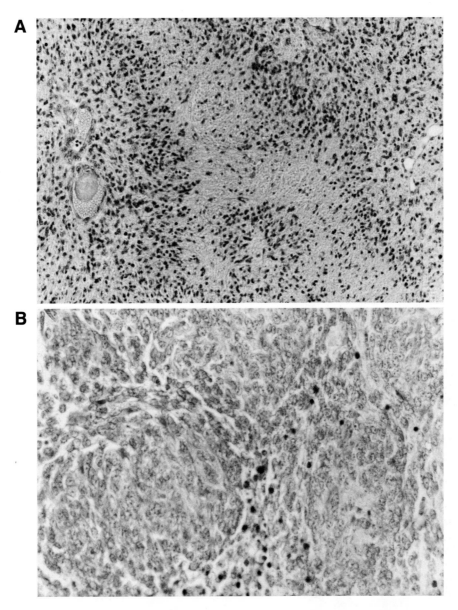

FIGURE   25–2
A. Circumscribed necrosis in a glioblastoma. H. E., X 200.   **B.** Small necrotic focus in medulloblastoma. H. E., X 400.

features of apoptosis (Schiffer *et al.*, 1994). It was observed that the apoptosis/mitosis ratio was 1:1. The interpretation of apoptosis in medulloblastoma was twofold: Apoptosis could act as a regulator of cell proliferation or it could represent the footprint of the embryonal tissue of origin where apoptosis is active in deleting cells during development.

Restricted Criteria of Apoptosis can Underestimate the Actual Number of Apoptotic Nuclei in Neuroepithelial Tumors

A study of apoptosis has been carried out in 200 neuro-epithelial tumors (Schiffer *et al.*, 1995). Apoptotic nuclei were recognized by their morphology at light- and elec-

tron-microscopy and by their positive staining with the ISEL technique (Box 25–1; Figure 25–3). An apoptotic index (AI) was calculated: It was high in embryonal tumors, such as medulloblastoma and ependymoma, and low in benign or differentiated tumors. The AI/MI ratio was very low in malignant tumors, high in benign tumors and intermediate in medulloblastoma. In the latter tumor this was due to the high AI. Of paramount importance is the observation that AI and AI/MI did not correlate with survival. On the contrary, a correlation has been found between MI and AI. This means either that the two phenomena, apoptosis and mitosis, are statistically correlated and, therefore, that apoptosis is a factor regulating cell proliferation, or that they are differently correlated through a complex link (Ucker, 1991; Lazebnik *et al.*,

The ISEL (*in situ* end labeling) Technique Helps Recognize Apoptotic Nuclei   **Box 25–1**
in Tissue Sections

Apoptotic nuclei can easily be recognized in cell cultures. Besides the morphological method of identification, other techniques can be employed such as DNA electrophoresis and flow cytometry (Darzynkiewicz *et al.*, 1992). However it is much more difficult to recognize apoptotic nuclei *in vivo* where morphology alone can be used and apoptotic nuclei may be indistinguishable from necrotic nuclei, lymphocytes or telophases (Wijsman *et al.*, 1993).

A technique widely used today to help recognize apoptotic nuclei in tissue sections is the *in situ* labeling of fragmented DNA by DNA polymerase (Gold *et al.*, 1993; Wood *et al.*, 1993; Wijsman *et al.*, 1993) and terminal deoxynucleotidyl transferase (TdT) (Gavrieli *et al.*, 1992). The TdT enzyme and DNA polymerase recognize the 3'-hydroxyl-recessed termini of DNA breaks produced by endonuclease and incorpo-

rate labeled nucleotides in these sites. Another name for the technique is TUNEL, which stands for Terminal Nucleotide End Labeling.

Although the ISEL/TUNEL technique is not specific for apoptosis, it has been applied to many tissues of nervous origin (Migheli *et al.*, 1994) appearing to be of great help (Figure 25–3). When counting apoptotic nuclei in sections, small necrotic foci are discarded, because the ISEL technique is positive also in necrotic nuclei. It must be borne in mind, however, that this is a restrictive precaution since small groups of condensed nuclei may also correspond to dying cells derived from a single progenitor and undergoing a common death program. It is likely, therefore, that by using restrictive criteria to recognize apoptosis, the number of apoptotic nuclei can be underestimated.

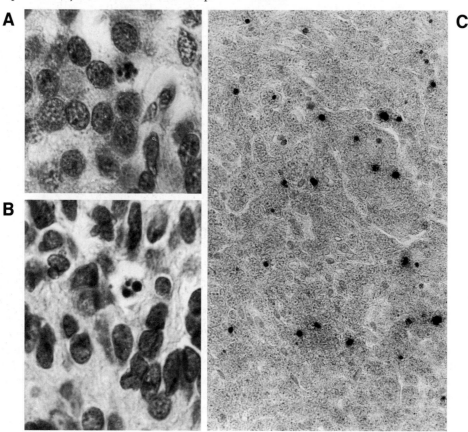

FIGURE 25–3

A and **B.** Ependymoma, apoptotic nuclei. H. E., X 400.

C. Medulloblastoma, apoptotic nuclei. *In situ* end-labeling (ISEL) technique, H.E., X 400.

1993). Also no significant correlation has been found between AI and AI/MI and labeling index (LI) of proliferative marker Ki-67 clone MIB-1.

In another study, carried out on 81 astrocytic tumors by Ellison and colleagues, AI was found to increase with anaplasia, showing a strong correlation with the growth fraction. However, no relationship came out with the expression of bcl-2 and p53 genes. Very likely, the regulation of apoptosis in astrocytic tumors is too complex and a direct correlation with two gene proteins which inhibit it cannot be identified. As a matter of fact, apoptosis has been considered as a possible prognostic factor in neuroepithelial tumors (Schelper and Anderson, 1994), and bcl-2 gene expression has been found to correlate with survival in medulloblastoma (Heck et al., 1994). However, in two studies such a correlation involving bcl-2 has not been found. In astrocytic tumors the degree of bcl-2 expression has been inversely related to the degree of malignancy, but no relationship was found with survival in glioblastomas and medulloblastomas (Nakasu et al., 1994). In our own series, bcl-2 was highly expressed in medulloblastomas and astrocytic tumors, with no correlation with survival and, therefore, of no prognostic value (Schiffer et al., 1996).

As in other tumors, also in medulloblastoma cells undergo radiation-induced apoptosis, which is mediated by p53. In cell lines, wild type p53 is required for high levels of apoptosis and cell lines in which p53 has been inactivated by mutation have very low levels of apoptosis. Besides, inactivation of wild type p53 decreases the level of radiation-induced apoptosis (Dee et al., 1995).

Another marker which can be used as a criteria of apoptosis is Fas/APO-1 antigen, which is a member of the TNF/NGF family whose activation induces apoptosis. The activation of Fas requires activation of an enzyme, ICE, homologous to the product of Caenorhabditis elegans cell-death gene ced-3 (Yuan et al., 1993). Conversely, inhibition of ICE suppresses Fas-induced apoptosis (Los et al., 1995). Fas has been immunohistochemically demonstrated in 70 percent of gliomas where it correlates with apoptosis, whereas bcl-2, bcl-x and bax were positive in 71 percent, 56 percent and 37 percent respectively in malignant brain tumors (Shiraishi et al., 1995). By RT-PCR, Fas in RNA was found to correlate with malignancy (Tachibana et al., 1995).

Using a polyclonal antibody, Fas/APO1 (CD 95) has been demonstrated in 87 percent of glioblastomas, in perinecrotic tumor cells; a role of Fas-mediated apoptosis in the pathogenesis of necrosis has, therefore, been suggested (Tachibana et al., 1996).

An Overall View

Apoptosis has been shown to regulate glial cell death during development. In addition, apoptosis can be viewed as a possible prognostic factor in neuroepithelial tumors (Schelper and Anderson, 1994) because dysregulation of apoptosis appears to be a basic mechanism leading to uncontrolled cell proliferation. A potentially revealing link of glial cell proliferation to apoptosis has been made that may guide new strategies for cancer therapy utilizing checkpoint controls to induce or establish apoptosis. Nevertheless, it is not yet known whether and how apoptosis influences cell loss in tumors. Further studies are needed in order to clarify this issue.

Selected Readings

Barr, P. J., and Tomei, L. D. 1994. Apoptosis and its role in human disease. Bio-Technol. 12:487–493.

Buja, L. M., Eigenbrodt, M. L., and Eigenbrodt, E. H. 1993. Apoptosis and necrosis. Basic types and mechanism of cell death. Arch. Pathol. Lab. Med. 117:1208–1214.

Buttke, T. M., and Sandstrom, P. A. 1994. Oxidative stress as a mediator of apoptosis. Immunology Today 15:7–10.

Carson, D. A., and Ribeiro, J. M. 1993. Apoptosis and disease. Lancet 341:1251–1254.

Ellis, H. M., Yuan, J., and Horvitz, H. R. 1991. Mechanisms and functions of cell death. Ann. Rev. Cell. Biol. 7:663–698.

Groothuis, D. R., and Vick, N. A. 1980. Radionecrosis of the central nervous system: the perspective of the clinical neurologist and neuropathologist. In: H. A. Gilbert, and A. R. Kagan (eds.) Radiation Damage to the Nervous System. Raven Press, New York, pp. 93–106.

Hickman, J. A. 1992. Apoptosis induced by anticancer drugs. Cancer Metastasis Rev. 11:121–139.

Hildebrand, C. 1971. Ultrastructural and light-microscopic studies of the developing feline spinal cord white matter II. Cell death and myelin sheath disintegration in the early postnatal period. Acta Physiol. Scand. Suppl. 354:109–144.

Hockenbery, D. 1995. Defining apoptosis. Am. J. Pathol. 146:16–19.

Hockenbery, D. M., Oltvai, Z. N., Yin, X. M., Milliman C. L., and Korsmeyer, S. J. 1993. Bcl-2 functions in an antioxidant pathway to prevent apoptosis. Cell 75:241–251.

Hoshino, T., Townsend, J. J., Muraoka, I., and Wilson, C. B. 1980. An autoradiographic study of human gliomas: growth kinetics of anaplastic astrocytoma and glioblastoma multiforme. Brain 103:967–984.

Hubbard, B. M., and Hopewell J. W. 1979. Changes in the neuroglial cell population of the rat spinal cord after local x-irradiation. Br. J. Radiol. 52:816–821.

Kane, D. J., Sarafian, T. A., Anton, R., Hahn, H., Gral, E. B., Valentine, J. S., Ord T., and Bredesen, D. E. 1993. Bcl-2 inhibition of neural death: decreased generation of reactive oxygen species. Science 262:1274–1277.

Kerr, J. F. R., Wyllie, A. H., and Curie, A. R. 1972. Apoptosis: a basic biological phenomenon with wide ranging implications in tissue kinetics. Br. J. Cancer 26:239–257.

Majno, G., and Joris, I. 1995. Apoptosis, oncosis, and necrosis. An overview of cell death. American J. Pathol. 146:3–15

Pannese, E., and Ferrannini E. 1967. Nuclear pyknosis in neuroglia cells of normal mammals. Acta Neuropathol. 8:309–319.

Rubin, L. L., Philpott, K. L., Brooks, S. F. 1993. The cell cycle and cell death. Curr. Biol. 3:394.

Smart, I., and Leblond, C. P. 1961. Evidence for division of neuroglia cells in the mouse brain, as derived from radioautography after injection of Thymidine-H3. J. Comp. Neurol. 116:349–367.

References

Allan, D. J., Howell, A., Roberts, S. A., et al. 1992. Reduction in apoptosis relative to mitosis in histologically normal epithelium accompanies fibrocystic change and carcinoma of the premenopausal human breast. J. Pathol. 167:25–32.

Barres, B. A., Hart, I. K., Coles, H. S. R., et al. 1992. Cell death and control of cell survival in the oligodendrocyte lineage. Cell 70:31–46.

Bissonette, R. P., Echeverri, F., Mahboubi, A., and Green, D. R. 1992. Apoptotic cell death induced by c-myc is inhibited by bcl-2. Nature 359:552–554.

Burger, P. C., Vogel, F. S., Green, S. B., and Strike, T. A. 1985. Glioblastoma multiforme and anaplastic astrocytoma: pathologic criteria and prognostic implications. Cancer 56:1106–1111.

Cotter, T. G., Lennon, S. V., Glynn, J. G., and Martin, S. J. 1990. Cell death via apoptosis and its relationship to growth. Development and differentiation of both tumour and normal cells. Anticancer Res. 10:1153–1160.

Darzynkiewicz, Z., Bruno, S., Del Bino G., et al. 1992. Features of apoptotic cells measured by flow cytometry. Cytometry 13:795–808.

Dee, S., Haaskogan, D. A., and Israel, M. A. 1995. Inactivation of p53 is associated with decreased levels of radiation induced apoptosis in medulloblastoma cell lines. Cell Death Differ. 2:267–275.

Del Vecchio, M. T., Leoncini, L., Buerki, K., et al. 1991. Diffuse centrocytic and/or centroblastic malignant non-Hodgkin's lymphomas: comparison of mitotic and pyknotic (apoptotic) indices. Int. J. Cancer 47:38–43.

Diemer, N. H., Jorgensen, M. B., Jensen, M. B., Bruhn, T., Valente, E., and Johansen, F. F. 1992. Involvement of excitatory transmitter systems in ischemia-induced damage to CA1 pyramidal cells, dentate hilus neurons, and Purkinje cells. In U. Ito, T. Kirino, T. Kuroiwa, and I. Klatzo (eds.) Maturation Phenomenon in Cerebral Ischemia. Springer, Berlin-Heidelberg-New York, pp. 95–105.

Eastman, A. 1993. Apoptosis: a product of programmed and unprogrammed cell death. Toxicol. Appl. Pharmacol. 121:160–164.

Ellison, D. W., Steart, P. V., Gatter, K. C., and Weller, R. O. 1995. Apoptosis in cerebral astrocytic tumors and its relationship to expression of the bcl-2 and p-53 proteins. Neuropathol. Appl. Neurobiol. 21:352–361.

Evan, G. I., Wyllie, A. H., Gilbert, C. S., et al. 1992. Induction of apoptosis in fibroblasts by c-myc protein. Cell 69:119–129.

Ferrer, I., Soriano, E., Del Rio, J. A., Alcantara, S., and Auladell, C. 1992. Cell death and removal in the cerebral cortex during development. Progr. Neurobiol. 39:1–43.

Ferrer, I., Tortosa, A., Macaya, A., et al. 1994. Evidence of nuclear DNA fragmentation following hypoxia-ischemia in the infant rat brain, and transient forebrain ischemia in the adult gerbil. Brain Pathol. 4:115–122.

Ferrer, I. 1992. The effect of cycloheximide on natural and X-ray-induced cell death in the developing cerebral cortex. Brain Res. 588:351–357.

Fesus, L., Davies, P. J. A., and Piacentini, M. 1991. Apoptosis: molecular mechanisms in programmed cell death. European J. Cell. Biol. 56:170–177.

Gavrieli, Y., Sherman Y., and Ben-Sasson, S. A. 1992. Identification of programmed cell death in situ via specific labeling of nuclear DNA fragmentation. J. Cell Biol. 119:493–501.

Gold, R., Schmied, M., Rothe, G., et al. 1993. Detection of DNA fragmentation in apoptosis: application of in situ nick translation to cell culture systems and tissue sections. J. Histochem. Cytochem. 41:1023–1030.

Gold, R., Schmied, M., Giegerich, G., et al. 1994. Differentiation between cellular apoptosis and necrosis by the combined use of in situ tailing and nick translation techniques. Lab. Invest. 71:219–225.

Hara, H., Sakamoto, T., and Kogure, K. 1993. Mechanism and pathogenesis of ischemia-induced neuronal damage. Progr. Neurobiol. 40:645–670.

Heck, K., Pyle, P., and Bruner, J. M. 1994. Bcl-2 expression in cerebellar medulloblastomas. Brain Pathol. 4:430 (abstract.)

Ikonomidcu, C., Price, M. T., Mosinger, J. L., et al. 1989. Hypobaric-ischemic conditions produce glutamate-like cytopathology in the infant rat brain. J. Neurosci. 9:1693–1700.

Jackson, K. F., and Duncan, I. D. 1988. Cell kinetics and cell death in the optic nerve of the myelin deficient rat. J. Neurocytol. 17:657–670.

Kaplan, M. S., and Hinds, J. W. 1977. Neurogenesis in adult rat. Electron microscopic analysis of light autoradiographs. Science 197:1092–1094.

Kawai, K., Saito, N., Xu, S., et al. 1992. Role of neuroexcitation in maturation of post-ischemic and post-traumatic injury. In U. Ito, T. Kirino, T. Kuroiwa, and I. Klatzo (eds.) Maturation Phenomenon in Cerebral Ischemia. Springer, Berlin-Heidelberg-New York, pp. 75–86.

Kerr, K. M., and Lamb, D. 1984. Actual growth rate and tumor cell proliferation in human pulmonary neoplasms. Br. J. Cancer 50:343–349.

Kleihues, P., Burger, P. C., and Scheithauer, B. W. 1993. Histological typing of tumors of the central nervous system. WHO Blue Book, 2nd ed. Springer, Berlin Heidelberg New York, pp. 1–37.

Knapp, P. E., Skoff, R. P., and Redstone, D. W. 1986. Oligodendroglial cell death in jimpy mice: an explanation for the myelin deficit. J. Neurosci. 6:2813–2822.

Korr, H., Schultre, B., and Maurer, W. 1973. Autoradiographic investigations of glial proliferation in the brain of adult mice. The DNA synthesis place of neuroglia and endothelial cells. J. Comp. Neurol. 150:169–176.

Korr, H., Schultre, B., and Maurer, W. 1975. Autoradiographic investigations of glial proliferation in the brain of adult mice. II Cycle time and mode of proliferation of neuroglia and endothelial cells. J. Comp. Neurol. 160:477–490.

Korsmeyer, S. J. 1992. Bcl-2: an antidote to programmed cell death. Cancer Surv. 15:105–118.

Lazebnik, Y. A., Cole, S., Cooke, C. A., et al. 1993. Nuclear events of apoptosis in vitro in cell-free mitotic extracts: a model system for analysis of the active phase of apoptosis. J. Cell Biol. 123:7–22.

Lewis, P. 1981. Cell proliferation in the postnatal nervous system and its relationship to the origin of gliomas. Semin. Neurol. 1:181–187.

Lipponen, P. K., and Aaltomaa, S. 1994. Apoptosis in bladder cancer as related to standard prognostic factors and prognosis. J. Pathol. 173:333–339.

Los, M., Van de Craen, M., Penning, L. C., et al. 1995. Requirement of an ICE/CED-3 protease for Fas/APO1-mediated apoptosis. Nature 375:81–83.

Meyn, R. E., Stephens, L. C., Ang, K. K., et al. 1993. Heterogeneity in the development of apoptosis in irradiated murine tumours of different histologies. Int. J. Radiat. Biol. 64:583–591.

Migheli, A., Cavalla, P., Marino S., and Schiffer D. 1994. A study of apoptosis in normal and pathologic nervous tissue after in situ end-labeling of DNA strands breaks. J. Neuropathol. Exp. Neurol. 53:606–616.

Moore, J. V. 1987. Death of cells and necrosis of tumors. In C.

S. Potten (ed.) Perspectives in Mammalian Cell Death. Oxford University Press, pp. 295–325.

Nakasu, S., Nakasu, Y., Nioka, H., Nakajima, M., and Handa, J. 1994. Bcl-2 protein expression in tumors of the central nervous system. Acta Neuropathol. 88:520–526.

Noetzel, H., and Rox, J. 1964. Autoradiographische Untersuchungen über Zellteilung und Zellentwicklung im Gehirn der erwachsenen Maus und des erwachsenen Rhesus-Affen nach Injektion von radioaktiven Thymidin. Acta Neuropathol. 3:326–342.

Paulus, W., Grothe, C., Sensenbrenner, M., et al. 1990. Localization of basic fibroblastic growth factor, a mitogen and angiogenic factor, in human brain tumors. Acta Neuropathol. 79:418–423.

Plate, K., Breier, G., and Risau, W. 1994. Molecular mechanisms of developmental and tumor angiogenesis. Brain Pathol. 4:207–218.

Ringertz, N., and Tola, J. H. 1954. Medulloblastoma. J. Neuropathol. Exp. Neurol. 9:354–372.

Schelper, R., and Anderson, M. 1994. Apoptosis in glial neoplasms: implications for tumors grading and future therapy. Brain Pathol. 4:436 (abstract.)

Schiffer, D., Cavalla, P., Migheli A. et al. 1995. Apoptosis and cell proliferation in human neuroepithelial tumors. Neurosci. Letters 195:81–84.

Schiffer, D., Cavalla, P., Migheli, A., Giordana, M. T., and Chiadò-Piat, L. 1996. Bcl-2 distribution in neuroepithelial tumors: an immunohistochemical study. J. Neuro-Oncol. 27:101–109.

Schiffer, D., Cavalla, P., Chió, A., Giordana, M. T., Marino, S., Mauro A., and Migheli A. 1994. Tumor cell proliferation and apoptosis in medulloblastoma. Acta Neuropathol. 87:362–370.

Schiffer, D., Chió, A., Giordana, M. T., Mauro, A., Migheli, A., and Vigliani, M. C., 1989. The vascular response to tumor infiltration in malignant gliomas. Morphometric and reconstruction study. Acta Neuropathol. 77:369–378.

Schiffer, D., Fabiani, A., Monticone, G. F., and Cognazzo, A. 1966. On the nature of the lymphocyte-like cells of medulloblastomata. Acta Neuropathol. 6: 290–297.

Shiraishi, T., Tabuchi, K., Toda, K., and Kawaguchi, S. 1995. Apoptotic cell death and apoptosis-related gene products in brain tumors. Proc. XIth Intern. Conf. Brain Tumor Res. Therap., Silverado.

Shweiki, D., Itin, A., Soffer D., and Keshet, E. 1992. Vascular endothelial growth factor induced by hypoxia may mediate hypoxia-initiated angiogenesis. Nature 359:843–845.

Sidman, R. L., Dickie M. M., and Appel, S. H. 1964. Mutant mice (quaking and jimpy) with deficient myelination in the central nervous system. Science 144:209–211.

Steel, G. G. 1977. Growth Kinetics of Tumours. Oxford University Press, Clarendon.

Sturrock, R. R. 1979. A quantitative lifespan study of changes in cell number, cell division and cell death in various regions of the mouse forebrain. Neuropathol. Appl. Neurobiol. 5:433–456.

Tachibana, O., Nakazawa, H., Lampe, J., Watanabe, K., Kleihues, P., and Ohgaki, H. 1995. Expression of Fas/APO-1 during the progression of astrocytomas. Cancer Res. 55:5528–5530.

Tachibana, O., Lampe, Kleihues, P., and Ohgaki, H. 1996. Preferential expression of Fas/APO1 (CD95) and apoptotic cell death in perinecrotic cells of glioblastoma multiforme. Acta Neuropathol. 92:431–434.

Ucker, D. S. 1991. Death by suicide: one way to go in mammalian cellular development. New Biologist 3:103–109.

Wijsman, J. H., Jonker, R. R., Keijzer, R., Van de Velde, C. J. H., Cornelisse C. J., and Van Dierendonck, J. H. 1993. A new method to detect apoptosis in paraffin sections: in situ end-labeling of fragmented DNA. J. Histochem. Cytochem. 41:7–12.

Wood, K. A., Dipasquale, B., and Youle, R. J. 1993. In situ labeling of granule cells for apoptosis-associated DNA fragmentation reveals different mechanisms of cell loss in developing cerebellum. Neuron 11:621–632.

Wyllie, A. H., Duvall, E., and Blow, J. J. 1984. Intracellular mechanisms in cell death in normal and pathological tissues. In I. Davies, and D. C. Sigee (eds.) Cell Ageing and Cell Death. Cambridge University Press, Cambridge, pp. 269–284.

Wyllie, A. H., Rose, K. A., Morris, R. G., Steel, S. M., Foster E., and Spandidos, D. A. 1897. Rodent fibroblast tumours expressing myc and ras genes. Growth, metastasis and endogenous oncogene expression. Br. J. Cancer 56:251–259

Wyllie, A. H. 1993. Apoptosis (The 1992 Frank Rose Memorial Lecture). Br. J. Cancer 67:205–208

Yuan, J., Shaham, S., Ledoux, S., Ellis, H. M., and Horvitz, H. R. 1993. The C. elegans cell death gene ced-3 encodes a protein similar to mammalian Interleukin-1ß-Converting Enzyme. Cell 75:641–652.

Zerban, H., Radig, S., Kopfschneider, A., and Bannash, P. 1994. Cell proliferation and cell death (apoptosis) in hepate preneoplastic and neoplasia are closely related to phenotypic cellular diversity and instability. Carcinogenesis 15:2467–2473.

Zülch, K. J. 1956. Biologie und Pathologie der Hirngeschwülste. In Handbuch der Neurochirurgie, Vol. 3. Springer, Berlin.

cent years much attention has been driven to age-related, presumably primary glial changes, and this has stressed the need to better characterize the glial changes.

What is necessary to characterize a glial change as primary? Such a characterization should be considered if the glial change is disproportionately prominent or appears earlier than other abnormalities. It is also indicated where the type of glial change is different from those occurring as secondary reactions. The *dissociation glio-myelinique* or massive subcortical glial proliferation seen in *progressive subcortical gliosis* and *Pick disease* are examples of the former condition, and examples of secondary reactions are numerous. The classification must be reviewed, however, in the light of recent developments of immunohistochemical or sensitive silver impregnation methods which have disclosed some new, unsuspected types of glial degeneration. Several cytoskeletal abnormalities have been reported recently in astrocytes and oligodendroglia; in 1992, *paired helical filaments* (PHF), which were long believed to occur only in neurons, have been found also in astrocytes by I. Nakano and colleagues and in astrocytic processes by our group, in advanced cases of Alzheimer disease. Reports on various abnormal argyrophilic structures in glial cells, most of which have also been shown to be immunoreactive with anti-tau antibodies, have shed new light on the concept of glial degeneration. Different glial cytoskeletal abnormalities appear to be related to the particular diseases in which they occur.

Reactive Gliosis is the Most Common of All Glial Changes

The most common of all glial changes is *reactive gliosis* occurring after neuronal damage. This reaction has a direct connection to the essential functions of glia, namely tissue support and restoration. In the acute stage of gliosis, the astrocytic reaction is characterized by a swelling of the nucleus without thickening of the nuclear membrane or hypertrophy of the cytoplasm. In a second stage, however, proliferation of astrocytes and hypertrophy of the cytoplasm occur. The appearance of a markedly eosinophilic cytoplasm, which is strongly positive for *glial fibrillary acidic protein* (GFAP), is a common finding at this stage. Subsequently, fibrillary gliosis takes place, with active proliferation of glial fibrils and reactive astrocytes with vigorous processes which finally yield the *glial scar*, the end stage of the process. At this stage, the nucleus and cytoplasm are no longer remarkable and the decrease in GFAP immunoreactivity indicates cessation of activity.

Abnormal Argyrophilic Inclusions in Glial Cells are Cytoskeletal Changes of Unknown Origin

In recent years, some types of abnormal argyrophilic structures or inclusions have been recognized in both astrocytes and oligodendroglia. The main epitope identified in most of these structures is abnormally phosphorylated tau, which may occur with or without ubiquitin. Tau-pro-

tein is found abundantly in axons in normal conditions, but its expression in glial cells has not been well studied so far (Binder *et al.*, 1985). In 1986, Yasuo Ihara and his colleagues showed that an abnormally phosphorylated tau is the basic constituent of PHFs in neurons. Ubiquitin, which combines with abnormal proteins and acts as a cytoplasmic marker in non-lysosomal proteolytic pathways (Chapter 7), has also been shown to be a constituent of PHFs by Mori and colleagues (1987). During formalin fixation, normal tau-protein immediately loses its immunogenicity, but abnormally phosphorylated tau maintains its immunoreactivity even after fixation. Any immunohistochemical trace of tau in formalin-fixed material, is therefore an evidence of some cytoskeletal abnormality. The presence of ubiquitin is also an important hallmark of the accumulation of abnormal intracellular proteins. For these reasons, argyrophilic and/or tau-positive glial inclusions have been regarded as glial cytoskeletal abnormalities; whether primary, secondary or both is still a matter of discussion. Tau-positive structures found in glial cells may represent either tangle formation, and thus be the glial counterpart to *neurofibrillary tangles* (Chapters 19 and 20), or simply the remnants of neuronal material which has been phagocytically resorbed by glial cells. Molecular biological studies using techniques such as *in situ* hybridization will be required to shed more light into this problem.

Meanwhile, structural and immunohistochemical studies of abnormal argyrophilic inclusions in glia have already begun; they have disclosed varied morphologies and immunohistochemical features, which have invariably led to multiple designations sometimes used for the same structure. A tentative classification is proposed in Table 26–1, with the preferred nomenclatures being those used in the first report of each abnormality. Using this tentative classification, each different type of inclusion will be discussed here, with particular emphasis on the diseases in which they seem to be important.

TABLE **26–1.**   Tentative classification of argyrophilic abnormal structures in glial cells.

I. Tau-positive

Glial fibrillary tangles (GFT)

Astrocytic
Tuft-shaped astrocyte
Thorn-shaped astrocyte

Oligodendroglial
Coiled bodies

Argyrophilic thread (AT)
(incl. neuronal origin)

II. Tau-negative

Glial cytoplasmic inclusions (GCI)

Tuft-shaped Astrocytes are Characteristically Found in Progressive Supranuclear Palsy

In 1990, Jean Jacques Hauw and colleagues reported on a peculiar argyrophilic fiber structure appearing in cases of *progressive supranuclear palsy* (PSP) (Chapter 20). They called the structures 'tufts of abnormal fibers', but did not mention the originating cells. Years later T. Yamada and colleagues investigated the same structure using both electron microscopic and immunohistochemical methods. They found 'star-like tufts of fibers radiating from an unstained central area' and reported on large, lucent, sometimes paired, nuclei in the central part of the tufts. The morphology of the affected cells resembled that of astrocytes, especially those which were positive for the antibody CD44 used in a study by H. Akiyama and coworkers in 1993. Actually, the abnormal argyrophilic tuft-bearing cells have been shown to react positively with CD44, all available tau- and PHF antibodies, but negatively with an anti-GFAP antibody. Immunoelectron microscopy revealed that tau-positive tufts consist of partially tubular structure but also partially exhibit an amorphous feature. T. Yamada found 20 to 25 nm smooth tubules in the cytoplasm.

M. Nishimura and coworkers (1992) observed the same tau-positive structures in PSP brain and proved ultrastructurally the coexistence, in some astrocytic perikarya, of glial fibrils and 15 nm smooth tubules, which were quite similar to the abnormal tubular constituent of neurofibrillary tangles (NFT). Based on their observations, they called them *glial fibrillary tangles* (GFT). However, it is not yet certain whether GFT have the same nature of NFT, whether GFT are really formed in glial cells or even if they are just byproducts of glial phagocytosis of neuronal NFT. In the report by Nishimura and coworkers there is also a picture of 'thorn-shaped' astrocytes, whose morphology appeared different from that of the tuft-shaped astrocytes. However, the distribution and further characterization of the thorn-shaped structures were not mentioned. From our observations, the tuft-shaped astrocytes

vary in the nature of their radiating processes; most of them are very fine and thin but some are rather thick (Figure 26–1, A-C).

Anyway, the tuft-shaped astrocytes are quite different from any other hitherto known pathological change involving astrocytes. Immunohistochemically, their main constituent is a form of full-length, non-ubiquitinated, phosphorylated tau (Figure 26–1, D, E). The majority of authors have pointed out that these are almost unique to PSP, but in 1993 we have reported on quite similar structures seen, though in smaller numbers, also in some cases of *postencephalitic parkinsonism of the Economo type* (Chapter 20). The distribution of the tuft-shaped astrocytes in PSP does not always coincide with the distribution of NFT. Tuft-shaped astrocytes are found in all cortical layers except the superficial one, where thorn-shaped astrocytes are occasionally found. The abnormal tufts are particularly abundant in the frontal cortex, a region usually unaffected by NFT in PSP, although they also occur in the *striatum*, *pallidum* and *thalamus* and, to a lesser degree, in the *Luys body*, the tectal area of the brainstem and the *substantia nigra*, all of which are regions of occurrence of NFT in PSP. However the temporal cortex, a predilection site of NFT, is scarcely affected by the GFT change. The partial topographical overlap between NFT and GFT in PSP might be regarded as evidence against the hypothesis that the astrocytic inclusions are a consequence of glial phagocytosis of neuronal material, or it might be seen under the general scope of a continuum of changes or spectral topographic distribution of degeneration (Chapter 20). However, the fact that tuft-shaped astrocytes are almost unique to PSP may relate to the special features of this disease. The so-called *subcortical dementia*, as described in 1974 by Albert and colleagues, is characteristic of PSP and may be related to the NFT pathology (Chapter 20). The PSP dementia resembles the frontal lobe syndrome; since GFT predominate also in the frontal lobe, we can speculate about a possible role of a primary astrocytic degeneration in this condition.

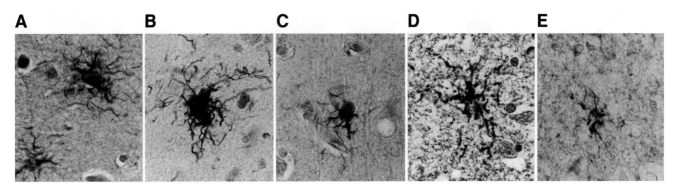

A   **B**   **C**   **D**   **E**

FIGURE   26–1

A-E. Many tuft-shaped astrocytes appear in progressive nuclear palsy and also, though in a small number, in other conditions. Most of them have 'tufts' of argyrophilic, fine, thin radiating fibers (A, B), while some others present rather short, thick processes (C). These argyrophilic fibers react against anti-tau anti-

bodies in variable degree (D, E). The origin of the abnormal structures is presumably astrocytic.
A-C. Modified Gallyas-Braak method counterstained by Kernechtrot X 460
D, E. Anti-tau immunostaining X 460.

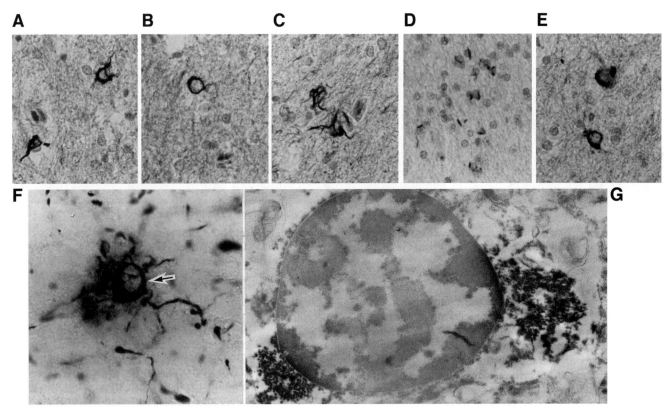

FIGURE   26–4

A-G. Coiled bodies were reported first in argyrophilic grain dementia and later in PSP and also in some other neurodegenerative diseases. Argyrophilic coiled, circular- or curved-shaped inclusions very often surround a small lucent nucleus (A-D). They consist of phosphorylated tau (E) without ubiquitination. Double immunostaining using tau- and C4d antibodies confirmed the coiled bodies to be of oligodendroglial origin. The dark colored tau-positive part (arrow) is originally purple, while the sur-

rounding light colored C4d-positive part is stained red (F). Immunoelectron microscopy reveals tau-positive tubular structure (G).
A-D. Modified Gallyas-Braak method counterstained by Kernechtrot X 460.
E. Anti-tau immunostaining X 460.
F. Anti-tau and anti-C4d double immunostaining X 820.
G. Immunoelectron microscopy without counterstaining X 12,000.

dendroglial microtubular masses. Recently, Wakabayashi and colleagues reported that coiled bodies in corticobasal degeneration are comprised of 15 nm smooth tubules, while we have revealed coiled bodies in SSPE with irregular woven tubules of approximately 14–25 nm in diameter. These findings require more detailed comparative studies.

According to the reports by the Braaks, the findings of Yamada and McGeer, a report by H. Ishizu and coworkers in 1992, a recent paper by Amano, and our own experience, coiled bodies appear in a relatively wide range of neurodegenerative diseases. Up to now, such inclusions have been reported in argyrophilic grain dementia, Alzheimer disease, Pick disease, PSP, corticobasal degeneration and subacute sclerosing panencephalitis (SSPE). However, they do not appear as extensively in these diseases as do GCIs in multiple system atrophy. Coiled bodies are observed in the cerebral white matter in argyrophilic grain dementia and corticobasal degeneration and in the cerebellar white matter, as well as some other regions, in PSP. In Pick disease, coiled bodies are seen only occasionally in cases presenting *Pick bodies*. A systematic survey of

such inclusions in each neurodegenerative disease is difficult because useful oligodendroglial markers applicable to paraffin embedded sections are not yet available. Such markers are required, for example, to help distinguish between neurofibrillary tangles located in granular nerve cells and coiled bodies located in oligodendroglia. They are also of great value for confirming the presence of coiled bodies in the white matter in a series of diseases featured by NFT. On this basis, it would be possible to ascertain the real meaning of this type of GFT in Alzheimer disease and related dementias, as well as in PSP, corticobasal degeneration and some cases of Pick disease and SSPE.

Argyrophilic Threads in Corticobasal Degeneration and in Progressive Supranuclear Palsy are Oligodendroglial Threads Resembling Neuropil Threads

Argyrophilic threads (AT) have some resemblance to the *neuropil threads* described in 1986 by Braak and coworkers in connection with neurofibrillary tangles, but appar-

A   **B**   **C**

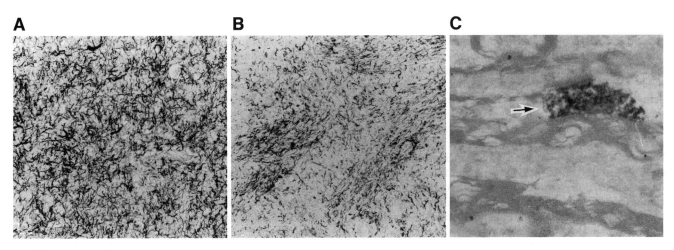

FIGURE 26–5

A-C. Argyrophilic thread structures (AT) are demonstrated by the modified Gallyas-Braak method but not by conventional Bodian staining. Fine thread-like fibrils form a prominent meshwork (A) or bundle (B) and are partially tau-positive. Immuno-electron microscopy reveals tau-positive AT (C, arrow) attached to myelin sheaths. AT are the essential findings of corticobasal degeneration but appear also in some cases of progressive supra-nuclear palsy in variable amounts.
A, B. Modified Gallyas-Braak method X 160.
C. Immunoelectron microscopy without counterstaining X 20,000.

ently differ in their distribution. Probst and colleagues reported on extensive neuropil threads in addition to neurofibrillary tangles in PSP. The antigenicity of these threads was very similar to that found in the subcortical neuronal pathology of PSP and in Alzheimer disease. However, AT have not been reported in any disease other than corticobasal degeneration and PSP. We have shown in 1994 that AT appear less intensely in some cases of PSP as compared to their extensive distribution in degenerating regions in corticobasal degeneration.

Corticobasal degeneration, originally reported in 1967 by Rebeiz and colleagues as *corticodentatonigral degeneration*, begins in the presenile age with motor disturbance and dementia and exhibits unique neuropathological features. Although AT are regarded as one of the hallmarks of this disease, they were not noticed in the reference paper by Gibb and colleagues (1989) because AT are difficult to detect using conventional silver impregnation methods. In modified Gallyas-Braak preparations however, AT appear as prominent meshworks or bundles of argyrophilic threads in both gray and white matters (Figure 26–5, A, B). Very often coiled bodies are found amidst the meshwork.

Immunohistochemically AT are partially positive with tau antibodies but negative with ubiquitin antibodies. Electron microscopy using the Gallyas-Braak method and tau-immunostaining revealed that AT are not a single structure. One common type of AT is the *tau-positive thread in myelin sheaths*, which is often encountered in the vicinity of coiled bodies (Figure 26–5, C). These threads occur mainly in the outer-, but sometimes also in the inner loop of the oligodendroglial processes of the myelin sheath enwrapping the axon. Despite the overwhelming abundance of this type of AT, as noted in the putamen and corticomedullary junction of the cerebrum,

it cannot be identified by routine electron microscopic examination. It can be visualized only by the Gallyas-Braak method or immuno-applied electron microscopy. The Gallyas-Braak- or tau-positive part of this type of AT is an amorphous structure, which may not be artificial because nearby coiled bodies are often composed of tau-positive tubules.

Another common type of AT is found as *tau-immunolabeled dendrites*, which contain normal-appearing cell organelles but consistently do not contain abnormal tubules. This type is supposed to be the dendritic part of pre-tangles, which in turn are regarded as early cytoskeletal alterations and are very abundantly observed in corticobasal degeneration and in some cases of PSP.

The detailed observation of AT in corticobasal degeneration and atypical PSP revealed that severe phosphorylated tau abnormality is extensive in both neurons and glia.

Glial Cytoplasmic Inclusions are Essential Degenerative Changes in Multiple System Atrophy

A particular type of argentophilic structure has been called *glial cytoplasmic inclusion* (GCI) by Papp and colleagues (1989), or *oligodendroglial microtubular tangles* (OMT), by Nakazato and coworkers (1990). GCIs appear widely and in an exclusive manner in cases of *olivopontocerebellar atrophy, striatonigral degeneration and Shy-Drager syndrome*, all three of which belonging to the group of diseases termed *non-hereditary multiple system atrophy* (MSA). According to Nakazato and coworkers, GCIs have never been found neither in hereditary spinocerebellar degeneration nor in any control cases including neurodegenerative diseases other than MSA. This evi-

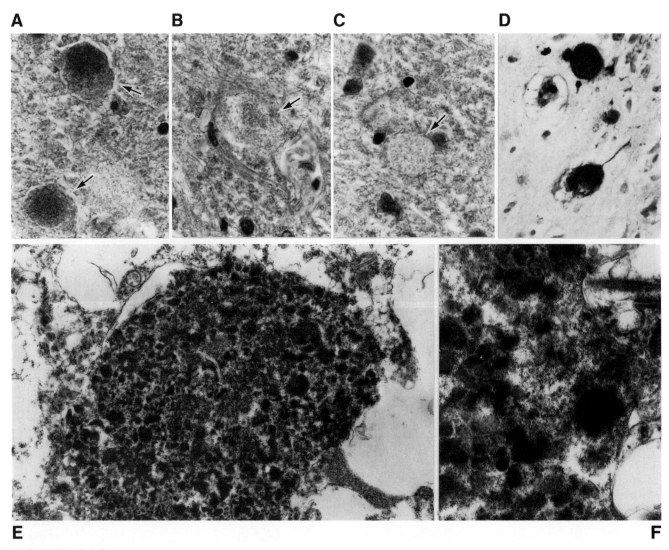

FIGURE 26–9

A-F. Foamy spheroid bodies (FSB) are named after their foamy
appearance (B-C, arrows). The faint eosinophilic bodies are either
filled compactly with coarse granules (A, arrow) or partially (B,
arrow). FSB present a positive iron reaction, especially those
found in the regions of superficial hemosiderosis or other foci
with hemorrhage (D). Such bodies have the nature of lipopigments; electron microscopically they are filled with dense
bodies, amorphous substance and ferritin-like granules (E, F).

However, different histochemical and ultrastructural features of
FSB, which are especially found in the reticular zone of substan-
tia nigra and pallidum, indicate their heterogenous origin and
nature.
A-C. H.-E. stain, X 660.
D. Purrcian blue, X 660
E. Routine electron microscopy, X 6,000.
F. Routine electron microscopy, X 20,000.

bodies do not always present with a foamy appearance
and their electron microscopic appearance, as well as their
histochemical and immunohistochemical features, are
rather complex. Furthermore, with regard to their formation, one must consider the possibility of some neuro-glial
interaction as well as that of an independent glial or neuronal origin.

An Overall View

The common glial cytoskeletal change occurring in the
form of an increase in glial fibrillary acidic protein is char-

acteristic of astrocytic gliosis which is thought to be a secondary, thus reactive change in astrocytes. A non-cytoskel-
etal type of reactive glial change is Alzheimer type II glia
found in metabolic disorders of the liver causing ammone-
mia. Interaction of brain ammonia and astrocytic glutamine synthetase may affect two important cellular organelles, namely ribosomes and mitochondria. Although
the pathogenesis of foamy spheroid bodies is not yet resolved, the excessive accumulation of lipopigment in
many of these inclusion bodies indicates that their formation can be induced by augmented iron uptake by astrocytes.

The most recent development related to glial degeneration is the identification of a variety of abnormal cytoskeletal structures in glial cells. Glial inclusions composed mainly of tau and, in some conditions, also ubiquitin, are thought to represent distinct types of glial cytoskeletal changes. From the observation of a variety of abnormally phosphorylated tau products in glial cells, we believe that some of them probably represent a kind of secondary degeneration. Tau-positive thorn-shaped astrocytes in superficial cortical regions, frequently observed in the boxer's brain but also non-specifically, though rarely, in other neurodegenerative diseases, are thought to be induced by a secondary astrocytic reaction. Multiple pathogenetic factors causing degeneration of neurons, such as recurrent head trauma, some kinds of viral infections and aging itself may interest glial cells in similar ways. The problem to ascertain whether these causes of neuronal degeneration are inducing glial degeneration directly, and not as a consequence of the neuronal degeneration, demands further studies, especially at the molecular biological level.

It is interesting that certain cytoskeletal glial abnormalities occur preferentially in some kinds of neurodegenerative diseases. Furthermore, the glial system involved and the degree of abnormality are different in each disease. In Alzheimer disease, glial degeneration is greatly limited to a common secondary reaction due to neuronal loss and other degenerative changes. Therefore, Alzheimer disease should be regarded as a mainly neuronal disease. On the other hand, a wide range of cytoskeletal abnormalities, including NFT and GFT in both astrocytes and oligodendroglia occur in PSP which appears to constitute an example of a disease involving primary neuro-glial degeneration. Corticobasal degeneration exemplifies another aspect of glial degeneration in addition to neuronal changes, namely the massive formation of argyrophilic threads (AT) in distal parts of oligodendroglial processes, and coiled bodies. Therefore corticobasal degeneration probably involves neurons as well as oligodendroglia. Since tau-negative oligodendroglial GCIs appear more extensively in the initial stage of multiple system atrophy than in the advanced stage, and their distribution coincides with degenerating systems in this class of diseases, GCIs in multiple system atrophy might be regarded as one example of primary glial degeneration.

The evidence presented in this chapter lead us to the conclusion that glial degeneration, likewise neuronal degeneration, must be taken into account in the study of neurodegenerative conditions. Cytoskeletal abnormalities of glia have not been enough investigated, and details about the range of diseases in which they appear, their different types and intensity in each disease, and their possible relationships to neuronal neurofibrillary changes remain to be elucidated. For the present suffice it to say that it is worthwhile to shift the concept of cytoskeletal abnormalities from a focus on neurons or glia alone to a focus on neuro-glia interactions. The accumulation of further evidence should cast new light on the whole question of glial degeneration.

Selected Readings

Albert, M. L., Feldman, R. G., and Willis, A. L. 1974. The subcortical dementia of progressive supranuclear palsy. J. Neurol. Neurosurg. Psychiatry 37:121–130.

Braak, H., and Braak, E. 1989. Cortical and subcortical argyrophilic grains characterize a disease associated with adult onset dementia. Neuropathol. Appl. Neurobiol. 15:13–26.

Cavanagh, J. B., Nolan, C. C., and Brown, A. W. 1990. Glial cell intrusions actively remove detritus due to toxic chemicals from within nerve cells. Neuro Toxicology 11:1–12.

Corsellis, J. A. N., Bruton, C. J., and Freeman-Browne, D. 1973. The aftermath of boxing. Psychol. Med. 3:270–303.

Ikeda, K., Akiyama, H., Haga, C. et al. 1992. Evidence that neurofibrillary tangles undergo glial modification. Acta Neuropathol. 85:101–104.

Minagawa, M., Shioda, K., and Shimizu, Y. et al. 1992. Inclusion bodies in cerebral cortical astrocytes. Acta Neuropathol. 84:113–116.

Norenberg, M. D., and Martinez-Hernandez, A. 1979. Fine structural localization of glutamine synthetase in astrocytes of rat brain. Brain Res. 161:303–310.

Phelps, C. H. 1975. An ultrastructural study of methionine sulphoximine-induced glycogen accumulation in astrocytes of the mouse cerebral cortex. J. Neurocytol. 4:478–490.

Sakai, M., Austin, J., Witmer, E., et al. 1970. Studies in myoclonus epilepsy (Lafora body form) II. polyglucosans in the systemic deposits of myoclonus epilepsy and in corpora amylacea. Neurology 20:161–176.

Seitelberger, F. 1970. General neuropathology of central neuroglia: The concept of glial syndromes. VIth International Congress of Neuropathology, Paris, pp 392–406.

Seitelberger, F. 1971. Neuropathological conditions related to neuroaxonal dystrophy. Acta Neuropathol. Suppl. V:17–29.

Yamamoto, T., Iwasaki, Y., Sato, H. et al. 1989. Astrocytic pathology of methionine sulfoximine-induced glycogen accumulation in astrocytes of the mouse cerebral cortex. Acta Neuropathol. 77:357–368.

References

Abe, H., Yagishita, S., Itoh, K., et al. 1992. Novel eosinophilic inclusions in astrocytes. Acta Neuropathol. 83:659–663.

Akiyama, H., Tooyama, I., Kawamata, T., et al. 1993. Morphological diversities of CD44 positive astrocytes in the cerebral cortex of normal subjects and patients with Alzheimer's disease. Brain Res. 632:249–259.

Albert, M. L., Feldman, R. G., and Willis, A. L. 1974. The subcortical dementia of progressive supranuclear palsy. J. Neurol. Neurosurg. Psychiatry 37:121–130.

Amano, N., Hanihara, S., Ito, K., et al. 1992. 33th Annual Meeting of Japanese Society of Neuropathology (abstract). Neuropathology (Jpn.) 12:106.

Amano, N. 1994. Glial fibrillary tangles and dementia. Dementia (Jpn.) 8:94–101.

Arai, N., Nishimura, M., Oda, M., et al. 1992. Immunohistochemical expression of microtubule-associated protein 5 (MAP 5) in glial cells in multiple system atrophy. J. Neurol. Sci. 109:102–106.

Arai, N., Yagishita, S., Misugi, K., et al. 1992. Peculiar axonal debris with subsequent astrocytic response (foamy spheroid body). Virchows Archiv A 420:243–252.

Arai, N., Mizutani, T., and Morimatsu, Y. 1993. Foamy spheroid bodies in the globus pallidus and the substantia nigra pars reticulata – an investigation on regional distribution in 56 persons without neurodegenerative diseases. Virchows Archiv A 422:307–311.

Binder, L. I., Frankfurter, A., and Rebhun, L. I. 1985. The distribution of tau in the mammalian central nervous system. J. Cell Biol. 101:1371–1378.

Braak, H., Braak, E., Grundke-Iqbal, I., et al. 1986. Occurrence of neuropil threads in the senile human brain and in Alzheimer's disease: a third location of paired helical filaments outside of neurofibrillary tangles and neuritic plaques Neurosci. Lett. 65:351–355.

Braak H., Braak E., Ohm T. G., et al. 1988. Silver impregnation of Alzheimer's neurofibrillary changes counterstained for basophilic and lipofuscin pigment. Stain. Technol. 63:193–200.

Braak, H., and Braak, E. 1989. Cortical and subcortical argyrophilic grains characterize a disease associated with adult onset dementia. Neuropathol. Appl. Neurobiol. 15:13–26.

Cavanagh, J. B., and Kyu, M. H. 1971. Type II Alzheimer change experimentally produced in astrocytes in the rat. J. Neurol. Sci. 12:63–75.

Cavanagh, J. B., Nolan, C. C., and Brown, A. W. 1990. Glial cell intrusions actively remove detritus due to toxic chemicals from within nerve cells. Neuro Toxicology 11:1–12.

Choi, D. W. 1988. Glutamate neurotoxicity and diseases of the nervous system. Neuron 1:623–634.

Corsellis, J. A. N., Bruton, C. J., and Freeman-Browne, D. 1973. The aftermath of boxing. Psychol. Med. 3:270–303.

Feany, M. B., and Dickson, D. W. 1995. Widespread cytoskeletal pathology characterizes corticobasal degeneration. Am. J. Pathol. 146:1388–1396.

Friede, R. L. 1975. Developmental Neuropathology. pp. 89–93. Springer, Wien-New York.

Gibb, W. R. G., Luthert, P. J., and Marsden, C. D. 1989. Corticobasal degeneration. Brain 112:1171–1192.

Greenfield, J. G. 1958. System degeneration of the cerebellum, brain stem and spinal cord. In J. G. Greenfield, W. Blackwood et al. (eds.) Greenfield's Neuropathology, 1st Ed., pp. 520–549. Edward Arnold, London.

Hamberger, A., Chiang, G. H., Sandoval, E., et al. 1979. Glutamate as a CNS transmitter. Regulation of synthesis in the releasable pool. Brain Res. 168:531–541.

Hauw, J. J., Verny, M., Delacre, P., et al. 1990. Constant neurofibrillary changes in the neocortex in progressive supranuclear palsy: basic differences with Alzheimer's disease and aging. Neurosci. Lett. 119:182–186.

Hof, P. R., Bouras, C., Buée, L., et al. 1992. Differential distribution of neurofibrillary tangles in the cerebral cortex of dementia pugilistica and Alzheimer's disease cases. Acta Neuropathol. 85:23–30.

Horoupian, D. S., and Dickson, D. W. 1991. Striatonigral degeneration, olivopontocerebellar atrophy and atypical Pick disease. Acta Neuropathol. 81:287–295.

Hughes, J. T., and Oppenheimer, D. R. 1969. Superficial siderosis of the CNS, a report of nine cases with autopsy. Acta Neuropathol. 13:56–74.

Ihara, Y., Nukina, N., Miura, R., et al. 1986. Phosphorylated tau protein is integrated into paired helical filaments in Alzheimer's disease. J. Biochem. 99:1807–1810.

Ikeda, K., Akiyama, H., Haga, C., et al. 1992. Evidence that neurofibrillary tangles undergo glial modification. Acta Neuropathol. 85:101–104.

Ikeda, K., Akiyama, H., Haga, C., et al. 1994. Argyrophilic thread-like structure in corticobasal degeneration and supranuclear palsy. Neurosci. Lett. 174:157–159.

Ikeda, K., Akiyama, H., Kondo, H., et al. 1993. Anti-tau-positive glial fibrillary tangles in the brain of postencephalitic parkinsonism of Economo type. Neurosci. Lett. 162:176–178.

Ikeda, K., Akiyama, H., Kondo, H., et al. 1995. Numerous glial fibrillary tangles in oligodendroglia in cases of subacute sclerosing panencephalitis with neurofibrillary tangles. Neurosci. Lett. 194:133–135.

Ikeda, K., Akiyama, H., Kondo, H. et al. 1996. Thorn-shaped astrocytes: possibly secondarily induced tau-positive glial fibrillary tangles. Acta Neuropathol. 90:620–625

Ikeda, K., Haga, C., Akiyama, H., et al. 1992. Coexistence of paired helical filaments and glial filaments in astrocytic processes within ghost tangles. Neurosci. Lett. 148:126–128.

Ishii, T. 1963. Neuropathological study of ammonia poisoning in dogs, with reference to pathogenesis of hepatocerebral disease (Inose type). Seishin Shinkeigaku Zasshi (Jpn.) 65:667–693.

Ishizu, H., Syomori, T., Kuroda, S., et al. 1992. 33th Annual Meeting of Japanese Society of Neuropathology (abstract). Neuropathology (Jpn.) 12:109–110.

Kato, S., Hirano, A., Umehara, T., et al. 1992. Immunohistochemical studies on the new type of astrocytic inclusions identified in a patient with brain malformation. Acta Neuropathol. 84:449–452.

Koeppen, A. H. W., and Barron, K. D. 1971. Superficial siderosis of the central nervous system. A histochemical and chemical study. J. Neuropathol. Exp. Neurol. 30:448–469.

Martinez-Hernandez, A., Bell, K. P., and Norenberg, M. D. 1977. Glutamine synthetase: glial localization in brain. Science 195:1356–1358.

Minagawa, M., Shioda, K., Shimizu, Y., et al. 1992. Inclusion bodies in cerebral cortical astrocytes. Acta Neuropathol. 84:113–116.

Mori, H., Kondo, J., and Ihara, Y. 1987. Ubiquitin is a component of paired helical filaments in Alzheimer's disease. Science 235:1641–1644.

Nakano, I., Iwatsubo, T., Otsuka, N., et al. 1992. Paired helical filaments in astrocyte: electron microscopy and immunohistochemistry in a case of atypical Alzheimer's disease. Acta Neuropathol. 83:228–232.

Nakazato, Y., Yamazaki, H., and Hirato, J. 1990. Oligodendroglial microtubular tangles in olivopontocerebellar atrophy. J. Neuropathol. Exp. Neurol. 49:521–530.

Nishimura, M., Namba, Y., Ikeda, K., et al. 1992. Glial fibrillary tangles with straight tubules in the brains of patients with progressive supranuclear palsy. Neurosci. Lett. 143:35–38.

Neumann, M. A., and Cohn, R. 1967. Progressive subcortical gliosis, a rare form of presenile dementia. Brain 90:405–418.

Oda, M., Ikeda, K., and Yamamoto, T. 1983. Immunohistochemistry of glutamine synthetase of the mouse and human brain. A preliminary study on pathogenesis of hepatic gliopathy. Neuropathology (Jpn) 4:19–30.

Oda, M. 1993. Astrocytes in liver diseases. Adv. Neurol. Sci. (Jpn.) 37:617–629.

Oppenheimer, D. R. 1976. Disease of the basal ganglia, cerebellum and motor neurons. In W. Brackwood, J. A. N. Corsellis, et al. (eds.) Greenfield's Neuropathology, 3rd Ed., pp. 699–747. Edward Arnord, London.

Papp, M. I., Kahn, J. E., and Lantos, P. L. 1989. Glial cytoplasmic inclusions in the CNS of patients with multiple system atrophy (striatonigral degeneration, olivopontocerebellar atrophy and Shy-Drager syndrome). J. Neurol. Sci. 94:79–100.

Probst, A., Langui, D., and Lautenschlager, C. 1988. Progressive supranuclear palsy: extensive neuropil threads in addition to neurofibrillary tangles. Very similar antigenicity of subcortical neuronal pathology in progressive supranuclear palsy and Alzheimer's disease. Acta Neuropathol. 77:61–68.

Rebeiz, J. J., Kolodny, E. H., and Richardson, E. P. 1967. Corticodentatonigral degeneration with neuronal achromasia: a progressive disorder of late adult life. Trans Am. Neurol. Assoc. 92:23–26.

Schaffer, K. 1918 Beiträge zur Histopathologie der protoplasmatischen Neuroglia. Zeitschr. Neurol. Psychiat. 38:85–110.

Tokuda, T., Ikeda, S., and Yanagisawa, N. 1991. Re-examination of ex-boxers' brains using immunohistochemistry with antibodies to amyloid á-protein and tau protein. Acta Neuropathol. 82:280–285.

Trétiakoff, C. 1919. Étude histopathologique du locus niger dans 54 cas de maladies du systeme nerveux. Contribution al étude de l'anatomie pathologique du locus niger. pp. 29–56. Thesis, Paris.

Wakabayashi, K., Oyanagi, K., Makifuchi, T., et al. 1994. Corticobasal degeneration: etiopathological significance of the cytoskeletal alterations. Acta Neuropathol. 87:545–553.

Wegiel, J. and Wisniewski, H. M. 1994. Rosenthal fibers, eosinophilic inclusions, and anchorage densities with desmosome-like structures in astrocytes in Alzheimer's disease. Acta Neuropathol. 87:355–361.

Yamada, T., and McGeer, P. L. 1990. Oligodendroglial microtubular masses: an abnormality observed in some human neurodegenerative diseases. Neurosci. Lett. 120:163–166.

Yamada, T., McGeer, P. L., and McGeer, E. G. 1992. Appearance of paired nucleated, Tau-positive glia on patients with progressive supranuclear palsy brain tissue. Neurosci. Lett. 135:99–102.

Yamada, T., Calne, D. B., Akiyama, H., et al. 1993. Further observations on tau-positive glia in the brains with progressive supranuclear palsy. Acta Neuropathol. 85:308–315.

Jürgen R. E. Bohl
Akira Hori

Vascular Changes

William Osler in 1901 declared that 'a man is only as old as his arteries'. This aphoristic sentence is particularly true for cerebral arteries and for the four arteries that supply the brain with blood. A progressive reduction of the cerebral blood supply may finally result in selective nerve cell losses, in complete infarcts and in an aggravating dementing process called multi-infarct dementia. The two most important vascular changes accounting for the reduction of cerebral blood supply are atherosclerosis and amyloid angiopathy.

Atherosclerosis is the Most Frequent Disease of Arteries Resulting in Brain Dysfunction

The term *atheroma* is derived from the Greek word 'athere', that means 'mush'. It describes the pultaceous or caseous material of high lipid content in circumscribed plaque-like thickenings of the interior portion of the wall of the vessel. This most common degenerative disease of arteries is named *atherosclerosis* to emphasize the sclerotic or fibrous tissue component of the pathologic alterations in the wall of arteries. The term *arteriosclerosis* is often used synonymously; indeed, the nomenclature of degenerative vascular diseases is confusing. Arteriosclerosis literally means sclerosis and hardening of arteries, as if these were a manifestation of aging independent of atherosclerosis. Generically speaking, arteriosclerosis includes atherosclerosis, *Mönckeberg sclerosis* and sclerotic age-related changes of large and small peripheral arteries. For the common degenerative chronic disease of arteries described here the term atherosclerosis should be preferred.

The severity of atherosclerotic lesions in intracranial and intracerebral arteries is not always the same as in the arteries of the whole body. In some cases of a severe general atherosclerosis there are nearly no changes in the cerebral arteries. There is currently no explanation for this strange phenomenon. Furthermore there is often no correlation between the severity of atherosclerotic alterations of intracranial and intracerebral arteries and the intensity and extension of cerebral vascular lesions; therefore sometimes there is no correlation between cerebral atherosclerosis and clinical symptoms. We have observed cases with cerebral atherosclerosis of highest degree, which had no apparent functional repercussion. The site, extension and severity of brain damage is not generally predictable, even when the site of the most severe lesion of the blood vessel wall is known. This is accounted for by the high variability of the cerebral arteries at the base of the brain. Only in rare cases the composition of the *circulus arteriosus Willisi* (Willis' ring) is the same as in textbooks of anatomy; variations are more common than the ideal standard. As once pointed out by Michel Serres, 'the essential, the invariant, is just the variation in diversity.'

Fatty Streaks, Fibrous Plaques and Complicated Lesions are the Principal Atherosclerotic Changes

During the development of atherosclerotic lesions the principal changes take place largely within the *intima* or the innermost layer of the wall of the vessel. In fact, atherosclerosis begins as a disease of the *intima*. The principal lesions of atherosclerosis are: The *fatty streak*, the *fibrous plaque*, and the *complicated lesion*.

Fatty streaks are thought to be one of the first signs of atherosclerosis. They are found in all regions of the arterial tree throughout the whole body. They can be found in all ages, even in children in early infancy and even at birth in some cultures, depending on dietary habits and life styles. They do not necessarily progress into fibrous plaques and more severe atherosclerotic lesions; some may clearly regress and disappear whereas others remain unchanged during the individual's lifetime. Fatty streaks consist mainly of monocyte-derived macrophages that have entered into the intima from the blood stream. These cells become foam cells and contain large amounts of lipid in the form of lipid droplets, which consist mainly of cholesterol ester. In advanced fatty streaks there are also variable numbers of lipid-filled smooth muscle cells derived from the *tunica media* of the blood vessel wall. Another early lesion in the pathogenesis of atherosclerosis is the so-called 'gelatinous lesion', containing a large amount of extracellular matrix relatively rich in proteoglycans. Numerous cells are found in this matrix, mainly macrophages and smooth muscle cells. Possibly some of these gelatinous lesions may become advanced fibrous plaques.

The *fibrous plaque*: When causal agents persist, a dense fibrous cap develops at the inner surface of the atherosclerotic lesion. This asymmetric fibrous cap contains thick bands of a collagen-rich connective tissue matrix surrounding numerous smooth muscle cells and some macrophages and covered towards the vessel lumen by endothelial cells.

The *complicated lesion* is probably a fibrous plaque that has become altered by calcification, and may develop cracks or fissures, undergo ulceration, or initiate the formation of hemorrhages and thrombosis. Intramural hemorrhage and obliterating thrombosis may lead to severe complications such as myocardial or cerebral infarction or gangrene. Beneath the dense fibrous cap varying numbers of smooth muscle cells and macrophages containing varying amounts of lipid, are often found. Sometimes there are abundant numbers of foam cells in these areas, particularly in hypercholesterolemic individuals. Another cellular component of complicated lesions may be an accumulation of *T-lymphocytes*. In progressing lesions all these cells undergo necrotic changes, resulting in large amounts of extracellular lipid debris and caseous masses. At the base of these plaques there may be large numbers of proliferated smooth muscle cells surrounded by connective tissue matrix. Further complications are calcifications, even ossifications, and very often cracks and fissures. These latter induce secondary intramural hemorrhages in larger arteries and lead to stenosis or obliteration of the vessel by formation of thrombosis. The occluding thrombus may become organized, thus the vessel becomes recanalized and the pathologic process may start again.

All these pathologic processes are mainly found in the internal layer of the blood vessel wall, in the *intima*. They induce secondary changes in the *tunica media* and alterations of the *lamina elastica interna*. Finally these secondary lesions in *the tunica media*, in the smooth muscle layer, result in a total breakdown of the blood vessel wall. Sometimes in final stages the blood vessels resemble totally calcified rigid tubes.

Different Cell Types Play Different Roles in Atherogenesis

To understand the dynamic process of atherogenesis we have to understand the functional roles of each cell, the alterations in each of the cells and especially the reciprocal interactions between the cells involved in the development of the lesion. These cells involved in atherogenesis are not only cells of the arterial blood vessel wall, i.e., endothelium and smooth muscle cells; but also circulating blood cells, including platelets, monocytes and macrophages as well as lymphocytes. Most important for the combined action of these cells are the various growth factors which are produced in response to different types of injury in order to repair cell or tissue damages, to maintain or to re-establish the life supporting function of the vascular system.

Normal *endothelial cells* are capable to perform a large number of different functions: The endothelium has a special capacity to modify and transport lipoproteins, to participate in the adherence of leucocytes, to form vasoactive substances, to participate in procoagulant and in anticoagulant activity and to produce growth factors. Endothelial cell turnover is reasonably low in most parts of the adult arterial system, except at sites where rheologic changes have an influence on this property. A wide range of injuries to endothelial cells at given anatomic sites, or exposure of the endothelium to cytokines such as *tumor necrosis factor*, can induce the endothelial cells to express mitogens such as *platelet-derived growth factor* (PDGF) and *interleukin*-1. Furthermore the exposure of endothelium to coagulant factors such as activated *factor X* or *thrombin* can induce early secretion of stored PDGF and later gene expression, synthesis and secretion of PDGF. Advanced lesions of atherosclerosis often become vascularized by *vasa vasorum* (vessels' own vessels) originating from the *adventitia*. Even these endothelial cells become a source of growth factors for further progression of the proliferating process, if they are appropriately stimulated.

Advanced lesions of atherosclerosis mainly consist of multiplicated *smooth muscle cells* and of new connective tissue. Smooth muscle cells are the principal source of connective tissue in the fibrous plaque. Additionally they also have the capacity to form growth factors, in particular PDGF A-chain. In some regions smooth muscle proliferation starts in a preexisting region of diffuse intimal thickening, that occurred during normal development and aging; in other regions, where the *intima* is very thin, there can be observed an acute migration of smooth muscle cells into the *intima*, associated with smooth muscle proliferation. This migration might be provoked by a localized traumatic rupture of the internal elastic membrane, resulting in a circumscribed fibrous plaque above the membrane defect, accompanied by a production of small splitted elastic membranes.

Monocytes are the precursor cells of *macrophages* in all tisues. When activated, macrophages can secrete growth factors for connective tissue cells, such as smooth muscle cells and fibroblasts, in the form of both chains of PDGF. Macrophages also form *fibroblast growth factor* (FGF), that is a potent angiogenic agent and can play a role in capillary formation as well as in connective tissue proliferation. Activated macrophages can secrete many more important and highly effective substances, e.g., *transforming growth factor-alpha* (TGF-alpha), a mitogen that can induce epithelial migration and proliferation; *transforming growth factor-beta* (TGF-beta) which is the most potent inhibitor of cell proliferation thus far known and one of the most potent inducers of collagen synthesis; *interleukin*-1 (IL-1), that can have an indirect and profound effect on lymphocyte proliferation; *colony stimulating factor*-1 (CSF-1) which acts in an autocrine fashion on macrophages or on stem cell precursors of the macrophages; and also *tumor necrosis factor* (TNF alpha or *cachectin*), that induces expression of PDGF by the endothelium.

Macrophages also act as scavenger cells and can induce free radical formation by oxidizing ingested lipids. Secretion of oxidized material together with other agents such as hydrolytic enzymes could be injurious to neighbouring cells. Thus macrophages could induce further tissue in-

jury and maintain the progression of atherosclerosis. Macrophages are probably the key cells responsible for mitogenic stimulation of smooth muscle and thus are critical in lesion formation and the progression of atherosclerosis.

Platelets produce multiple growth factors and mitogens. Activated platelets release PDGF and also secrete large amounts of an *epidermal growth factor* (EGF)- like substance, TGF-beta, and furthermore a specific growth factor for arterial endothelial cells. Platelets also play a major role in the coagulation process and in the formation of thrombosis. Usually fresh thrombi are organized by ingrowth and proliferation of smooth muscle cells, which induce deposition of new connective tissue. This process is stimulated by the wealth of growth factors that have been released from the aggregated and degranulated platelets.

Focal accumulations of *T-lymphocytes* in advanced lesions of atherosclerosis suggest that immune or auto-immune responses may be involved in atherogenesis (Stemme *et al.*, 1991, 1992). Many of the T-cells located in fibrous plaques were found to be activated, based on their ability to express *class II HLA surface antigens*. L. Capron (1993) suggested that the auto-immune mechanisms of vasculitis and sclerotic plaques might be regarded as foci of chronic inflammation. The role of T-cells in the process of atherogenesis is yet poorly understood. Little is known about the risk factor-associated phenomena that could result in auto-immunity in atherosclerosis. Some drugs – such as *cyclosporin*, that inhibit the immune response of T-helper cells have been observed to produce a decrease in the incidence and size of lesions formed in experimentally induced atherosclerosis.

Several Risk Factors for Atherogenesis Have Been Identified

Many epidemiologic studies as well as conscientious experimental investigations have discovered several risk factors for atherogenesis, e.g.: Hypercholesterolemia; hypertension; cigarette smoking; diabetes mellitus and several less common diseases such as homocystinuria, among others.

Hypercholesterolemia is considered to be the major risk factor associated with the increased incidence of atherosclerosis in many industrial countries. Human plasma lipoproteins are composed of several classes of particles, including: *Chylomicrons*; VLDL (*very-low-density lipoprotein*); IDL (*intermediate-density lipoprotein*); LDL (*low-density lipoprotein*); and HDL (*high-density lipoprotein*). These different lipoprotein particles are bound to cells by their apoproteins (e.g., ApoA, ApoB, ApoC and ApoE), each of which binds to specific receptors on cells such as endothelium, smooth muscle and macrophages. Circulating plasma lipoproteins are derived from two sources: Exogenous dietary fat and endogenous fat of hepatic origin. Hyperlipoproteinemia reflects a defect in the metabolism of lipoproteins. High plasma levels can occur from overproduction, deficient removal, or from a combination thereof. Additionally there is a number of forms of genetic hyperlipidemias, that are either monogenic or polygenic. Some of these genetic disorders are, e.g.: *Familial hypercholesterolemia; multiple lipoprotein hyperlipidemia; familial hypertriglyceridemia; familial dysbetalipoproteinemia* and *cholesterolester storage disease*, among others. In all these disorders a high incidence of a severe atherosclerosis can be observed. More common than these hereditary diseases are other disorders that result secondarily in hyperlipoproteinemia, such as diabetes mellitus, renal disease, alcoholism, treatment with corticosteroids or estrogens, hypothyroidism and the dysglobulinemias.

Experimental studies as well as clinical trials with pharmacological agents have shown unequivocally that decreasing cholesterol levels will lead to a decrease in the incidence of clinical sequelae directly attributable to advanced lesions of atherosclerosis. Plasma cholesterol levels should be below 200 mg/dl. Levels between 200 and 240 mg/dl should be treated by diet and above 240 mg/dl by diet and cholesterol-lowering agents.

Epidemiologically *hypertension* correlates with an increased incidence of coronary heart disease, cerebrovascular disease and accelerated atherogenesis, but the mechanisms by which hypertension causes the cellular changes leading to atherosclerosis are not yet clear. Perhaps the mechanism is similar to that in hypercholesterolemia: Increased monocyte adherence and intimal localization of monocyte-derived macrophages. Of high importance in the process of atherogenesis might also be humoral mediators of blood pressure, such as angiotensin and renin and many drugs and poisons, and last but not least, altered hemodynamic properties. Complex adaptive cellular interactions finally result in proliferative intimal smooth muscle lesions.

Cigarette smoking (or smoking in general) is undoubtedly one of the most important risk factors for the development of atherosclerosis. The complex mechanisms are not yet fully understood. One theory stresses the role of a series of tobacco glycoproteins, inducing an immune response within the artery wall and initiating a proliferation of intimal smooth muscle cells. If smokers could stop smoking, there would be a decrease of the risk for the development of the clinical sequelae of atherosclerosis.

In individuals with *diabetes mellitus* the fast progression of atherosclerosis might have several causes: Many diabetic individuals are hypercholesterolemic; some demonstrate decreased levels of HDL and often are hypertensive, associated with hyperglycemia. Controlling diabetes by careful diet and therapy usually lowers the risk for further progression of atherosclerosis.

A recent epidemiological study showed a correlation between higher frequencies of preclinical atherosclerosis, as assessed by intimal-medial thickening of the carotid arteries, and low socioeconomic state. The intimal-medial wall thickening has been associated with established coronary heart disease risk factors and with increased risk of acute coronary events (Diez-Roux *et al.*, 1995).

Various Theories and Hypotheses Try to Explain the Different Types and Ways of Atherogenesis

Considering all these epidemiologically proven risk factors for the development of a severe atherosclerosis, there have been proposed a number of theories and hypotheses to explain the different types and ways of atherogenesis, e.g., the 'lipid hypothesis', the 'lipid autoxidation theory', the 'thrombogenic theory of atherogenesis', the 'intimal injury hypothesis', the 'monoclonal hypothesis' (concerning smooth muscle cells), the 'mechanical or hemodynamic hypothesis' and the 'fatigue hypothesis' and most recently the 'Chlamydia pneumoniae-infection hypothesis'... One theory tries to combine different elements of others: The 'response to injury hypothesis'. This theory suggests that some types of injury to the endothelium lining result in a sequence of events, finally leading to a migration, accumulation and proliferation of intimal smooth muscle cells. This injury might be a very subtle event (e.g., radiation injury; electro-magnetic influences? side-effects of drugs?) inducing merely functional alterations. The consequences might be increased monocyte and lymphocyte adhesion to the endothelium, accompanied by chemotactic attraction of these cells into the subendothelial space. One of the first events possibly could be an increased endothelial turnover, inducing the expression of genes for growth factors in the endothelium, or resulting in a generation of chemotactic factors for monocytes. Once the production of growth factors by both macrophages and activated endothelial cells has started, the proliferating process of smooth muscle cells continues and ends in the formation of an advanced typical atherosclerotic plaque. Therapeutic strategies could be designed so as to prevent the formation of this lesion by protecting the endothelium or by preventing selectively the monocyte adherence and conversion to macrophages within the arterial wall.

Atherosclerosis may be Reversible Under Certain Circumstances

Several clinicians have reported that chronological serial angiographic examinations can demonstrate a decrease in arteriosclerotic changes (Blankenhorn, 1981). According to G. F. Sholler and colleagues (1984), arterial calcification may disappear completely in cases of *idiopathic arterial calcification in infancy* – IACI (Chapter 30). Blankenhorn (1981) recognized three conditions for the regression of early arteriosclerotic changes: major reduction of blood lipid level, rigid control of hypertension, and non-smoking.

According to the 'response to injury hypothesis' the atherogenic process could be interpreted as an adaptive process aiming at a functional and structural adaptation to an altered mechanical or chemical strain of the blood vessel wall. Like in other diseases, this adaptive process could, under special circumstances, result in structural changes that even worsen the injurious effect on the artery wall. Thus, the initially adaptive process turns into a self-destructive, steadily progressing disorder. In early

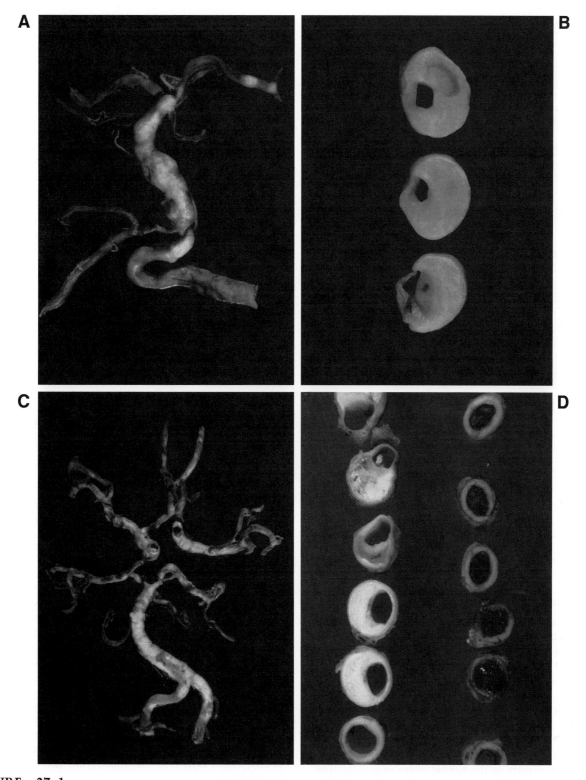

FIGURE   27–1

Atherosclerosis of basal cerebral arteries.
A. Basilar and vertebral arteries with severe atherosclerotic changes.
B. Cross sections of the basal artery with a high grade stenosis.

C. Basal arteries including Willis' ring (*Circulus arteriosus Willisi*) with severe atherosclerosis.
D. Cross sections of the basal and vertebral arteries show stenosis and obliterating thrombosis.

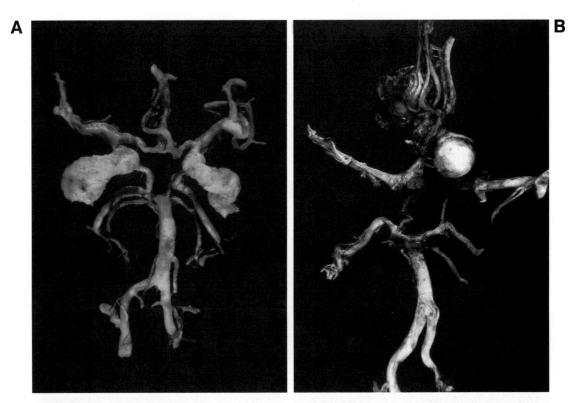

FIGURE   27–2
Atherosclerosis and its sequelae.
A. Basal cerebral arteries with severe atherosclerosis and fusi-
form dilatation of both internal carotid arteries.

B. Basal cerebral arteries with atherosclerotic changes and two
huge berry-like aneurysms at the anterior communicating artery.

stages of the disease a regression of the lesions might be
possible and has been observed. But beyond a point of no
return the disease gains a self-perpetuating dynamic character.

Consequences of Cerebral Atherosclerosis

Consequences of cerebral atherosclerosis (Figures 27–
1,2,3) include secondary changes in the artery wall leading to the formation of angiectasia, infarction, cortical
atrophy, and leukoencephalopathy.

Fusiform aneurysms may be observed in elderly people
and are formed on the basis of atherosclerotic arteries.
The morphology of this state is nothing else than *sclerotic angiectasia* and not a true aneurysm. Due to enlargement and atheromatous degeneration of the arterial wall,
this 'aneurysm' may rupture or manifest as space-occupying lesion, frequently in the basilar artery or middle cerebral artery. Atherosclerotic aneurysms are not only fusiform but also, though infrequently, *saccular* (Figure 27–
2). Another kind of saccular aneurysm is observed independently of atherosclerosis, typically at the branching
portions of the peripheral artery; clinical manifestations
beginning with sudden severe headache are due to rupture of the aneurysm, usually seen in adults.

*Clinical Symptoms Depend on Location of the Brain
Lesions and not on the Vascular Change Itself*

Atherosclerosis may result in narrowing or obliteration
of the vessel lumina or formation of thrombi followed by
circulatory disturbances in irrigated organ/tissue areas.
Thrombosis occurs at the site of the plaques either due to
plaque rupture, intramural hemorrhage at the plaque, or
thrombosis without plaque rupture or *intramural hemorrhage* (Ogata *et al.*, 1994). One of the most frequent consequences of atherosclerotic changes are an infarction due
to thrombosis. Cerebral (arterial) infarctions are typically
seen in the territory of main cerebral arteries, namely in
territories of anterior, middle, and posterior cerebral arteries. Thrombosis of the internal carotid artery results in
infarctions mainly in the territory of the middle cerebral
artery since the anterior and posterior arterial territories
are irrigated by the collateral blood stream through the
Willis' ring. Territorial infarctions are demonstrated in
Figure 27–3.

Clinical manifestations depend greatly on the location
of infarctions. They are usually produced as a functional
deficit of the destroyed structures. However, further
pathological development of the once damaged tissue
may later cause additional symptoms such as vascular or
multi-infarct dementia. Astrocytes, for example, do not

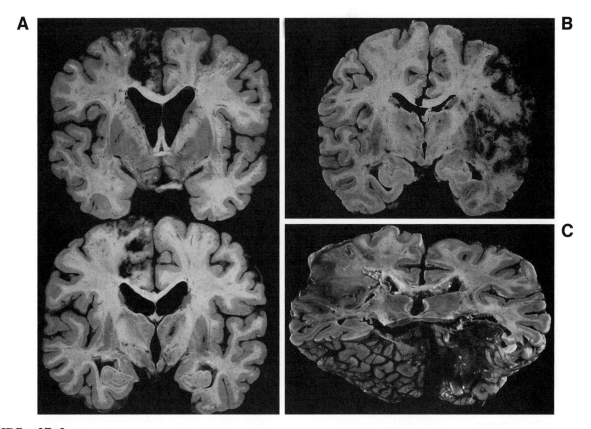

FIGURE   27–3

Atherosclerosis and its sequelae.

A. Recent hemorrhagic infarction of the anterior cerebral arterial territory on the left; an old watershed infarction between the anterior and middle cerebral arterial irrigation is seen on the right of the upper brain slice.

B. On the right, a recent hemorrhagic infarction due to throm-

boembolism in the middle cerebral arterial territory with diffuse swelling of the brain.

C. Oblique view of the posterior half of the brain showing an old lefthemispheric, anemic infarction of the posterior cerebral arterial territory and a righthemispheric recent anemic infarction of the middle cerebral arterial territory.

express immunoreaction against *endothelin-1* in normal states; however, in pathological states such as reactive gliosis in Alzheimer disease, *Binswanger disease* (see below), or infarctions, reactive astrocytes express high amounts of endothelin-1. It is therefore hypothesized that endothelin-1 produced by reactive astrocytes may reach intracerebral arterioles inducing long-lasting vasoconstriction (Zhang *et al.*, 1994).

There are some data on the relationship between infarctions in young adults and atherosclerosis. Lanziano and coworkers (1991) found atherosclerosis to be a cause of cerebral infarction in 31 percent of 155 ischemic stroke patients of 16–45 years of age, whereas H. P. Adams and colleagues (1986) found cerebral infarction in 26.4 percent of 144 patients between 15 and 45 years. However, Barinagarrementeria and coworkers (1996) reported a lower frequency of premature atherosclerosis (only 3 percent among 300 patients under 40 years of age) and commented that atherosclerosis was an uncommon cause of cerebral infarction in young patients.

Lacunar infarctions: Multiple microinfarction is called morphologically *lacunar state*. The nomenclature has been introduced by Pierre Marie indicating *état lacunaire* in the gray matter, while *status cribrosus* (Oscar Vogt) or *état criblé* (M. Durant-Fardel) indicated an equivalent state in the white matter. However, lacunar and cribrate states are often confused and used as synonyms. (The term *lacune* was used for the first time by Amédée Dechambre in 1838 after Román, 1986; further historical background of the nomenclatures has been reviewed by Poirier and Derouesné, 1985). *Lacunar infarcts* are defined as 'infarcts that lie in the deeper noncortical parts of the cerebrum and brainstem' (basal ganglia, internal capsule, thalamus, pons, etc.) and result from occlusion of penetrating branches of the larger cerebral arteries; the infarcts range in size from 3–4 mm to 1.5–2.0 cm in diameter. This state is observed in patients with hypertension and hyalinotic and atheromatous degeneration of the vessels. Clinical manifestations largely depend on the location of the infarcts; even parkinsonism due to basal ganglia lacunar states was described in the literature. Fisher

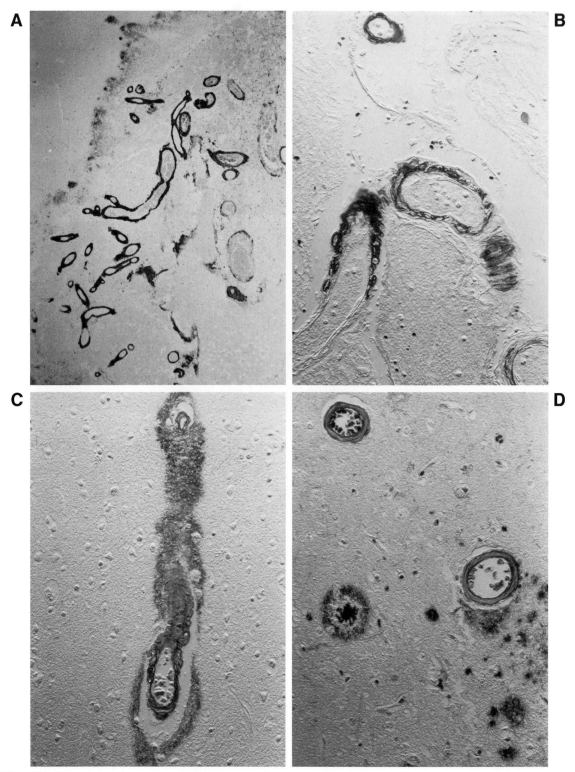

FIGURE   27–4

Cerebral amyloid angiopathy in old age and senile dementia of Alzheimer type. Silver staining according to Campbell, Switzer and Martin.

A. Severe amyloid angiopathy in leptomeningeal blood vessels, arteries and veins. In the adjacent cortical brain tissue there are diffuse amyloid deposits of ßA4 type. 40 X.

B. The amyloid depositions are not equally distributed in the whole vessel wall. Note the amyloid loops around smooth mus-cle cells in the arterial wall. 100 X.

C. Small cortical vessel with amyloid angiopathy. In the surrounding brain tissue there are diffuse amyloid deposits at the rim of the Virchow Robin spaces. 100 X.

D. In most cases of senile dementia of Alzheimer type cortical amyloid angiopathy, senile plaques with a dense amyloid core and small diffuse amyloid deposits occur simultaneously. 100 X.

(1982) listed possible clinical symptoms and Poirier and Derouesné (1985) proposed the differentiation of the infarcts from hemorrhages and simple dilatation of the perivascular spaces. It is important to know that the lacunar state in the brain represents largely a late stage of infarction (stage 3 or cystic stage of infarction) and does not correspond to the clinically recent 'lacunar strokes.'

Granular atrophy of the cortex: In the chronic stage of small cortical infarctions, lesions are substituted by reactive gliosis; the multiple gliotic micro-scars result in multiple small shrinkages forming a granular appearance of the gyral surface. The distribution of this *cortical granular atrophy* corresponds, in the majority of the cases, to the 'watershed' areas, territorial border zones of irrigation between the anterior, medial, and posterior cerebral arteries. Watershed infarctions (Figure 27–3A) are seen in patients who experienced hypotonic episodes (patients with cardiac arrhythmia or chronically hypertonic patients with hypotonic episodes) as well as in patients with hypertensive vascular narrowing or *thromboangiitis obliterans*. Granular atrophy is not only a result of arteriosclerotic vascular changes.

Vasculogenic leukoencephalopathy (Binswanger subcortical encephalopathy): The Binswanger 'disease' has its roots in a peripheral description on differential diagnosis of the progressive paralysis in a very long lecture record of Otto Binswanger in 1894 in which the author apparently did not intend to propose or describe a new disease entity. Due to degeneration (thickening, hyalinosis, fibrosis) of arterioles, the cerebral white matter is damaged as perivascular demyelinating lesions – usually with additional axonal damage – converge, while subcortical *U-fibers (arcuate fibers)* are preserved. The lesions are focused mainly in frontal and/or occipital areas. Concomitant *lacunar changes* (p. 365 and Chapter 28) in the basal ganglia and pons are often found. Atherosclerosis is not an essential factor for the disorder and it has been assumed that the encephalopathy is due to hypertensive *arteriolopathy*. While a 'pure subcortical arteriosclerotic encephalopathy' has been recorded as Binswanger disease (Olszewski, 1962; Fredriksson *et al.*, 1992; Brun *et al.*, 1992), patients without chronic arterial hypertension have also been reported. There are several fundamental discussions about the definition or validity of Binswanger disease (see Rosenberg, 1986; Hachinski, 1991). The cause(s) and underlying mechanisms of the peripheral vascular changes are still obscure. Some disorders which may be associated with Binswanger disease or may cause changes similar to Binswanger disease include hypertension, cerebral amyloid angiopathy (see below), CADASIL (*Cerebral Autosomal Dominant Arteriopathy with Subcortical Infarcts and Leukoencephalopathy*) (Ragno *et al.*, 1995; Ruchoux *et al.*, 1995), *pseudoxanthoma elasticum*, and *antiphospholipid antibody syndrome*, among others. Additionally, an entity of vascular leukoencephalopathy due to glycosaminoglycan degeneration of the cerebral vessels was demonstrated by Torack and Morris (1989). The '*Binswanger type encephalopathy*' might therefore be a better nomenclature than 'Binswanger disease'. The

semantics discussion notwithstanding, there are several reports on Binswanger type encephalopathy of young patients and/or familial Binswanger disease (Yamamura *et al.*, 1987; Davous and Fallet-Bianco, 1991; Berthier *et al.*, 1992; Gutiérrez-Molina *et al.*, 1994): Yamamura's cases may possibly belong to a distinct disease; the others to CADASIL. A detailed family study of 'Binswanger type encephalopathy' without hypertension was carried out by Maeda and colleagues in 1976, when they discussed the differential diagnostic problems on various forms of vasculitis from the clinico-pathological aspect although this case, to our today's knowledge, also belongs to CADASIL.

In patients with Binswanger 'disease', the clinical differential diagnosis between vascular and degenerative dementia is usually difficult if neuroimaging tools are not applied, even though several patients manifest acute strokes or signs of lacunar syndromes.

Cerebral Amyloid Angiopathy is Caused by the Accumulation of Extracellular Amyloid Protein Within Blood Vessels

Amyloid depositions in human cerebral blood vessel walls are a very common finding in old age and also seen in age-related degenerative conditions such as Alzheimer disease (Figure 27–4). The term amyloid here is restricted to extracellular deposits of amyloid fibrils. These fibrils are derived from soluble circulating or diffusely spreading proteins, that are processed by partial proteolysis and polymerization to convert them into insoluble deposits, that may be remote from the sites of synthesis of these circulating or diffusing proteins. These amyloid fibrils are straight and non-branching, measure 7–10 nm in diameter, have an affinity for *Congo red stain*, demonstrate thereafter a green birefringence in polarized light and show an x-ray diffraction pattern of *ß-pleated sheets* (Figure 27–5). These fibrillar protein deposits are associated with the *P-component*, a normal serum glycoprotein with a molecular weight of 180–220 kDa, that shows a striking structural homology with *C-reactive protein*, an acute-phase reactant. The P-component consists of doughnut-shaped pentagonal structures that measure 9 nm in external diameter and contain globular subunits. Other common components of amyloid deposits are sulfated proteoglycans. The interactions of these two additional components of amyloid deposits with the formation of amyloid fibrils are not known. Obviously in most types of amyloidosis the favorite sites of deposition are in close vicinity to basement membranes. In cerebral amyloid angiopathy the fibrillar amyloid deposits occur at the outer surface of the endothelial basement membrane of capillaries, at the basement membrane of pericytes and mainly at the basement membranes surrounding the smooth muscle cells of veins and arteries. Additionally the astrocytic basement membranes at the surface of the brain and surrounding the Virchow-Robin spaces are the favorite sites of amyloid depositions.

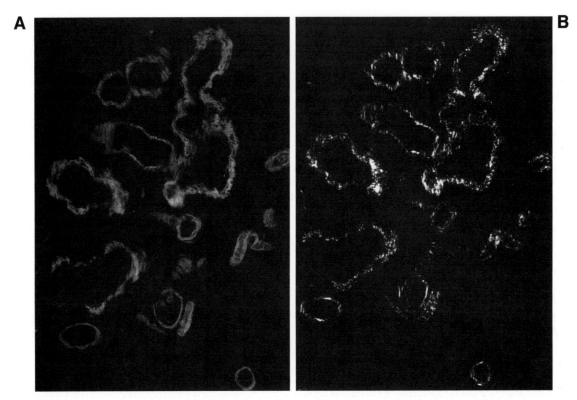

FIGURE   27–5

Cerebral amyloid angiopathy in old age (senile dementia of Alzheimer type). Intense amyloid deposits (ßA4 type) in leptomeningeal and cortical blood vessels (arteries and veins) as stained by Congo red. 40 X.

A. Photomicrograph taken in a fluorescence microscope.
B. Photomicrograph of the same area as (A), in polarized light (birefringence).

Cerebral Amyloid Angiopathy is Usually Observed in the Gray Matter Regions of the Brain, but not in the White Matter

In cerebral amyloid-angiopathy all types of blood vessels could be involved: Capillaries, veins and arteries, but not in all regions of the brain. Cerebral amyloid angiopathy can be observed only in the leptomeninges and in gray matter regions, mainly in the cerebral or cerebellar cortex. White matter regions are normally free of amyloid deposits. Little is known about the involvement of the spinal cord and the surrounding leptomeninges in cases of severe cerebral amyloid angiopathy.

Increasing amounts of amyloid deposits around capillaries finally result in an obliteration of the capillary lumen. Often the center of a senile amyloid plaque consists of remnants of an obliterated capillary. In arterial and venous vessel walls the continuously growing amyloid masses surrounding smooth muscle cells finally lead to degenerative alterations and to cell necrosis in the *tunica media* of the blood vessel wall. The formation of small aneurysms, focal thromboses and not seldom of sudden hemorrhages are the consequences (Figure 27–6). In some cases multiple small cortical hemorrhages can be observed (so called 'globe-shaped' hemorrhage: *Kugelblutung*, in German). In other cases a spontaneous intracerebral mass hemorrhage is the first clinical manifestation of this disease (Haan *et al.*, 1994a). In a characteristic manner these intracerebral hematomas occur mainly in temporal and/or occipital regions, where the amyloid angiopathy usually is most severe. In the pons-region and in the cerebellum hemorrhages due to an amyloid-angiopathy are rare, though amyloid deposits in cerebellar blood vessels are a common finding.

The cerebral amyloid angiopathy accounts for approximately 10 percent of all spontaneous intracerebral hemorrhages, typically in the cortex and subcortical white matter of the occipital lobes. Diagnosis is made *post mortem* by an autopsy or during lifetime by investigating the neurosurgically removed blood clots with remnants of the surrounding brain tissue. The structural changes of amyloidotic blood vessel walls in the brain increase the fragility of the vessel wall and result in severe disturbances of the blood supply. In severe cases the final stage is vascular dementia (Silbert *et al.*, 1995). Sudden mass hemorrhages on the basis of an amyloid angiopathy might also be triggered by severe (or even mild) traumatic lesions of the skull and brain. In cerebral amyloid angiopathy the amyloidogenic proteins are believed to result from the metabolism of the nervous system. In cases of generalized amyloidoses with

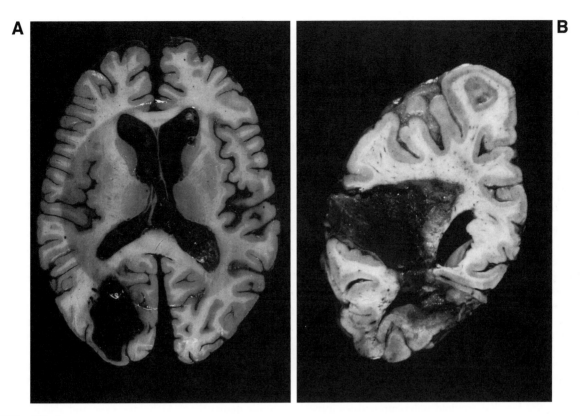

FIGURE 27–6

Atypical intracerebral mass hemorrhage due to amyloid angiopathy.

A. Acute intracerebral hemorrhage in the occipital lobe with involvement of the ventricular system. Horizontal section of the

brain (after plastination).

B. Subacute intracerebral hemorrhage in the temporal and occipital lobe after neurosurgical intervention. Frontal section of the left occipital lobe.

widespread amyloid angiopathy in many regions of the whole body the cerebral blood vessels are normally spared. In cases of a generalized amyloidosis the intracerebral or intracranial blood vessel walls are involved only in those regions of the brain, where the normal *blood brain barrier* is absent or insufficient (Bohl *et al.*, 1989). These are: the *plexus chorioideus*, the *infundibulum* and the pituitary stalk, the *epiphysis* (pineal gland), the *area postrema* and the *eminentia mediana*, as well as the subcommissural organ (the so-called circumventricular organs), and the neurohypophysis (posterior lobe of the pituitary gland). In addition the blood vessels of the cerebral *dura mater* normally are involved in systemic amyloidosis. Special types of amyloidoses prefer the pericollagen location for deposition, e.g. the $\beta 2$ microglobulin-amyloid.

Other regions of the brain are involved in rare cases of a generalized amyloidosis only when the blood brain barrier in these regions is defect or insufficient as a consequence of another different brain disease. In cases of generalized amyloidoses the amyloidogenic proteins are coming from the blood, and from inside the blood vessel. Therefore the amyloid deposits begin in the inner portions of the blood vessel wall, i.e. at the inner surface of the *tunica media*. In primary cerebral amyloidoses with

an amyloid angiopathy the process of amyloid deposition is noticed first in outer portions of the *tunica media*. This phenomenon sustains the hypothesis that the amyloid precursor proteins (APP) or the amyloidogenic protein fragments are floating in the cerebrospinal fluid and are diffusing from outside into the vessel wall. This pathogenetic mechanism could be reproduced experimentally by using leptomeninges of old dogs with a severe amyloid angiopathy. The question arises, why amyloid deposits could be abundant in leptomeningeal blood vessels and why they are never observed in *Pacchionian arachnoid granulations*. The fact that in these arachnoid granulations there are no basement membranes could perhaps explain this strange phenomenon.

There Are Different Types of Amyloidoses

In humans more than 30 different types of amyloidoses are known (Natvig *et al.*, 1991). According to the location of the amyloid deposits and to the distribution in the whole body, localized and generalized types are differentiated. The nomenclature and classification of amyloidoses is difficult and not yet completed. If possible, the basis for classification and naming of the disease should be the fibrillar protein producing the amyloid deposits.

Among the systemic generalized amyloidoses at least 7 types are known (Stehbens and Lie, 1995):

AL amyloidosis (often referred to as primary amyloidosis), in which the amyloid deposits are derived from immunoglobulins and are associated with immunocyte dyscrasias (idiopathic, i.e., primary, or myeloma- or macroglobulinemia-associated). The letter 'A' stands for 'Amyloid' or 'Amyloidosis' and 'L' means immunoglobulin 'Light' chain, e.g. type kappa or lambda.

AH amyloidosis is a consequence of increased immunoglobulin 'Heavy' chain production. The precursor protein is IgG1 (gamma 1).

AA amyloidosis (sometimes called reactive systemic amyloidosis or secondary amyloidosis) is associated with chronic inflammatory conditions, especially rheumatoid arthritis, in which the amyloid deposits are derived from a serum precursor known as SAA, i.e., 'Serum Amyloid Associated protein', which is synthesized in the liver and circulates in association with the HDL3 subclass of lipoproteins (apo SAA).

Aβ2M amyloidosis is associated with chronic hemodialysis, in which the deposits are derived from circulating β2 microglobulins. These amyloid depositions are mainly found in bones, joints and in connective tissues (pericollagen deposition).

ATTR amyloidosis; these are hereditary amyloidoses including, e.g., the familial amyloid polyneuropathies (type 1: Andrade or Portuguese type; type 2: Rukovina type; type 3: Van Allen type and type 4: Meretoja type). This group also includes the familial amyloid cardiomyopathy (Danish type) and the systemic senile amyloidosis (previous ASc). The precursor proteins are mutant forms of transthyretin (TTR), a plasma protein that migrates electrophoretically in the prealbumin fraction and functions as a carrier for circulating thyroxine and retinol. At least 20 different mutations are known to involve the structure of transthyretin, mostly single amino acid substitutions.

AGel amyloidosis is a familial disease described for the first time in Finnish families. The amyloid precursor protein is a mutant gelsolin (Asn 187).

AApoAI amyloidosis is another type of familial amyloid polyneuropathy (type Iowa). The precursor protein is a mutant apolipoprotein AI (Arg 26).

Sometimes an involvement of intracranial structures in these types of systemic generalized amyloidoses can be observed. An amyloid angiopathy may occur in all those regions mentioned above where the blood brain barrier is absent, insufficient or damaged. Furthermore the peripheral portions of all cranial nerves may be involved in familial amyloid polyneuropathies.

Besides these generalized amyloidoses there are localized forms in the brain and in the anterior lobe of the pituitary gland. Most important and most common is the Aβ or *βA4 amyloidosis* connected with old age, with dementia of the Alzheimer type (DAT) or Alzheimer disease (AD) (Chapters 7 and 8). The precursor protein of this amyloidosis is one of the best known proteins of the human brain: The 'Amyloid Precursor Protein' (APP), a transmembrane protein of nerve cells and other cells, too.

Short fragments of this precursor protein aggregate spontaneously in the extracellular space and initiate the formation of insoluble fibrillar amyloid deposits, named Aβ, βA4 or simply A4. Obviously the main source of these amyloidogenic proteins (APP) are nerve cells and their processes (neurites and dendrites), for amyloid deposits are found only in gray matter regions and in cortical and leptomeningeal blood vessels. Amyloidogenic proteins are transported along the Virchow Robin spaces (perivascular spaces) to the subarachnoid space and induce amyloid deposition in external portions of the blood vessel walls. There are experimental hints that smooth muscle cells of the vessel wall may also be involved in the processing of these precursor proteins (Wisniewski *et al.*, 1995), but the main source of these proteins is probably nerve cells and their metabolism (perhaps glial cells additionally). Blood vessels in the white matter and vessels in regions with an absent blood brain barrier are nearly never involved in this type of Aβ amyloid angiopathy.

βA4 amyloid angiopathy is a very common finding in old age, not only in human brains, but also in dogs, horses, monkeys and bears. It is not always combined with clinical signs. In most cases this angiopathy is combined with plaque-like amyloid deposits in the cerebral gray matter. Thus this type of amyloid angiopathy is a common finding in all cases of Alzheimer disease and senile dementia of Alzheimer type and also in trisomy 21 (Down Syndrome). The question whether amyloid deposits of the βA4 type are an essential event in the pathogenesis of Alzheimer disease cannot be answered with certainty till now; the amyloid hypothesis is not yet generally accepted (Terry *et al.*, 1994). Another hypothesis believes an abnormal metabolism of the Tau-protein to be the primary disturbance in Alzheimer disease. How these two phenomena (βA4 amyloid and abnormal tau) could be connected one with the other is not clear (Nicolini *et al.*, 1993), though the hypothesis of a general slowing of the protein breakdown with aging has been considered (Chapter 9). Sporadic cases of a severe amyloid angiopathy combined with a typical Alzheimer pathology are a very common finding in old age.

Some rare familial diseases with cerebral amyloid angiopathy are caused by genetic abnormalities. *Hereditary Cerebral Hemorrhage With Amyloidosis of Dutch type* (HCHWA-D) has been described in four families from two coastal villages in the Netherlands. The disease is characterized by amyloid depositions in small leptomeningeal and cortical arteries, leading to dementia, hemorrhage and early death. In addition, plaque-like amyloid deposits in the cortical gray matter could be found, resembling preamyloid lesions and early plaques in Alzheimer disease (Maat Schieman *et al.*, 1994). Only few neuritic plaques occurred; neurofibrillary tangles were absent. Sequence analysis of genomic DNA in HCHWA-D patients demonstrated a point mutation, cytosine for guanine at position 1852 of the APP gene, which causes a single amino acid substitution (glutamine for glutamic acid) corresponding to position 22 of the amyloid protein and residue 618 of the precursor protein.

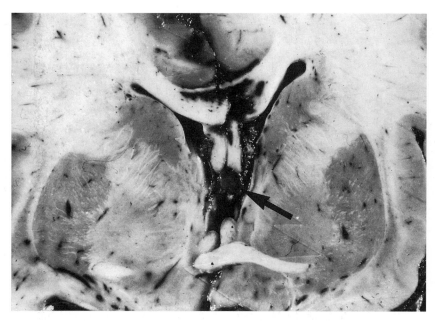

FIGURE   27–7
Amyloidoma in the subfornical region (arrow) incidentally found at necropsy as a small mass of opaque color in a

33-year-old male patient with traumatic injury of the corpus callosum.

Recently a British type of familial cerebral amyloid angiopathy has been described, probably due to a novel amyloid protein (Ghiso *et al.*, 1995).

A third type of Hereditary Cerebral Hemorrhage With Amyloidosis was first described in Iceland: HCHWA-I. It is a dominantly inherited disorder, featured by a *cystatin* C amyloid angiopathy with dementia, paralysis and death from cerebral hemorrhage in early adult life (Haan *et al.*, 1994b). A variant of the cysteine proteinase inhibitor cystatin C is deposited as amyloid in several tissues not only in the brain, and the spinal fluid level of cystatin C is abnormally low. The amyloid protein in this disease is homologous to cystatin C but it lacks the first ten amino terminal residues and there is an amino acid substitution at position 58 (glutamine for leucine).

All types of cerebral amyloid angiopathies may induce dementia (vascular dementia) and are combined with a high incidence of spontaneous atypical intracerebral hemorrhage.

Apart from the plaque like βA4 amyloid deposits in cerebral gray matter, there are only two other diseases with similar amyloid deposits. In *Creutzfeldt-Jakob disease* (CJD) and in *Gerstmann-Sträussler-Scheinker disease* (GSSD) the amyloid precursor protein is called *Prion protein* (PrP). The morphology of intracerebral PrP amyloid deposits is in most cases different from the βA4 amyloidosis. In rare cases of CJD and GSSD an amyloid angiopathy has been observed; but the amyloid deposits in vessel walls proved to be βA4 amyloid (Gray *et al.*, 1994). In GSSD a co-localization of PrP- and βA4 protein amyloid has been observed in plaque-like lesions, but not in blood vessel walls (Ikeda *et al.*, 1994). In rare cases a similar co-

localization of βA4 amyloid and AL 'amyloid' has been shown immunohistologically in cerebral blood vessels, but it could not be proven, that this is due to a concomitant generalized AL amyloidosis. Probably this should be interpreted as a side effect of a blood brain barrier damage.

Nowadays specific immunohistological and/or molecular genetic methods are requested to define the type of amyloidosis, especially when different types of amyloidoses occur simultaneously. In old age this is not an uncommon finding (Störkel *et al.*, 1983).

Focal Amyloid Accumulation

Cerebral amyloid angiopathy may exceptionally be present as a mass lesion (Briceno *et al.*, 1987). Indepedent of systemic amyloid angiopathy, a focal accumulation of amyloid substance as a space-occupying and/or tissue destroying process is defined as an *amyloidoma*. Amyloid masses of non-neoplastic character may accumulate everywhere in the body, both in soft tissues as well as in the skeleton. Amyloidomas are, again, not related to amyloid angiopathy, amyloid deposition in Alzheimer disease, or any aging processes. In the field of neurosurgery and neuropathology there are several single case reports of amyloidomas in the nervous system, including peripheral nerves (Gabet *et al.*, 1989), spine (Cloft *et al.*, 1995; Mandl, 1924), dura mater (Toyokuni *et al.*, 1992), spinal cord (McAnena *et al.*, 1982), orbit (Cohen and Lessel, 1979; Sevestre *et al.*, 1987), skull or skull base (Barr and Lampert, 1972; Ünal *et al.*, 1992), trigeminal nerves and ganglia (O'Brien *et al.*, 1994), choroid plexus (Lampert, 1958), and

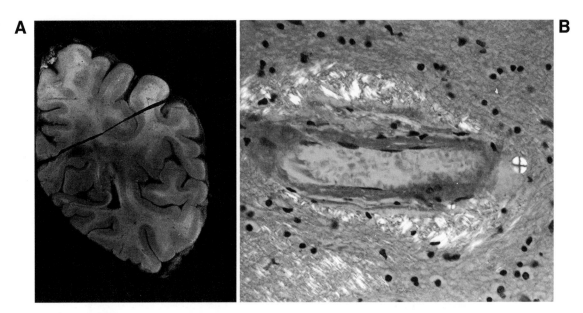

FIGURE   27–8

Asymptomatic, incidentally found amyloid accumulation in the cerebral parenchyma of a 60 year-old male patient who suffered from a bronchial carcinoma.
A. The lesion is grossly seen as a small brownish focus in the medial occipital subcortical white matter.
B. The accumulated substance was histologically birefringent

after Congo-red staining; this was also found in the basal ganglia as shown in the picture. Note that the amyloid accumulation is found in the parenchyma but not in the vessel wall. X 400 (From Hori *et al.*, 1988; reproduced by permission of Springer-Verlag.)

cerebrum (Cohen *et al.*, 1992; Hori *et al.*, 1988; Spaar *et al.*, 1981; Vidal *et al.*, 1992).

There are symptomatic and asymptomatic amyloidomas of different sizes. Amyloidomas in the brain can be detected by CT as increased density and T_1-weighted MRI sequences (Lee *et al.*, 1995). Accumulation of amyloid in the nervous system may present as a mass (Figure 27–7) or an accumulation in parenchyma without mass effect (Figure 27–8). The types of amyloid in amyloidomas are not yet sufficiently established although Krishnan and coworkers (1993) found that 10 of 14 soft tissue amyloidomas could be classified as immunocytic dyscrasia-associated AL-amyloidosis and four as reactive (secondary) AA-amyloidosis. Patients with the latter type of amyloidomas had better prognosis.

Amyloid deposits in the pituitary gland were found in high frequency in aged individuals (80 percent of patients over 84 years of age). Chronic obstructive pulmonary disease correlated to the occurrence and amount of amyloid deposits in the pituitary (Röcken *et al.*, 1995). The high amount of interstitial accumulation of amyloid in the pituitary gland also correlated to the clinical non-insulin-dependent diabetes mellitus, although this correlation is not yet understood.

Amyloid deposits in different neoplasms, particularly in pituitary *prolactinomas*, have repeatedly been described (Delafontaine *et al.*, 1982; Kubota *et al.*, 1986; Landolt *et al.*, 1987; Saeger *et al.*, 1983). Amyloid deposits were observed sporadically in other neoplasms (Foschini *et al.*, 1993; Olsen and Westermark, 1994). Although the

cause of focal amyloid accumulation is unknown, an altered focal metabolic state of the tissue may well be responsible for the amyloid deposits.

An Overall View

Progressive reduction of the blood supply to the brain may cause or aggravate nerve cell loss and dysfunction. Atherosclerosis is one of the most frequent diseases of arteries resulting in brain dysfunction. Different cells play different roles in atherogenesis, including cells of the wall of the arteries, i.e., endothelium and smooth muscle cells; and also circulating blood cells, including platelets, monocytes and macrophages, as well as lymphocytes. Several risk factors and pathogenetic mechanisms for atherogenesis have been identified and discussed (e.g., hypercholesterolemia, hypertension, autoimmune reactions, smoking, and diabetes mellitus) and various theories and hypotheses to account for atherogenesis have been advanced. In addition to atherosclerosis, the accumulation of extracellular amyloid proteins of different classes can cause amyloid angiopathy mainly in the gray matter, though not in white matter regions of the brain. Both conditions, atherosclerosis and amyloid angiopathy, may result in infarcts and dementing processes such as multi-infarct dementia. In addition, as a presumable cause of chronic hypoxia, vascular changes may play an important role in the development and progression of chronic dementing conditions.

Selected Readings

Adams, J. H., and Duchen, L. W. (eds.) 1992. Greenfield's Neuropathology, Fifth Edition. Edward Arnold, London.

Iqbal, K., Wisniewski, H. M., and Winblad, B. (eds.) 1989. Alzheimer's Disease and Related Disorders. Progr. Clin. Biol. Res., Vol. 317. Alan R. Liss, Inc., New York, pp. 857–1059.

Iqbal, K., Mortimer, J. A., Winblad, B., and Wisniewski, H. M. (eds.) 1995. Research Advances in Alzheimer's Disease and Related Disorders. John Wiley & Sons, Chichester.

Stehbens, W. E., and Lie, J. T. (eds.) 1995. Vascular Pathology. Chapman & Hall Medical, London.

References

Adams, H. P. Jr., Butler, M. J., Biller, J., and Toffol, J. 1986. Nonhemorrhagic cerebral infarction in young adults. Arch. Neurol. 43:793–796.

Barinagarrementeria, F., Figueroa, T., Huebe, J., and Cantú, C. 1996. Cerebral infarction in people under 40 years. Etiologic analysis of 300 cases prospectively evaluated. Cerebrovasc. Dis. 6:75–79.

Barr, R., and Lampert, P. 1972. Intrasellar amyloid tumor. Acta Neuropathol. 21:83–86

Berthier, E., Broussolle, E., Garciajacquier, M., Tommasi, M., and Chazot, G. 1992. Juvenile arteriosclerotic leukoencephalopathy. Clinico-pathological study of one case. Rev. Neurol. 148:146–149.

Binswanger, O. 1894. Die Abgrenzung der allgemeinen progressiven Paralyse. Berl. Klin. Wochenschr. 31:1103–1105, 1137–1139, 1180–1186.

Blankenhorn, D. H. 1981. Will atheroma regress with diet and exercise? Am. J. Surg. 142:644–645.

Bohl, J., Störkel, S., and Steinmetz, H. 1989. Involvement of the central nervous system and its coverings in different forms of amyloidosis. In K. Iqbal, H. M. Wisniewski, and B. Winblad (eds.) Alzheimer's Disease and Related Disorders. Progr. Clin. Biol. Res., Vol. 317, pp.1007–1019. Alan R. Liss, Inc., New York.

Briceno, C. E., Resch, L., and Bernstein, M. 1987. Cerebral amyloid angiopathy presenting as a mass lesion. Stroke 18:234–239

Brun, A., Fredriksson, K., and Gustafson, L. 1992. Pure subcortical arteriosclerotic encephalopathy (Binswanger's disease). A clinicopathologic study.2. Pathologic features. Cerebrovasc. Dis. 2:87–92

Capron, L. 1993. Immunity, inflammation and atherosclerosis. Rev. Neurol. 149:751–754.

Cervós-Navarro, J., and Ferszt, R. (eds.) 1989. Klinische Neuropathologie. Georg Thieme Verlag, Stuttgart.

Cloft, H. J., Quint, D. J., Markert, J. M., et al. 1995. Primary osseous amyloidoma causing spinal cord compression. Am. J. Neuroradiol. 16:1152–1154.

Cohen, M., Lanska, D., Roessmann, U., et al. 1992. Amyloidoma of the CNS. 1. clinical and pathologic study. Neurology 42:2019–2023.

Cohen, M. M., and Lessel, S. 1979. Amyloid tumor of the orbit. Neuroradiology 18:157–159.

Davous, P., and Fallet-Bianco, C. 1991. Démence sous-corticale familiale avec leucoencéphalopathie artériopathique. Observation clinico-pathologique. Rev. Neurol. 147:376–384.

Delafontaine, P., Ochsner, F., and Pizzolato, G. P. 1982. Pitui-

tary adenoma with amyloid deposits and hyperprolactinemia. Case report and review. Acta Neuropathol. 57:81–84.

Diez-Roux, A. V., Nieto, F. J., Tyroler, H. A., et al. 1995. Social inequalities and atherosclerosis: The atherosclerosis risk in communities study. Am. J. Epidemiol 141:960–972.

Fisher, C. M. 1982. Lacunar strokes and infarcts: a review. Neurology 32:871–876.

Foschini, M. P., D'Adda, T., Bordi, C., and Eusebi, V. 1993. Amyloid stroma in meningiomas. Virchows Arch. [A] 422:53–59.

Fredriksson, K., Brun, A., and Gustafson, L. 1992. Pure subcortical arteriosclerotic encephalopathy (Binswanger's disease). A clinicopathologic study. 1. Clinical features. Cerebrovasc. Dis. 2:82–86

Gabet, J. Y., Durand, D. V., Bady, B., et al. 1989. Pseudo-tumeur amyloide du nerf sciatique. Rev. Neurol. 145:872–876.

George, B., and Laurian, C. 1987. The Vertebral Artery. Pathology and Surgery. Springer-Verlag, Wien.

Ghiso, J., Plant, G. T., Revesz, T., Wisniewski, T., and Frangione, B. 1995. Familial cerebral amyloid angiopathy (British type) with nonneuritic amyloid plaque formation may be due to a novel amyloid protein (letter). J. Neurol. Sci. 129:74–75.

Gray, F., Chretien, F., Cesaro, P., et al. 1994. Creutzfeldt-Jakob disease and cerebral amyloid angiopathy. Acta Neuropathol. 88:106–111.

Gutiérrez-Molina, M., Rodriguez, A. C., Garcia, C. M., et al. 1994. Small arterial granular degeneration in familial Binswanger's syndrome. Acta Neuropathol. 87:98–105.

Haan, J., Maat Schieman, M. L., and Roos, R. A. 1994a. Clinical aspects of cerebral amyloid angiopathy. Dementia 5:210–213.

Haan, J., Maat Schieman, M. L., van Duinen, S. G., Jensson, O., Thorsteinsson, L., and Roos, R. A. 1994b. Co-localization of beta/A4 and cystatin C in cortical blood vessels in Dutch, but not in Icelandic hereditary cerebral hemorrhage with amyloidosis. Acta Neurol. Scand. 89:367–371.

Hachinski, V. 1991. Binswanger's disease – Neither Binswanger's nor a disease. J. Neurol. Sci. 103:1.

Hori, A., Kitamoto, T., Tateishi, J., Hann, P., and Friede, R. L. 1988. Focal intracerebral accumulation of a novel type of amyloid protein. An early stage of cerebral amyloidoma? Acta Neuropathol. 76:212–215.

Ikeda, S. I., Yanagisawa, N., Allsop, D., and Glenner, G. G. 1994. Gerstmann-Sträussler-Scheinker disease showing beta-protein type cerebellar and cerebral amyloid angiopathy. Acta Neuropathol. 88:262–266.

Krishnan, J., Chu, W. S., Elrod, J. P., and Frizzera, G. 1993. Tumoral presentation of amyloidosis (amyloidomas) in soft tissues: a report of 14 cases. Am. J. Clin. Pathol. 100:135–144.

Kubota, T., Kuroda, E., Yamashima, T., et al. 1986. Amyloid formation in prolactinoma. Arch. Pathol. Lab. Med. 110:72–75

Lampert, P. 1958. Tumor forming atypical amyloidosis of the choroid plexus with invasion of the cerebral white matter. J. Neuropathol. Exp. Neurol. 17:604–611.

Landolt, A. M., Kleihues, P., and Heitz, P. U. 1987. Amyloid deposits in pituitary adenomas. Arch. Pathol. Lab. Med. 111:453–458.

Lanziano, G., Andreoli, A., Di Pascoale, G., et al. 1991. Etiopathogenesis and prognosis of cerebral ischemia in young adults. A survey of 155 treated patients. Acta Neurol. Scand. 84:321–325.

Lee, J., Krol, G., and Rosenblum, M. 1995. Primary amyloidoma of the brain: CT and MR presentation. Am. J. Neuroradiol. 16:712–714.

Ma, K. C., Lundberg, P. O., Lilja, A., and Olsson, Y. 1992. Binswanger's disease in the absence of chronic arterial hypertension. A case report with clinical, radiological and immunohistochemical observations on intracerebral blood vessels. Acta Neuropathol. 83:434–439.

Maat Schieman, M. L., Radder, C. M., van Duinen, S. G., et al. 1994. Hereditary cerebral hemorrhage with amyloidosis (Dutch): a model for congophilic plaque formation without neurofibrillary pathology. Acta Neuropathol. 88:371–378.

Maeda, S., Nakayama, H., Isaka, K., Aihara, Y., and Nemoto, S. 1976. Familial unusual encephalopathy of Binswanger's type without hypertension. Folia Psychiat. Neurol. Jpn. 30:165–177.

Mandl, J. 1924. Über lokales Amyloid im Bereiche der Brustwirbelsäule. Virchows Arch. [A] 253:639–655.

McAnena, O. J., Feely, M. P., and Keaky, W. F. 1982. Spinal cord compression by amyloid tissue. J. Neurol. Neurosurg. Psychiatry 45:1067–1069.

McGee, J. O'D., Isaacson, P. G., and Wright, N. A. (eds.) 1992. Oxford Textbook of Pathology. Oxford University Press, Oxford.

Natvig, J. B., Forre, O., Husby, G., et al. (eds.) 1991. Amyloid and Amyloidosis 1990. Kluwer Academic Pub., Dordrecht.

Nicolini, M., Zatta, P. F., and Corain, B. (eds.) 1993. Alzheimer's Disease and Related Disorders. Adv. Biosci., Vol. 87. Pergamon Press, Oxford.

O'Brien, T. J., Mckelvie, P. A., and Vrodos, N. 1994. Bilateral trigeminal amyloidoma: An unusual case of trigeminal neuropathy with a review of the literature. Case report. J. Neurosurg. 81:780–783.

Ogata, J., Masuda, J., Yutani, C., and Yamaguchi, T. 1994. Mechanisms of cerebral artery thrombosis: a histopathological analysis on eight necropsy cases. J. Neurol. Neurosurg. Psychiatry 57:17–21.

Olsen, K. E., and Westermark, P. 1994. Amyloid in basal cell carcinoma and seborrheic keratosis. Acta Dermatol. Venereol. [Stockh.] 74:273–275.

Olszewski, J. 1962. Subcortical arteriosclerotic encephalopathy: review of the literature on the so-called Binswanger's disease and presentation of two cases. World Neurol. 3:359–375.

Poirier, J., Derouesné, C. 1985. Le concept de lacune cérébrale de 1838 a nos jours. Rev. Neurol. 141:3–17.

Ragno, M., Tournierlasserve, E., Fiori, M. G., et al. 1995. An Italian kindred with cerebral autosomal dominant arteriopathy with subcortical infarcts and leukoencephalopathy (CADASIL). Ann. Neurol. 38:231–236.

Röcken, C., Saeger, W., Fleege, J. C., and Linke, R. P. 1995. Interstitial amyloid deposit in the pituitary gland. Morphometry, immunohistology, and correlation to diseases. Arch. Pathol. Lab. Med. 119:1055–1060.

Román, G. C. The original description of lacunes. Neurology 36:85.

Rosenberg, G. A. 1986. Binswanger's disease. (Letter) Arch. Neurol. 43:641.

Ruchoux, M. M., Guerouaou, D., Vandenhaute, B., et al. 1995. Systemic vascular smooth muscle cell impairment in cerebral autosomal dominant arteriopathy with subcortical infarcts and leukoencephalopathy. Acta Neuropathol. 89:500–512.

Saeger, W., Gerigk, C., Missmahl, H. P., and Lüdecke, D. K. 1983. Amyloidablagerungen in Hypophysenadenomen: polarisationsoptische, immunhistochemische, und elektronenmikroskopische Untersuchungen. Pathologe 4:183–189.

Sevestre, H., Betermiez, P., Deramond, H., et al. 1987. Amylose orbitaire pseudotumorale. Ann. Pathol. 7:231–233.

Sholler, G. F., Yu, J. S., Bale, P. M., et al. 1984. Generalized arterial calcification of infancy: three case reports, including spontaneous regression with long-term survival. Pediatrics 105:257–260.

Silbert, P. L., Bartleson, J. D., Miller, G. M., et al. 1995. Cortical petechial hemorrhage, leukoencephalopathy, and subacute dementia associated with seizures due to cerebral amyloid angiopathy. Mayo Clin. Proc. 70:477–480.

Spaar, F. W., Goebel, H. H., Volles, E., and Wickboldt, J. 1981. Tumor-like amyloid formation (amyloidoma) in the brain. J. Neurol. 224:171–182.

Stehbens, W. E., and Lie, J. T. (eds.) 1995. Vascular Pathology, pp. 157–161. Chapman & Hall, London.

Stehbens, W. E. 1972. Pathology of the Cerebral Blood Vessels. C. V. Mosby, St.Louis.

Stemme, S., and Hansson, G. K. 1992. T-lymphocytes in human atherosclerotic plaques are memory cells expressing CD45RO and the integrin VLA-1. Arterioscler. Thromb. 12:206–211.

Stemme, S., Rymo, L., and Hansson, G. K. 1991. Polyclonal origin of T lymphocytes in human atherosclerotic plaques. Lab. Invest. 65:654–660.

Störkel, S., Bohl, J., and Schneider, H.-M. 1983. Senile amyloidosis: principles of localization in a heterogeneous form of amyloidosis. Virchows Arch. B 44:145–161.

Terry, R. D., Katzman, R., and Bick, K. L. (eds.) 1994. Alzheimer Disease. Raven Press, New York.

Torack, R. M., and Morris, J. C. 1989. Vascular glycosaminoglycans in periventricular leukoencephalopathy. Acta Neuropathol. 78:492–496.

Toyokuni, S., Ebina, Y., Okada, S., et al. 1992. Report of a patient with POEMS/Takatsuki/Crow-Fukase syndrome associated with focal spinal pachymeningeal amyloidosis. Cancer 70:882–886.

Ünal, F., Hepgul, K., Bayindir, C., et al. 1992. Skull base amyloidoma. J. Neurosurg. 76:303–306.

Vidal, R. G., Ghiso, J., Gallo, G., et al. 1992. Amyloidoma of the CNS. 2. immunohistochemical and biochemical study. Neurology 42:2024–2028.

Wisniewski, H. M., Frackowiak, J., and Mazur Kolecka, B. 1995. In vitro production of beta-amyloid in smooth muscle cells isolated from amyloid angiopathy-affected vessels. Neurosci. Lett. 183:120–123.

Yamamura, T., Nishimura, M., Shirabe, T., and Fujita, M. 1987. Subcortical vascular encephalopathy in a normotensive, young adult with premature baldness and spondylitis deformans. A clinicopathological study and review of the literature. J. Neurol. Sci. 78:175–188.

Zhang, W. W., Badonic, T., Hoog, A., et al. 1994. Structural and vasoactive factors influencing intracerebral arterioles in cases of vascular dementia and other cerebrovascular disease: A review – Immunohistochemical studies on expression of collagens, basal lamina components and endothelin-1. Dementia 5:153–162

Hartmut Becker

Imaging the Aging Brain

CT and MRI Resolve Gray and White Matter

Age-related Gray Matter Changes Such as Polio-araiosis and Changes in the Chemical Composition are Best Observed with MRI

Leuko-araiosis Comprises a Group of Age-related White Matter Changes Characterized by Hypodensities on CT and Hyperintensities on MRI

Enlargement of CSF Spaces is not an Inevitable Consequence of Advancing Age

CT Exceeds Conventional Skull Radiography in the Detection of Calcified Vasculature

CT and MR are Reliable Methods to Diagnose and Stage Neurodegenerative Diseases *in vivo*

The Consequences of Toxic and Metabolic Diseases to the Brain Tissue can be Identified by Neuroimaging

Imaging of CSF Related Diseases is Mainly Based Upon the Findings at CT and MR

Different Imaging Techniques are Necessary to Recognize Vascular Diseases

CT and MRI Have Improved the Angiographic Technique

An Overall View

Advances in sophisticated and sensitive imaging techniques such as *computerized tomography* (CT), *magnetic resonance imaging* (MRI) *and digital subtraction angiography* (DSA) have revolutionized the study of the living aging brain. These techniques have greatly amplified and refined the means by which specific age-related changes can be clearly visualized in the different regions of the living brain: The cerebral gray and white matters, the adjacent cerebrospinal fluid (CSF) space, and the brain vasculature.

In this chapter we shall examine some age-related changes as observed by CT, MRI and DSA, both in normal aging and in neurodegenerative conditons. The use of *positron emission tomography* (PET) in the study of the regional biochemical changes of the aging brain will be examined in the next chapter.

CT and MRI Resolve Gray and White Matter

In contrast to conventional radiography, the *X-ray computerized tomography* (CT) allows us to distinguish gray and white matter. The vast majority of today's CT fan-beam scanners are designed according to the continuous rotation principle. They have stationary, ring-shaped detectors surrounding the patient in which only the X-ray tube has to be moved. A CT scanner measures the attenuation of X-rays in tissue. The radiodensities of each voxel are calculated by the computer from thousands of radiation intensity measurements and visually displayed as dark and light areas. Computer-analyzed X-ray transmission profiles are able to resolve gray and white matter, blood, and cerebrospinal fluid, despite very small differences in radiodensity. Intravenous injection of iodinated radiopaque material further enhances the contrast between tissue constituents in regions that have either increased vasculature or impaired blood-brain barrier functions.

Magnetic resonance imaging (MRI) is based on computerized tomography and can be used to explore function as well as structure, but with much better spatial resolution. MRI is better suited to the study of age-related changes in brain morphology. Relative to CT, MRI provides more accurate structural information because of the absence of bone-hardening artifact, and the capability to image in the coronal and sagittal plane, which provides an optimal view of the cerebral anatomy with less volume-averaging artifacts.

Magnetic resonance technology was originally developed to measure the atomic constituents of chemical samples. When elements with odd atomic weight, such as hydrogen, are exposed to a strong static homogeneous magnetic field, the nuclei behave as spinning magnets and develop a net alignment of their spin axes along the direction of the applied field. The alignment can be perturbed by a brief pulse of radio waves, which cause a gyroscope-like motion of the nuclei, called *precession*. When the pulse is turned off, the nuclei tend to return to their original orientation, and in doing so release energy in the form of radio waves with distinct frequencies for different atomic species as well as for a given atomic nucleus in different chemical or physical environments.

Different nuclear species absorb energy from radio waves of a particular frequency. The ability of the atomic nuclei to absorb energy from radio waves is called nuclear magnetic resonance. The atomic nuclei, having absorbed energy from the externally applied radio waves, then release it as a signal as they return to a lower-energy state. The rate at which nuclei return to a lower-energy state is called *relaxation* and is usually described by its time constant (T). There are two types of relaxation of importance in MRI at present: *Spin-lattice relaxation time* (T_1), and *spin-spin relaxation time* (T_2). MR images can be generated by emphasizing either one of these two types of relaxation in a cross section of tissue, or the actual concentration of a particular atomic nucleus in the tissue section. For example, the difference between gray and white matter is best visualized by images emphasizing T_1, whereas cerebrospinal fluid is greatly enhanced on images emphazising T_2. An MR image of the brain based on T_2 can reveal minute differences in tissue water concentration which is particularly interesting, as most structural disease processes expand the extracellular space, and the brain has the smallest extracellular space of all organs (approximately 20 percent of volume).

Age-related Gray Matter Changes Such as Polio-araiosis and Changes in the Chemical Composition are Best Observed with MRI

MRI allows an excellent differentiation of the gray and white matter. Owing to the many different physical param-

eters contributing to the generation of a MR image, the information acquired with this modality is superior to that provided by CT alone. The MRI contrast between gray and white matter appears to be higher in young normal subjects than in older patients. There is a close relation between T_1, spin density and T_2 values of white and gray matter with aging. Such a phenomenon is possibly due to an increased water content in the white matter and the progressive neuronal shrinkage (Chapter 18) or neuronal loss in the gray matter that occurs with age. Meyer and colleagues (1994) have measured changes in cerebral gray and white matter tissue densities associated with normal aging, using cross-sectional plain CT. In their measurements they also recorded cerebral blood flow values during *stable xenon inhalation* (Xenon-CBF-CT). Their results led to the conclusion that cortical gray matter tissue densities progressively decline after age 60. This progressive decreased in the cortical gray matter tissue densities, called *polio-araiosis* (Greek *polios* = gray + *araios* = thin, meaning 'gray matter thinning') is coupled with regional hypoperfusion but not with cortical atrophy.

De Leon and coworkers (1989) demonstrated that thin-slice axial CT images obtained parallel to the temporal lobe provide a unique view of the medial and perihippocampal anatomy, permitting a rapid and sensitive assessment of the region's structural integrity. This is based on a characteristic appearance of the dilated transverse fissure and adjacent choroidal and hippocampal fissures as seen in the axial plain. MR-studies confirm that the enlargement of these fissures is directly related to parenchymal volume losses in the hippocampus, subiculum, and parahippocampal gyrus. The prevalence of hippocampal atrophy increases significantly with age and is more common in male than in female subjects. It is a common feature of normal aging. CT and MR can detect atrophic changes of the perihippocampal region in a high percentage of cognitively normal and medically healthy, elderly persons. Especially coronal MRI scans are able to show very precise hippocampal changes.

MRI provides some information on the changes in the chemical composition of the central nervous system during life. Heavily T_2 weighted spin echo sequences show substantial, age-dependent low intensity in two different groups of brain structures. The first, characterized by shortening of the T_1 and T_2 relaxation times with age, includes myelinated pathways. The shortening is caused by increasing myelination and simultaneously decreasing water content. The second group, characterized by shortening of T_2 but not of T_1 relaxation times with age, include the nuclei of the extrapyramidal system such as the *globus pallidus, substantia nigra, red nucleus,* and *putamen* as well as the caudate, dentate and subthalamic nuclei. The decrease in signal in the extrapyramidal nuclei is obviously age-dependent and appears likely to result from the corresponding iron concentration. Schenker and colleagues (1993) found that the curves of T_2 relaxation time in the basal ganglia are congruent with published curves of iron concentration, indicating a high probability that the changes in T_2 relaxation times and the low signal in the basal ganglia result from the local, age-dependent iron deposition (Figure 28–1).

Leuko-araiosis Comprises a Group of Age-related White Matter Changes Characterized by Hypodensities on CT and Hyperintensities on MRI

In 1987, Hachinski and coworkers proposed the designation *leuko-araiosis* (LA) (Greek *leuko*, white; *araios*, thin, thus meaning 'white matter thinning') for the white matter changes identified by CT and MRI, and characterized by a decrease in the white matter representation density, as indicated by white matter *hypodensities* on CT and *hyperintensities* on MRI. These lesions are more frequently observed on MRI than on CT. They frequently occur apparently without any clinical counterpart, in normal elderly persons as well as in pathological conditions (Verny et al., 1991), and appear to be associated with vascular changes.

Neuropathologically, CT and MR studies suggest that even elderly individuals without neurologic deficits have focal abnormalities in the cerebral white matter. MR has a greater sensitivity compared with CT in detecting white matter abnormalities of the aging brain. With this increased sensitivity, however, problems with specificity sometimes arise. The foci of abnormalities are found in several different locations: subcortical, central, and periventricular.

Spotty white matter hyperintensities are distributed in areas of perforating ectatic vessels with enlargement of surrounding perivascular spaces. The perivascular or *Virchow-Robin Space* (VRS) is an extension of the subarachnoid space. High-field MR permits routine visualization of normal VRS. They are found with increasing frequency with advancing age (Figure 28–2). On MR VRS are isointense to CSF on all pulse sequences. They enlarge as the subarachnoid space does elsewhere in the brain with aging. Age related vascular changes may contribute to enlarged VRS. Occasionally, it is difficult to differentiate them from lacunar infarcts, especially when widening of the VRS is observed in the white matter (Ogawa et al., 1995).

Periventricular hyperintense white matter lesions are contiguous with the margin of the lateral ventricles. Different types of such lesions are seen on the T_2 weighted MR images in elderly patients: (i) Triangle-shaped 'caps' around the frontal horns. In this location, myelin is more loosely compacted and there is an increase in periependymal fluid (Sze et al., 1986). (ii) Thin, smooth periventricular rims. These are characterized by subependymal gliosis and higher concentrations of interstitial water at the ventricular lining. (iii) Patchy, periventricular hyperintensities due to enlarged VRS, atrophy of axons and myelin with associated gliosis. (iv) Triangular-shaped regions posterior and superior to the trigones. These are thought to represent delayed myelination of the fiber tracts. (v) Hyperintensity of the posterior internal capsule possibly owing to less heavy myelination of the parietopontine tract.

White matter lesions can be found in regions outside the periventricular region such as in the *corona radiata*, *centrum semiovale*, and subcortical region (Bowen et al., 1990). They increase in number and extent with increasing age and range from punctuate to larger patchy, irregular lesions. These white matter lesions are hyperintense to brain parenchyma on the long TR sequences and not visible on the short TR sequence. The number of lesions identified is greater with the FLAIR (*Fluid Attenuated Inversion Recovery*) sequence. This heavily T_2-weighted inversion recovery technique nulls fluid such as CSF. Thus, subtle white matter lesions stand out against a background of black CSF and hypointense white matter (Figure 28–3). Their precise histologic correlate is uncertain. The results of several pathologic investigations suggest that these foci are predominantly a spectrum of lesions ranging from ischemic foci to infarctions (Braffman et al., 1988). They were found to be associated with arteriosclerosis, dilated perivascular spaces, and vascular ectasia. Awad and colleagues (1986) are of the opinion that subcortical parenchymal lesions may represent an index of chronic cerebrovascular diseases. However, some authors found no correlation of risk factors for cerebrovascular disease (Hendrie et al., 1989; Meguro et al., 1993).

It is often difficult to determine if white matter signal hyperintensities on MR represent normal aging or neurological disease. Multiple sclerosis and other demyelinating diseases, cerebrovascular disease and human immunodeficiency virus infection are also associated with patchy white matter lesions.

Enlargement of CSF Spaces is not an Inevitable Consequence of Advancing Age

Enlargement of sulci, cisterns, and ventricles is part of the normal aging process, and indicates a mixed age-related central and cortical volume loss. Numerous studies have been performed with CT to analyze the limits of normalcy in healthy, elderly individuals. CT allows an easy and safe noninvasive study of the functioning brain; the technique has been especially useful in helping to establish the age-related width of the ventricular system. However actual quantification of cortical atrophy has been difficult with CT because of technical limitations such as partial volume averaging, and bone-hardening artifact at the cerebral convexities and at the temporal and posterior fossae. Despite the fact that MRI circumvents such CT artifacts, up to now there are no statistically proven age-related, generally accepted norms for the CSF-spaces.

Beginning about the fourth decade, gradual widening of the third ventricle, Sylvian and interhemispheric fissures, superficial sulci, and basal cisterns have been reported to occur. Enlargement of the lateral ventricles is most striking after the sixth decade of life (LeMay, 1984). Sandor and colleagues (1990) found that specific regions in the brain change with age. Age-related changes in mean CT attenuation values of brain tissue were analyzed by an objective, automated technique. On the med-

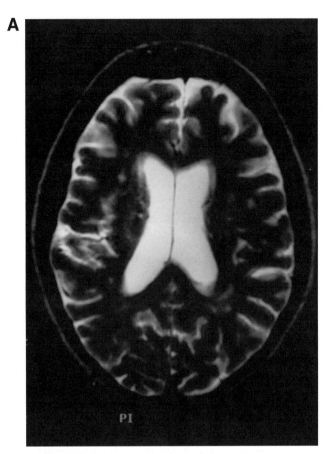

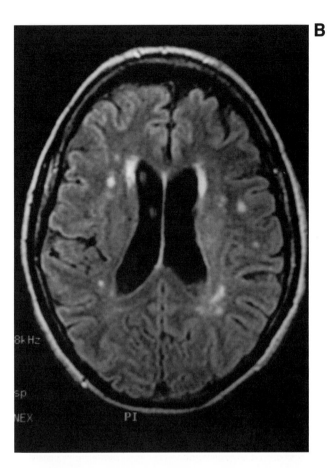

FIGURE   28–3
White matter lesions. **A.** Fast Spin Echo (SE) T$_2$-weighted MRI.

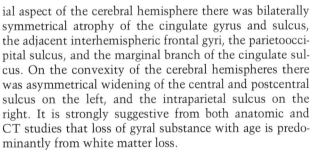

B. FLAIR (fluid attenuated inversion recovery). The FLAIR image gives much better lesion definition than T$_2$-weighted SE image.

ial aspect of the cerebral hemisphere there was bilaterally symmetrical atrophy of the cingulate gyrus and sulcus, the adjacent interhemispheric frontal gyri, the parietoocci-pital sulcus, and the marginal branch of the cingulate sulcus. On the convexity of the cerebral hemispheres there was asymmetrical widening of the central and postcentral sulcus on the left, and the intraparietal sulcus on the right. It is strongly suggestive from both anatomic and CT studies that loss of gyral substance with age is predominantly from white matter loss.

On the basis of MR-data of 76 adult healthy volunteers, increasing age is associated with decreasing volumes of the cerebral hemispheres (0.23 percent per year), increasing volumes of the third ventricle (2.8 percent per year) and the lateral ventricles (3.2 percent per year), and increasing odds of cortical atrophy (8.9 percent per year). These changes were typically mild. However, many elderly subjects did not exhibit cortical atrophy or lateral ventricular enlargement, indicating that such changes are not inevitable consequences of advancing age (Coffey et al., 1992).

On the other hand prominent sulci, cisterns, and ventricles are usual findings on imaging studies, particularly in patients over 70 years of age. The width of the external

and internal CSF-spaces can not be used to predict the presence or progression of dementia in individual cases.

CT Exceeds Conventional Skull Radiography in the Detection of Calcified Vasculature

Age is an important risk factor for stroke. Neuropathologic study of cerebral arteries and clinical study of occlusive cerebral vascular lesions generally show trends for increasing severity of atherosclerosis with advancing age (Chapter 27). The distribution of cerebrovascular disease by age has not been a primary focus in most recent angiographic reports. However, in an ultrasonography study, of all known risk factors, age has the strongest association with atherosclerotic lesions of all arteries, including the carotid artery (Handa et al., 1990; Gorelick, 1993).

Calcification of arterial walls of the large arteries at the base of the brain is considered a sign of atherosclerosis. Radiographic calcification of the carotid artery siphon is frequent. Di Chiro and Libow (1971) found diminished cerebral blood flow in healthy patients with intimal carotid siphon calcification. CT exceeds conventional skull radiography in the detection of calcified structures, because of its high density resolution (Becker et al., 1977).

Marked calcification of the carotid siphon is readily recognized on skull radiographs, but calcification of intracranial vertebral artery is difficult to detect due to the overlap of dense petrous bones and air-filled sinuses. CT can avoid the interference by means of axial sections (Katada et al., 1983).

CT and MR are Reliable Methods to Diagnose and Stage Neurodegenerative Diseases *in vivo*

Alzheimer disease is the commonest degenerative disease of the brain and the most common form of dementia. Volumetric analysis is one method to study structure-function relation in Alzheimer patients and healthy aging. CT and MR imaging studies show diffusely enlarged ventricles and widened sulci; the volumetric measurements by using CT in patients with senile dementia of Alzheimer type demonstrated greater cerebral atrophy. The annual rate of ventricular enlargement is significantly greater than in age-matched control subjects (De-Carli et al., 1990; Wippold II et al., 1991). The degree of atrophy generally increases parallel to the progress of the clinical stage (De Leon et al., 1989) and correlates with the severity of dementia (Hentschel et al., 1995). The gray matter is reduced, especially in the temporal lobes (Figure 28–4) with disproportionate volume loss in the anterior temporal lobe, particularly the hippocampal formation (Jack et al., 1990, 1992; Rusinek et al., 1991). The temporal horns and Sylvian cisterns, as well as the choroid and hippocampal fissures, appear enlarged (Kido et al., 1989; George et al., 1990).

MRI studies have shown the volumetric atrophy of the hippocampus to be a sensitive indicator early in the course of Alzheimer disease. MR-based hippocampal volumetry is accurate in differentiating dementia of Alzheimer type from cognitively normal elderly individuals (Jack et al., 1992). Some Alzheimer disease patients show areas of high signal intensity affecting hippocampal and Sylvian cortex on long TR MR-images. It is likely that abnormalities reflect the histopathological features of Alzheimer disease, such as a disturbed quantitative relationship of neurons to glia and associated degenerative changes (neuritic plaques and neurofibrillary tangles) (Fazekas et al., 1987).

Many, but not all MR and CT studies found white matter lesions more commonly in Alzheimer disease patients than in normal elderly controls. Patients with prominent subcortical white-matter lesions are more likely to have a diagnosis of vascular- rather than Alzheimer dementia (Bowen et al., 1990).

Subtle gyral bands of hypointensity on T_2-weighted MR-images, particularly in the parietal region, were noted in approximately 50 percent of the patients with Alzheimer disease and most likely represent iron accumulation as reported in pathologic studies (Drayer, 1988). To detect regional differences in accompanying metabolic changes, *^{1}H-Magnetic Resonance Spectroscopic Imaging* (MRSI) was performed in patients with Alzheimer disease. The observed elevation of choline compounds in the hippo-campus supports the hypothesis that alterations in the cholinergic system play an important role in Alzheimer disease. The reduction of N-acetylaspartate is explained by neuronal degeneration (Block et al., 1995).

Pick disease is another, but much less frequent, neurodegenerative dementing disease. Presenile onset is common. Pick disease is characterized by fronto-temporal atrophy, whereas the parietal and occipital lobes are relatively spared. The frontal lobe atrophy is dominant medial and inferiorly, while temporal lobe atrophy begins anteriorly to involve the inferior and middle temporal gyri. CT is a valuable tool in the evaluation of specific, localized atrophy consistent with Pick disease (Figure 28–5). Knopmann and colleagues found marked frontal pole or temporal pole atrophy on CT, which clearly differed from the pattern of cerebral atrophy seen in the Alzheimer patients. In families with dominant hereditary disease, CT aids in the detection of the disease in family members before clinical signs appear (Groen et al., 1982). Mild hyperintense signal of the cortex and adjacent white matter is seen additionally on long TR MR-images (Braffman et al., 1988).

Huntington disease shows characteristic atrophy of the caudate nuclei and the putamina, as well as cortical atrophy, usually beginning in frontal regions and progressing posteriorly. Typical is an enlargement of the frontal horns of the lateral ventricles with loss of the usual bulge of the inferolateral border created by the head of the caudate nucleus. Striatal atrophy can be imaged with both CT and MRI (Figure 28–6). MR is superior to CT for imaging morphologic changes (Simmons et al., 1986). Aylward and colleagues (1994) found MRI volume reductions of the *caudate*, *putamen*, and *globus pallidus* in a group of presymptomatic individuals who carry the Huntington disease gene, suggesting that basal ganglia atrophy begins before clinical symptoms. MR also shows signal changes of the *corpus striatum* on T_2 weighted images. Savoiardo and colleagues (1991) observed high signal intensity especially in cases with the rigid variant of Huntington disease.

In *Parkinson disease* MRI shows decreased width of the *pars compacta* of the *substantia nigra* (Huber et al., 1990) (Figure 28–7). This probably reflects selective loss of neuromelanin-containing cells, but may also be due to iron deposition. Hyperintense foci may be seen, possibly due to gliosis that accompanies cell loss. Most Parkinson disease patients do not have putaminal hypointensity on long TR images that are greater than expected from age. The use of gradient echoes allows more sensitive detection than did spin echoes of susceptibility changes in the putamina and substantia nigra (Braffman et al., 1988). Although nigral changes are detected in different studies, technical factors such as slice thickness, image averaging, and positioning make it difficult to define these abnormalities with certainty in all cases. Subcortical and cortical atrophy is more common in patients with Parkinson's disease than in controls (Becker et al., 1979).

Besides Parkinson disease, other age-related degenerative changes in the striatonigral system may play a role in

A

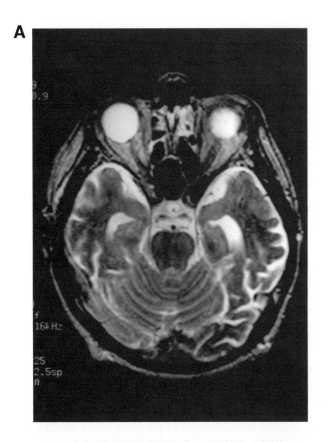

B

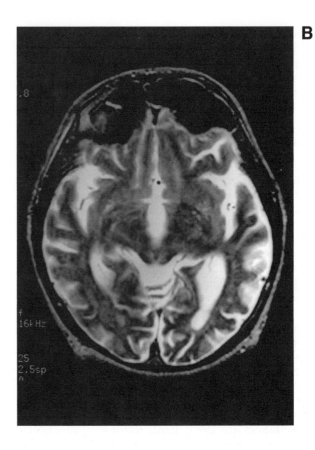

C

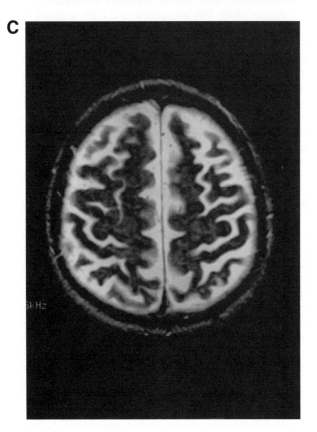

FIGURE   28–4

Alzheimer disease on MRI showing markedly enlarged ventricles and sulci. The temporal horns (A) and sylvian fissures (B) are severely affected, as demonstrated by the white color (hyperintensity) indicating space occupied by CSF. Subtle gyral bands of hypointensity (darkening) can be seen in the parietal region (C) on T_2-weighted MRI.

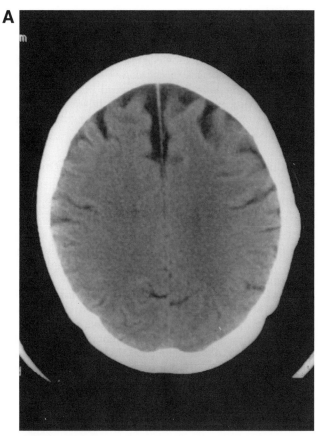 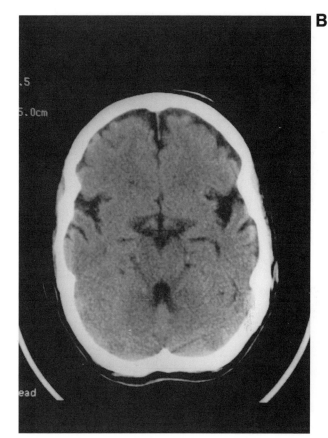

FIGURE   28–5
Pick disease. CT shows circumscribed frontal (A) and temporal (B) lobar atrophy.

the pathogenesis of parkinsonism, including striatonigral degeneration, Shy-Drager syndrome, and progressive supranuclear palsy. Striatonigral degeneration may be associated with olivopontocerebellar degenerations and or Shy-Drager syndrome in multiple system atrophy. In cases of *striatonigral degeneration* neuroimaging shows atrophy of the *corpus striatum*. On T$_2$ weighted MRI, at 1.5 Tesla magnetic field strength, the putaminal hypointensity is equal or more evident than pallidal hypointensity. This may be accompanied by a thin rim of hyperintense signal. These changes of the putamen vary with the magnetic field strength. With a lower strength magnet, the putamina are hyperintense on T$_2$ weighted images, likely caused by increased amounts of water due to gliosis and or cell loss. At 1.5 Tesla, magnetic susceptibility effects predominate.

Shy-Drager syndrome is characterized by orthostatic hypotension, urinary incontinence and inability to sweat. Hypointensity in T$_2$-weighted images is increased in all nuclei. The hypointensity in the *putamen* is superior or equal to that of the *pallidum* in patients examined with a 1.5 Tesla MR unit. At low or intermediate field strength, there was absence of magnetic susceptibility effect in the putamen, which appeared hyperintense (Savoiardo *et al.*, 1989).

Imaging studies in *progressive supranuclear palsy* (Steele-Richardson-Olszewski disease) demonstrate midbrain and tectal atrophy with a dilated cerebral aqueduct and enlarged perimesencephalic cisterns. Some patients show superior collicular focal atrophy and slight hyperintensive signal on T$_2$-weighted MRI of the periaquaductal gray matter. In general there is no uniformity of findings and MRI appears unable to consistently support the clinical diagnosis (Savoiardo *et al.*, 1989).

CT and MR imaging studies of *olivo-ponto-cerebellar degeneration* show small inferior olives and medulla, a small flattened pons, and substantial atrophic cerebellar hemispheres and vermis with marked enlargement of the fourth ventricle (Figure 28–8). Slight hyperintensity on T$_2$-weighted MRI is often seen in the transverse pontine fibers ventral to the *tegmentum*, the raphe, and the anterior and anterolateral contours of the pons where transverse pontine fibers merge with the abnormal signal of middle cerebellar peduncles. Striatonigral degeneration and/or Shy-Drager syndrome occasionally coexist with olivo-ponto-cerebellar degeneration.

Amyotrophic lateral sclerosis (ALS) is characterized by degeneration of the corticospinal tract and by involvement of both upper and lower motor neurons. On MR, corresponding hyperintense foci on T$_2$-weighted images

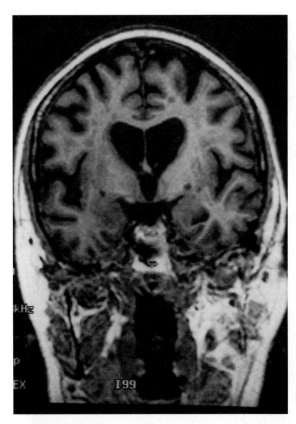

FIGURE 28–6
Huntington disease. Coronal MRI shows atrophic caudate
nuclei with frontal horn enlargement.

of the corticospinal tract, as well as atrophy of the spinal
cord is seen. Atrophy, with flattening of the anterior and
lateral portions of the spinal cord, is presumably caused
by loss of motor neurons (anterior horn cells) (Sherman *et
al.*, 1987; Friedman *et al.*, 1993). Low signal intensity in
the precentral cortex bilateral has been noted on conventional T_2-weighted Spin-echo images. Abnormal iron deposition associated with the degenerative process could
be the source of T_2 shortening in the motor cortex (Oba
et al., 1993) (Figure 28–9). However, T_2 shortening of the
motor cortex was seen frequently in older normal individuals and in patients with cerebrovascular disease. These
findings are compatible with those of histochemical studies of normal iron deposition of the motor cortex (Hirai *et
al.*, 1996).

Creutzfeldt-Jakob disease (spongiform encephalopathy)
is a transmissible neurodegenerative disease caused by
prion protein that usually affects older adults. Rapidly
progressive atrophic changes on serial CT of the brain are
highly suggestive of the disease (Rao *et al.*, 1977). Ventricular enlargement, especially of the frontal horns due to
atrophy of the basal ganglia, is more characteristic than
sulcal enlargement (Zieger *et al.*, 1981). MRI findings are
not uniform. Several groups have described increased signal intensity in the basal ganglia on T_2-weighted images
(Milton *et al.*, 1991; Barboriak *et al.*, 1994; Gertz *et al.*,

1988). There have also been reports of extensive white
matter involvement, with cortical atrophy and severe periventricular high signal (Krüger *et al.*, 1990; Uchino *et al.*,
1991). Follow-up MRI showed that the high signal region
on T_2-weighted images in the cortex of the left frontal,
parietal and temporal lobes had spread in the right cerebral cortex and into the basal ganglia bilaterally. Frontal
cortical atrophy was apparent on T_1-weighted images
(Ishida *et al.*, 1995).

*The Consequences of Toxic and Metabolic Diseases
to the Brain Tissue can be Identified by
Neuroimaging*

The CNS effects of chronic alcoholism include *Wernicke
encephalopathy*, *Marchiafava-Bignami disease*, *central
pontine myelinolysis*, and cerebral atrophy. These consequences of ethanol intoxication can be identified by neuroimaging.

Wernicke encephalopathy is associated with the classical triad of ataxia, oculomotor disorders, and confusion.
Most of the patients exhibit the selective disturbance of
Korsakoff amnestic syndrome. The characteristic lesions
occur symmetrically in the medial thalamic nuclei, *massa
intermedia*, third ventricular floor, and mamillary bodies.
The periaquaeductal region, midbrain reticular formation,
and the posterior *corpora quadrigemina* are typically affected (Yokote *et al.*, 1991). In general, MRI appears to be
more sensitive than CT in detecting abnormalities (Hoffman *et al.*, 1988; Osterthun *et al.*, 1990). CT may show
bilateral low density areas in the thalamic region. Kitaguchi and coworkers (1987) found contrast-enhancing
lesions bilaterally in hypothalamus, thalamus and in the
floor of the fourth ventricle. On T_2-weighted MRI, there
are hyperintense areas that surround the third ventricle
and aqueduct with atrophic changes in the superior
vermis and the mamillary bodies (Galluci *et al.*, 1990).
Mamillary body atrophy, which is a relatively specific
pathologic abnormality, can be easily imaged by MRI on
T_1-weighted sagittal and coronal images. Post-contrast
T_1-weighted images may show enhancement around the
third ventricle, cerebral aqueduct, and fourth ventricle.
The enhancement disappears after successful thiamine
therapy (Schroth *et al.*, 1988).

Marchiafava-Bignami syndrome is an uncommon disease of demyelination or necrosis of the *corpus callosum*
and adjacent subcortical white matter, which occurs predominantly in poorly nourished alcoholics. It is marked
by dementia, spasticity, dysarthria, inability to walk, and
disturbances of consciousness. CT may demonstrate hypodense areas in portions of the *corpus callosum*. MR
scans typically show hyperintensities in T_2-weighted
images and diffuse swelling of the *corpus callosum* in the
acute stage. In the chronic stage, in addition to atrophy,
focal necrosis can be observed in the *corpus callosum*
(Becker *et al.*, 1992; Chang *et al.*, 1992).

Central pontine myelinolysis is characterized by regions
of demyelination throughout the brain, but are most prominent in the pons. It affects alcoholics, but it has been

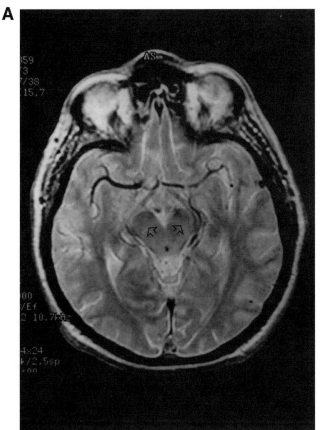
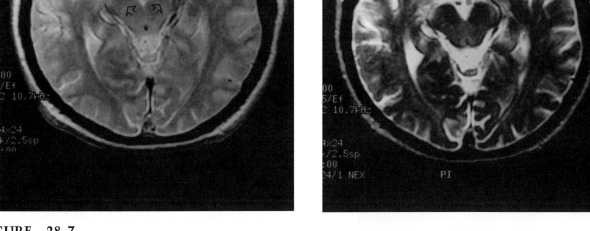

FIGURE   28–7

Parkinson disease. The width of the pars compacta (arrows) of the substantia nigra is diminished, visible on proton density-

weighted MRI (A) and on T$_2$-weighted MRI (B).

also found in patients with electrolyte abnormalities, such as hyponatremia, liver disease, malnutrition and *Addison disease*. The symptoms include spastic quadriparesis, pseudobulbar palsy, and acute changes of consciousness. MRI is more sensitive than CT in imaging the lesions. CT sometimes demonstrates hypodensities in the pons. However, the CT is often normal or artifacts obscure subtle changes. The most common MR finding is an area of decreased T$_1$ signal and increased T$_2$ signal within the base of the pons (Figure 28–10). The lesions are usually triangular- or trident-shaped (Miller *et al.*, 1988). Koch and Smith observed peripheral ringlike contrast enhancement. Serial MRI studies indicate the initial MR images may appear normal, particularly within 1 week after symptoms onset. Approximately 1–2 weeks later, the lesion within the pons may be quite large. With time, as the acute process subsides, the lesion becomes smaller and better defined. Residual focal signal abnormalities may persist. Extrapontine lesions in the *thalamus, putamen*, caudate nucleus, *globus pallidus*, cerebellar peduncles, periventricular white matter, and corticomedullary junction have also been detected by MR in patients having central pontine myelinolysis. However, Gallucci and colleagues (1990) also found white matter lesions in

40 percent of the patients who did not have neurologic complications of alcoholism.

CT and MRI studies show enlargement of the ventricles and sulci in the majority of alcoholics. However, in abstinent patients, marked decrease of cerebrospinal fluid space enlargement is visible (Artmann *et al.*, 1981). It has been hypothesized that changes in brain parenchyma such as the rise of protein synthesis and a subsequent increase in dendritic growth may account for the reversible radiographic abnormalities of alcoholics. It cannot be due to de- and rehydration of the brain solely (Schroth *et al.*, 1988). Reversible brain shrinkage has been seen also in *anorexia nervosa* and *Cushing syndrome*.

Imaging of CSF Related Diseases is Mainly Based Upon the Findings at CT and MR

Normal pressure hydrocephalus is characterized by the triad of dementia, gait disturbance, and urinary incontinence. It is uncommon before the age of 60. It has been suggested that normal pressure hydrocephalus results from deficient CSF absorption due to obstruction within the basal cisterns, in the subarachnoid space over the convexities or at the level of the arachnoid granulations (com-

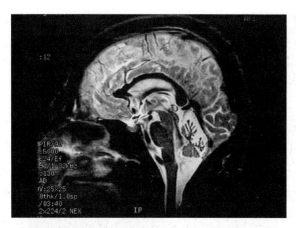

FIGURE 28–8
Olivo-ponto-cerebellar degeneration. Sagittal T_2-weighted MRI shows marked atrophy of the vermis, pons and medulla.

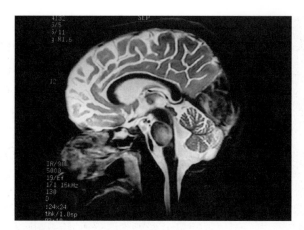

FIGURE 28–10
Central pontine myelinolysis. The pons appears hyperintense on sagittal T_2-weighted MRI.

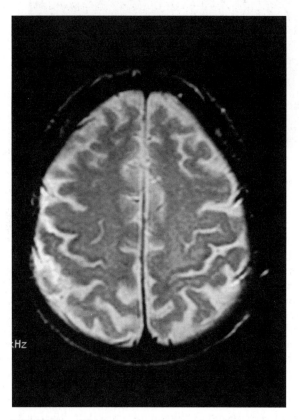

FIGURE 28–9
Amyotrophic lateral sclerosis. Hypointense signal in the precentral cortex bilateral on conventional T_2-weighted SE MRI.

municating hydrocephalus with obstruction distal to the foramina of the forth ventricle). It is thought to result most commonly from previous hemorrhage or meningeal infection. In some cases no cause can be determined. The disturbed CSF circulation leads to increased pressure and reflux within the ventricular system and transependymal

flow of CSF into the periventricular white matter. CSF pressure may be normal after ventricular dilatation and due to equilibration between CSF production and absorption. The symptoms can be reversible with shunting.

Imaging is mainly based upon the findings at CT and MR. There is generally a discrepancy between the dilated ventricles (especially frontal and temporal horn dilatation) and the appearance of the cisterns and sulci. In typical cases the parasagittal sulci are poorly visible or absent (Figure 28–11). Lateral ventricular distention causes smooth thinning of the *corpus callosum*. Because of the superior sensitivity of MRI in detecting white matter changes, MR shows the interstitial edema due to transependymal egress of CSF better than CT does. This is shown on proton density- and T_2-weighted images throughout the periventricular white matter. This finding is not specific. However, Jack and colleagues (1987) found that periventricular hyperintensity was more often seen in normal pressure hydrocephalus than in other forms of dementia.

CSF flow in *normal pressure hydrocephalus* causes a to and fro motion of CSF through the ventricular system. The hyperdynamic flow through the third ventricle, cerebral aqueduct and fourth ventricle produces a marked 'flow void' on sagittal and axial MR images (Bradley *et al.*, 1991; Jack *et al.*, 1987; Schroth *et al.*, 1992).

The distinction on CT or MRI of atrophy due to aging or neurodegenerative diseases from normal pressure hydrocephalus is often a difficult problem.

Different Imaging Techniques are Necessary to Recognize Vascular Diseases

Cerebral vascular disease is the third commonest cause of death. Approximately 85 percent of cerebrovascular diseases are caused by ischemia. Intracerebral hematoma and subarachnoid hemorrhage account for the remaining 15 percent (Holtas, 1993). Imaging techniques are useful to confirm the diagnosis, to detect complications and to provide a differential diagnosis.

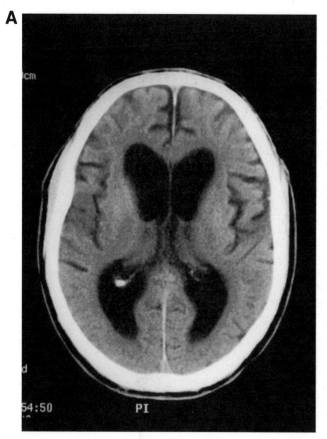

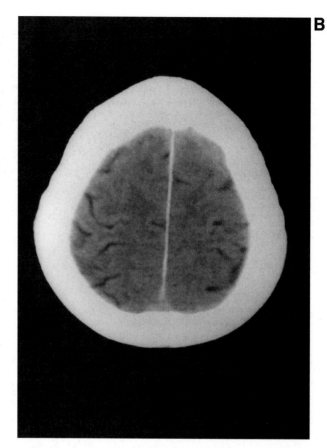

FIGURE 28–11
Normal pressure hydrocephalus. Note the difference of enlarged ventricles (A) compared to the quite normal parietal sulci (B) on CT.

Infarcts are caused by cardiac emboli, large vessel disease and small vessel disease. Cerebral embolism of cardiac origin accounts for 25–30 percent of strokes. Large vessel disease accounts for 25–35 percent of cerebrovascular disease. Most cerebral emboli arise from ulcerated arteriosclerotic plaques of the common carotid bifurcation, but occasionally hemodynamic effects can contribute to symptoms in patients with severe stenosis or arterial occlusion. Small vessel occlusion causing *lacunar infarcts* accounts for approximately 20 percent of cerebrovascular disease and is caused by local changes in arterioles. These lesions are found in areas of the brain with long penetrating end arteries, such as the basal ganglia, internal capsule and pons. Brain infarcts can also be seen in some other conditions, such as *vasculitis* and following arterial dissection.

Since the *acute cerebral infarction* is imaged as hypodense in CT, a definitive differential diagnostic delimitation from *fresh intracerebral hemorrhage*, which is imaged as hyperdense, is possible. CT scans are quite good at showing hemorrhages. Acute hematomas are not as easy to diagnose on MRI. Different imaging techniques are necessary to recognize that a hemorrhage has occurred. The MRI characteristics of hemorrhage are deter-

mined predominantly by hemoglobin and its breakdown products (Janick *et al.*, 1991). Although CT detects acute hemorrhage more accurately than MRI, the latter is much more sensitive for identification of subacute and chronic hemorrhage.

After about 24 hours, the cerebral infarction can be delimited unequivocally in CT, but a more diffuse reduction in density in the infarct region can already be seen after 6 hours. A minor swelling and unsharp margins between the gray and white matter can be observed, if carefully looked for (Figure 28–12). Attention has also to be paid to the large basal arteries of the brain in fresh infarction, as fresh thrombosis is imaged as a hyperdense structure (v. Kummer *et al.*, 1995).

The cerebral infarction is not always hypodense in CT. In the second and third week, there is the 'fogging effect' (Becker *et al.*, 1979). At this time, the infarct can be isodense, so that it is not detected in plain CT. The infarct can be delimited only after intravenous administration of contrast medium, since a maximum disorder of the blood-brain-barrier is then present. Around the 10th day, there is withdrawal of fluid of the edema. The signs of space occupation thus disappear, and the infarct becomes isodense. The infarct becomes hypodense again in

A

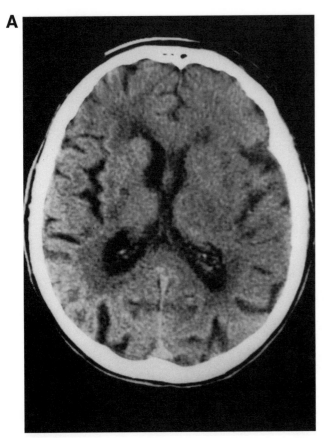

B

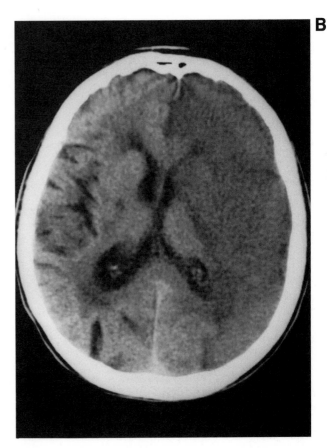

FIGURE   28–12

Acute cerebral infarction. **A.** CT shows a minor swelling and a poor differentiation between the gray and white matter on the left few hours after the acute onset. **B.** A large infarcted area of the middle and anterior cerebral arteries is seen 24 hours later.

the context of phagocytosis with occurrence of lipid granule cells, and then passes into the chronic stage of cysts and glial scar with intensive hypodensity after six weeks (Figure 28–13).

The reaction of the infarcted area to contrast medium is time-dependent also. The first contrast enhancement is patchy and, for the most part, peripheral. Marked, more streaky contrast enhancement is seen on the seventh day. The cerebral infarct with 'fogging effect' regularly has an intensive homogeneous contrast enhancement. When the 'fogging effect' has disappeared, patchy contrast enhancement with decreased intensity can be observed. After six weeks the cerebral infarctions reveal no reaction after contrast medium.

There may be associated secondary hemorrhage of the infarct. The hemorrhagic component is confined predominantly to the gray matter. Small areas of hemorrhagic infarction are frequently missed by CT due to partial volume effects with radiolucent non-hemorrhagic infarction. MRI is much more sensitive than CT in diagnosing hemorrhagic infarction.

CT can reveal typical patterns in some types of infarcts, indicating the etiology. Emboli from the heart or large vessels give cortical infarcts of varying size, most of-ten in the distribution area of the middle cerebral artery or posterior cerebral artery. *Lacunar infarcts* are seen in basal ganglia and internal capsule after occlusion of the lenticulostriate arteries. Occlusion of the small perforating branches of the basilar artery result in mesencephalic, pontine, or medullary infarctions of the lacunar type. Similar small infarcts, frequently called *lacunae* as well, occur in the *centrum semiovale*.

Ischemic changes in patients with severe stenosis or vascular occlusion and hypoxic events are seen in the watershed area between different vascular territories. *'Watershed' infarcts* occur most commonly at the territorial junction of the anterior and middle cerebral arteries, less often at the junction of the middle and posterior cerebral territories.

Subcortical arteriosclerotic encephalopathy is a white matter disorder as a result of arteriosclerosis of the medullary arteries. It causes severe psychoorganic disorders with transient but frequently recurrent neurologic deficits and is called *Binswanger disease*. CT is moderately sensitive to subcortical arteriosclerotic encephalopathy. Symmetrical diminished densities are seen in the white matter, particularly around the frontal horns and trigones.

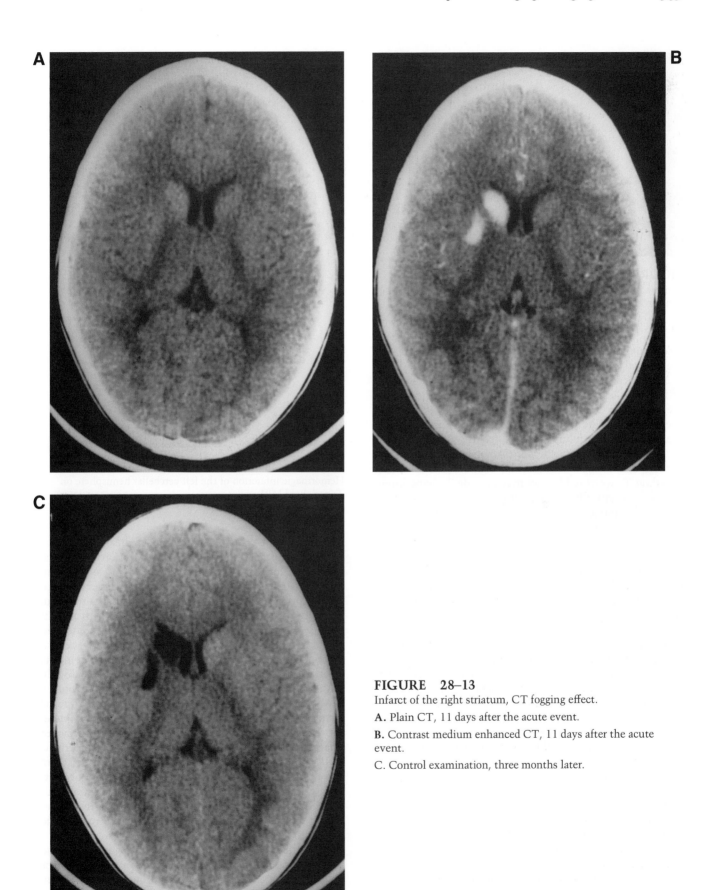

FIGURE   28–13
Infarct of the right striatum, CT fogging effect.

A. Plain CT, 11 days after the acute event.

B. Contrast medium enhanced CT, 11 days after the acute event.

C. Control examination, three months later.

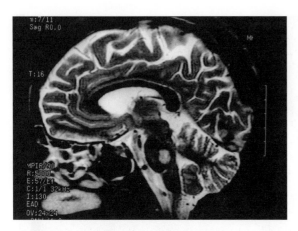

FIGURE 28–14
Pontine infarction. Note the posterior fossa without any artifacts on T_2-weighted MRI.

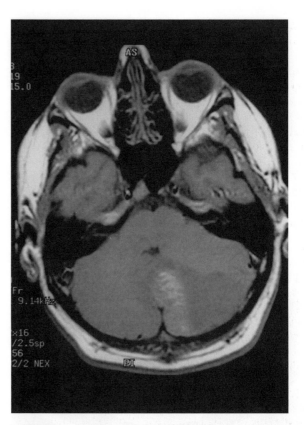

FIGURE 28–15
Hemorrhagic infarction of the left cerebellar hemisphere on T_1-weighted MRI.

Additional changes include dilated ventricles and moderate cortical brain atrophy (Zeumer *et al.*, 1980).

MRI has a significant higher sensitivity in the detection of ischemic lesions than CT, especially when the lesions are located in the posterior fossa (Figure 28–14) or near the skullbase. The first MR signs of cortical ischemia are seen within a few hours of vessel occlusion. The changes include sulcal effacement, blurring of gray-white matter borders and loss of intravascular signal voids. Swelling noted on T_1-weighted images may precede T_2 hyperintensity, which typically develops at 6 to 12 hours post ictus. The fresh infarct can only be recognized well in the T_2-weighted images, whereas it is poorly delimitable in the T_1-weighted images. Old brain infarcts have an increased signal on T_2-weighted images and a low signal on T_1-weighted images.

Like CT, MR yields an image of cerebral infarct that varies with time during the first six weeks. The time-dependent changes of cerebral infarct in MRI can also be easily correlated with the pathological anatomical stages.

The *edema* is fundamental for MRI. It can be depicted in the acute stage of necrosis and the subacute stage of resorption until approximately the 10th day after which it is mobilized. At this time no more signs of space occupying process are visible. The T_2 contrasts show an initial temporary decline followed by a significant increase at the time of transition to the chronic stage.

Petechial bleedings within the infarct region can be detected with T_1-weighted image (Figure 28–15) that are not visible in the CT scan. As the blood-brain-barrier loses integrity, petechial gyral hemorrhage may appear as bands of hyperintensity that follow cortical contours on unenhanced T_1-weighted images. They appear during the second week after the acute incident and can be observed about 10 weeks and more.

MR *contrast agents* may improve the detection, delineation and dating of cerebral infarcts in T_1-weighted images. The enhancement pattern seen on MR images closely matches that known from contrast-enhanced CT.

There are some other abnormalities in the acute phase of the large cortical infarction after injection of contrast medium. The 'intravascular enhancement sign' is produced by slow flow within vessels supplying an acute cerebral infarction. The sign disappears after about 1 week. An 'abnormal meningeal enhancement' can be frequently seen next to the infarct up to 1 week after the acute onset of the infarct (Elster, 1993).

The early morphologic changes seen in *cortical infarcts* are generally absent in *subcortical infarcts*, probably due to differences in vascular supply and tissue architecture.

MR measurements of the diffusion of water protons have been shown to be a highly sensitive way to detect the early changes of *ischemia*. With diffusion-weighted images, *cytotoxic edema* can be visualized directly on MRI as a change in signal intensity. The changes observed in acute infarction reflect distribution of water from the extracellular to the more restrictive intracellular space. Diffusion-weighted imaging also helps in differentiating reversibly versus irreversibly damaged tissue (Spielman *et al.*, 1995).

With the advent of *echo-planar imaging* in MRI, observation of the first pass through a tissue of a contrast agent bolus became possible. It causes time-dependent signal changes. By measuring the signal-intensity variations during bolus transit, tissue perfusion can be assessed. Perfusion imaging made it possible the measurement of regional cerebral blood volume on MRI and improved the detectability of *acute cerebral ischemia* (Kucharczyk *et al.*, 1993).

Proton MR spectroscopic imaging studies show considerable promise as a method for detection of ischemic brain regions. When infarction occurs spectroscopic images obtained at 24 hours after symptom-onset demonstrate localized elevation of lactate levels. The presence of lactate in the infarct indicates anaerobic glycolysis due to ischemia (Duijn *et al.*, 1992). In the chronic stage the infarct is associated with reduced N-acetylaspartate levels, increased choline levels, and absence of lactate (Barker *et al.*, 1994).

On MRI white matter lesions that may represent *subcortical arteriosclerotic encephalopathy* are common findings in elderly patients (Figure 28–16). Lesions are more numerous and more easily recognizable on MRI and frequently also appear larger than on CT. Typical subcortical arteriosclerotic encephalopathy manifests on T_2-weighted images as well defined patches of high signal intensity scattered throughout the white matter with a predilection for the periventricular and subcortical regions, which however on T_1-weighted images are iso- to mildly hypointense. In advanced cases the abnormalities become

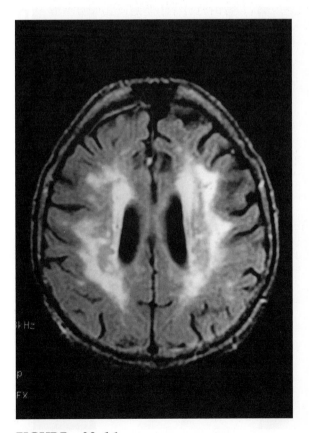

FIGURE   28–16
Subcortical arteriosclerotic encephalopathy. Extensive subcortical lesions and large, confluent periventricular hyperdensities on T_2-weighted MRI.

confluent. Although in the proper clinical setting the described MR findings are likely to represent subcortical arteriosclerotic encephalopathy, they are far from being specific (Caplan, 1995). Similar abnormalities may be seen on MR in elderly patients without apparent cerebrovascular disease. They also occur in several other conditions affecting the white matter, especially *multiple sclerosis*, various toxic and metabolic disorders, disseminated infectious processes, specifically HIV-encephalitis and *progressive multifocal leukoencephalopathy*.

CT and MRI Have Improved the Angiographic Technique

MR angiography (MRA) has been shown to be capable of producing selective images of both the extra- and intracranial vessels. It provides a non-invasive modality for imaging the vasculature. MRA is used in clinical practice as part of the diagnostic work-up of patients with extracranial dissection, arterial occlusive disease, vertebrobasilar ischemia, intracranial aneurysms, vascular malformations, and venous occlusive disease. However, MRA also has its limitations. It consistently overestimates the degree of *stenosis* (Figure 28–17). Rapid and turbulent flow distal to the stenosis itself results in marked dephasing of flowing spins. As a consequence, vascular signal is lost and the extent of the stenosis tends to be exaggerated. MRA technology is still evolving (Atlas, 1994).

Spiral CT opened a new possibility of vascular imaging. The patient is scanned while being drawn through the CT gantry, resulting in the generation of a continuous volume of cross-sectional data. With intravenous injection of contrast medium, 2-D *multiplanar maximal intensity projections* (MIP) and 3-D *shaded surface display images* of the vessels can be produced. *CT angiography* (CTA) can be used to image aneurysm, stenosis or occlusion of intra- and extracranial vessels. The short examination time and clear depiction of arterial lumen in areas of stenosis are significant advantages of CTA compared with MRA. Rotating the vessel in space allows the stenosis to be judged accurately. CTA can show plaque morphology. Calcification within plaques are differentiated from contrast-filled lumen. This is best accomplished through the use of MIP displays (Figure 28–17). Calcium can potentially interfere with the visualization of vascular anatomy. Particularly in older or diabetic patients, plaques may contain calcium, which can obscure the bifurcation. Disadvantages of CTA over other noninvasive imaging techniques, for instance *sonography* and MRA, include the requirement of an intravenous contrast injection and ionizing radiation (Schwartz, 1994).

Only *digital subtraction angiography* (DSA) can depict the status of the extra- and intracranial vessels completely. The improvement in angiographic technique has simplified and reduced the risk of the examination. Catheter technique via femoral artery using non ionic contrast medium is the best method. Biplane high-resolution DSA-equipment should be used (Becker *et al.*, 1991). A fast information of the vessels is obtained biplane without

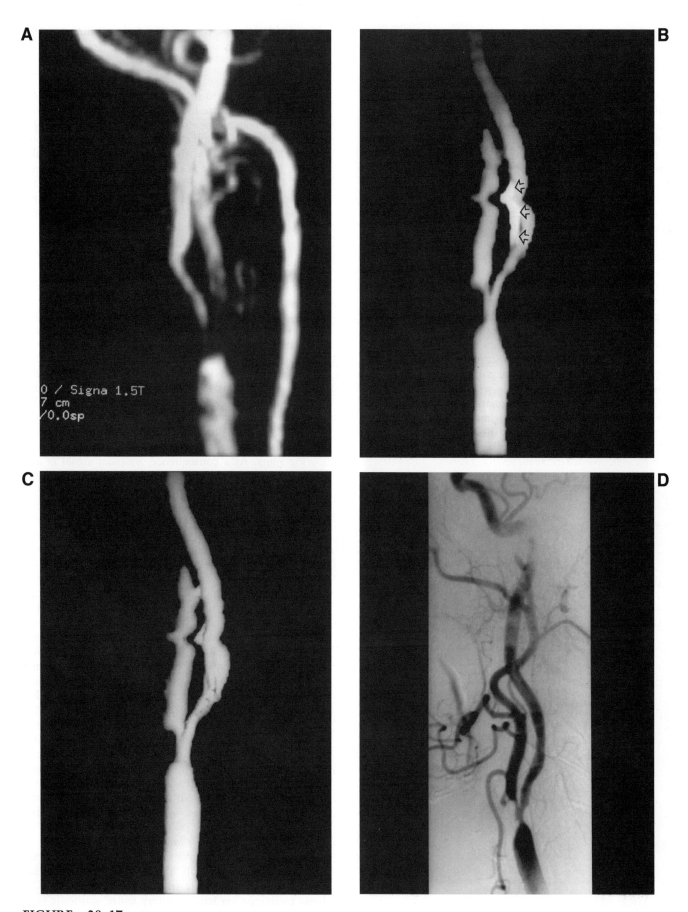

FIGURE   28–17

Stenosis of the carotid bifurcation, as seen with different imaging techniques: **A.** MRA. **B.** CTA: MIP image – note the calcified plaque (arrows) in the internal carotid artery. **C.** CTA: 3-D image. **D.** DSA.

changing the arrangement of the C-arm system. Examination time and consumption of contrast medium can be reduced by half. In the carotid area the most frequent causes of ischemia are emboli originating from arteriosclerotic plaque located prevalently at the carotid bifurcation and in the first segment of the internal carotid artery (Figure 28–17). These plaques have an ulcerative character being the source of emboli. Arteriosclerotic plaques lead to stenosis which can progress to occlusion due to the growth of the plaque or to a secondary thrombus.

Views of the intracranial vessels are also necessary. Peripheral intracranial branch occlusion and delayed washout of contrast medium with evidence of collateral flow to the territory of the involved vessels are the hallmarks of embolic or thrombotic infarction of the brain by angiography.

Arch aortography is also part of the thorough angiographic work-up of ischemic cerebrovascular disease and may increase the safety factor if done first, by showing the proximal vessel orifices through which selective catheterization will ensue.

Angiography should be performed in patients with transient ischemic attacks as soon as possible. In patients with complete stroke the brain parenchyma is already damaged. Since carotid surgery is generally not done in the face of an acute infarction, angiography can be delayed for six weeks after the event, when there is no severe disturbance of the blood-brain-barrier any more. If the patient is seen within the first few hours of the event, however, intraarterial thrombolysis can be indicated, especially in cases of an acute thrombosis of the basilar artery.

Although DSA remains the gold standard for vascular evaluation, risks from the invasive procedures are present, including bleeding, dissection and thromboembolism, especially in elderly patients. It is generally accepted that patients suffering from arteriosclerotic cerebral vascular disease reveal a higher angiographic risk than other patients. It should be recognized, however, that when performed by a neuroradiologist, cerebral angiography is a relatively safe procedure and has, in fact, become much safer with the improvement in equipment, contrast agents, and techniques. Definitive neurological deficits occurred in 0.09 percent, transient deficits were observed in 0.45 percent after selective cerebral intraarterial DSA (Grzyska *et al.*, 1990).

An Overall View

Modern imaging techniques such as CT and MR have revolutionized the study of the aging brain *in vivo*. These techniques are promising because they are noninvasive and provide accurate approaches to structure and function in health and disease. In addition, by providing an *in vivo* chemical analysis, MRI can detect metabolic processes, but *positron emission tomography* (PET) (Chapter 29) is currently more sensitive than MRI for detecting small concentrations of a labeled compound. Although DSA still is the gold standard for evaluation of cervical and cranial vessels, the accurate evaluation using noninvasive techniques remains an important challenge. By combining the different imaging methods we have obtained new insights into the aging processes in the brain, which enabled us to develop therapies to deal with them more adequately.

Selected readings

Brant-Zawadzki, M., Fein, G., Van Dyke, C., Davenport, L., and de Groot, J. 1985. MR imaging of the aging brain: patchy white-matter lesions and dementia. Am. J. Neuroradiol. 6:675–682.

Fukuda, H., Kobayashi, S., Koide, H., *et al.* 1990. Age-related changes in cerebral white matter measured by computed cranial tomography. Comput. Med. Imag. Graph. 14:79–84.

George, A. E., de Leon, M. J., Stylopoulos, L. A., *et al.* 1990. CT diagnostic features of Alzheimer disease: importance of the choroidal/hippocampal fissure complex. Am. J. Neuroradiol. 11:101–107.

George, A. E., de Leon, M. J., Gentes, C. I., *et al.* 1986. Leukoencephalopathy in normal and pathologic aging: 1. CT of brain lucencies. Am. J. Neuroradiol. 7:561–566.

George, A. E., de Leon, M. J., Kalnin, A., *et al.* 1986. Leukoencephalopathy in normal and pathologic aging: 2. MRI of brain lucencies. Am. J. Neuroradiol. 7:567–570.

Golomb, J., de Leon, M. J., Kluger, A., *et al.* 1993. Hippocampal atrophy in normal aging. Arch. Neurol. 50:967–973.

Hendrie, H. C., Farlow, M. R., Austrom, M. G., *et al.* 1989. Foci of increased T2 signal intensity of brain MR scans of healthy elderly subjects. Am. J. Neuroradiol. 10:703–707.

Kobari, M., Meyer, J. S., and Ichijo, M. 1990. Leuko-araiosis, cerebral atrophy, and cerebral perfusion in normal aging. Arch. Neurol. 47:161–165.

Magnaldi, S., Ukmar, M.,Vasciaveo, A., *et al.* 1993. Contrast between white and grey matter: MRI apparearance with ageing. Eur. Radiol. 3:513–519.

Martin, J. H., Brust, J. C. M., and Hilal, S. 1991. Imaging the living brain. In E. R. Kandel, J. H. Schwartz, and T. M. Jessel (eds.) Principles of Neural Science. 3rd Ed., Elsevier, New York and Amsterdam. pp. 309–324.

Meyer, J. S., Takashima, S., Terayama, Y., *et al.* 1994. CT changes associated with normal aging of the human brain. J. Neurol. Sci. 123:200–208.

Moonen, C. T. W., Van Zijl, P. C. M., Frank, J. A., *et al.* 1990. Functional magenetic resonance imaging in medicine and physiology. Sience 250:53–61.

Rosenbusch, G., Oudkerk, M., and Ammann, E. 1995. Radiology in Medical Diagnostics. Blackwell, Oxford.

Rydberg, J. N., Hammond, C. A., Grimm, R. C., *et al.* 1994. Initial clinical experience in MR imaging of the brain with a fast fluid-attenuated inversion-recovery pulse sequence. Radiology 193:173–180.

Sandor, T., Albert, M., Stafford, J., and Kemper, T. 1990. Symmetrical and asymmetrical changes in brain tissue with age as measured on CT scans. Neurobiol. Aging 11:21–27.

Sartor, K. 1992. MR Imaging of the skull and brain. Springer, Berlin.

Wippold II, F. J., Gado, M. H., Morris, J. C., *et al.* 1991. Senile dementia and healthy aging: a longitudinal CT study. Radiology 179:215–219.

References

Aylward, E. H., Brandt, J., Codori, A. M., et al. 1994. Reduced basal ganglia volume associated with the gene for Huntington's disease in asymptomatic at-risk persons. Neurology 44:823–828.

Artmann, H., v. Gall, M., Hacker, H., and Herrlich, J. 1981. Reversible enlargement of cerebral spinal fluid spaces in chronic alcoholics. Am. J. Neuroradiol. 2:23–27.

Atlas, S. W. 1994. MR angiography in neurologic disease. Radiology 193:1–16.

Awad, I. A., Spetzler, R. F., Hodak, J. A., Awad, C. A., and Carey, R. 1986. Incidental subcortical lesions identified on magnetic resonance imaging in the elderly. I. correlation with age and cerebrovascular risk factors. Stroke 17:1084–1089.

Awad, I. A., Johnson, P. C., Spetzler, R. F., and Hodak, J. A. 1986. Incidental subcortical lesions identified on magnetic resonance in the elderly. II. postmortem pathological correlations. Stroke 17:1090–1097.

Barboriak, D. P., Provenzale, J. M., and Boyko, O. B. 1994. MR diagnosis of Creutzfeldt-Jacob disease: significance of high signal intensity of the basal ganglia. Am. J. Neuroradiol. 162:137–140.

Barker, P. B., Gillard, J. H., van Zijl, P. C. M., et al. 1994. Acute stroke: evaluation with serial proton MR spectroscopic imaging. Radiology 192:723–732.

Becker, H., Grau, H., and Hacker, H. 1977. Endokranielle Verkalkungen in der Computer-Tomographie – Ein Vergleich zum Röntgenbild. Fortschr. Röntgenstr. 126:509–512.

Becker, H., Desch, H., Hacker, H., and Pencz, A. 1979. CT fogging effect with ischemic cerebral infarcts. Neuroradiology 18:185–192.

Becker, H., Schneider, E., Hacker, H., and Fischer, P.-A. 1979. Cerebral atrophy in Parkinson's disease – represented in CT. Arch. Psychiatr. Nervenkr. 227:81–88.

Becker, H., and Brassel, F. 1991. 2 Ebenen DSA für die diagnostische und interventionelle Neuroradiologie. Klin. Neuroradiol. 1:229–236.

Becker, T., Hofmann, E., Struck, M., et al. 1992. Marchiafava-Bignami-Syndrom: CT- und MR-Befunde in einem atypischen Fall. Klin. Neuroradiol. 2:24–27.

Block, W., Träber, F., Kuhl, C. K., et al. 1995. 1H-MR-Spektroskopische Bildgebung bei Patienten mit klinisch gesichertem Morbus Alzheimer. Fortschr. Röntgenstr. 163:230–237.

Bowen, B. C., Barker, W. W., Loewenstein, D. A., Sheldon, J., and Duara, R. 1990. MR signal abnormalities in memory disorder and dementia. Am. J. Neuroradiol. 11:283–290.

Bradley, W. G. Jr., Whittemore, A. R., Watanabe, A. S., et al. 1991. Association of deep white matter infarction with chronic communicating hydrocephalus: implication regarding the possible origin of normal-pressure hydrocephalus. Am. J. Neuroradiol. 12:31–39.

Braffman, B. H., Zimmerman, R. A., Trojanowski, J. Q., et al. 1988. Brain MR: pathologic correlation with gross and histopathology. 2. Hyperintense white-matter foci in the elderly. Am. J. Neuroradiol. 9:629–636.

Braffman, B. H., Grossman, R. I., Goldberg, H. I., et al. 1988. MR imaging of Parkinson disease with spin-echo and gradient-echo sequences. Am. J. Neuroradiol. 9:1093–1099.

Braffman, B. H. 1993. Invecchiamento cerebrale e patologia neurodegenerativa. Rivista di Neuroradiologia 6 (Suppl.1):121–134.

Caplan, L. R. 1995. Binswanger's disease – revisited. Neurology 45:626–633.

Chang, K. H., Cha, S. H., Han, M. H., et al. 1992. Marchiafa-va-Bignami disease: serial changes in corpus callosum on MRI. Neuroradiology 34:480–482.

Coffey, C. E., Wilkinson, W. E., Parashos, I. A., et al. 1992. Quantitative cerebral anatomy of the aging human brain. Neurology 42:527–536.

DeCarli, C., Kaye, J. A., Horwitz, B., and Rapoport, S. I. 1990. Critical analysis of the use of computer-assisted transverse axial tomography to study human brain in aging and dementia of the Alzheimer type. Neurology 4:872–883.

DeLeon, M. J., George, A. E., Reisberg, B., et al. 1989. Alzheimer's disease: longitudinal CT studies of ventricular change. Am. J. Roentgenol. 152:1257–1262.

DeLeon, M. J., George, A. E., Stylopoulos, L. A., et al. 1989. Early marker for Alzheimer's disease: the atrophic hippocampus. Lancet 2:672–673.

Di Chiro, G., and Libow, L. S. 1971. Carotid siphon calcification and cerebral blood flow in the healthy aged male. Radiology 99:103–107.

Drayer, B. P. 1988. Imaging of the aging brain. Part II. pathological conditions. Radiology 166:797–806.

Duijn, J. H., Matson, G. B., Maudsley, A. A., et al. 1992. Human brain infarction: proton MR spectroscopy. Radiology 183:711–718.

Elster, A. D. 1993. MR imaging of cerebral infarction: patterns of contrast enhancement. Advances in MRI Contrast 2:2–12.

Fazekas, F., Chawluk, J. B., Alavi, A., Hurtig, H. I., and Zimmerman, R. A. 1987. MR signal abnormalities at 1.5 T in Alzheimer's dementia and normal aging. Am. J. Neuroradiol. 8:421–426.

Friedman, D. P., and Tartaglino, L. M. 1993. Amyotrophic lateral sclerosis: hyperintensity of the corticospinal tracts on MR images of the spinal cord. Am. J. Roentgenol. 160:604–606.

Gallucci, M., Amicarelli, I., Rossi, A., et al. 1989. MR imaging of white matter lesions in uncomplicated chronic alcoholism. J. Comput. Assist. Tomogr. 13:395–398.

Galluci, M., Bozzao, A., Splendiani, A., Masciocchi, C., and Passariello, R. 1990. Wernicke encephalopathy: MR findings in five patients. Am. J. Neuroradiol. 11:887–892.

Gertz, H. J., Henkes, H., and Cervós-Navarro, J. C. 1988. Creutzfeldt-Jacob disease: correlation of MRI and neuropathologic findings. Neurology 38:1481–1482.

Gorelick, P. B. 1993. Distribution of atherosclerotic cerebrovascular lesions. Stroke (Suppl.I) 24:I-16- I-19.

Groen, J.J., and Hekster, R. E. M. 1982. Computed tomography in Pick's disease: findings in a family affected in three consecutive generations. J. Comput. Assist. Tomogr. 6:907–911.

Grzyska, V., Freitag, J., and Zeumer, H. 1990. Selective arterial intracerebral DSA: complication rate and control of risk factors. Neuroradiology 32:296–299.

Hachinski, V. C., Potter, P., and Merskey, H. 1987. Leuko-araiosis. Arch. Neurol. 44:21–33.

Handa, N., Matsumoto, M., Maeda, H., et al. 1990. Ultrasonic evaluation of early carotid atherosclerosis. Stroke 21:1567–1572.

Hentschel, F., Zerfaß, R., and Förstl, H. 1995. Morphometrische Unterschiede im kranialen Computertomogramm zwischen Patienten mit Alzheimer-Demenz und normalem Altern. Klin. Neuroradiol. 5:61–70.

Hirai, T., Korogi, Y., Sakamoto, Y. et al. 1996. T_2 shortening in the motor cortex: Effect of aging and cerebrovascular disease. Radiology 199:799–803.

Hofmann, E., Friedburg, H., Raseneck, J., Ott, D., and Wimmer, B. 1988. Die Wernicke-Enzephalopathie im CT und MR. Fortschr. Röntgenstr. 148:97–98.

Holtas, S. 1993. The role of CT and MRI in ischemic lesions. Rivista di Neuroradiologia 6 (Suppl. 2):85–91.

Huber, S. J., Chakeres, D. W., Paulson, G. W., and Khanna, R. 1990. Magnetic resonance imaging in Parkinson's disease. Arch. Neurol. 47:735–737.

Ishida, S., Sugino, M., Koizumi, N., et al. 1995. Serial MRI in early Creutzfeldt-Jacob disease with a point mutation of prion protein at codon 180. Neuroradiology 37:531–534.

Jack, C. R. Jr., Petersen, R. C., O'Brien, P. C., and Tangalos, E. G. 1992. MR-based hippocampal volumetry in the diagnosis of Alzheimer's disease. Neurology 42:183–188.

Jack, C. R. Jr., Bomey, C. K., and Zinsmeister, A. R. 1990. MR imaging-based volume measurements of the hippocampal formation and anterior lobe: validation studies. Radiology 176:205–209.

Jack, C. R. Jr., Mokri, B., Laws, E. R., et al. 1987. MR findings in normal pressure hydrocephalus: significance and comparison with other forms of dementia. J. Comput. Assist. Tomogr. 11:923–931.

Janick, P. A., Hackney, D. B., Grossman, R. I., and Asakura, T. 1991. MR imaging of various oxidation states of intracellular and extracellular hemoglobin. Am. J. Neuroradiol. 12:891–897.

Katada, K., Kanno, T., Sano, H., Shinomiya, Y., and Koga, S. 1983. Calcification of the vertebral artery. AJNR 4:450–453.

Kido, D. K., Caine, E. D., Le May, M., et al. 1989. Temporal lobe atrophy in patients with Alzheimer disease: a CT study. Am. J. Neuroradiol. 10:551–555.

Kitaguchi, T., Kobayashi, T., Tobimatsu, S., Goto, I., and Kuroiwa, Y. 1987. Computed tomography and magnetic resonance imaging in a young patient with Wernicke's encephalopathy. J. Neurol. 234:449–450.

Knopman, D. S., Christensen, K. J., Harbaugh, R. E., et al. 1989. The spectrum of imaging and neuropsychological findings in Pick's disease. Neurology 39:362–368.

Koch, K. J., and Smith, R. R. 1989. Gd-DTPA enhancement in MR imaging of central pontine myelinolysis. Am. J. Neuroradiol. 10:58.

Krüger, H., Meesmann, C., Rohrbach, E., Müller, J., and Mertens, H. G. 1990. Panencephalopathic type of Creutzfeldt-Jacob disease with primary extensive involvement of the white matter. Eur. Neurol. 30:115–119.

Kucharczyk, J., Vexler, Z. S., Roberts, T. P., et al. 1993. Echoplanar perfusion-sensitive MR imaging of acute cerebral ischemia. Radiology 188:711–717.

LeMay, M. 1984. Radiologic changes of the aging brain and skull. Am. J. Neuroradiol. 5:269–275.

Meguro, K., Yamaguchi, T., Hishinuma, T., et al. 1993. Periventricular hyperintensity on magnetic resonance imaging with brain ageing and atrophy. Neuroradiology 35:125–129.

Miller, G. M., Baker, H. L., Okazaki, H., and Whisnant, J. P. 1988. Central pontine myelinolysis and its imitators: MR findings. Radiology 168:795–802.

Milton, W. J., Atlas, S. W., Lavi, E., and Mollman, J. E. 1991. Magnetic resonance imaging of Creutzfeldt-Jacob disease. Ann. Neurol. 29:438–440.

Oba, H., Araki, T., Ohtomo, K., et al. 1993. Amyotrophic lateral sclerosis: T_2 shortening in motor cortex at MR imaging. Radiology 189:843–846.

Ogawa, T., Okudera, T., Hashimoto, M., et al. 1995. Unusual widening of Virchow-Robin-spaces: MR appearance. Am. J. Neuroradiol. 16:1238–1242.

Osterthun, B., Dewes, W., Hanisch, E., and Harder, T. 1990. MR-Tomographie und Computertomographie von alkoholtoxischen Hirngewebsveränderungen. Fortschr. Röntgenstr. 152:87–90.

Rao, C. V. G. K., Brennan, T. G., and Garcia, J. H. 1977. Computed tomography in the diagnosis of Creutzfeldt-Jacob disease. J. Comput. Assist. Tomogr. 1:211–215.

Rusinek, H., de Leon, M. J., George, A. E., et al. 1991. Alzheimer disease: measuring loss of cerebral gray matter with MR imaging. Radiology 178:109–114.

Savoiardo, M., Strada, L., Girotti, F., et al. 1989. MR imaging in progressive supranuclear palsy and Shy-Drager syndrome. J. Comput. Assist. Tomogr. 13:555–560.

Savoiardo, M., Strada, L., Oliva, D., Girotti, F., and D'Incerti, L. 1991. Abnormal MRI signal in the rigid form of Huntington's disease. J. Neuro. Neurosurg. Psychiatry 54:888–891.

Schenker, C., Meier, D., Wichmann, W., Boesiger, P., and Valavanis, A. 1993. Age distribution and iron dependency of the T_2 relaxation time in the globus pallidus and putamen. Neuroradiology 35:119–124.

Schroth, G., Naegele, T., Klose, U., Mann, K., and Petersen, D. 1988. Reversible brain shrinkage in abstinent alcoholics, measured by MRI. Neuroradiology 30:385–389.

Schroth, G., Wichmann, W., and Valavanis, A. 1991. Blood-brain-barrier disruption in acute Wernicke encephalopathy: MR findings. J. Comput. Assist. Tomogr. 15:1059–1061.

Schroth, G., and Klose, U. 1992. Cerebrospinal fluid flow, III: pathological cerebrospinal fluid pulsations. Neuroradiology 35:16–24.

Schwartz, R. B. 1994. Neuroradiological applications of spiral CT. Seminars in Ultrasound, CT, and MRI, 15:139–147.

Sherman, J. L., Clawson, L. L., Citrin, C. M., et al. 1987. MR evaluation of amyotrophic lateral sclerosis (ALS). Am. J. Neuroradiol. 8:941.

Simmons, J. T., Pastakia, B., Chase, T. N., and Shults, C. W. 1986. Magnetic resonance imaging in Huntingon disease. Am. J. Neuroradiol. 7:25–28.

Spielman, D., Butts, K., de Crespigny, A., and Moseley, M. E. 1995. Diffusion-weighted imaging of clinical stroke. Int. J. Neuroradiol. 1:44–55.

Sze, G., De Armond, S. J., Brant-Zawadzki, M., et al. 1986. Foci of MRI signal (pseudo lesions) anterior to the frontal horns: histologic correlations of a normal finding. Am. J. Neuroradiol. 7:381–387.

Uchino, A., Yoshinaga, M., Shiokawa, O., Hata, H., and Ohno, M. 1991. Serial MR imaging in Creutzfeldt-Jacob disease. Neuroradiology 33:364–367.

Verny, M., Duyckaerts, C., Pierot, L., and Hauw, J.-J. 1991. Leuko-Araiosis. Dev. Neurosci. 13:245–250.

von Kummer, R., Bozzao, L., and Manelfe, C. 1995. Early CT diagnosis of hemispheric brain infarction. Springer, Berlin.

Yokote, K., Miyagi, K., Kuzuhara, S. Yamanouchi, H., and Yamada, Y. 1991. Wernicke encephalopathy: follow-up study by CT and MR. J. Comput. Assist. Tomogr. 15:835–838.

Zeumer, H., Schonsky, B., and Sturm, K. W. 1980. Predominant white matter involvement in subcortical arteriosclerotic encephalopathy (Binswanger disease). J. Comput. Assist. Tomogr. 4:14–19.

Zieger, A., Vonofakos, D., and Gräfin Vitzthum, H. 1981. Creutzfeldt-Jakobsche Krankheit: Das Computertomogram in Korrelation zu klinischen, elektroenzephalographischen und neuropathologischen Befunden. Nervenarzt 52:685–691.

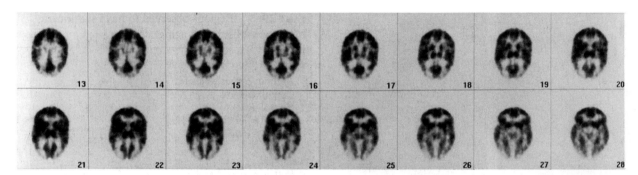

FIGURE 29–4

This figure shows multiple transaxial FDG-PET images of a normal elderly subject. The images extend from the frontal-parietal region (top left) to the temporal region (bottom right). Of note is decreased activity in the frontal regions compared to the parietal regions in all planes. The visual cortex is prominent and symmetric. (Reprinted with permission from Loessner *et al.*, 1995.)

It appears that there are no significant differences between men and women with regard to regional cerebral glucose metabolism (Miura *et al.*, 1990). Furthermore, there has been no report of differences between the sexes in cerebral metabolism with advancing age (Loessner *et al.*, 1995). The lack of difference in cerebral metabolism is interesting given the observed structural differences between males and females. A study by Gur and colleagues (1991) indicated that there is significantly increased cerebrospinal fluid volumes in elderly males compared to elderly females (Gur *et al.*, 1991).

While the initial studies showed a decrease in cerebral glucose metabolism with increasing age, it was thought that this finding might be related to the rate with which the radiopharmaceutical, fluorodeoxyglucose, is transported into the brain or is phosphorylated once inside the neurons. However, several reports (Kuhl *et al.*, 1984; Hawkins *et al.*, 1983) showed that the decrease in cerebral metabolism was not related to these rate constants. Thus, the decrease in FDG uptake correlated with an actual decrease in brain metabolism.

Dastur (1985) reported no difference in the global cerebral metabolic rate of oxygen ($CMRO_2$) with normal aging. However, PET studies using the ^{15}O inhalation method have found decreases in $CMRO_2$ in the gray matter with increasing age (Pantano *et al.*, 1984; Yamaguchi *et al.*, 1986). Similarly, a significant decrease in the mean $CMRO_2$ has been observed in subjects over age 51 years compared to subjects under 50 years of age (Takada *et al.*, 1992). Particular areas found to have a significant decrease in oxygen metabolism with age were the putamen bilaterally, the left supratemporal, left infrafrontal, and left parietal cortices. As described above, decreases in cerebral blood flow have been observed in normal aging. Other studies have not found a significant decrease in blood flow with aging (Takada *et al.*, 1992) or have found that the decreases could not account for the extent of the decreased oxygen metabolism (Frackowiak and Gibbs, 1983). It has been hypothesized that oxygen extraction increases with age which partly compensates for the observed decrease in cerebral blood flow. This maintains the oxygen metabolic rate at a higher level than would be ex-

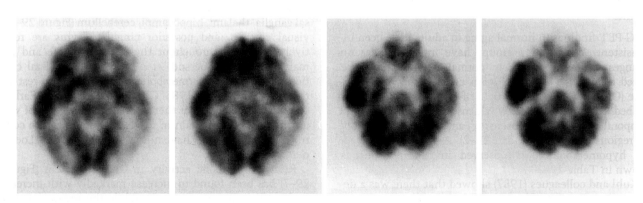

FIGURE 29–5

FDG-PET images at the level of the upper and middle temporal lobes show mild asymmetry in the metabolic activity of the cerebral hemispheres. The left temporal lobe is less active than the right which is found consistently through all ages of subjects. (Reprinted with permission from Loessner *et al.*, 1995.)

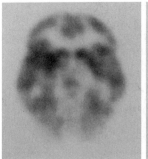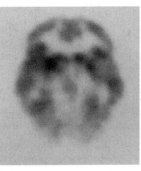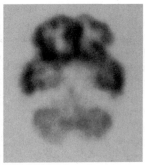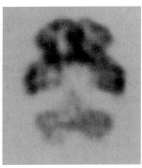

FIGURE   29–6

FDG-PET images at the level of the temporal lobe and cerebellum have occasionally shown marked hypometabolism in the cerebellum. This is infrequently found in normal subjects and has an unknown etiology. (Reprinted with permission from Loessner *et al.*, 1995.)

pected if oxygen extraction remained constant or decreased with aging (Frackowiak and Gibbs, 1983).

One concern regarding the accuracy of PET studies involves the effects of age-related brain atrophy on the measurement of cerebral metabolism. The problem is that the resolution of PET causes averaging of signals from the brain tissue and inactive CSF spaces. Therefore, if a subject has marked atrophy, measured mean cerebral metabolism by PET would appear lower than real values. Several reports have appeared in the literature which deal with normal aging and brain volume using MR imaging. Tanna and colleagues (1991) measured absolute ventricular and sulcal volumes in healthy elderly subjects and correlated these volumes with age. The best correlations were seen between age and ventricular volumes, and age and total brain volumes. Sulcal volumes correlated less well with age. As described above, Gur and colleagues studied the relation of gender differences in the effect of age on brain atrophy using the same methodology. Healthy males had larger brain and CSF volumes compared to age-matched females. Age correlated with decreasing brain and increasing CSF volumes with steeper regression slopes in males compared to females, suggesting more atrophy with age in males. The greatest degree of atrophy in elderly men occurred in the left hemispheres while women had symmetrical changes.

Since brain atrophy might account for a reduction in cerebral metabolism, it has been suggested that changes in brain volume need to be accounted for when considering the results from PET (Clark *et al.*, 1987; Schlageter *et al.*, 1987). While atrophy correction of cerebral metabolism has been done in patients with Alzheimer disease and other types of dementia, it has not been done as part of a study of normal aging. However, while both CT and MRI studies have found marked atrophy in the frontal lobes during aging (Wahlund *et al.*, 1990; Pfefferbaum *et al.*, 1990; Chawluk *et al.*, 1990), it is unclear whether this atrophy accounts for the hypometabolism in the frontal region that is associated with normal aging (Chawluk *et al.*, 1990).

The results obtained with atrophy correction in various types of dementia must also be considered with regard to normal aging. In several studies in which Alzheimer dementia (AD), multi-infarct dementia (MID), and *primary progressive aphasia* (PPA), the actual changes in cerebral metabolism when corrected for atrophy yielded different information regarding the metabolic nature of the dementia. For example, in patients with AD, several studies have shown that while whole brain metabolism is significantly reduced compared to age-matched controls, this decrease is not significant when the metabolic rates are corrected for atrophy (Alavi *et al.*, 1993; Tanna *et al.*, 1991). Thus, in AD, it appears that the hypometabolism is related to the absence of brain tissue while the existing brain tissue has a metabolism comparable to controls. The same appears to be true in subjects with primary progressive aphasia (PPA). These subjects, who suffer from a slowly progressive aphasia without signs of a generalized dementia, have significant hypometabolism throughout the left hemisphere and particularly in the temporal lobe

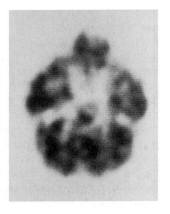

FIGURE   29–7

FDG-PET images of normal aging show moderate uptake in the brainstem which is anterior to the cerebellum. The cerebellum is noted to have similar tracer uptake compared to the temporal lobes. (Reprinted with permission from Loessner *et al.*, 1995.)

where the language center exists. As in AD patients, the PPA patients have cerebral metabolic rates in both hemispheres similar to that of controls once corrected for atrophy (Newberg et al., 1992). MID patients, on the other hand, have been found to have significant whole brain hypometabolism compared to age-matched controls even after atrophy correction (Alavi et al., 1992). Thus, MID patients have cerebral hypometabolism that is out of proportion to brain atrophy. This suggests that the process leading to dementia in MID patients is metabolically different than that in AD.

Yoshii and colleagues (1988) used a large number of healthy volunteers to determine the effects of gender, age, brain volume, and cerebrovascular risk factors on CMRGlc values as determined by the FDG-PET method. When brain atrophy was not considered, mean CMRGlc values were lower in older patients, particularly in the frontal, parietal, and temporal regions. Also women had significantly higher mean CMRGlc than men. When covariate analysis was used to account for brain atrophy, since brain volume was highly correlated with age, the effects of age and gender on CMRGlc were no longer significant. Cerebrovascular risk factors in this population did not have any effect on CMRGlc. Brain atrophy accounted for only 21 percent of the variance in CMRGlc.

Neurotransmitter Function with Age can be Studied Using PET and SPECT in a Large Number of Neurotransmitter Systems

In addition to measuring changes in cerebral blood flow and metabolism with age, both PET and SPECT can measure neurotransmitter activity, which may also change with age. A large number of neurotransmitter systems can be studied using PET and SPECT (see Tables 29–1 and 29–2). There have been only a limited number of reports utilizing neurotransmitter analogues in the study of the aging brain.

The nigrostriatal dopaminergic pathways have been studied with both PET and SPECT imaging. This pathway is important with regards to extrapyramidal symptoms that occur in the elderly. This system also has particular significance in the study of Parkinson disease (Chapter 32). Changes in both D_2 and D_1 receptors levels with age have been studied in vitro (Rinne, 1987, 1990; Morgan et al., 1987). D_2 receptor levels have been generally shown to decrease with age. However, studies measuring D_1 receptor numbers have found inconsistent results with some suggesting a decrease, some no change, and some an increase with age. The results from neuroimaging studies, which can measure the dopaminergic pathway in vivo, have also been inconsistent.

Several PET studies have shown that the uptake of [^{18}F]-fluorodopa (FD) decreases with age. Cordes and coworkers (1994) found a 21 percent decrease in FD uptake when comparing the uptake in grandparents (ages range from 70 to 80 years) to that in their grandchildren (ages range from 18 to 29 years). This study corroborates earlier studies by the same group which indicated similar decreases in FD uptake with age (Bhatt et al., 1991; W. Martin et al., 1989). Further, the authors suggest that this decrease is consistent with the decline in the number of nigral dopaminergic neurons with age. In fact the average decrease per year of 0.35 percent in FD uptake is similar to the mean decrease in nigral neurons of 0.6 percent per year (McGeer et al., 1977; Gibb and Lees, 1991). Other studies have not found a decrease in FD uptake with age (Sawle et al., 1990; Eidelberg et al., 1993). This inconsistency may be related to the relatively small number of subjects in each study and how regions of interest (ROIs) were drawn. For example, in a related study, ROIs that span the entire striatum showed a relationship of FD uptake to age while small ROIs did not yield the same correlation (Vingerhoets et al., 1994). Several PET studies using a different radiopharmaceutical, [^{11}C] raclopride which binds to post-synaptic D_2 receptor sites, found a decrease in receptor density (Rinne et al., 1993; Antonini and Leenders, 1993). Antonini and Leenders reported that after 30 years of age, there was a 0.6 percent decline per year in raclopride binding. D_1 receptor density has also been found to decrease with age using PET imaging (Suhara et al., 1991).

Radioligands that can measure the dopamine transporter system that removes dopamine from the neuronal synapse into the terminal for storage have also been developed. One PET study by Tedroff and colleagues (1988) showed a decline with age of the dopamine transporter using [^{11}C] nomifensine.

SPECT studies have also been utilized to measure changes in the dopaminergic system with age. A study by Woda and associates (1992) measured the age-related changes in IBZM uptake (a D_2 receptor agonist). The results indicated that with increasing age, there was a significant decrease in the basal ganglia to cerebellum uptake ratio. However, there was no correlation between age and the uptake ratio between the basal ganglia and either the frontal, parietal, or occipital lobes. Another study, using the cocaine analog 2βcarbomethoxy-3β-(4-iodophenyl)tropane (β-CIT), indicated an age related decrease in β-CIT uptake of approximately 8 percent per decade from the age of 18 (van Dyck et al., 1995). This decrease likely reflects a decrease in the activity of the dopamine transporter with age. Specifically, this decrease may result from a loss of dopaminergic nerve terminals rather than a 'downregulation' of the dopamine transporter. However, β-CIT has also been found to have a high affinity for the serotonin transporter. Thus, the decrease in uptake must be distinguished between the dopamine and serotonin transporters. Fortunately, in the striatum, the dopamine transporter has been found to be almost exclusively responsible for β-CIT uptake. Furthermore, in vitro studies have shown that the serotonin transporter density is relatively preserved with increasing age (Severson et al., 1987).

Given the list of radioligands available for both PET and SPECT imaging (see Table 29–1 and 29–2), it seems that these techniques may have vast applications in the study of the neurotransmitter effects that result from normal aging. Several studies have been mentioned above, but there remains a significant amount of neurotransmitter systems which have yet to be explored.

Amino Acid Transport

Neutral amino acids (NAAs) are transported across the blood-brain barrier (BBB) via a competitve carrier system. Using positron emitting labeled NAA analogs, investigators have been able to measure the NAA transport across the BBB with PET imaging.

PET imaging with $[^{11}C]$ l-methionine in pediatric patients showed increased transfer of the amino acid across the blood-brain barrier compared to adults (O'Tuama *et al.*, 1991). This finding suggests that during developmental periods, the brain allows for a greater influx of amino acids. Thus, PET might be useful in the study of various inborn errors of metabolism. Preliminary studies of disorders such as adrenoleukodystrophy (Volkow *et al.*, 1987), mitochondrial disorders (Frackowiak *et al.*, 1988), and adenylosuccinase deficiency (DeVolder *et al.*, 1988) have been initiated by various groups which may yield interesting results.

In adults, O'Tuama and colleagues (1991) used $[^{11}C]$ l-methionine to study amino acid transport changes with normal aging. They found a decrease in amino acid transport with increasing age. The frontal lobes were found to be particularly affected. Unfortunately, the labeling of natural amino acids with positron emitting isotopes has been found to reduce the accuracy of the kinetic rate to be measured with this technique. Koeppe and colleagues (1990) found no significant decrease in uptake of the synthetic amino acid $[^{11}C]$-*aminocyclohexanecarboxylate* (ACHC). This may more accurately reflect amino acid transport since ACHC is not metabolized in the brain and allows for simplification of kinetic models. A PET study by Ito and colleagues (1995) using L-(2-^{18}F)-fluorophenylalanine (^{18}F-Phe) corroborated the findings with ACHC such that there was no observed decrease in amino acid uptake in the brain with increasing age. Interestingly, they found an increase with aging in the rate constant for the transport of ^{18}F-Phe from the brain to the blood. This may indicate decreased competition between ^{18}F-Phe and natural amino acids due to a decreased concentration of intracellular amino acids.

Biochemical Changes that Occur in the Aging Brain can be Studied by Magnetic Resonance Spectroscopy

MR spectroscopy has had limited use in the study of biochemical changes with aging. This technique uses the magnetic spin of various biologically active isotopes such as ^{1}H, ^{13}C, and ^{31}P to measure the concentration of these isotopes and the related molecules. Specifically, ^{1}H MRS can be used to study the concentrations of various molecules such as amino acids, creatine, myo-inositol, lactate, etc. ^{31}P MRS can detect the concentrations of various phosphate containing molecules such as ATP, ADP, and AMP. Initial *in vivo* findings have indicated a decreased level of phosphomonoesters (PMEs) and an increased level of phosphodiesters (PDEs) with normal aging. This finding is consistent with the loss of neuritic processes associated with aging (McClure *et al.*, 1995). MRS is now used in the study of various neurodegenerative disorders such as Alzheimer disease, but MRS may also play a larger role in the study of the biochemical changes that occur in the brain during normal aging.

An Overall View

Functional imaging using SPECT and PET have provided detailed *in vivo* measurements of cerebral biochemical changes that occur with aging. Alterations have been noted in cerebral blood flow, glucose and oxygen metabolism, neurotransmitter concentrations, and amino acid metabolism. Additional studies will be needed as newer techniques become available such as functional MRI. Further, functional neuroimaging is an important complementary tool to *in vitro* studies in the measurement of the biochemical activity of the human brain. Functional neuroimaging may also be able to measure the effects of various pharmacological and non-pharmacological interventions to modify and decelerate the aging process. Thus, functional neuroimaging will play a key role as a powerful research modality to study the biochemical changes that occur in the human brain with aging.

Selected Readings

Alavi, A. 1989. The aging brain. J. Neuropsychiatry 1 (suppl.):S51–S56.

Alavi, A., and Hirsch, L. J. 1991. Studies of central nervous system disorders with single photon emission computed tomography and positron emission tomography. Evolution over the past 2 decades. Semin. Nucl. Med. 21:58–81.

Altman, D. I., and Volpe, J. J. 1991. Positron emission tomography in newborn infants. Clin. Perinatol. 18:549–562.

Baron, J. 1992. PET studies of neuroreceptors in the human frontal cortex. Adv. Neurol. 57:465–470.

Chawluk, J. B., Alavi, A., Dann, R., *et al.* 1987. Positron emission tomography in aging and dementia. Effect of cerebral atrophy. J. Nucl. Med. 28:431–437.

Chugani, H. T., Phelps, M. E., and Mazziotta, J. C. 1987. Positron emission tomography study of human brain functional development. Ann. Neurol. 22:487.

Chugani, H. T., and Phelps, M. E. 1986. Maturational changes in cerebral function in infants determined by [18]FDG positron emission tomography. Science 231:840.

Cordes, M., Snow, B. J., Cooper, S., *et al.* 1994. Age-dependent decline of nigrostriatal dopaminergic function: A positron emission tomographic study of grandparents and their grandchildren. Ann. Neurol. 36:667–670.

DeLeon, M., George, A., Tomanelli, J., *et al.* 1987. Positron emission tomography studies of normal aging, a replication of PET III and 18-FDG using PET IV and II-CDG. Neurobiol. Aging 8:319–323.

Fazekas, F., Alavi, A., Chawluk, J. B., *et al.* 1989. Comparison of CT, MR and PET in Alzheimer's dementia and normal aging. J. Nucl. Med. 30:1607–1615.

Fazekas, F., Chawluk, J. B., Alavi, A., *et al.* 1987. MR signal ab-

phy: the effects of age and Parkinson's disease. Acta Neurol. Scand. 77:192–201.

Ter-Pogossian, M. M., Phelps, M. E., Hoffman, E. J. et al. 1975. A positron emission transaxial tomography for nuclear medicine imaging (PET). Radiology 114:89–98.

The Workshop Panel. 1990. Advances in clinical imaging using positron emission tomography. National Cancer Institute Workshop Statement. Arch. Intern. Med. 150:735–739.

Therapeutic and Technology Assessment Subcommittee of the American Academy of Neurology. 1991. Assessment. positron emission tomography. Neurology 41:163–167.

van Dyck, C. H., Seibyl, J. P., Malison, R. T., et al. 1995. Age-related decline in striatal dopamine transporter binding with iodine-123-β-CIT SPECT. J. Nucl. Med. 36:1175–1181.

Vingerhoets, F. J. G., Snow, B. J., Schulzer, M. J., et al. 1994. Reproducibility of fluorine-18-6-fluorodopa positron emission tomography in normal human subjects. J. Nucl. Med. 35:18–24.

Volkow, N. D., Patchell, L., Kulharni, M. C., et al. 1987. Adrenoleukodystrophy: Imaging with CT, MRI, and PET. J. Nucl. Med. 28:254.

Wahlund, L. O., Agartz, I., Almqvist, O., et al. 1990. The brain in healthy aged individuals. MR imaging. Radiology 174:675–679.

Waldemar, G., Hasselbalch, S. G., Andersen, A. R., et al. 1991. 99mTc-d,l-HMPAO and SPECT of the brain in normal aging. J. Cereb. Blood Flow Metab. 11:508–21.

Woda, A., Alavi, A., Mozley, D., and Galloway, S. 1992. Effects of age on dopamine receptors as measured with SPECT and IBZM. J. Nucl. Med. 33:897 (abstract).

Yamaguchi, T., Kanno, I., Nemura, K., et al. 1986. Reduction in regional cerebral metabolic rate of oxygen during human aging. Stroke 17:1220.

Yoshii, F., Barker, W. W., Chang, J. Y., et al. 1988. Sensitivity of cerebral glucose metabolism to age, gender, brain volume, brain atrophy, and cerebrovascular risk factors. J. Cereb. Blood Flow Metab. 8:654–661.

Akira Hori

Aging in Childhood

Precocious aging is known as *progeria* (Latin *pro-*, before + Greek *geras*, old age). The term *progeria* is misleading, as pointed out by Hall and Denneny (1993), because the reported cases of progeria have not manifested most physical or biochemical aspects of old age. Yet, some of the progeroid aspects are indeed similar to normal aging, therefore the study of progeria is instructive for the understanding of aging.

In this chapter, the literature is reviewed on *progeric syndromes*, symptoms, and further elementary degenerative processes (usually observed in senile neurodegenerative conditions such as Alzheimer disease, thus 'Alzheimerization'), affecting neonates, infants, children and young adults.

Progeric Syndromes are Mesodermal Disorders

The terms progeria or progeric syndromes are used in this chapter indicating the syndromes of Wiedemann-Rautenstrauch, Hutchinson-Gilford, and Werner.

Congenital or Neonatal Progeria (Wiedemann-Rautenstrauch Syndrome)

Wiedemann-Rautenstrauch syndrome is a congenital or neonatal type of progeroid anomaly originally reported by Rautenstrauch in 1977, and by Wiedemann in 1979. Up to now less than 20 cases have been recorded in the literature. The majority of children were born later than term or at term. Babies with progeroid face already have incisors at birth although dentition is generally delayed and deficient; the patients are small for date and show slow growth rate. The following features are noted: hydrocephaloid skull, widely open suture and persistent open fontanels, reduced ossification of calvarium, scarce scalp hair, prominent scalp veins, diminution of subcutaneous fat (paradoxical cushions of subcutaneous fat in the finger joints) and dysplastic skin. In the majority of cases, mental retardation is present. One case showed elevated maternal serum alpha-fetoprotein in the 16th gestational week (Hagadorn *et al.*, 1990); this child additionally manifested congenital heart defects and urinary reflux.

Rautenstrauch and colleagues (1994) followed up a patient to the age of 16 years. The stigmata were unchanged. In addition to a psychomotor retardation, considerable atactic movement developed. The metabolic anomaly of proteoglycan, remarkable in infancy, was no longer detectable. There was no description of *dementia* (= *deterioration* of mental ability in contrast to *retardation*), and the child was apparently able to write a friendly letter to the doctor (though very atactic), as illustrated in the original report. Rudin and colleagues (1988) suggested that intracranial hemorrhage is a frequent finding in patients of Wiedemann-Rautenstrauch syndrome, although this was not justified by the review of further cases. Prognosis of this syndrome is indefinite.

Autosomal recessive inheritance is believed to be involved in the syndrome, but Hagadorn and colleagues (1990) considered it a heterogenic phenotype. Fibroblasts taken from patients and grown in culture had a reduced growth rate and life span as compared to the controls; collagen studies showed normal collagenous protein production and secretion, and normal proportions of the collagen components (Rudin *et al.*, 1988). Chessa and colleagues (1992) found increased tetraploidy in 80 percent of fibroblasts *in vitro*. Mazzarerro and colleagues (1992) confirmed a decrease of thymidine kinase activity in about 60 percent of fibroblasts. Alteration of thymidine kinase activity could produce a deoxyribonucleotide pool imbalance with possible mutagenic effect.

Based on their investigation on the fibroblast analysis of a female patient of Rautenstrauch (1977, 1994), Beavan and colleagues (1990) proposed that reduced *decorin* (a small proteoglycan species) expression may contribute to the formation of an abnormal matrix and hence contributing to the pathogenesis of the disorder. Additionally the authors found that fibroblasts from a patient with *Hutchinson-Gilford syndrome* (see below) were almost completely deficient in decorin. Slight reduction in decorin mRNA and concomitant increase in biglycan mRNA indicated that the alteration occurs at the transcriptional level of protein expression. *In vitro* treatment by interleukin 1β stimulated the transcription of decorin in fibroblasts up to 3-fold. Beavan and colleagues claimed that the reduced decorin expression may be responsible for the main clinical features of connective tissue abnormalities.

A 5-year-old girl with normal karyotype and retarded psychomotor development, previously reported by Devos and colleagues (1981) when the patient was 4 years of age, was studied neuropathologically by J. J. Martin and colleagues (1984). The main feature in this patient was *sudanophilic leukodystrophy* and micropolygyria in small parts of deep cerebral sulci. The authors maintained that Wiedemann-Rautenstrauch syndrome shared with *Cockayne syndrome* (see below) the association of a peculiar somatic appearance with a form of sudanophilic leukodystrophy. However, there were too many clinical and neuropathological differences to assimilate both conditions. Sudanophilic leukodystrophy is, admittedly, one of the phenotypes of different metabolic anomalies. Castiñeyra and colleagues (1992) described two sisters with neuropathological findings; the one who died on the 7th postnatal month, had *Dandy-Walker anomaly* and growth retardation and the other, whose intrauterine life was terminated at the 28th fetal week, had ventriculomegaly and cortical atrophy.

Hagadorn and coworkers (1990) reported on a girl born in the 35th gestational week with progeric appearance, early dentition, and fat accumulation in the buttocks, who died on the 104th postnatal day (4-month-old). Her brain weighed 529 g and showed normal cellular architecture with no evidence of a demyelinating process (no leukodystrophy). There have been no further neuropathological studies of Wiedemann-Rautenstrauch syndrome. Precocious aging or complications of the central nervous system are not obligatory in this syndrome; no specific changes in nervous system are expected.

Progeria in Infants (Hutchinson-Gilford Syndrome)

Hutchinson-Gilford syndrome is characterized by precocious and accelerated senescent appearances in early childhood; at birth the patients show no progeric symptom. About 100 case records are found in the literature. The early report of 'pseudo-senilism' by Grossman and coworkers (1955) may be grouped in this section. The incidence of Hutchinson-Gilford syndrome is estimated at 1:8 million births. Age at onset of the disease is in the first year of life.

The clinical manifestations mainly consist of growth retardation and accelerated degenerative changes of the cutaneous, musculoskeletal and cardiovascular systems: short stature, micrognathia, a disproportionately large head, sculptured nose, alopecia, prominent scalp veins, prominent eyes, absence of earlobes, faint midfacial cyanosis, loss of subcutaneous fat, sclerodermatous skin, brownish-yellow spots over the skin, delayed dentition, delayed closure of fontanels, dystrophic nails, prominent joints, skeletal hypoplasia and dysplasia, horse-riding stance, hyperlipidemia, early arteriosclerosis and high-pitched voice. Evidence for bioinactive growth hormone was presented, and treatment with growth hormone was suggested (Brown *et al.*, 1990). Another patient had no endocrinological manifestations (Matsuo *et al.*, 1994). In a case studied by Erdem and colleagues (1994), total lipid was 748 mg/dl (normal range 170–450 mg/dl) and triglyceride 245 mg/dl (normal range 5–40 mg/dl) while total cholesterol was normal. Arteriosclerosis is one of the frequent complications; consequently also cerebral infarctions. For example, in a 7-year-old boy with an incomplete type of Hutchinson-Gilford syndrome a previous infarction of the right putamen was detected by MRI (Smith *et al.*, 1993). The existence of arteriosclerotic lesions was assumed. Wagle and colleagues (1992) recorded a 14-year-old girl with an infarction in the distribution of the superior division of the right middle cerebral artery (detected by MRI), resulting in left hemiparesis.

Orthopedically, bilateral talus deformities of the feet, bilateral dislocation of the hips, *pes planus*, a fractured femur, aseptic necrosis in the nuclear head of the femur, bilateral fixed hip flexion deformities, bone dysplasia, osteoporosis and osteolysis have been described (Fernandez-Palazzi *et al.*, 1992). This syndrome is, though rare, distributed world-wide (Naganuma *et al.*, 1990).

Genetic studies suggested that a sporadic autosomal dominant mutation of the fertilizing sperm or ovum is the most likely mode of inheritance (Stables and Morley, 1994). The gene may be located on chromosome 1 (Erdem *et al.*, 1994).

Marked reduction of insulin receptor gene expression was found by Briata and colleagues (1991) and this might account for the severe insulin resistance presented by their female patient of 15 years of age. Brown (1992) confirmed elevated levels of hyaluronic acid excretion, normal levels of growth hormone but very low insulin-like growth factor I along with very high basal metabolic rates. Growth hormone treatment resulted in a marked increase

of linear growth and paradoxical drop in basal metabolic rates, suggesting a bioinactive form of growth hormone and a lack of vasculogenesis caused by excess hyaluronic acid. After Erdem and colleagues skin fibroblast culture exhibited 76 percent DNA-repair capacity compared with the normal controls.

Progeria of Young Adult Onset (Werner Syndrome)

Werner syndrome is a pathologic and premature aging syndrome with onset age generally between the 1st and 3rd decades (average age when the symptoms were recognized is 38.7 years) and is said to be observed in 'all' organs and systems. However, description on aging of central nervous system in this syndrome is lacking. The clinical features include short stature with characteristic habitus, slender extremities, senile appearance, early graying and loss of the hair, alteration of the voice (high-pitched, hoarse voice), cataracts, atherosclerosis, cardiac problems (Carrel *et al.*, 1994), diabetes mellitus, osteoporosis, skin hyperkeratosis with trophic ulcers of the extremities, hypogonadism (including early cessation of menstruation) as well as predisposition to malignancy. Occurrence of flat feet was also frequent in a review of 15 Japanese patients (Goto *et al.*, 1978). According to Epstein and colleagues (1966) approximately 1/3 of 125 patients reviewed showed mild neurological symptoms, predominantly involving loss of distal tendon reflexes. Three patients (two females and one male) had meningiomas. Intelligence was commented on in 19 patients: 9 of these were retarded, but there is also a description of an 'intelligent woman'. Two were psychotic. There is no clear description on dementia in the literature.

According to the review of Epstein and colleagues, average morbid age of this syndrome was 47 years (31–63 years) and the main causes of death were malignancies and vascular accidents (myocardial and cerebrovascular); other causes were 'diabetes', 'liver trouble', anemia, and 'cachexia, edema and anemia'.

Werner syndrome is also inherited in a recessive autosomal manner. Chromosome and genomic instability at the cellular level was established (Hoehn *et al.*, 1975; Fukuchi *et al.*, 1990; Romero and Aznares, 1992) and the defective gene has recently been identified (Yu *et al.*, 1996) in the chromosome 8p11.1–21.1 region. The affected gene responsible for Werner syndrome is a *helicase*, an enzyme responsible for unwinding the DNA double helix and thought to play an integral role in some forms of DNA repair. In the absence of such repair processes the chromosomes of Werner syndrome patients exhibit multiple chromosome abnormalities and deletions which are correlated with the clinical syndrome.

In this syndrome, as in other progeric syndromes, research has been centered on fibroblast function and characteristics. Fibroblasts derived from the patients demonstrate severely limited capacity of dividing, similar to, though more extreme than, those from normal aged people. Slow growth and a reduced life span of the fibroblasts *in vitro* has also been observed. A reduced rate of DNA replication (Fujiwara et al., 1977; Takeuchi et al., 1982) was reported while DNA repair was normal (Fujiwara et al., 1977; Higashikawa and Fujiwara, 1978; Thompson and Holliday, 1983).

Cerebral atrophy was recorded in at least five cases of 125 patients reviewed by Epstein and colleagues. However, detailed histological data of the brain are not available. Sumi (1985) and Haustein and coworkers (1989) reported unspecific changes such as neuronal lipofuscinosis and arteriolosclerosis. Again, 3 out of 125 patients had meningiomas, including a Japanese patient (Kobayashi et al., 1980). An astrocytoma is known in one patient (Laso et al., 1989). In a 39-year-old male, a subclinical pituitary adenoma (subclinical microtumors are dubbed as 'incidentalomas') was recorded. Frequency of the pituitary incidentalomas has been reported between 2.7 and 27 percent of routine necropsy series; the reported frequencies were different according to the method of examination. In two Werner syndrome patients, acidophilic and chromophobic invasion of the adenohypophyseal cells into the posterior lobe was documented. Well known is basophilic (= ACTH positive cells) invasion which is frequently observed as proportionate to increasing age, whereas invasion of other cell components is exceptional (Kuebber et al., 1990).

Subjective progeric appearance of patients of different disorders alone provides no reason to compare with the progeric syndromes or related conditions. For example, Seckel syndrome was also referred to as having progeric symptoms by some authors. This syndrome comprises microcephalus, receding forehead with protruding nose without frontonasal angle, intrauterine hypotrophy, and postnatal developmental retardation. Pathogenetically, early ceasing of matrix cell production in the cerebrum in fetal life and hypopituitarism have been considered as responsible for the microcephalus and hypotrophy (Hori et al., 1987). However, the physiognomy itself is no longer a diagnostic criteria, and cytogenetic and further modern diagnostic tools are today required.

Progeric Manifestations in Central Nervous System Disorders

Patients of Down syndrome show neuropathological changes similar to Alzheimer disease earlier in their adult life than the Alzheimer patients. Patients of Cockayne syndrome are known to show senescent external features already at the beginning of the disease in early childhood.

Down Syndrome

Down syndrome is due to trisomy 21, including mosaicism. Patients with Down syndrome over the age of 35 years are at high risk of manifesting neuropathological changes identical with Alzheimer disease and consequently dementia, superimposed to the preexisting mental retardation. (Fig. 30–1). An increased rate of births with Down syndrome is known in families of Alzheimer disease patients (Heston et al., 1981; Heyman et al.,

1983). The clinical pathological relationship between both disorders have been proven genetically when the gene coding for the APP (β-amyloid precursor protein) has been found on chromosome 21q11–22. In fact, the mutation in this gene was proven in patients of familial early onset Alzheimer disease (Chapters 8 and 9).

Down syndrome is not only a disorder of the brain. Patients with Down syndrome manifest congenital heart diseases and/or gastrointestinal abnormalities. Associations with different disorders such as leukemia, syringomas, Moyamoya disease, Hirschsprung disease, autoimmune diseases and many other kinds of disorders including apparently incidental combinations have been reported. Intensive investigations in neural aging in Down syndrome are in contrast to the few studies on progeric syndromes. It is well known that patients with Down syndrome show progeric features externally, even in young adult age. A. J. Holland (1994) introduced the results of Brooksbank and Balazs which showed increased activity of superoxide dismutase (SOD) activity in Down syndrome. SOD gene is localized on the distal part of chromosome 21q, and a SOD gene dosage effect presumably results in 'premature aging' due to increased membrane permeability and disorders of oxidation. Another study reported the strongly impaired AP-1 DNA binding activity in lymphocytes in Down syndrome, suggesting the same molecular mechanisms of proliferation cessation in fibroblasts characterized by replicative senescence (Sikora et al., 1993).

Cockayne Syndrome

This syndrome is characterized by external progeric appearance and neuronal degeneration in form of leukodystrophy. Up-to-date molecular genetic investigations of this disorder are still insufficient.

Boys are more frequently affected than girls (Rowlatt, 1969). The disease begins around 2 years of age after normal postnatal development. Although the birth weight is usually normal, the somatic and speech development are retarded (dwarfism). In addition to the congenital dysmorphic features such as microcephaly and low set ears, dried skin, scanty facial subcutaneous fat, and deeply set eyes give an impression of progeric appearance. Additionally, crippling from flexion deformities and kyphosis become more marked. Extensive retinal pigmentary anomaly and optic atrophy (Levin et al. 1983; Traboulsi et al. 1992), hypoplastic and carious teeth, and coarse voice are observed. Photosensitivity of skin, especially to the lethal effects of 254-nm UV (Leech et al., 1985; Proops et al., 1981) and deafness of different degrees are further manifestations. Precocious puberty, recognized as early menarche, may be exceptional. Renal anomalies were described by Ohno and Hirooka (1966): thickening of glomerular basal membrane, poor vascularization and hyalinization of glomeruli, atrophy in some tubules and interstitial fibrosis. Epidermis was histologically atrophic and hair follicles showed fetal features (Sugarman et al., 1977).

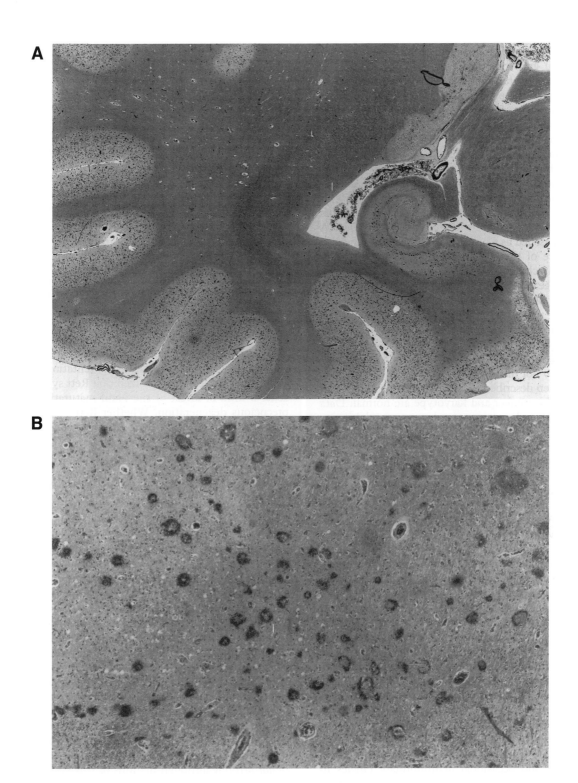

FIGURE   30–1

Neuritic plaques seen in a 57-year-old female patient with Down syndrome. Numerous plaques were even grossly recognizable on the histological slide; the plaques were distributed not only in the neocortex and archicortex but also in the caudate nucleus as well as in the pulvinar thalami. In this patient, the number of plaques in Ammon's horn was rather small and neurofibrillary tangles were rarely observed in the whole brain areas. Staining by Bielschowski method. Original magnification: X1 (**A**) and photomicroscopic enlargement: X70 (**B**).

1993; Gieron *et al.,* 1995; Holtzman *et al.,* 1992; Pemde *et al.,* 1995; Pratap-Chand *et al.,* 1995; Tomoda *et al.,* 1991).

An interesting contribution was made by Golden and colleagues (1995) in a case report on a mentally retarded 35-year-old man with *Williams syndrome* (see p. 419). The patient's later life was complicated by convulsions which were treated temporarily with phenobarbital. I.Q. scores ranged between 18 and 36. In his medical history, hepatitis B infection (at age 10), *Hodgkin disease* (at age 15 with chemotherapy; later on recurrence additionally radiotherapy), gastric rupture, recurrent urinary infections, anemia as well as diabetes mellitus were documented. At necropsy infection as a cause of death and malformations of several organs were found. In the brain of this patient, Alzheimer pathology was found including neuritic plaques containing βA4 amyloid in the neocortex as well as in the entorhinal cortex and neurofibrillary tangles in the hippocampus, amygdala and entorhinal cortex and to a lesser extent in the neocortex; these alterations were ascertained histochemically and immunohistochemically.

As discussed in Chapter 20, if we consider the relationship between Lewy bodies and neurofibrillary tangles, the early onset of *diffuse Lewy body disease* should be considered here. Diffuse Lewy body disease in an unusually young patient (onset at 27, death at 32 years of age) was reported by Opeskin and colleagues (1993) and they summarized further 4 cases of young onset of diffuse Lewy body disease recorded in the literature. Peculiar is furthermore, that the symptoms manifested immediately at postpartum in 3 of 5 patients.

'Alzheimerization' in Non-aging Processes and in Young Age

Neurofibrillary Tangles in Dysplastic Neurons

Some reports describe neurofibrillary tangles in dysplastic neurons, occasionally associated with further changes of *granulovacuolar degeneration* or neuritic plaques.

Bedwell and Lindenberg (1961) may be the first authors who discussed the relationship between the changes of Alzheimer disease and hypothalamic ganglionic hamartoma. They described the 'dendritic' reaction with glomerular proliferation of the ganglionic cells of the hamartoma which was similar to the neuritic plaques of Alzheimer disease. However, the authors did not find neurofibrillary tangles in the ganglionic cells. Neurofibrillary tangles in the ganglionic cells of the hypothalamic hamartoma were described later by Janota and colleagues (1974), and then confirmed by Beal and colleagues (1981) and Kudo and colleagues (1986). In addition to the neurofibrillary tangles the former authors also found granulovacuolar degeneration as well as argentophilic bodies (Pick bodies) in tumorous ganglionic cells but no neuritic plaques.

In *tuberous sclerosis* lesion in a 13-year-old girl examined by Hirano and colleagues (1968), abundant Pick bodies were found in addition to neurofibrillary tangles

and granulovacuolar degeneration in abnormal ganglionic cells.

Morán and colleagues (1995) found neurofibrillary tangles localized in neurons at the site of the *verrucose dysplasia.* Considering that the morphogenetic mechanisms of verrucose state and micropolygyria are similar and that a local defect of blood supply is widely accepted as pathogenetic of the latter, the authors discussed the relationship between the neurofibrillary tangles and ischemia. The ischemia hypothesis may be interesting in the context of *dementia pugilistica* (Corsellis *et al.,* 1973; Grahman and Ule, 1957), a disorder identical to Alzheimer disease, triggered by chronic repetitive head trauma such as in professional boxing.

There are three cases documented in the literature in which neurofibrillary tangles were found in the neuronal tumor cells in gangliogliomas (Oberc-Greenwood *et al.,* 1984; Hori *et al.,* 1988; Soffer *et al.,* 1995) (Figure 30–3); granulovacuolar changes were also occasionally observed (Hori *et al.,* 1988). Upon electron microscopic examination, the tangles consisted of paired helical filaments (Soffer *et al.,* 1995). Gangliogliomas are mixed tumors with astrocytic and ganglionic components. Intracranial gangliogliomas are frequently found in the temporal region in young patients (Demierre *et al.,* 1986). They are usually benign; however, if malignant alteration occurs, it is seen in glioma cells as a form of anaplastic astrocytomas. Ganglionic tumor cells are polymorphic and occasionally multinucleated, so that they seem to be neoplastic. A recent report, however, revealed that the cerebral cortical structure near the ganglioglioma is dysgenetic (Prayson *et al.,* 1995). Gangliogliomas may therefore arise on a maldevelopmental basis, like hypothalamic ganglionic hamartomas or tuberous sclerosis.

Duong and coworkers (1994) examined dysplastic hyperplastic neuronal cells of the patients with focal cerebral dysplasia and hemimegalencephaly by immunohisto-

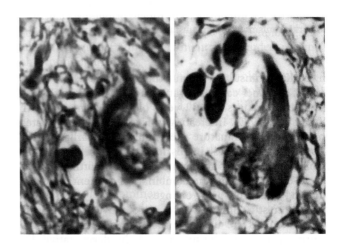

FIGURE   30–3

Neurofibrillary tangles in ganglionic tumor cells of a ganglioglioma. The patient was 49-year-old. (from Hori *et al.* 1988; reproduced with permission of the American Medical Association.

chemical methods and identified the tangles ('neurofila-mentous tangles') which immunoreacted positively to the antisera of neurofilaments, phosphorylated and non-phos-phorylated, ubiquitin as well as tau, similar to the neuro-fibrillary tangles seen in Alzheimer disease patients. The neurofilamentous tangles, however, did not react to the PHF (paired helical filament)-antibody. The authors sug-gested some similarities of the pathological processes lead-ing to the formation of neurofilamentous tangles in corti-cal dysplasia and neurofibrillary tangles in Alzheimer disease, but the neurofilamentous tangles are not com-posed of the paired helical filaments so that they are not identical to the neurofibrillary tangles. The authors' group previously studied abnormal neurons in cortical dysplasias electron microscopically and identified no paired helical filaments (De Rosa *et al.*, 1992).

Review of the literature revealed that there is some rela-tionship between appearance of neurofibrillary tangles and the developmental disposition of neuronal cells although discrepancy between paired helical filaments and neurofilamentous tangles should, in some cases, be considered. The occasional association of neuritic plaques and further degeneration may or may not be incidental (Chapter 19).

Neurofibrillary Tangles in Niemann-Pick Disease, Subacute Sclerosing Panencephalitis (SSPE), Leukodystrophy, and Other Conditions

Neurofibrillary tangles have been recognized in *Nie-mann-Pick disease* type C, a nosologically distinct storage disease. Suzuki and colleagues (1995) reviewed 10 pa-tients, including 7 of their own, whose ages ranged be-tween 18 and 53 years. The authors reported that the pa-tients under 20 years of age showed no tangles but axonal dystrophy. They concluded that the formation of tangles and axonal spheroids had an inverse relationship. Axonal dystrophy is frequently observed in the posterior columns and Goll and Burdach nuclei of the spinal cord in aging (Fujisawa, 1968; Fujisawa and Shiraki, 1978). Love and colleagues (1995) studied 5 patients whose ages ranged from 17 to 33 years and found that the distribution of tangles fairly correlated to that of storage substance, as similarly described by Suzuki and colleagues (1995). Both groups could not find any βA4-protein or neuritic plaques in these patients. According to Auer and colleagues (1995) paired helical filaments in Niemann-Pick disease type C are indistinguishable from those in Alzheimer disease if tested immunohistochemically by anti-PHFtau. In further congenital metabolic disease groups, only *Kuf disease* is known to present neurofibrillary tangles (Korn-feld, 1972).

Since the 1950s it is known that tangles are observed in neurons of different brain areas in *subacute sclerosing panencephalitis* (SSPE) patients (about one fifth of cases). The patients of SSPE with neurofibrillary tangles are al-most all young children or teenagers and 20s/30s are rare. Neurofibrillary tangles are not accompanied by neuritic plaques in these cases; granulovacuolar degeneration was

seldom found (Mandybur *et al.*, 1977). Pathogenetically, the measles virus may play a role in the formation of tan-gles, but tangles were not restricted to the nerve cells car-rying viral antigen. Bancher and coworkers (1996) dis-cussed that tangles are not induced directly by measles virus at the individual cellular level but due to some kind of response of the neuronal network to a specific type of tissue injury in certain vulnerable neuron populations. This hypothesis might also explain that only one fifth of SSPE patients with longer disease duration develops tan-gles and that not all tangle-bearing neurons are necessary to be infected by the virus.

Neurofibrillary tangles are also found in cases of *leuko-dystrophy*. In a boy of 7 years and 10 months of age with sudanophilic leukodystrophy, abundant neurofibrillary tangles (paired helical filaments) were widely distributed in the cerebral cortex, basal ganglia including Meynert's basal nucleus, hypothalamus, and brainstem (Harada *et al.*, 1988).

Takada reviewed different disease states including Cockayne syndrome and Hallervorden-Spatz disease as well as different brain malformations (age of patients was under 44 years) in which only neurofibrillary tangles and no neuritic plaques or Lewy bodies were found.

There is a special type of congenital muscular dystro-phy with mental retardation (Fukuyama *et al.*, 1981), known as *Fukuyama type congenital muscular dystrophy* (FCMD) featured by cerebral cortical as well as cerebellar cortical dysgeneses. This syndrome, originally found in the Japanese population, was also reported from Western countries (Goebel *et al.*, 1983). In young adult patients of FCMD, neurofibrillary tangles were observed in the Mey-nert's nucleus and the locus caeruleus (Takada *et al.*, 1986); the tangles were ultrastructurally paired helical fi-laments, but they were not found in the hippocampus or cerebral cortex where some dysgenesis was recognized. Neuritic plaques and further 'aging degenerative hall-marks' were not found. Takada and coworkers discussed the possible presence of degenerative processes in FCMD on the one hand, and viral infection as one of the possible pathogenetic factors of neurofibrillary tangles on the other, even though the pathogenesis of FCMD is still un-known.

In patients of *myotonic dystrophy* between 35 and 56 years of age, Kikuchi and coworkers (1991) observed neu-rofibrillary tangles (paired helical filaments) distributed mainly in the parahippocampal gyrus and not in the hip-pocampus. In their oldest patient, they observed tangles also in the hippocampus. However, they did not find any neuritic plaques. Myotonic dystrophy is a dominantly in-herited disorder; G. M. Martin (1978) considered this dis-order to be one of the progeric diseases since it may be ac-companied by aging phenomena such as cataracts, frontal baldness, and atrophy of the testes. Kikuchi and col-leagues discussed the neurofibrillary tangle distribution which was different from that of Alzheimer disease but was similar to that of 'physiological' aging. Additionally, the intensity of the tangle appearance in their patients correlated to mental deterioration which is usually observed in myotonic dystrophy patients. It is, however, still uncertain whether or not the 'Alzheimerization' in this disorder represents an aspect of precocious aging.

Neurotoxicity and Neurofibrillary Tangles?

The hypothesis of a toxic cause of tangles by neuroleptics is controversial. In elderly schizophrenic patients, the incidence of neurofibrillary tangles was twice as high in the patient group with long-term neuroleptic treatment as in that without (Wisniewski et al., 1994). On the contrary, Niizato and Ikeda (1996) reported that even high dosis of major tranquilizers (chlorpromazine) for duration of decades did not promote the development of Alzheimer pathology. Additionally, non-demented hypertensive population had a higher incidence of neurofibrillary tangles than critical cardiac disease and non-cardiac disease groups (Sparks et al., 1995).

Neurofibrillary tangles were also found in a brain of a child with lead intoxication (Niklowitz et al., 1975). In chronic alcoholics with thiamine deficiency, neurofibrillary tangles were found in the nucleus basalis of Meynert followed by loss of neurons in this nucleus (Cullen and Halliday, 1995).

Lewy Bodies, Pick Bodies, and Plaque-like Structures in the Brains of Children and Young Adults

We already reviewed the literature describing the appearance of neurofibrillary tangles in cases of subacute sclerosing panencephalitis (SSPE), and the chemical and morphological similarity between neurofibrillary tangles and Lewy bodies (Chapter 20). Worth stressing is the observation by Gibb and colleagues (1990) of Lewy bodies in two male patients of 27 and 19 years of age who died of SSPE. Both patients suffered from SSPE for 3 and 10 years, respectively. In these patients, Lewy bodies were found in the substantia nigra and in one patient additionally in the locus coeruleus, with coexistent neurofibrillary tangles. But Lewy bodies were never found in the dorsal vagal nucleus, Meynert's nucleus, cerebral cortex, or spinal sympathetic ganglia. The authors discussed that Lewy bodies might rather be a by-product of attempted regeneration and not of degeneration. This calls in mind, however, the similarity of Lewy bodies and neurofibrillary tangles (Chapter 20). The coexistence of both of these types of inclusions in cases of SSPE is difficult to regard as coincidental.

In classical psychiatry, Alzheimer disease and Pick disease belong to typical, idiopathic senile and/or presenile dementia spectrum. In addition to precocious Alzheimer pathology or 'Alzheimerization' in a variety of disorders, a unique report should be mentioned here, since this case again raises the question as to whether the 'Pick body' may be regarded as one of the hallmarks of the 'aging process'. De León reported a 7-week-old female infant, born at 37 weeks of gestation with hypotrophy, clinical manifestations of psychomotor retardation, lethargy, and akinesia. Laboratory data showed hormonal disequilibrium and electrolyte imbalance. Neuropathological findings were characterized by diffuse distribution of Pick cells (mostly with accumulation of eosinophilic material) with central chromatolysis in the cerebral cortex and Pick argentophilic bodies, confirmed at electron microscopy. There was no cortical atrophy but the brain was rather large. The authors classified the case as a unique type of encephalopathy and not as a precocious aging process.

It is probably incorrect that the plaque-like structures to be described here, are interpreted as an 'Alzheimerization'; however, it is worth discussing these structures in comparison to the morphological characteristics in neuronal aging. Crain and coworkers (1995) found argyrophilic plaque-like deposits in the neocortex and cerebellar cortex in children. The deposits could be demonstrated by different silver impregnation methods applied to stain the 'senile' plaques; the deposits had the same size, shape and distribution as the diffuse neuritic plaques commonly seen in older adults (Chapter 19), but these structures were not accompanied by amyloid deposits. The authors observed the deposits not only in a child with Down syndrome but in 10 children between 5½ months to 10 years who had very different neurological disorders with primary neuropathological changes. The authors additionally observed the same deposits in 6 otherwise 'normal' children. The definitive morphology, including ultrastructure and the relationship between these structures and neuritic plaques, and their origin, pathogenesis or functional significance are unknown, although Crain and colleagues thought these may represent some subtle brain injury.

Does Precocious Brain Development Correlate to Neural Aging?

This author recently observed intrauterine precocious cerebral development (abnormally early gyration) associated with agenesis of the corpus callosum (Hori, 1996). The clinical significance and prognosis of this anomaly is unknown. There is no evidence that the brain with agenesis of the corpus callosum may show precocious aging. However, in the brains of this entity, a very small number of differentiated neuronal cells were found in the periventricular matrix cell zone in the second trimester of fetal age. It should be noted that 'premature' neurons (not Cajal-Retzius cells, see below) may be sporadically found, though extremely rare, in the matrix cell zone in fetal brains, even near the physiological neuroblastic mitotic activity.

Cajal-Retzius cells are neuronal cells which exist only in later fetal age in the molecular layer of the cerebral cortex. In contrast to the still undifferentiated neuroblasts in the fetal cerebral cortex, Cajal-Retzius cells differentiate early. The cell number decreases in reverse relation to the increasing brain weight during later fetal life (unpublished own data). They disappear probably by cell death during the neonatal period. They are essential in corticogenesis (neuronal migration). 'Alzheimerization' of these cells has not been observed. These cells are seen to persist in patients with clinically pathological conditions such as mental retardation or epilepsy.

Pubertas praecox is known in cases of hypothalamic ganglionic hamartomas, and is caused by anomaly of the hypothalamo-hypophyseal axis. In this disorder, the pathogenetic factors are found in the abnormal ganglionic cells. In contrast, precocious gyration is rather a gross anomaly and it is difficult to discuss its possible pathogenetic relationship to the 'premature neurons'. The prematurity of the brain or of individual neurons will be one of the future topics in research on neural aging.

Congenital, Neonatal and Childhood Vascular Disorders

Congenital Arteriosclerosis is not Atherosclerosis

Moschkowitz and Strauss (1963) reported a baby born at term and died 36 hours after birth with 'congenital' pulmonary arteriosclerosis. The baby had complete transposition of the aorta and pulmonary artery with intact ventricular septum, cardiac enlargement with right and left ventricular hypertrophy and dilatation, small foramen ovale, and obliterated *ductus arteriosus*. Although the authors discussed the multifactorial pathogenesis of the arteriosclerosis, they stressed the altered arterial pressure (even during the intrauterine life) resulting in intima fibrosis and further degeneration of pulmonar artery and muscular proliferation of its terminal arteries.

Congenital arteriosclerosis is occasionally observed in connection with chromosome anomalies. Rosenfield and colleagues (1962) described for the first time arteriosclerosis in trisomy 18. They observed sclerosis in aorta, inferior mesenteric, iliac, and femoral arteries, in the latter also calcification and thrombi in a 4-month-old male baby. Histologically this change consisted of fragmentation of the internal elastic lamina and elastic fibers of the media with an increase of medial ground substance. They stressed that these findings are compatible with the 'infantile' medial arteriosclerosis and differed from the atherosclerosis. The authors discussed genetic failure in establishing the damage to lamina elastica as a pathogenetic factor. According to their review of the literature on typical idiopathic infantile arteriosclerosis, one out of 6 patients was stillborn with encephalocele, cystic kidneys and polydactyly (Meckel-Gruber syndrome? – according to the present author's estimation), three others apparently had central nervous system damage (two with cerebral hemorrhage and one with prolonged jaundice), and the remaining two had either an umbilical hernia or cryptorchidism. In further documents on infantile arteriosclerosis, the authors found association of uremia, hypercalcemia, or inherited connective tissue disorders. It is difficult to elucidate whether or not congenital arteriosclerosis in these cases is related to central nervous system damages or to any malformations other than cardiovascular ones.

In contrast to the above cited case, a 24-year-old woman with *Turner's syndrome* reported by Reske-Nielsen and colleagues, who died of a ruptured aneurysm of the posterior cerebral artery, showed typical atherosclerotic plaques of both internal carotid artery and additional multiple small infarctions in both cerebral hemispheres. Taken together these findings, diagnostic problems should be considered differentiating from systemic vascular diseases such as vasculitis (Chapter 27), independent of Turner syndrome.

Congenital arteriosclerosis in form of fibrosis is also known in a syndrome described by Williams and colleagues and by Beuren and colleagues in the early 1960's. Clinical characteristics of the *Williams syndrome* (*Williams-Beuren syndrome*) comprise distinctive facial appearance, cardiovascular disease (typically supravalvular aortic and/or pulmonary stenosis), infantile hypercalcemia, physical growth rate along the lower percentiles, and/or failure to thrive, and renal, dental, and musculoskeletal abnormalities. Ophthalmologically, strabismus and stellate pattern of the iris are observed frequently and retinal vascular tortuosity may occasionally be detected (Pankau et al.,1996). Patients may have altered cognitive abilities and/or mental retardation. I.Q. scores of the patients vary from the normal range to severe mental retardation (Golden et al., 1995). Neurological analysis of 24 patients of Williams syndrome (Chapman et al., 1995) revealed lowered cognitive level in areas of language, attention and imitative-constructional praxis, hypotonia in a younger group of patients (ages between 2 and 8 years) and hypertonia rather in an older group (ages between 12 and 30 years). Parallel examinations revealed no correlating morphologic abnormalities of the central nervous system. Neuropsychologically linguistic abilities are preserved although they show a characteristic pattern of intellectual strength and weakness and substantial impairment of visual-spatial abilities (Bellugi et al., 1990). The incidence of this syndrome is thought to be 1:10,000. Genetically, microdeletion in the chromosomal region of 7q11.23 (elastin gene) was explored (Ewart et al., 1994). Mari and colleagues (1995) analyzed an intragenic restriction fragment length polymorphism and gene dosage of elastin. In 54 out of 60 patients, they were able to demonstrate the deletion of the elastin gene and could not confirm the diagnosis of Williams syndrome in the rest of the 6 patients who had not shown the deletion. This regional deletion was also confirmed as a cause of Williams syndrome in Japanese (Hirota et al., 1996). Further chromosomal anomaly (chromosome 4q) was also discussed (Jefferson et al., 1986).

Patients with Williams syndrome manifest multiple arterial stenoses due to intimal fibrosis (Figure 30–4). Stenosis of cerebral arteries may be followed by strokes in childhood (Kaplan et al., 1995; Putman et al., 1995; Soper et al., 1995). Besides, cerebral arterial stenosis may result in *Moyamoya disease* (Kawai et al., 1993). A 'senile degeneration' of the brain in form of Alzheimer disease in a 35-year-old patient with Williams syndrome was already described (p. 416).

A

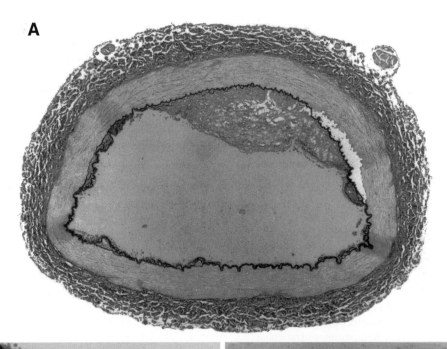

B

C

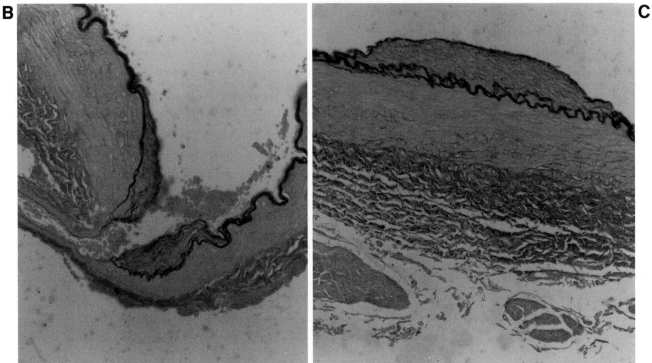

FIGURE   30–4

Arteriosclerosis in a 8-month-old boy with Williams syndrome. Prominent focal intima fibrosis of the right vertebral artery (**A**, X70), left posterior cerebral artery (**B**, X200) and left internal carotid artery (**C**, X130) stained by elastica-van Gieson method. Fibrosis is observed at the site of the arterial branching as well as in the inner surface where there is no branching.

In summary, congenital arteriosclerosis is not an extremely rare disorder. Pathomorphologically, the arteriosclerosis consists of intimal and medial fibrosis and is fundamentally different from atheromatous changes. One of the main pathogenetic factors may be an altered hemodynamics, mainly due to associated cardiovascular malformation.

Idiopathic Arterial Calcification in Infancy (IACI) may be Due to Inflammation

One of the earliest descriptions of infantile arterial calcification is that by Schopper (1934) who reported on an 8-week-old infant who died suddenly. Histological examination revealed medial necrosis and calcification with chronic adventitial inflammatory infiltrate, intimal fibrosis, and proliferation of elastic fibers of coronary arteries. The cause of death was myocardial necrosis (infarction).

Idiopathic arterial calcification of infancy (IACI) is seen within the first six months of life and is usually fatal. Intrauterine diagnosis by ultrasound is possible (Bellah *et al.*, 1992). Longer survival is the exception; in this circumstance, however, calcification may disappear completely as observed radiologically (Sholler *et al.*, 1984). Usual cause of death is myocardial ischemia and/or infarction. The disease was therefore previously called 'medial coronary sclerosis' of infancy. Intracranial calcification is usually not found (Maayan *et al.*, 1984). Since familial occurrence has been frequently observed, some hereditary predisposition is apparent but inheritance does not follow (1985) a Mendelian pattern although possible autosomal recessive inheritance is discussed.

Anderson and colleagues reviewed 12 cases of IACI newborn infants less than 40 weeks of gestation including two of their own female sibling cases. They observed extensive aorta and arterial (both of elastic and muscular arteries) calcification in different organs including cutaneous tissue. In several arteries they found acute inflammatory infiltrates in the intima and media which were accompanied by mild adventitial lymphocytic infiltrate. There was also non-arterial parenchymal calcification. Intimal proliferation was also present in different arteries and the aorta in association with calcification. In one patient, the karyotype was proven to be normal and a third sibling was healthy. Laboratory examination of viral and bacterial culture was negative; syphilis was also not present. The authors concluded that IACI was a result of intrauterine *arteriitis* (*panarteriitis*). The fibrosis of vessel walls (in relation to arteriosclerosis) is apparently the result of vasculitis. Anderson and colleagues additionally revealed a unique pathogenetic mechanism of calcification with altered iron metabolism. Results of molecular genetic studies of IACI are expected.

IACI should, as understood from the above review, be excluded from the category of primary congenital or infantile arteriosclerosis and rather be discussed within the concept of vasculitis although this disease should be referred to child arteriosclerosis. As a matter of fact, calcification of carotid siphon and iliac arteries in infancy and childhood is rather a common finding due to hemodynamic stress according to the opinion of Meyer and Lind (1972).

Arteriosclerosis in Children due to Neurogenic Factors

One theory explaining the arteriosclerosis in childhood is that of *neurogenic atherosclerosis*, in which the arteriosclerosis may be induced by chronic central nervous system injury in childhood. R. H. Chaney (1987) investigated 812 autopsied patients under 21 years of age of an institutionalized population of mentally handicapped. After excluding all cases predisposing to childhood arteriosclerosis, the remaining 65 patients 'were analyzed and compared with a control group. The author found a preponderance of epilepsy in the arteriosclerosis group. The majority of these patients had poor nutrition, retarded physical growth and development, cranial anomalies and requirement for nursing care. One hypothesis put forward was that epilepsy may cause arterial changes. The background of this theory is the promotion of sympathoadrenal overstimulation by seizures which may underlie early atherogenesis. Supporting this notion is the finding of Gutstein and colleagues (1987) who ascertained electron microscopically the occurrence of secondary atherosclerosis in the aorta and coronary arteries after electric stimulation in the lateral hypothalamus in normally fed, unrestrained rats. Their results imply possible neurogenic development of human atherosclerotic lesions.

Chaney (1987) also observed arteriosclerosis in Down syndrome patients under 21 years of age, slightly more frequently (8.9 percent) than in other mentally retarded patients (7.9 percent). The author discussed the factors influencing the atherosclerosis in Down syndrome patients from those of unexpected atherosclerosis groups in mentally retarded young patients. Because of the different sets of variables for predisposition of or protection from atherosclerosis and the different subgroups of Down syndrome, the results should have remained unexplained.

Atherosclerosis in Children, Children at Risk for Later Atherosclerosis, Familial Hypercholesterolemia

About the risk factors of atherosclerosis the readers are referred to Chapter 27 of this book. Hypertension in childhood correlates with arteriosclerotic disorder in an early stage (Newman *et al.*, 1986). Among pediatric hypertension, essential hypertension is most common and various renal disorders and others including Williams syndrome are the causes of secondary hypertension (Ogborn and Crocker, 1987). Hypertensive encephalopathy in childhood symptomatologically resembles that of adults (Kandt *et al.*, 1995).

Ten percent of 10- to 14-year-old children in Europe are considered to suffer from fibrous plaques in their coronary arteries (Strasser, 1982). The statistic data from obese lowteens showed unfavorable potentially atherogenic lipoprotein profile: high-density-lipoprotein, cholesterol and triglycerides (Flodmark *et al.*, 1994). Kupke and colleagues (1983) examined 497 German kindergarten children in three groups (reference, overweight, and socially underprivileged), stressing the importance of early detection of risk group children. The authors considered hypercholesterolemia and elevated β- against α-lipoprotein ratio to be risk factors. Isolated decrease of β-lipoprotein was also interpreted as an early indicator of metabolic disorders in obese young children. Obesity is thought to be a risk factor of coronary heart diseases since these are associated with increased cholesterol synthesis and enhanced cholesterol elimination mechanisms. As etiologic factors for the arterial lesions leading to childhood atherosclerosis, Schaffner and Cottier (1982) suggested mechanical stress, immune complexes, infection, toxic products, and hyperlipidemia.

Based on the report that fatty streaks are seen in the aortae even of three-year-olds (Holman *et al.*, 1958) and appear in the coronary arteries during the second decades of life (Strong and McGill, 1962), Newman and colleagues (1986) studied 35 necropsied patients under 24 years of age (mean age at death 18 years) and found that aortic fatty streaks were strongly correlated to levels of both total and low-density-lipoprotein cholesterol. Coronary artery fatty streaks were correlated to the levels of very-low-density-lipoprotein cholesterol. The authors recommended an early preventive approach in risk group children against cardiovascular diseases.

For the early therapy of the pediatric hyperlipidemia to prevent later atherosclerosis, Widhalm (1982) indicated that polygenetic and combined familial hyperlipidemias should be treated by diet alone whereas familial hypercholesterolemias need drug treatment. Familial hypercholesterolemia is an autosomal dominantly inherited disorder which is based on a mutation in the low-density-lipoprotein receptor gene. The defect of the gene results in deficient binding of low-density-lipoprotein to receptors in hepatocytes and other cell membranes that normally bind these lipids for transport into the cells (Brown and Goldstein, 1986).

Cerebral Amyloid Angiopathy in Childhood

Cerebral amyloid angiopathy is described in Chapter 27, therefore only a unique, exceptional case of cerebral amyloid angiopathy seen in a child, reported by C. M. Shaw (1979) will be cited here. The patient was a 14-year-old boy with a clinical course of 3–4 years beginning with intellectual deterioration and incoordination. He developed spasticity, limited upward gaze, hyperreflexia, ataxia, positive Babinski signs, and showed electroencephalographic anomalies (abnormal slow and epileptiform discharges). His mental deterioration further progressed to frequent yawing and chewing movements without any motility, and contractures. He responded to deep pain and could follow an object with his eyes. The seizures, which had meanwhile developed, were well controlled by antiepileptics until he died due to bronchopneumonia. Neuropatho-

logical examination revealed mild to moderate atrophy of the cerebral white matter and pyramids in the medulla oblongata while the histological changes were more severe in the gray matter than in the white matter. Capillaries were thickened and contained Congo-red positive birefringent material; this substance was also found continuously radiating from the vessel wall and free in the gray matter. Degenerated neurites in the periphery of plaques were sometimes thick and formed small cones, suggesting a portion of a neuron with neurofibrillary tangles; however, tangles in the whole neurons were never found. In other organs, there was mild congophilia in occasional arterial walls only in the spleen and renal medulla. The author interpreted the plaque-like amyloid deposits in the parenchyma as of vascular origin and thought they were not the neuritic plaques typically seen in Alzheimer disease. The primary occurrence of the amyloid angiopathy can thus be observed in childhood.

An Overall View

What we can say from the review of the progeric syndromes, is that these syndromes are no primary central nervous system diseases but essentially a disease of mesodermal tissues. Central nervous system lesions are occasionally observed such as leukodystrophy but this is the exception. Vascular accidents in the central nervous system are also a secondary phenomenon due to mesodermal disorders. In this sense, the criticism of Hall and Denneny is correct and the term *progeria* stands only for some aspects of the aging processes. Thus, to the question whether the precocious aging syndromes are a partial expression or a simple acceleration of the 'normal' senescence, one should answer by 'neither nor'. Senescence is a generalized and complex process in humans; we observe in so-called progeric syndromes only the mesodermal aspect of age dependent degeneration and not in the central nervous system, for example. On the contrary, the mesodermal aspect of aging processes alone is insufficient to account for disorders such as Down syndrome. In Down syndrome, neural aging changes typical of Alzheimer pathology are observed in young patients.

By the review of the literature which dealt with neurofibrillary tangle appearance in different disorders, it was shown that pathogenesis of neurofibrillary tangles is multifactorial. The fact that they are observed in connection with genetic predisposition, in dysgenetic neurons, in conditions of metabolic anomaly, ischemic state, viral infection or others indicates that neurofibrillary tangles alone should not be regarded as a hallmark of neural aging. Neurofibrillary tangles may even be found in neonatal life. Early appearance of neurofibrillary tangles in conjunction with neuritic plaques and eventually further neuronal degeneration featured by Lewy bodies, granulovacuolar neuronal degeneration, and amyloid angiopathy, in Down syndrome, Fukuyama type congenital muscular dystrophy, and some patients with 'aging' disposition (for example Williams syndrome) deserve discussion on the 'true' precocious aging of nervous system.

Other neural degenerative products such as Lewy bodies or Pick bodies may also be observed in various pathological developmental conditions. In other aspect, there are indeed pathological conditions in which an accelerated neural aging process may be observed. Careful clinical observation and laboratory investigation of individual cases are required to solve the problems of the neural aging processes.

Arteriosclerosis including atherosclerosis and intimal and medial fibrosis in infancy and childhood is etiopathogenetically kaleidoscopic: genetic disposition, cardiovascular malformation, hypertension, hyperlipidemia and other anomalies of lipid metabolism, physical changes such as brain damages, inflammation, and others are only some examples of the possible multifactorial pathogeneses. Arteriosclerosis is not considered a disease only related to aging. So far as arteriosclerosis is generally not regarded as an aspect of various aging phenomena, it should not be taken for granted that infants and children with arteriosclerosis reflect an aging process, even though they may suffer from strokes. What appears to be reasonable is that atherosclerosis in children is generally believed to be an early stage of a lesion which may develop to atherosclerosis of adult or advanced age. Therefore, early detection of risk group or candidate patients and the appropriate preventive therapy is recommended.

Selected Readings

Beuren, A. J., Apitz, J., and Harmjanz, D. 1962. Supravalvular aortic stenosis in association with mental retardation and a certain facial appearance. Circulation 26:1235–1240.

Cockayne, E. A. 1936. Dwarfism with retinal atrophy and deafness. Arch. Dis. Child. 11:1–8.

Cockayne, E. A. 1949. Dwarfism with retinal atrophy and deafness. Arch. Dis. Child. 21:52–54.

Duong, T., De Rosa, M. J., Poukens, V., Vinters, H. V., and Fisher, R. S. 1994. Neuronal cytoskeletal abnormalities in human cerebral cortical dysplasia. Acta Neuropathol. 87:493–503.

Holland, A. J. and Oliver, C. 1995. Down's syndrome and the links with Alzheimer's disease. J. Neurol. Neurosurg. Psychiatry 59:111–114.

Nance, M. A., and Berry, S. A. 1992. Cockayne syndrome: review of 140 cases. Am. J. Med. Genet. 42:68–84.

Williams, J. C. P., Barratt-Boyes, B. G., and Lowe, J. B. 1961. Sypravalvular aortic stenosis. Circulation 24:311–318.

Yu, C. E., Oshima, J., Fu, Y. H., et al. 1996. Positional cloning of the Werner's syndrome gene. Science 272:258–262.

References

Anderson, K. A., Burbach, J. A., Fenton, L. J., et al. 1985. Idiopathic arterial calcification of infancy in newborn siblings with unusual light and electron microscopic manifestations. Arch. Pathol. Lab. Med. 109:838–842.

Armstrong, D. D. 1995. The neuropathology of Rett syndrome – Overview 1994. Neuropediatrics 26:100–104.

Auer, I. A., Schmidt, M. L., Lee, V. M. Y., et al. 1995. Paired he-

lical filament tau (PHFtau) in Niemann-Pick type C disease is similar to PHFtau in Alzheimer's disease. Acta Neuropathol. 90:547–551.

Bancher, C., Lettner, H., Jellinger, K. et al. 1996. On the relationship between measles virus and Alzheimer neurofibrillary tangles in subacute sclerosing panencephalitis. Neurobiol. Aging 17:527–733.

Bawle, E. V., Kupsky, W. J., Damato, C. J., et al. 1995. Familial infantile olivopontocerebellar atrophy. Pediat. Neurol. 13:14–18.

Beal, M. F., Kleinman, G. M., Ojemann, R. G., and Hochberg, F. H. 1981. Gangliocytoma of third ventricle: hyperphagia, somnolence, and dementia. Neurology 31:1224–1228.

Beavan, L. A., Quentin-Hoffmann, E., Schonherr, E., et al. 1993. Deficient expression of decorin in infantile progeroid patients. J. Biol. Chem. 268:9856–9862.

Bedwell, S. F., and Lindenberg, R. 1961. A hypothalmic hamartoma with dendritic proliferation and other neuronal changes associated with 'blastomatoid' reaction of astrocytes. J. Neuropathol. Exp. Neurol. 20:218–236.

Bellah, R. D., Zawodniak, L., Librizzi, R. J., and Harris, M. C. 1992. Idiopathic arterial calcification in infancy: prenatal and postnatal effects of therapy in infant. J. Pediatr. 121:930–933.

Bellugi, U., Bihrle, A., Jernigan, T., et al. 1990. Neuropsychological, neurological, and neuroanatomical profile of Williams syndrome. Am. J. Med. Genet. (Suppl.) 6:115–125.

Bergmann, M., Kuchelmeister, K., Kryne-Kubat, B., et al. 1994. Infantile multiple system atrophy with cytoplasmic amd intranuclear glioneural inclusions. Acta Neuropathol. 87:642–647.

Bugiani, O., Berio, A., Di Stefano, A., et al. 1978. Early degeneration of the cerebellar cortex, particular the granular cells. J. Neurol. 219:177–183

Beuren, A. J. 1964. Ein neues Syndrom: supravalvuläre Aortenstenose, multiple periphere Pulmonalstenosen, geistige Retardierung, ähnliche Gesichtszüge und identische Zahnmißbildungen. Monatschr. Kinderheilk. 112:218–221.

Briata, P., Bellicinii, C., Bignolo, M., and Gherzi, R. 1991. Insulin receptor gene expression is reduced in cells from a progeric patient. Molec. Cell. Endocrinol. 75:9–14.

Brown, M. S., and Goldstein, J. L. 1986. A receptor-mediated pathway for cholesterol homeostasis. Science 232:34–47.

Brown, W. T. 1992. Progeria: a human-disease model of accelerated aging? American J. Clin. Nutr. 55 (Suppl. 6):1222S-1224S.

Brown, W. T., Abdenur, J., and Goonewardena, P. 1990. Hutchinson-Gilford progeria syndrome: clinical, chromosomal and metabolic abnormalities. Am. J. Hum. Genet. 47 (Suppl):A50 (abstract)

Carrel, T., Pasic, M., Tkebuchava, T., et al. 1994. Aortic homograft and mitral valve repair in a patient with Werner's syndrome. Ann. Thorac. Surg. 57:1319–1320.

Castiñeyra, G., Panal, M., Lopez-Presas, H., et al. 1992. Two sibs with Wiedemann-Rautenstrauch syndrome: possibilities of prenatal diagnosis by ultrasound. J. Med. Genet. 29:4343–436.

Chaney, R. H. 1987. Neurogenic atherosclerosis in mentally retarded persons. J. Ment. Defic. Res. 31:235–240.

Chang, Y., Twiss, J. L., Horoupian, D. S., et al., 1993. Inherited syndrome of infantile olivopontocerebellar atrophy, micronodular cirrhosis, and renal tubular microcysts:review of the literature and a report of an additional case. Acta Neuropathol 86:399–404

Chapman, C. A., du Plessis, A., and Pober, B. R. 1995. Neurologic findings in children and adults with Williams syndrome. J. Child Neurol. 11:63–65.

Chessa, L., Bastianon, V., Del Porto, G., Nardo, T., and Stefanini, M. 1992. Cytogenetic and DNA repair studies in a patient affected by the neonatal progeroid syndrome. Ann. N. Y. Acad. Sci. 663:423–425.

Civantos, F. 1961. Human chromosomal abnormalities. Bull. Tulane Med. Fac. 20:241–253.

Corsellis, J. A. N., Bruton, C. J., and Freeman-Browne, D. 1973. The aftermath of boxing. Psychol. Med. 3:270–303.

Crain, B. J., McPhatter, L., Croom, D. W. II, and Hulette, C. M. 1995. Argyrophillic plaque-like deposits in children. Acta Neuropathol. 89:42–49.

Czeizel, A. E. and Marchalkó, M. 1995. Cockayne syndrome type III with high intelligence. Clin. Genet. 48:331–333.

De León, G. A., Breningstall, G., and Zaeri, N. 1986. Congenital Pick cell encephalopathy: a distinct disorder characterized by diffuse formation of Pick cells in the cerebral cortex. Acta Neuropathol. 70:235–242.

Demierre, B., Stichnoth, F. A., Hori, A., and Spoerri, O. 1986. Intracerebral ganglioglioma. J. Neurosurg. 65:177–182.

De Rosa, M. J., Secor, D. L., Barsom, M., Fisher, R. S., and Vinters, H. V. 1992. Neuropathologic findings in surgically treatred hemimegalencephaly: immunohistochemical, morphometric, and ultrastructural study. Acta Neuropathol. 84:250–260.

Devos, E. A., Leroy, J. G., Frijns, J. P., and Van de Berghe, H. 1981. The Wiedemann-Rautenstrauch or neonatal progeroid syndrome. Report of a patient with consanguineous parents. Eur. J. Pediatr. 136:245–248.

Elizan, T. S., and Casals, J. 1991. Astrogliosis in von Economo's and postencephalitic Parkinson's diseases supports probable viral etiology. J. Neurol. Sci. 105:131–134.

Epstein, C. J., Martin, G. M., Schultz, A. L., and Motulsky, A. G. 1966. Werner's syndrome. A review of its symptomatology, natural history, pathologic features, genetics and relationship to the natural aging process. Medicine (Baltimore) 45:177–221.

Erdem, N., Gunes, A. T., Avci, O., and Osma, E. 1994. A case of Hutchinson-Gilford progeria syndrome mimicking scleroderma in early infancy. Dermatology 188:318–321.

Ewart, A. K., Jin, W., Alkinson, D., Morris, C. A., and Keating, M. T. 1994. Supravalvular aortic stenosis associated with a deletion disrupting the elastin gene. J. Clin. Invest. 93:1971–1077.

Fernandez-Palazzi, F., McLaren, A. T., and Slowie, D. F. 1992. Report in a case of Hutchinson-Gilford Progeria, with special reference to orthopedic problems. Eur. J. Pediatr. Surg. 2:378–382.

Flodmark, C. E., Sveger, T., and Nilssonehle, P. 1994. Waist measurement correlates to a potentially atherogenic lipoprotein profile in obese 12–14-year-old children. Acta Paediat. 83:941–945.

Fujisawa, K. 1968. An unique type of axonal alteration (so-called axonal dystrophy) as seen in Goll's nucleus of 277 cases of controls. A contribution to the pathology of abeing process. Acta Neuropathol. 8:255–275.

Fujisawa, K. and Shiraki, H. 1978. Study of axonal dystrophy. I. Pathology of the neuropil of the gracile and the cuneate nuclei in ageing and old rats: a stereological study. Neuropathol. Appl. Neurobiol. 4:1–20.

Fujiwara, Y., Higashikawa, T., and Tatsumi, M. 1977. AS retarded rate of DNA replication and normal level of DNA re-

pair in Werner's syndrome fibroblasts in culture. J. Cell Physiol. 92:365- 374.

Fukuchi, K., Tanaka, K., Kumahara, Y., et al. 1990. Increased frequency of 6-thioguanine-resistant peripheral blood lymphocytes in Werner syndrome patients. Hum. Genet. 84:249–252.

Fukuyama, Y., Osawa, M., and Suzuki, H. 1981. Congenital progressive muscular dystrophy of the Fukuyama type – clinical, genetic and pathological considerations – Brain Dev. 3:1–29.

Gibb, W. R. G., Scaravilli, F., and Michaud, J. 1990. Lewy bodies and subacute sclerosing panencephalitis. J. Neurol. Neurosurg. Psychiatry 53:710–711.

Gieron, M. A., Gilbert-Barness, E., Vonsattel, J. P., and Korthals, J. K. 1995. Infantile progressive striato-thalamic degeneration in two siblings: A new syndrome. Pediat. Neurol. 12:260–263.

Goebel, H. H., Fidzianska, A., Lenard, H. G., et al. 1983. A morphological study of non-Japanese congenital muscular dystrophy associated with cerebral lesions. Brain Dev. 5:292–301.

Golden, J. A., Nielsen, G. P., Pober, B. R., and Hyman, B. T. 1995. The neuropathology of Williams syndrome: Report of a 35- year-old man with presenile beta/A4 amyloid plaques and neurofibrillary tangles. Arch. Neurol. 52:209–212.

Goto, M., Horiuchi, Y., Tanimoto, K., et al. 1978. Werner's syndrome: analysis of 15 cases with a review of the Japanese literature. J. Am. Geriat. Soc. 36:341–347.

Grahman, H., and Ule, G. 1957. Beitrag zur Kenntnis der chronischen cerebralen Krankheitsbilder bei Boxern. (Dementia pugilistica und traumatische Boxer-Encephalopathie). Psychiat. Neurol. 134:261–283.

Greally, J. M., Boone, L. Y., Lenkey, S. G., et al. 1992. Acrometageria: a spectrum of 'premature aging' syndromes. Am. J. Med. Genet. 44:334–339.

Grossman, H. J., Pruzansky, S., and Rosenthal, I., M. 1955. Progeroid syndrome. Report of a case of pseudo-senilism. Pediatrics 15:413–423.

Gutstein, W. H., Harrison, J., Parl, F., Kiu, G., and Avitable, M. 1978. Neural factors contribute to atherogenesis. Science 199:449–451.

Hagadorn, J. I., Wilson, W. G., Hogge, W. A., et al. 1990. Neonatal progeroid syndrome: more than one disease? Am. J. Med. Genet. 35:91–94.

Hall, J. W., and Denneny, J. C. 1993. Audiologic and otolaryngologic findings in progeria. J. Am. Acad. Audiol. 4:116–121.

Harada, K., Krucke, W., Mancardi, J. L., and Mandybur, T. I. 1988. Alzheimer's tangles in sudanophilic leukodystrophy. Neurology 38:55–59.

Haustein, J., Pawlas, U., and Cervos-Navarro; J. 1989. The Werner syndrome: a case study. Clin. Neuropathol. 8:147–151

Heston, L. L., Mastri, A. R., and Anderson, V. E. 1981. The genetics of Alzheimer's disease. Association with hematological malignancy and Down syndrome. Arch. Gen. Psychiatry 34:976–981.

Heyman, A., Wilkinson, W. E., Hurwitz, B. J. et al. 1983. Alzheimer's disease: genetic aspects and associated clinical disorders. Ann. Neurol. 14:507–516.

Higashikawa, T., and Fujiwara, Y. 1978. Normal level of unscheduled DNA synthesis in Werner's syndrome fibroblasts in culture. Exp. Cell Res. 113:438–442.

Hirano, A., Tuazon, R., and Zimmerman, H. M. 1968. Neurofibrillary changes, granulovacuolar bodies and argentophilic globules observed in tuberous sclerosis. Acta Neuropathol. 11:257–261.

Hirota, H., Matsuoka, R., Kimura, M., Imamura, S., Joh-o, K., Ando, M., Takano, A., Momma, K. 1996. Molecular cytogenetic diagnosis of Williams syndrome. Am. J. Med. Genet. 64:473–477.

Hoehn, H., Bryant, E. M., Au, K., *et al.* 1975. Variegated translocation mosaicism in human skin fibroblast cultures. Cytogenet. Cell Genet. 15:282–298.

Holland, A. J. 1994. Down's syndrome and dementia of the Alzheimer type. In A. Burns, and R. Levy (eds.) Dementia, pp. 695–708. Chapman & Hall, London.

Holman, R. L., McGill, H. C. Jr, Strong, J. P., and Geer, J. C. 1958. The natural history of atherosclerosis: the early aortic lesions as seen in New Orleans in the middle or the 20th century. Am. J. Pathol. 34:209–235.

Holtzman, D., Hedleywhite, E. T., Krishnamoorthy, K. S., Davis, K. R., Young, AB., Kosofsky, B. 1992. Progressive neurodegenerative disease in a young boy. Infantile striatonigral degeneration, with cerebellar degeneration, familial. N. Engl. J. Med. 327:261–268.

Hori, A. 1996. Precocious cerebral development associated with agenesis of the corpus callosum in mid-fetal life: a transient syndrome? Acta Neuropathol. 91:120–125.

Hori, A., Tamagawa, K., Eber, S. W., *et al.* 1987. Neuropathology of Seckel syndrome in fetal stage with evidence of intrauterine developmental retardation. Acta Neuropathol. 74:397–401.

Hori, A., Weiss, R., and Schaake, T. 1988. Ganglioglioma containing osseous tissue and neurofibrillary tangles. Arch. Pathol. Lab. Med. 112:653–655.

Houston, C. S., Zaleski, W. A., and Rozdilsky, B. 1982. Identical male twins and brother with Cockayne syndrome. American J. Med. Genet. 13:211–223.

Hudson, A. J., and Rice, G. P. A. 1990. Similarities of Guammanian ALS/PD to post-encephalitic Parkinsonism/ALS: possible viral cause. Canadian J. Neurol. Sci. 17:427–433.

Inoue, K., Hanyu, N., Takatsu, M., *et al.* 1978. The Cockayne's syndrome with benign clinical course. A study of four cases from two families. Rinsho Shinkei Gaku 18:477–485 (in Japanese.)

Ishitsu, T., Chikazawa, S., and Matsuda, I. 1985. Two siblings with microcephaly associated with calcification of cerebral white matter. Japanese J. Hum. Genet. 30:213–217.

Janota, I. 1974. Neurofibrillary tangles, granulovacuolar degeneration, and argentophilic bodies in a third ventricle tumor. Acta Neuropathol. 29:367–369.

Jefferson, R. D., Burn, J., Gaunt, K. L., Hunter, S., and Davison, E. V. 1986. A terminal deletion of the long arm of chromosome 4 (46,XX, del[4][q33]) in an infant with phenotypic features of Williams syndrome. J. Med. Genet. 23:474–480.

Kandt, R. S., Caoili, A. Q., Lorentz, W. B., and Elster, A. D. 1995. Hypertensive encephalopathy in children: Neuroimaging and treatment. J. Child Neurol. 10:236–239.

Kaplan, P., Levinson, M., and Kaplan, B. S. 1995. Cerebral artery stenoses in Williams syndrome cause strokes in childhood. J. Pediatr. 126:943–945.

Kawai, M., Nishikawa, T., Tanaka, M., *et al.* 1993. An autopsied case of Williams syndrome complicated by moyamoya disease. Acta Paediatr. Jpn. 35:63–67.

Kikuchi, A., Otsuka, N., Namba, Y., *et al.* 1991. Presenile appearance of abundant Alzheimer's neurofibrillary tangles without senile plaques in the brain in myotonic dystrophy. Acta Neuropathol. 82:1–5.

Kitt, C. A. and Wilcox, B. J. 1995. Preliminary evidence for neu-

rodegenerative changes in the substantia nigra of Rett syndrome. Neuropediatrics 26:114–118.

Knisely, A. S. 1993. Idiopathic arterial calcification of infancy – genetic studies. J. Pediatr. 122:836.

Kobayashi, S., Gibo, H., and Sugita, K. 1980. Wener's syndrome associated with meningioma. Neurosurgery 7:517–520.

Kornfeld, M. M. 1972. Generalized lipofuscinosis (generalized Kuf's disease). J. Neuropathol. Exp. Neurol. 31:668–681.

Kudo, M. 1986. Hypothalamic gangliocytoma: selective appearance of neurofibrillary changes, granulovacuolar degeneration, and argentophilic bodies. Acta Pathol. Jpn. 36:1225–1229.

Kuebber, S., Ropte, S., and Hori, A. 1990. Proliferation of adenohypophyseal cells into posterior lobe. Their normal anatomical condition and possible neoplastic potentiality. Acta Neurochir. 104:21–26.

Kupke, I. R., Heller, B., Weiss, P., *et al.* 1983. Early indicators for the risk of atherogenesis. A field test of a new methodology on Kindergarten children in Düsseldorf. Atherosclerosis 48:29–48.

Laso, F. J., Vasquez, G., Pastor, I., Procel, C., and Santos-Briz, A. 1989. Werner's syndrome and astrocytoma. Dermatológica 178:118–120.

Leech, R. W., Brumback, R. A., Miller, R. H., *et al.* 1985. Cockayne syndrome: clinicopathologic and tissue culture studies of affected siblings. J. Neuropathol. Exp. Neurol. 44:507–519.

Levin, P. S., Green, R., Victor, D. I., and MacLean, A. L. 1983. Histopathology of the eye in Cockayne's syndrome. Arch. Ophthalmol. 101:1093–1097.

Love, S., Bridges, L. R., and Case, C. P. 1995. Neurofibrillary tangles in Niemann-Pick disease type C. Brain 118:119–129.

Lowry, R. B. 1982. Early onset of Cockayne syndrome. Am. J. Med. Genet. 13:209–210.

Maayan, C., Peleg, O., Eyal, F., *et al.* 1984. Idiopathic infant arterial calcification: a case report and review of the literature. Eur. J. Pediatr. 142:211–215.

Mandybur, T. I., Nagpaul, A. S., Pappas, Z., and Niklowitz, W. J. 1977. Alzheimer neurofibrillary change in subacute sclerosing panencephalitis. Ann. Neurol. 1:103–107.

Mari, A., Amati, F., Mingarelli, R., *et al.* 1995. Analysis of the elastin gene in 60 patients with clinical diagnosis of Williams syndrome. Hum. Genet. 96:444–448.

Martin, G. M. 1978. Genetic syndromes in man with potential relevance to the pathobiology of aging. Birth Defects 14:5–39.

Martin, J. J., and Ceuterick, C. M. 1984. The Wiedemann-Rautenstrauch or neonatal progeroid syndrome. Neuropathological study of a case. Neuropediatrics 15:43–48.

Matsuo, S., Takeuchi, Y., Hayashi, S., Kinugasa, A., and Sawada, T. 1994. Patient with unusual Hutchinson-Gilford syndrome (progeria). Pediatr. Neurol. 10:237–240.

Mazzarello, P., Verri, A., Mondello, C., *et al.* 1992. Enzymes of DNA metabolism in a patient with the Wiedemann-Rautenstrauch progeroid syndrome. Ann. N.Y. Acad. Sci. 663:440–441.

Meyer, W. W., and Lind, J. 1972. Calcification of carotid siphon – a common finding in infancy and childhood. Arch. Dis. Child 47:355–363.

Meyer, W. W., and Lind, J. 1972. Calcifications of the iliac arteries in newborn and infants. Arch. Dis. Child 47:364–372.

Morán, M. A., Probst, A., Navarro, C., and Gómez-Ramos, P. 1995. Alzheimer's disease-type neurofibrillary degeneration in verrucose dysplasias of the cerebral cortex. Acta Neuropathol. 90:356–365.

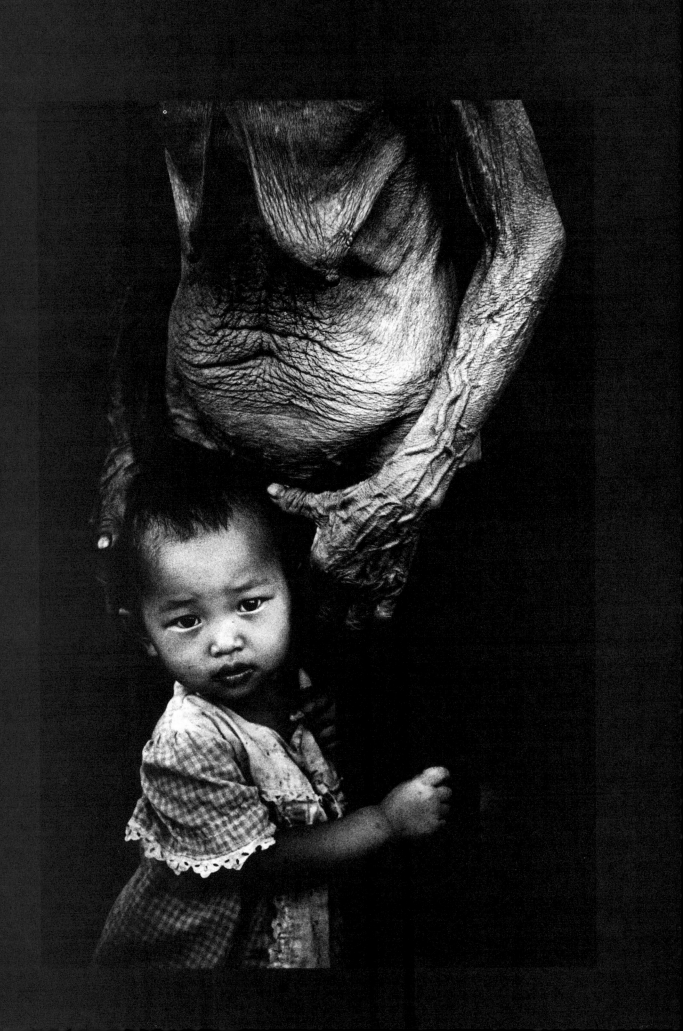

IV

Neural Aging, From Perception to Behavior

implicated by many studies in the younger adult population.

Another neurohumoral abnormality long known to be associated with, while not specific for, major depression is an elevation in blood plasma of the hormone, *cortisol*, as well as an disturbance in the feedback inhibition loop regulating the release of this hormone that is clinically assessed by the *dexamethasone-suppression test* (DST). These findings have been extended to depression in the elderly. Plasma cortisol levels were found to be elevated not only in comparison to non-depressed elderly subjects (Schleifer *et al.*, 1989), but also relative to younger depressed patients (Ferrier *et al.*, 1988). A correlation was found between post-DST cortisol level and severity of depression (Molchan *et al.*, 1990) and depression-induced cognitive impairment ('pseudo-dementia', Siegal *et al.*, 1989). However, outside of research, the lack of specificity makes the DST not very useful: Skare and colleagues summarised data demonstrating that the DST did not discriminate between major depression and dementia.

Imaging Studies Revealed that Brain Atrophy Correlates with Depression

Several studies using CT imaging have concluded that the *ventricle-brain ratio* (VBR), a measure of brain atrophy, is increased in depression (Pearlson *et al.*, 1989). Correlations have been found in some studies between VBR and degree of cognitive impairment (Kellner *et al.*, 1986), age of onset (Alexopoulos *et al.*, 1989) and the DST (Alexopoulos, 1989). In one study, elderly patients with larger VBR were less likely to profit from antidepressant drug treatment (Alexopoulos, 1989). While the findings of CT have, by and large, been confirmed by newer imaging modalities such as MRI (Chapter 28), an additional feature that has come into focus are lesions in the white matter of the brain, easily depicted as hyperintensities in appropriate MRI sequences (Chapters 21 and 28). In depressed elderly patients, the number of white matter lesions has been found to correlate with later onset, lack of response to pharmacotherapy, presence of psychotic features, and cognitive impairment (Lesser *et al.*, 1991). Of special interest is the finding that lesion location influences the liability for depression, the basal ganglia being especially implicated (Coffey *et al.*, 1993).

Functional imaging studies of depressed patients, while controversial in detail (Biol. Psychiatry editorial, 1996), have demonstrated a frontocaudal metabolic gradient commonly interpreted as frontal hypometabolism (Mayberg *et al.*, 1990). This may be of value in clinical differential diagnosis since dementing disorders, especially Alzheimer disease, show a different pattern.

Organic Brain Disease may Present as Depression in the Elderly

Since the prevalence of organic brain disease increases with age and many of these may present or be associated with depressive symptoms, it is mandatory that these disorders be considered in the elderly depressed patient.

While estimates vary, most authors find that about one quarter of all patients with Alzheimer disease are depressed (Teri and Wagner, 1992). Due to the presence of cognitive impairment in this disease, diagnosis may be difficult. Interesting in the context of the neurobiochemical hypotheses outlined above is the finding that serotonin and its metabolite 5-HIAA as well as norepinephrine were found lowered in the cerebrospinal fluid of depressed, compared to non-depressed, Alzheimer patients. In vascular dementia, about one-quarter of patients are depressed (Fischer *et al.*, 1990). It was noted above that white matter lesions have been found to be associated with severity of depression.

In Parkinson disease, up to one-half of patients may be severely depressed during the course of their illness (Cummings, 1992), and depression may precede motor symptoms in about 40 percent of these (Mayeux *et al.*, 1981), indicating that depression may not be a response to, but rather an expression of the illness. Since psychomotor and vegetative features of Parkinson disease bear similarities to the clinical picture of depression, diagnosis is difficult. The DST, while more often abnormal in depressed than non-depressed Parkinsonian patients (Kostic *et al.*, 1990), is not specific enough to aid in differential diagnosis. The serotonin metabolite, 5-HIAA, was lowered in the CSF of depressed patients with Parkinson disease when compared to euthymic patients (Mayeux *et al.*, 1988). Using PET imaging, Mayberg and colleagues demonstrated hypometabolism in the caudate and in orbitofrontal cortex in depression.

Robinson and colleagues (1990) showed that in the weeks following a stroke, about 45 percent of patients are depressed, a figure that falls to 14 percent two years after the insult. Of neurobiological interest is the linkage of lesion location to depressive symptoms. Several studies have demonstrated that depression is more likely to occur following left- than right-sided strokes. Many, but not all studies have found that in left-sided lesions, severity of depression is increased as the lesion nears the frontal pole (House *et al.*, 1990). This fits into the neurotransmitter hypotheses since the serotonin- and norepinephrine-containing projections travel via the medial forebrain bundle and the basal ganglia to the frontal cortex, implicating that massive depletion of these substances might result following a stroke at the frontal subcortical area (Robinson *et al.*, 1984). Lesion size is also important, greater lesions being associated with more emotional lability (House *et al.*, 1989). DST non-suppression is increased in post-stroke depression (Lipsey *et al.*, 1985).

Other brain disorders, such as Huntington disease (Chapter 32), may also be associated with depression, as may be cardiovascular (Rabins *et al.*, 1985), metabolic (Reynolds *et al.*, 1970) and endocrine diseases. Hypothyroidism is especially important in the elderly population and must be ruled out in all depressed elderly patients.

Late Life-Onset Psychoses

While the peak incidence for *schizophrenia* is in the second and third decade of life, late-life onset of psychosis is by no means a rare event, accounting for up to 10 percent of psychiatric hospital admissions of elderly patients (Siegel and Goodman, 1987). Many old age psychoses do not resemble full-blown schizophrenia but may show symptoms restricted to simple paranoia or may resemble more confusional states with delusions of poor systemic content. Depending on how narrowly the syndrome is defined, up to 50 percent of these patients may have an identifiable organic brain disease. Thus, late-life onset psychoses are a heterogeneous group of diseases comprising *'symptomatic' psychoses* due to degenerative or vascular disease, and a core group that might be aptly called *'late-life schizophrenia'*. The following account refers to a more narrowly defined disease. In these patients, the clinical picture does not differ much from the early onset-cases, although *persecutory delusions* may be especially common (Pearlson *et al.*, 1989) and negative symptoms rarer than in younger patients. Neuropsychological test performance also tends to be similar in early- and late-onset psychoses (Miller *et al.*, 1991).

The Stress-Vulnerability Concept

One of the best-documented facts in psychiatric research is that schizophrenia is a disease with a strong hereditary component. Kendler and colleagues have shown that first degree-relatives of schizophrenic patients have a risk of falling ill that is about 18 times that of the general population. Monozygotic twins, which are genetically identical, are concordant for the disease in 59 percent pooled over all studies, whereas dizygotic twins, which share only half of their genome, have a concordance rate of only 15 percent. These results have been repeatedly confirmed in study designs such as cross-adoption studies, that have been careful to control for environmental similarities as usually arise when siblings are reared together. For elderly patients suffering from late-life psychoses, a hereditary component has also been confirmed. Kay (1972) found 3.4 percent affected relatives of index patients with late-onset schizophrenia, a rate significantly higher than that in the general population, but lower than the rate in the relatives of early-onset schizophrenia (5.8 percent in this study).

On the other hand, it is as obvious from the findings cited above that schizophrenia is not purely determined by genetic factors. The fact that more than 40 percent of genetically identical individuals are discordant for schizophrenia testifies that environmental factors have a large role to play in the manifestation and maybe also in the pathogenesis of the disease.

In view of these facts, the stress-vulnerability theory of J. Zubin and B. Spring (1977) has found wide clinical acceptance as a framework for understanding the pathogenesis of schizophrenia and the onset of clinically manifest symptoms. It states that the pathophysiology underlying schizophrenic illness renders afflicted individuals more vulnerable to events in the environment that a healthy person could normally cope with. The afflicted patient cannot handle the stressful stimuli and becomes manifestly ill. In other words, there has to be a balance between vulnerability (which may be genetically determined) on the one hand, and the amount of stressful events one can take: This can mean that for a highly vulnerable subject, even a normal family situation may be too much to process and react to; which is why most schizophrenic episodes do not have an identifiable 'reason', in the sense of a single traumatic event, as laymen often erroneously presume.

The attractiveness of the stress-vulnerability model in a clinical setting is that it not only accounts for the abovementioned genetic data, but that it also suggests immediate clinical consequences: To help the patient, you have to reduce his or her vulnerability (by antipsychotic medication or individual psychotherapy, say) and remove stressors (e.g. by hospitalization or family therapy).

Can Zubin's model be applied to late-life psychosis? If so, it should be possible to (i) identify stressors that are related to old age and that may precipitate psychosis and/or (ii) to find results from neurobiochemistry or neuromorphology that point towards an increased vulnerability in the elderly. This evidence will now be reviewed.

Stressors and Risk Factors in Late-Life Psychosis

While much research remains to be done in this area, some data point towards the identification of stressors increasing the risk for late-life psychosis. Several studies have identified sensory deficits as a risk factor that is much more common in later life. Visual deficits caused by cataracts and auditory deficits caused by conductive deafness are the most common (Cooper *et al.*, 1974; Pearlson *et al.*, 1989). Treating the deafness may improve the psychosis in some patients (Eastwood *et al.*, 1981).

Patients with late-life onset psychoses have been reported to suffer from more social isolation than age matched-controls. Women, for example, are less likely to be married and have children (Kay and Roth, 1961). F. Post (1966) also found a trend towards lower socioeconomic status in patients. The rate of premorbid personality disorders is increased (mainly *schizoid* and *paranoid personality disorder*), a finding that may explain in part the low marriage rates and social isolation.

Evidence From Neurotransmitter Findings

The recognition that the neuroleptic agents effective in schizophrenia such as chlorpromazine, butyrophenones and phenothiazines were blocking dopaminergic activity (Seeman *et al.*, 1975; Snyder, 1976) led to the hypothesis that schizophrenia may be a disturbance of the dopaminergic system, reflecting a hyperdopaminergic state (Matthysse, 1973). In its initial, simple form, the hypothesis is no longer tenable as it cannot account for the effect of new, so-called atypical antipsychotic substances with low dopamine receptor affinity and relatively higher affinity to many other receptors (Meltzer, 1991). Revisions of the dopamine hypothesis have been proposed (Weinberger, 1987; Carlsson, 1988; Meltzer, 1988). However, newer evidence and lines of thought including *cognitive theories* suggest a more complex model in which interactions of various transmitter systems and substructures of the brain are considered. For example, involvement of the *noradrenergic* (van Kammen, 1991), *GABAergic* (Benes *et al.*, 1991; Roberts, 1972) and *serotonergic* transmitter systems has been proposed. Interest in serotonin metabolism has been strengthened by the recognition that several new antipsychotic agents exert part of their influence through the blockade of a subclass of serotonin receptors, the 5-HT2 receptors (Meltzer, 1991).

Finally, the last decade has witnessed a surge of interest in the role of the *excitatory amino acids* in brain disease (Ulas and Cotman, 1993). Schizophrenia research is no exception. Interest in these transmitter systems in psychiatry is founded in the observations that the excitatory amino acids, especially glutamate, have an important role in the phenomenon called *long-term potentiation*, a process believed to be central in learning and memory (Teyler and Discenna, 1987), and in the observation that potent psychotogenic drugs such as *phencyclidine* ('angel dust') act as non-competitive antagonists at a subclass of glutamate receptors (Sircar *et al.*, 1987). Important for the understanding of schizophrenia is the concept of excitotoxin-mediated neurotoxicity (Chapter 32), which states that overstimulation of neurons may lead, via a cascade of intraneuronal biochemical pathways triggered by glutamate-mediated calcium entry, to neuronal damage and death (Javitt and Zukin, 1991). This mechanism has been linked to a variety of diseases of the nervous system (Young *et al.*, 1988). In fact, glutamatergic hyperexcitation has been suggested as the primary cause of maladjustment in schizophrenia. According to this view defended by P. Riederer, dopaminergic overstimulation, which causes a disturbance in the focusing process, occurs in reaction to the disturbance in the glutamatergic system.

Of importance for our subject, there is evidence from both animal and human research that NMDA receptors decline with age (Kitamura *et al.*, 1992, Piggot *et al.*, 1992) and that this may be a process that is specific for the subcortical structures (Tamaru *et al.*, 1991).

Some Morphological Changes in Schizophrenia Have Been Elucidated

While initial lack of success has given rise to the mock phrase of schizophrenia as 'the graveyard of neuropathology', careful research has demonstrated both gross and fine-structure morphological alterations in schizophrenia. Decreases in volume and weight, presumably from atrophy, have been found in a variety of structures such as the dorsolateral frontal lobe (Stevens, 1982), the hippocampus (Conrad, 1991), the nucleus accumbens and other components of the limbic system-Papez circuit. Of relevance to the present discussion, most of the neuropathological studies performed have been on elderly individuals suffering from schizophrenia and dying from 'natural' causes. It is an unsettled question whether the atrophic changes result from accelerated neuronal loss, a form of 'accelerated aging', whether they reflect a form of prenatal disturbance or are a consequence of an ongoing damaging, e.g. inflammatory process. Most authorities in the field argue against the latter view since no glial reaction is found in the brains of schizophrenics. Some have even conceptualized that the time point at which schizophrenia becomes first symptomatic is determined by the initial effects of neural aging, thought to 'unmask' a defect that had been compensated before (Waddington, 1993).

Of interest are also the fine-structure alterations in schizophrenia. Various groups have found evidence for the occurrence of abnormal cell sprouting in several structures such as the hippocampus (Conrad *et al.*, 1991) and the entorhinal cortex (Arnold *et al.*, 1991). It is tempting to conclude that this 'miswiring' of circuits results in some sort of impairment of brain information processing.

Imaging Studies

Compared to matched controls, an increased VBR in patients with late-onset psychosis was demonstrated by several studies in CT (Pearlson *et al.*, 1987) and MRI imaging (Krull *et al.*, 1991; Pearlson *et al.*, 1993), but not confirmed by all (Burns *et al.*, 1989). White matter changes have also been demonstrated in several MRI studies in patients with late-onset psychoses (Miller *et al.*, 1991; Lesser *et al.*, 1991).

Functional imaging perfusion studies show that patients with late-onset psychoses have a relative excess of multiple areas with reduced flow (Lesser *et al.*, 1993). In one study (Miller *et al.*, 1992), more than 80 percent of psychotic patients had an area of hypoperfusion in the frontal or temporal area.

A PET neuroimaging study of dopamine D_2 receptor density in late-onset psychosis (Pearlson *et al.*, 1993), using the methodology of Wong and colleagues (1986), gave evidence for an increased number of postsynaptic dopamine receptors in psychosis, a finding consistent with findings in drug-naive younger schizophrenics, thus in support of a contribution of dopaminergic mechanisms in the pathogenesis of schizophrenia in old age too.

A Multimodal Model of Schizophrenia

The diversity of the morphological and biochemical data summarized so far call for a multimodal model of schizophrenia. Ideally, it should offer not only a way to integrate findings from the basic sciences, but lend itself also to an understanding of the way in which disturbances on a cellular or biochemical level lead to the symptoms of schizophrenia. Any such model is hypothetical at present, and the gap is wide between clinical manifestations such as thought disorder, delusions, hallucinations or blunted affect and the analysis of brain structure and physiology.

Therefore, a model is required that is situated on a theoretical ground between clinical psychiatry and basic science: A model of disturbed information processing and reality shaping in schizophrenia (Braff, 1993).

Patients suffering from schizophrenia cannot adjust to and process complex cognitive tasks properly. Disorders of information processing had already been detected by the clinicians who first defined the disease in the beginning of this century, namely Bleuler, and Kraepelin. Such disorders have been consistently found to be associated with schizophrenia (Holzmann, 1987), and are found in sub-clinically ill patients and unaffected family members (Siever, 1991), pointing towards an association with the genetic basis of the disease. Information processing disturbances have been found to be improved by medication in schizophrenic patients (Meyer-Lindenberg et al., 1997). Several clinical symptoms of schizophrenia have been found to correlate with information processing dysfunction, such as negative symptoms (Braff, 1989), blunted affect and withdrawal (Bernstein, 1987). These results have been found to be specific and not related to non-specific symptomatology (Nuechterlein, 1977).

In a top-bottom approach, a model of impaired information processing can be used to understand the evolution of schizophrenic symptoms. A patient unable to screen out irrelevant information and select data important for his present state may present with thought disorder and may be highly vulnerable to stressful interpersonal interaction (Braff, 1993). Blunted affect may result from an inability to screen enteroceptive and emotional information, and so on.

In the bottom-up approach, knowledge of the brain mechanisms involved in information processing allow an integration of data from the basic sciences. Cognitive stimuli cause an excitatory arousal in the brain. This more unspecific response to incoming signals causes a modulatory reaction which includes both excitatory and inhibitory responses that shape the information content to its proper weight which then represents the reality to which we adjust our responses. This reality shaping process involves a delicately balanced interaction between cortical and subcortical structures of the brain, as well as a balance between excitatory and inhibitory circuits necessary for an optimal level of arousal. A *cortico-striato-pallido-thalamic circuit* has been identified that subserves information processing, modulation and screening in several paradigms, such as pre-pulse inhibition (Braff et al., 1992). Data from neuropathological studies confirm this concept (Goldmann-Rakic, 1988), and abnormalities of the cortico-striato-pallido-thalamic circuit have also been found in imaging studies (Jernigan et al., 1991). Multiple neurotransmitter functions are involved in this circuit, mediating both excitatory (glutamatergic and noradrenergic) and inhibitory (GABAergic) functions. Animal studies support a prominent role for dopaminergic mechanisms in this circuit, with special emphasis on the *nucleus accumbens* (Swerdlow et al., 1986). The neuroanatomic and neurobiochemical properties of the dopaminergic system allow, in information-processing terms, a conceptualization of dopamine

as a modifier that sharpens and focuses ongoing neuronal network activity (Cohen and Servan-Schreiber, 1992).

The presence of information-processing disturbances in elderly patients with late-life psychosis has been confirmed (Miller et al., 1991). The model presented allows for an integration of several findings reported above, such as the disturbance in dopamine D_2-receptors in PET (Pearlson et al., 1993) and the morphological alterations found in various components of the cortico-striato-pallido-thalamic circuit (Benes et al., 1991; Arnold et al., 1991). The increased incidence of white-matter lesions in elderly patients with late-life psychosis (Miller et al., 1991; Lesser et al., 1991) may also be hypothesized to result from an additive effect of several small lesions in the information-processing circuitry. In the context of the stress-vulnerability paradigm, it is conceivable that patients with impaired information processing are especially challenged by having to cope with a sensory deficit, such as conduction deafness, or with living alone.

An Overall View

The data reviewed in this chapter show that, while much work remains to be done, the gap between basic science and clinical psychiatry is starting to be filled. It is probable that not only the understanding of the pathophysiology of mental diseases, but also the health of the elderly population, will profit from this.

Selected Readings

Bogerts, B. 1993. Recent advances in the neuropathology of schizophrenia. Schizophr. Bull. 19:431–445.

Busse, W. W., and Blazer, D. G. (eds.) 1996. The American Psychiatric Press Textbook of Geriatric Psychiatry. Washington, London, The American Psychiatric Press.

Carlesimo, G. A., and Oscar-Berman, M. 1992. Memory deficits in Alzheimer's patients: a comprehensive review. Neuropsychol. Rev. 3:119–169.

Coffey, C. E., and Cummings, J. L. (eds.) 1994. The American Psychiatric Press Textbook of Geriatric Neuropsychiatry. Washington, London, The American Psychiatric Press.

Grady, C. L., McIntosh, R. A., Horwitz, B., et al. 1995. Age-related reductions in human recognition memory due to impaired encoding. Science 269:218–221.

Jarvitt, D. C., and Zukin, S. R. 1991. Recent advances in the phencyclidine model of schizophrenia. Am. J. Psychiatry 148:1301–1308.

Kovelmann, J. A., and Scheibel, A. B. 1984. A neurohistological correlate of schizophrenia. Biol. Psychiatry 19:1601–1621.

Lang, C. 1994. Demenzen: Diagnose und Differential-diagnose. Chapman & Hall GmbH, Weinheim, Germany.

Schaie, K. W. 1989. The hazards of cognitive aging. Gerontologist 29:484–493.

van Kammern, D. P. 1991. The biochemical basis of relapse and drug response in schizophrenia: Review and hypothesis. Psychol. Med. 21:881–895.

Wallin, A., and Blennow, K. 1992. Neurologic motor signs in early and late onset Alzheimer's disease. Dementia 3:314–319.

References

AFAR – American Federation for Aging Research. 1995. Putting Aging on Hold: Delaying the Diseases of Old Age. AFAR and Alliance for Aging Research, Washington, DC, USA.

APA – American Psychiatric Association. 1987. Diagnostic and Statistical Manual of Mental Disorders. 3rd ed. rev. American Psychiatric Press, Washington, DC.

Arnold, S. E., Hyman, B. T., Van Hosen, G. W., and Damasio, A. R. 1991. Some cyroarchitectural abnormalities of the entorhinal cortex in schizophrenia. Arch. Gen. Psychiatry 48:625–632.

Benes, F. M., McSparren, J., Bird, E. D., San Giovanni, J. P., and Vincent, S. L. 1991. Deficits in small interneurons in prefrontal and cingulate cortices of schizophrenic and schizoaffective patients. Arch. Gen. Psychiatry 48:996–1001.

Benes, F. M., Sorensen, I., and Bird, E. D. 1991. Reduced neuronal size in posterior hippocampus of schizophrenic patients. Schizophr. Bull. 17:597–608.

Bernstein, A. S. 1987. Orienting response research in schizophrenia: Where we have come and where we might go. Schizophr. Bull. 13:623–641.

Bleuler, E. 1911. Dementia praecox oder die Gruppe der Schizophrenien.

Braff, D. L. 1989. Sensory input deficits an negative symptoms in schizophrenic patients. Am. J. Psychiatry 146:1006–1111.

Braff, D. L. 1993. Information processing and attention dysfunctions in schizophrenia. Schizophr. Bull. 19:233–259.

Braff, D. L., Grillon, C., and Geyer, M. A. 1992. Gating and habituation of the startle reflex in schizophrenic patients. Arch. Gen. Psychiatry 49:206–215.

Burns, A., Carrik, J., Ames, D., et al. 1989. The cerebral cortical appearance in late paraphrenia. Int. J. Geriat. Psychiatry 4:31–34.

Carlsson, A. 1988. The current status of the dopamine hypothesis of schizophrenia. Neuropsychopharmacology 1:179–186.

Coffey, C. E., Wilkenson, W. E., Weiner, R. D., et al. 1993. Quantitative cerebral anatomy in depression: a controlled magnetic resonance imaging study. Arch. Gen. Psychiatry 50:7–16.

Cohen, J. D., and Servan-Schreiber, D. 1992. Context, cortex, and dopamine: a connectionist approach to behaviour and biology in schizophrenia. Psychol. Rev. 99:45–77.

Cooper, A. F., Kay, D. W. K., Curry, A. R., et al. 1974. Hearing loss in paranoid and affective psychoses of the elderly. Lancet 2:851–861.

Eaton, W. W., Kramer, M., Anthony, J. C., et al. 1989. The incidence of specific DIS/DSM-III mental disorders: data from the NIHM Epidemiologic Cathement Area program. Acta Psychiatr. Scand. 79:163–178.

Ferrier, I. N., Pascual, J., Charlton, B. G., et al. 1988. Cortisol, ACTH and dexamethasone concentrations in a psychogeriatric population. Biol. Psychiatry 23:252–366.

Fischer, P., Simamyi, M., and Daniekczyk, W. 1990. Depression in dementia of the Alzheimer type and in multi-infarct dementia. Am. J. Psychiatry :1484–1487.

House, A., Dennis, M., Molyneux, A., et al. 1989. Emotionalism after stroke. Br. Med. J. 289:992–994.

House, A., Dennis, M., Warlow, G., et al. 1990. Mood disorders after stroke and their relation to lesion location. Brain 113:1113–1129.

Kane, L. R. 1990. Introduction. In L. R. Kane, J. Evans, and D. MacFayden (eds.) Improving the health of older people: a world view, pp. 15–18. Oxford, Oxford University Press.

Kay, D. W. K. 1972. Schizophrenia and schizophrenia-like states in the elderly. Br. Hosp. Med. 8:369–379.

Kay, D. W. K., and Roth, M. 1961. Environmental an hereditary factors in the schizophrenias of old age ('late paraphrenia') and their bearing on the general problem of causation in schizophrenia. J. Mental Sci. 107:649–686.

Kendler, K. S., and Diehl, S. R. 1993. The genetics of schizophrenia: a current, genetic-epidemiologic perspective. Schizophr. Bull. 19:261–285.

Kostic, V. S., Covickovic-Sternic, N., Belsac-Bubasirevic, L., et al. 1990. Dexamethasone suppression test in patients with Parkinson's disease. Mov. Disord. 5:23–26.

Lesser, I. M., Miller, B. L., Boone, K. B., et al. 1991. Brain injury and cognitive function in late-onset psychotic depression. J. Neuropsychiatry Clin. Neurosci. 3:33–40.

Lesser, I. M., Miller, B. L., Swartz, J. R., et al. 1993. Brain imaging in late-life schizophrenia and related psychoses. Schizophr. Bull. 19:773–782.

Lipsey, J. R., Robinson, R. G., and Pearlson, G. D. 1985. Dexamethasone suppression test an mood following stroke. Am. J. Psychiatry 142:318–323.

Mayberg, H. S., Starkstein, S. E., Sadzot, B., et al. 1990. Selective hypometabolism in the interior frontal lobe in depressed patients with Parkinson's disease. Ann. Neurol. 28:57–64.

Meltzer, H. Y. 1988. New insights into schizophrenia through atypical antipsychotic drugs. Neuropsychopharmacology 1:193–196.

Meltzer, H. Y. 1991. The mechanism of action of novel antipsychotic drugs. Schizophr. Bull. 17:263–287.

Meyer-Lindenberg, A., and Rao, M. L. 1993. Interrelationship between blood serotonin levels and affinity of platelet imipramine binding sites in healthy subjects. Pharmacopsychiatry 26:15–19.

Meyer-Lindenberg, A., Gruppe, H., Bauer, et al. 1997. Improvement of cognitive function in schizophrenic patients receiving clozapine or zotepine: results from a double-blind study. Pharmacopsychiatry 30:35–42.

Miller, B. L., Lesser, I. M., Boone, K. B., et al. 1991. Brain lesions and cognitive function in late-life psychosis. Br. J. Psychiatry 158:76–82.

Molchan, S. E., Hill, J. L., Mellow, A. M., et al. 1990. The dexamethasone suppression test in Alzheimer's disease and major depression: relationship to dementia severity, depression and CSF monoamines. Int. Psychogeriatry 2:99–122.

Nuechterlein, K. H. 1977. Reaction time and attention in schizophrenia: a critical evaluation of the data and theories. Schizophr. Bull. 3:373–436.

Pearlson, G. D., Garbacz, D. J., Tompkins, R. H., et al. 1987. Lateral cerebral ventricular size in late onset schizophrenia. In N. E. Miller, and G. D. Cohen (eds.) Schizophrenia and Aging, New York, Guilford. pp. 246–248.

Pearlson, G. D., Kreger, L., Rabins, P. V., et al. 1989. A chart review study of late-onset and early onset schizophrenia. Am. J. Psychiatry 146:1568–1574.

Pearlson, G. D., Rabins, P. V., Kim, W. S., et al. 1989. Structural brain changes and cognitive deficits in elderly depressives with and without reversible dementia ('pseudodementia'). Psychol. Med. 19:573–584.

Pearlson, G. D., Tune, L. E., Wong, D. F., et al. 1993. Quantitative D_2 dopamine receptor PET and structural MRI changes in late onset schizophrenia: a preliminary report. Schizophr. Bull. 18:783–795.

Post, F. 1966. Persistent Persecutory States of the Elderly. London, Pergamon.

Rabins, P. V., Harvis, K., and Koven, S. 1985. High fatality rates of late-life depression associated with cardiovascular disease. J. Affect. Disord. 9:165–167.

Reynolds, E. H., Preece, J. M., Bailey, J., et al. 1970. Folate deficiency in depressive illness. Br. J. Psychiatry 117:287–292.

Robinson, R. G., Kubos, K. L., Starr, L. B., et al. 1984. Mood disorders in stroke patients: importance of location of lesion. Brain 107:82–93.

Schaie, K. W. 1989. Perceptual speed in adulthood: cross-sectional and longitudinal studies. Psychol. Aging 4:443–453.

Schleifer, S. J., Keller, S. E., Bond, R. B., et al. 1989. Major depressive disorder and immunity. Arch. Gen. Psychiatry 46:81–87.

Siegel, C. E., and Goodman, A. B. 1987. Mental illness among the elderly in a large state psychiatric facility: a comparison with other age groups. In N. E. Miller, and G. D. Cohen (eds.) Schizophrenia and Aging, New York, Guilford. pp. 23–34.

Swerdlow, N. R., Braff, D. L., Geyer, M. A., and Koob, G. F. 1986. Central dopamine hyperactivity in rats mimics abnormal acoustic startle response in schizophrenics. Biol. Psychiatry 21:23–33.

Teyler, T. J., and Discenna, P. 1987. Long-term potentiation. Ann. Rev. Neurosci. 10:131–161.

Ulas, J., and Cotman, C. W. 1993. Excitatory amino acid receptors in schizophrenia. Schizophr. Bull. 19:105–117.

Waddington, J. L. 1993. Neurodynamics of abnormalities in cerebral metabolism and structure in schizophrenia. Schizophr. Bull. 19:55–69.

Weinberger, D. R. 1987. Implications of normal brain development for the pathogenesis of schizophrenia. Arch. Gen. Psychiatry 44:660–669.

Wong, D. F., Gjedde, J., Wagner, H. N. Jr, et al. 1986. Quantification of neuroreceptors in the living human brain, II: assessment of receptor density and affinity using inhibition studies. J. Cereb. Blood Flow Metab. 6:147–153.

Wong, D. F., Wagner, H. N. Jr., Tune, L. E., et al. 1986. Positron emission tomography reveals elevated D_2 dopamine receptors in drug-naive schizophrenics. Science 234:1558–1563.

Young, A. B., Greenamyre, J. T., Hollingworth, Z., et al. 1988. NMDA receptor losses in putamen from patients with Huntington's disease. Science 241:0981–983.

Zubin, J. 1975. Problem of attention in schizophrenia. In M. L. Kietzman, S. Sutton, and J. Zubin (eds.) Experimental Approaches to Psychopathology, New York, NY: Academic Press. pp. 139–166.

Zubin, J, and Spring, B. 1977. Vulnerability – a new view of schizophrenia. J. Abnorm. Psychol. 86:103–26.

Fabio Blandini
Cristina Tassorelli
J. Timothy Greenamyre

32

Movement Disorders

P roper execution of voluntary movements results from the correct processing of sensory-motor information in the brain. This task is carried out, in part, by the nuclei of the basal ganglia, whose anatomical and functional organization has received considerable attention in the last decade. This functional organization undergoes profound alterations in two age-related chronic, neurodegenerative diseases, *Parkinson disease* and *Huntington disease*. These diseases, in which the capacity to control voluntary movements is impaired, are referred to as movement disorders.

Functional Anatomy of Basal Ganglia

Improved understanding of the anatomy, physiology and neurotransmission of the basal ganglia has led to formulation of increasingly refined models of this circuitry. Currently, the basal ganglia are viewed as a circuit in which signals received from the cerebral cortex flow through the different nuclei, being processed and integrated at each level, until the result of this processing is transmitted, via the motor thalamus, back to the cortex (Figure 32–1). The main input nucleus of basal ganglia is the *corpus striatum* (Str), which receives a dense input from dopaminergic neurons of the *substantia nigra pars compacta* (SNc), and excitatory, glutamatergic, projections from virtually all regions of cerebral cortex and from the thalamus. Str projects to both segments of *globus pallidus*, medial globus pallidus (MGP) and lateral globus pallidus (LGP) and to the *substantia nigra pars reticulata* (SNr). Striatal projection neurons are GABAergic and appear to be segregated into two distinct subpopulations. Neurons projecting to

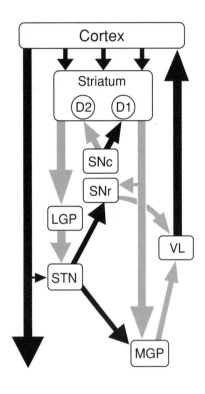

FIGURE   32–1

Highly simplified schematic diagram of basal ganglia circuitry. Gray arrows denote inhibitory pathways; black arrows represent excitatory pathways. The main input nucleus of this circuitry is the striatum, which receives excitatory, glutamatergic, projections from virtually all regions of cerebral cortex and a dense dopaminergic input from SNc. Striatal neurons are connected to the output nuclei of the basal ganglia, the medial segment of globus pallidus (MGP) and the substantia nigra pars reticulata (SNr), by two different pathways: a direct pathway, consisting of direct projections of striatal neurons to MGP and SNr, and an indirect pathway, wherein the striatum projects to the lateral segment of the globus pallidus (LGP) which, in turn, sends projections to the subthalamic nucleus (STN); STN then projects to MGP and SNr. Both the direct and indirect striatal projections, as well as the pathway from LGP to STN, are GABAergic, therefore inhibitory. The direct pathway is thought to originate from striatal neurons containing GABA and substance P, and expressing predominantly D_1 dopamine receptors, whereas neurons giving rise to the indirect pathway contain GABA and enkephalin and express primarily D_2 receptors. In contrast, the pathways from STN to MGP and SNr are excitatory and glutamatergic. MGP and SNr send GABAergic projections to the ventral anterior and ventral lateral nuclei of the thalamus (VL) which then closes the loop from cortex by sending excitatory (presumably glutamatergic) projections back to the motor cortex. Thus, inputs from the cortex are processed in the basal ganglia, and the output signal, which results from a balance between GABAergic and glutamatergic circuits, modulates the activity of thalamocortical feedback, allowing normal execution of movement.

MGP and SNr contain substance P as a co-transmitter and express predominantly D_1 dopamine receptors, while neurons projecting to LGP contain enkephalin as a co-transmitter and express primarily D_2 receptors. LGP sends GABAergic projections to the *subthalamic nucleus* (STN) which, in turn, sends glutamatergic projections to MGP, SNr, and back to LGP. Thus, striatal output reaches MGP and SNr both *directly* and *indirectly*, with LGP and STN as intermediary stations. Recently, this picture has been further complicated by the finding that LGP sends GABAergic projections to MGP, as well (Parent and Hazrati, 1995), and that Str might be able to affect STN neurons, directly (Kaatz and Albin, 1995). MGP and SNr, which are considered the *output nuclei* of the basal ganglia, send GABAergic projections to the ventral anterior and ventral lateral nuclei of the thalamus which, in turn, send excitatory (presumably glutamatergic) projections back to the motor cortex, thus closing the loop (Aldes, 1988). In conclusion, the processing of inputs from the cortex which takes place in the basal ganglia results in an output signal which modulates the activity of thalamocortical feedback, allowing normal execution of movement.

Role of Glutamate in Basal Ganglia Neurotransmission

As mentioned above, dopamine, GABA, glutamate and acetylcholine are the main neurotransmitters in the basal ganglia. In recent years, growing attention has been focused on glutamate, which mediates neural signaling at crucial points in this circuitry, such as cortical input to Str and subthalamic modulation of basal ganglia output,

which are involved in the pathophysiology of movement disorders.

Glutamate is the most abundant excitatory neurotransmitter in the central nervous system (CNS). It exerts its physiological actions by activating several classes of receptors, which are primarily located on postsynaptic neurons, and which are present in virtually all areas of the CNS. Glutamate receptors are classically classified into *ionotropic receptors*, whose activation leads to opening of associated ion channels, and *metabotropic receptors*, which are linked to *G proteins*, and whose activation produces changes in cyclic nucleotides or phosphoinositol metabolism. Ionotropic receptors, which have received most attention, have been divided into NMDA (N-methyl-D-aspartate) and non-NMDA receptors. Non-NMDA receptors have been further divided into those preferring α-amino-3-hydroxy-5-methylisoxazole propionic acid (AMPA) or kainic acid as agonists (Greenamyre and Porter, 1994).

The recent recognition of gene families encoding the subunits that compose these receptors has led to a deeper understanding, in particular, of NMDA and AMPA receptor function. Both NMDA and AMPA receptors are multimeric heteromers whose pharmacological and physiological properties depend on the specific subunits of which they are composed. For the NMDA receptor, two families of subunits – NMDAR1 and NMDAR2 – have been identified. There are multiple splice variants of the NMDAR1 subunit. The second family consists of four members, NMDAR2A through NMDAR2D, which share only 18–20 percent amino acid sequence homology to NMDAR1. As for the AMPA receptor, four subunits, GluR1 – GluR4 (also known as GluR A – GluR D) have been cloned (Hollman *et al.*, 1991; Keinanen *et al.*, 1990); each exists in two alternatively spliced forms termed 'flip' and 'flop'.

Glutamate receptors are present in all basal ganglia nuclei, although they are differentially distributed. The highest density of basal ganglia glutamate receptors is in the Str which, as mentioned above, receives dense glutamatergic inputs from neocortex and thalamus. In the Str, NMDA receptors are the most abundant glutamate receptor type and appear to be selectively enriched in projection neurons as opposed to intrinsic interneurons (Tallaksen-Greene *et al.*, 1992). As described by Landwehrmeyer and colleagues (1995), striatal projection neurons also differ from interneurons in terms of the specific NMDAR subunit mRNAs they express. AMPA receptor subunits show a differential expression in projection neurons and interneurons, as well; in particular, the GluR1 subunit does not appear to be expressed on projection neurons, at least in rodents (Tallaksen-Greene and Albin, 1994). Striatal glutamatergic tone seems to be modulated by nigrostriatal dopaminergic projections (Calabresi *et al.*, 1993). In addition, NMDA receptor activation stimulates striatal acetylcholine release (Anderson *et al.*, 1994).

Binding studies indicate that AMPA receptors have a higher relative density than NMDA receptors in STN, SNr, and in the rodent homologs of LGP and MGP, namely globus pallidus (GP) and entopeduncular nucleus (EP) (Albin *et al.*, 1992). AMPA receptors may have a larger role than NMDA receptors in motor-related synaptic transmission in MGP/EP and SNr, as suggested by the fact that intrapallidal infusion of the AMPA/kainate receptor antagonist, NBQX, reduces the firing rate of GP neurons significantly, whereas no effect is observed when the NMDA antagonist MK-801 is injected (Soltis *et al.*, 1994). However, the pharmacology of glutamatergic synapses in these nuclei, as well as the cellular localization of AMPA and NMDA receptor subunits, remain to be defined.

The importance of glutamate in basal ganglia neurotransmission is further suggested by the fact that STN, which directly influences basal ganglia output (Tzagournissakis *et al.*, 1994; Blandini and Greenamyre, 1995) is glutamatergic (Robledo and Feger, 1990; Brotchie and Crossman, 1991).

Parkinson Disease

Parkinson disease (PD) was first described almost 200 years ago by the English physician, James Parkinson, who called the disease *paralysis agitans* (shaking palsy), to define a clinical picture which includes muscular rigidity, slowness of movement (bradykinesia) and tremor at rest. Because PD is associated with a general paucity and slowness of movement, it is known as a hypokinetic movement disorder. Although motor symptoms are the prominent features of PD, cognitive impairment and depression are common. Aging is a major risk factor for development of PD. It typically begins insidiously in middle or old age and progresses over a period of 10–20 years. Juvenile onset, under age 30, is possible, but uncommon. Although

it is generally believed that PD affects about 1 percent of the population over age fifty and 2 percent of the population over age 70, it may be underdiagnosed. A recent community population study carried out by Bennet and colleagues (1996) found that the prevalence of parkinsonism was 14.9 percent for people 65–74 years of age, 29.5 percent for those 75–84, and 52.4 percent for those 85 or older.

The pathological hallmark of PD is the degeneration of pigmented, melanin-containing neurons in SNc. The degenerative process is characterized by cytoskeletal changes which include the formation of Lewy bodies, which are intraneuronal inclusions. Since the pigmented neurons in SNr use dopamine as their neurotransmitter, nigral degeneration leads, as first reported in 1960 by Ehringer and Hornykiewicz, to profound dopamine depletion in the striatum. Whether dopaminergic degeneration involves retrograde 'dying back' of nigrostriatal dopamine nerve terminals, or is primarily a disorder of the cell body is uncertain. The degenerative process is not restricted to SNc, but can also involve other brain areas, such as locus coeruleus, ventral-tegmental area, and pedunculopontine tegmental nucleus (Jellinger, 1989).

Pathogenesis

Notwithstanding the progress made in understanding the pathophysiology of PD in the past three decades, the *primum movens* of nigral degeneration is still unknown. In recent years, increasing evidence has suggested that impairment of neuronal energy metabolism, possibly related to *mitochondrial defects*, and *oxidative stress* might play a pivotal role in the process that leads to SNc degeneration. A pathogenic role has also been proposed for *glutamate* which, under certain circumstances, is neurotoxic.

Mitochondrial Defects

A fundamental contribution to the understanding of PD pathophysiology came in the early 1980's, when it was observed that unintentional self-administration of *1-methyl-4-phenyl-1,2,3,6-tetrahydropiridine* (MPTP), a by-product of the illicit synthesis of meperidine analogs, caused a PD-like syndrome (Langston *et al.*, 1983) as a result of selective nigral degeneration. As it was subsequently shown, MPTP, once in the brain, is oxidized to *1-methyl-4-phenylpyridinium* (MPP$^+$), the active toxin, by monoamine oxidase type B (Markey *et al.*, 1984; Chiba *et al.*, 1984). MPP$^+$ is then taken up selectively by nigral neurons, via the dopamine transporter, and further accumulated in mitochondria, where it inhibits mitochondrial respiration (Figure 32–2) by binding to the rotenone-sensitive site of complex I (NADH:ubiquinone oxidoreductase), the proximal component of the electron transport chain (Nicklas *et al.*, 1985; Ramsay and Singer, 1986). The same phenomenon occurs in human blood platelets (Blandini and Greenamyre, 1995). The discovery of reduced complex I activity in the SNc and, to a lesser extent, in platelets of PD patients (refer to selected readings) has lent further support to the role that a complex I defect might play in PD pathophysiology.

Together, the mechanism of action of MPP^+, and the fact that complex I activity is reduced in PD patients, have prompted extensive investigation into the role of mitochondrial dysfunction in PD pathogenesis. Mutations in mitochondrial DNA (mtDNA), which encodes part of complex I, have been proposed to explain the enzymatic defect. However, despite the increased occurrence of spontaneous mutations with aging (Chapters 3 and 6), no preferential incidence of mutations or deletions has been reported in brain mtDNA of PD patients with respect to age-matched controls. Instead, more convincing evidence suggests that oxidative damage to mtDNA, or to complex I itself, might account for the degenerative process which takes place in the SNc. Aging is associated with a decline in mitochondrial function, possibly due to accumulation of mtDNA oxidative damage, which results from the increase in free radicals formation that parallels aging (Mecocci et al., 1993). This process, for reasons that are discussed below, is likely to be pathologically enhanced in PD. In fact, a higher degree of oxidative damage to mtDNA is present in SNc and Str of PD patients with respect to age-matched controls (Sanchez-Ramos, 1994). Complex I, being the largest and most complicated of the electron-transferring complexes, is highly vulnerable to oxidative damage (Allen et al., 1995). In addition, partial inhibition of complex I leads to free radical formation, which may cause irreversible damage to the enzyme complex (Cleeter et al., 1992). Sorting out whether a complex I defect is the cause or consequence of excessive oxidative stress will be one of the keys to understanding the pathogenesis of PD.

Oxidative Stress

The SNc is exposed to a high degree of oxidative stress, which results from the high rate of free radical formation that characterizes this area (Coyle and Puttfarcken, 1993; Jenner, 1994). Considerable oxidative stress comes from the metabolism of catecholamines: the activities of tyrosine hydroxylase, the rate-limiting enzyme of catecholamine synthesis, and monoamine oxidase, which catabolizes catecholamines, cause the formation of H_2O_2 as a normal byproduct. In addition, auto-oxidation of dopamine, which leads to the production of melanin, also yields H_2O_2. H_2O_2, toxic per se, slowly decomposes to .OH, the most reactive free radical. Furthermore, these reactions are accelerated in the presence of iron (particularly in the free, ferrous form, Fe^{++}), which is abundant in the SNc. In experimental animals, local injection of iron causes selective damage to nigral neurons, while the iron chelator desferrioxamine prevents the toxic effect of 6-hydroxydopamine on nigral dopaminergic neurons (Ben-Shachar, 1991; Youdim, 1993). In PD patients, abnormally elevated levels of iron have been reported in the SNc, but opposite changes in ferritin, the protein which binds Fe^{++}, have been found (Jellinger et al., 1993). Thus, it is unclear whether this increase is ascribable to higher levels

of free or ferritin-bound iron. However, since similar increases in iron levels have also been described in other neurodegenerative diseases, this phenomenon may be a consequence, rather than a cause of the degenerative process observed in PD.

Impaired activities of endogenous scavengers of cytotoxic free radicals, in particular glutathione, have also been suggested to play an important role in PD pathophysiology. *Glutathione*, in its reduced form (GSH), acts as an electron donor in the reduction of H_2O_2 to $H_2O + O_2$ catalyzed by *glutathione peroxidase*. As a result, glutathione is transformed into *oxidized glutathione* (GSSG), then rapidly reduced back to GSH by glutathione reductase. GSH can also scavenge singlet oxygen and .OH nonenzymatically. Decreased levels of total glutathione (GSH + GSSG), and GSH have been reported in the substantia nigra of PD patients (Perry et al., 1986; Sofic et al., 1992; Sian et al., 1994), while reduced levels of GSSG and a reduced GSSG/GSH ratio have been reported in the cerebrospinal fluid (Tohgi et al., 1995). Interestingly, it has been demonstrated by Mithöfer and colleagues (1992) that treatment of hepatic cells in vitro with mitochondrial poisons causes a rapid loss of both GSH and GSSG. In addition, intracerebral microinjection of the mitochondrial inhibitor, malonate, depletes GSH by 40 percent within 4 hours (Halpern and Greenamyre, unpublished data). Thus, the loss of GSH reported in PD might be due to impairment of mitochondrial energy production, possibly related to the complex I defect. In contrast to the changes in iron levels, these alterations appear to be specific to PD.

Glutamate Neurotoxicy: Synergism With Bioenergetic Defects

John Olney coined the term *excitotoxicity* after he correlated the neurotoxic and the excitatory properties of various glutamate analogs. He demonstrated that excessive stimulation of glutamate receptors by agonists can, under some circumstances, lead to neuronal damage and death. Neurotoxicity mediated by the NMDA receptor is apparently caused by a massive influx of extracellular Ca^{++} (Meldrum and Garthwaite, 1990). The increase in cytoplasmic Ca^{++} activates a number of Ca^{++}-dependent enzymes involved in the catabolism of proteins, phospholipids and nucleic acid, which lead to cell death through different pathways. Excitotoxic cell death is usually of the necrotic type, with swelling of organelles, cytolysis and subsequent inflammatory reaction. However, glutamate receptor-mediated overload of Ca^{++} might also trigger apoptosis (Chapter 17).

Mitochondria represent one of the main targets of excitotoxic injury. They sequester Ca^{++} in a rapid and reversible fashion when cytoplasmic levels rise abnormally, such as following NMDA receptor activation (Peng et al., 1995). They also are the site of NMDA receptor-induced free radical formation (Reynolds and Hastings, 1995). Prolonged activation of the NMDA receptor impairs the reversibility of mitochondrial Ca^{++} sequestration, and this

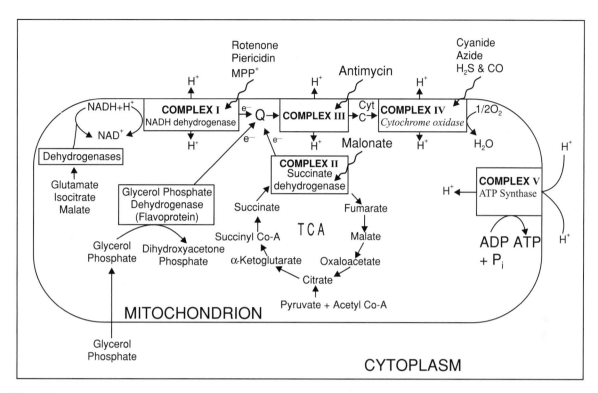

FIGURE 32–2

Schematic diagram of the mitochondrial electron transport chain and TCA (Krebs) cycle. Complex I is the site of action of MPP$^+$, the toxic metabolite of MPTP. Complex I may also be defective in Parkinson disease.

may contribute to the mitochondrial dysfunction associated with excitoxicity. Moreover, as discussed below, mitochondrial damage may sensitize neurons to further excitotoxic challenges.

The 'Indirect Excitotoxic Hypothesis'

Although excitotoxicity has been suggested to play a role in the pathophysiology of numerous neurologic diseases, a direct toxic action of glutamate in the pathophysiology of chronic, neurodegenerative disorders such as PD seems unlikely. In fact, the brain is remarkably resistant to very high concentrations of glutamate; in addition, no consistent evidence of changes in the extracellular levels or in the inactivation mechanisms of glutamate, capable per se of overcoming the adaptive defenses of the brain, has ever been provided for PD.

Any impairment in neuronal energy production, however, enhances the vulnerability to glutamate toxicity. This is related to certain properties of the NMDA receptor which, at normal resting membrane potential, is blocked by extracellular Mg^{++} (Figure 32–3). Because this blockade is voltage-dependent, it is reduced as a neuron becomes depolarized for any reason. Therefore, when a neuron is depolarized, the Mg^{++} block is relieved, and binding of glutamate leads to a large Ca^{++} influx.

The ability to maintain membrane polarity and, hence, Mg^{++} block of the NMDA receptor, depends on func-

tional ion pumps, in particular, the Na$^+$/K$^+$ ATPase (Glynn and Karlish, 1975). The Na$^+$/K$^+$ ATPase, in turn, depends on an adequate supply of ATP, more than 90 percent of which is derived from mitochondrial oxidative metabolism. Impaired mitochondrial function depletes ATP, disrupts Na$^+$/K$^+$ ATPase activity, and causes depolarization (Erecinska and Dagani, 1990). It ensues that, in this circumstance of depolarization, even non-toxic levels of glutamate may become lethal (Novelli *et al.* 1988).

This has led to formulation of the 'weak' or 'indirect excitotoxic hypothesis' (Albin and Greenamyre, 1992; Beal *et al.*, 1993), according to which any process that impairs a neuron's ability to maintain normal membrane potential can be expected to enhance its vulnerability to the toxic effects of glutamate. This hypothesis has been substantiated by the experimental demonstration that substances inhibiting oxidative phosphorylation, Na$^+$/K$^+$ ATPase or mitochondrial respiration produce 'excitotoxic' lesions. These lesions can be prevented by NMDA antagonists (Beal, 1992; Greene *et al.*, 1993; Greene *et al.*, 1995), which are also protective against the neurotoxic effects of MPP$^+$ (Turski *et al.*, 1991). Of particular interest to PD pathogenesis is the observation that cultured mesencephalic dopaminergic neurons are selectively vulnerable to the combined effects of complex I inhibition and NMDA receptor activation (Marey-Semper *et al.*, 1995).

In conclusion, it appears that the degeneration of SNc, which leads to the clinical manifestations of PD, might result from a multifactorial process. This process includes age-related mitochondrial (bioenergetic) defects and age-related excessive free radical formation, as well as excitotoxicity and depletion of GSH, all of which are intimately related. Impaired mitochondrial function can lead indirectly to NMDA receptor-mediated excitotoxicity, and activation of NMDA receptors can lead to mitochondrial dysfunction. In addition, both NMDA receptor activation and mitochondrial dysfunction generate free radicals which, in turn, may lead to depletion of GSH. On the other hand, a primary loss of GSH may account for excessive levels of free radicals, which damage components of the mitochondrial electron transport chain. The initiating event, which could be at the level of the mitochondrion, the NMDA receptor, or elsewhere, starts a self-perpetuating cycle which leads to neuronal damage and death in the SNc.

Functional Modifications of Basal Ganglia Circuitry in PD

Dopaminergic denervation of the striatum causes a cascade of complex alterations in the activity of basal ganglia nuclei (Figure 32–4). The main consequence of this cascade is overactivity of the basal ganglia output nuclei, MGP and SNr, which results from two simultaneous but distinct mechanisms. Firstly, as a consequence of nigrostriatal dopamine depletion, striatal GABAergic neurons projecting directly to MGP and SNr become underactive, thus causing disinhibition of these GABAergic nuclei. Secondly, striatal GABAergic neurons projecting to LGP become overactive. Therefore, LGP is overinhibited and cannot maintain its normal control over STN. STN, freed from the pallidal inhibition, overstimulates MGP and SNr via its glutamatergic projections. The further result is that neurons of the ventrolateral (motor) thalamus receiving this enhanced inhibitory input from MGP and SNr become underactive and reduce their outflow to the motor cortex. This mechanism is believed to underlie many of the clinical manifestations of PD (Albin et al., 1989; DeLong, 1990).

Glutamate plays a pivotal role in these functional modifications. Release of glutamate in striatum is enhanced after striatal dopamine depletion or chronic D_2 receptor blockade (Calabresi et al., 1993; Yamamoto and Cooperman, 1993). In a rodent model of unilateral DA denervation, there is a down-regulation of striatal NMDA receptors, but not AMPA receptors (Porter et al., 1994). These results complement the work of Klockgether and Turski (1993), which showed that microinjection of nontoxic doses of NMDA, but not AMPA, into the anterior striatum produces signs of parkinsonism in rats. Downstream from the striatum, overactivity of the excitatory glutamatergic projections from STN to the basal ganglia output nuclei appears to play a major role in the pathophysiology of parkinsonian motor signs (Bergman et al., 1990; Hamada and DeLong, 1993; Limousin et al., 1995; Mitchell et al., 1989). In rodents, striatal dopaminergic denervation leads to metabolic activation of the basal ganglia output

nuclei (Porter et al., 1994). This is presumably due to increased excitatory input from STN, because in normal animals, selective lesions of STN reduce metabolic activity in these nuclei (Blandini and Greenamyre, 1995; Blandini et al., 1995). Moreover, in dopamine-depleted rats, STN lesions normalize metabolic activity in the basal ganglia output nuclei (Blandini et al., in press). In the rodent model of unilateral dopamine depletion, there also is a selective down-regulation of AMPA receptors, but not NMDA receptors, in the basal ganglia output nuclei, consistent with the hypothesized importance of AMPA receptors in these regions. These results are also consonant with the work of Klockgether and Turski showing that microinjection of AMPA, but not NMDA, into the basal ganglia output nuclei induces parkinsonism in rats.

In conclusion, it appears that AMPA and NMDA receptor systems in the basal ganglia regulate differently in response to dopaminergic denervation of the striatum. Whether there is the same relationship between striatal NMDA receptors and output nuclei AMPA receptors in the primate brain remains to be investigated. Understanding the molecular basis of this glutamate receptor regulation will be important for developing new therapeutic agents for PD.

Symptomatic and Neuroprotective Treatments

Conventional treatment of parkinsonian symptoms is based on the fact that there is profound depletion of striatal dopamine in PD. Replacement therapy with dopamine itself is not feasible because dopamine does not cross the blood-brain-barrier. The immediate biosynthetic precursor of dopamine, levodopa, is used instead. Levodopa is generally used in combination with an inhibitor of peripheral dopa decarboxylase in order to prevent conversion to dopamine in the bloodstream. Today, thirty-five years after its introduction, levodopa remains the single most effective drug for treating the motor manifestations of Parkinson's disease. Unfortunately, levodopa is associated with several dose-related side effects including hallucinations and psychosis. In addition, with disease progression and increased duration of treatment, response fluctuations and abnormal involuntary movements (dyskinesias) become frequent.

Another conventional method for treating the symptoms of PD is to use direct-acting agonists of striatal dopamine receptors. For unknown reasons, none of the available dopamine agonists is as effective as levodopa. A more recent strategy for symptomatic treatment is to inhibit the enzymes responsible for dopamine metabolism, thereby prolonging its effects.

It may also be possible to treat PD by manipulating the glutamatergic system (Greenamyre, 1993). Studies in MPTP-treated parkinsonian monkeys indicate that selective NMDA and AMPA receptor antagonists have antiparkinsonian effects (Greenamyre et al., 1994; Klockgether et al., 1991). In addition, glutamate antagonists synergize with dopaminergic agents, so it may be possible to use very low doses of a dopaminergic drug and a glutamate

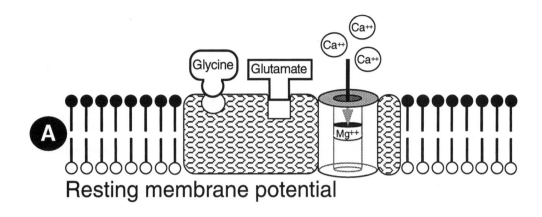

Resting membrane potential

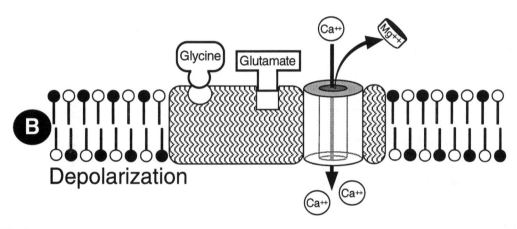

Depolarization

FIGURE   32–3

Schematic diagrams of the NMDA receptor complex at normal membrane potential (**A**) and in the setting of partial membrane depolarization (**B**). At normal membrane potential, the NMDA receptor ion channel is blocked by magnesium and there is little calcium flux into the neuron. The magnesium blockade is vol-

tage-dependent, so when the neuron is depolarized for any reason, the magnesium is extruded. Consequently, ambient concentrations of glutamate and glycine can activate the receptor and allow calcium to flow inward. Membrane depolarization can occur as a result of a bioenergetic defect.

antagonist in combination to treat PD effectively, while avoiding dose-related side effects.

In addition to symptomatic treatment, neuroprotective treatment has been devised. By defining the mechanisms involved in neurodegeneration in PD, it is hoped that new targets for therapeutic intervention will be identified. For example, it is anticipated that agents that bolster mitochondrial function, quench free radicals, block excitotoxicity or increase GSH levels would protect neurons from relevant pathogenic mechanisms and slow disease progression. Given the efficacy of glutamate antagonists in treating PD symptoms, these drugs are especially attractive since they should also be able to block excitotoxic events. In this regard, there is preliminary evidence suggesting that the use of *amantadine*, a weak blocker of the NMDA receptor channel, is an independent predictor of improved survival in PD patients (Uitti *et al.*, 1993).

Huntington Disease

Huntington disease (HD), first described by George Huntington in 1872, is a hereditary, neurodegenerative disease characterized by abnormal, involuntary movements, cognitive impairment and behavioral changes. Although the incidence of HD is age-related, it usually begins in early middle age. The age of onset peaks at about 35–39 years of age, and is distributed more or less normally. After onset, symptoms progress relentlessly to death over a period of 10 to 25 years. Juvenile onset (before the age of 20) occurs in a restricted percentage of cases. The prevalence of HD is between 5 and 10 per 100,000 population (Conneally, 1984).

In contrast to PD, HD is a hyperkinetic disorder, the clinical picture being characterized by quick, random, involuntary movements (*chorea*), which can evolve into disabling, violent movements, potentially affecting all parts of the body. With disease progression, sustained, prolonged movements or postures (*dystonia*) supervene. Superimposed chorea and dystonia result in writhing and dance-like patterns of movement, called *choreoathetosis*. Parkinsonian features, such as rigidity, bradykinesia and dystonia are common in the later stages of the illness (Shoulson, 1982). Although HD is most commonly thought of as a motor disorder, dementia, behavioral disturbances and depression are very common, and may result in more disability than the motor symptoms.

HD is an autosomal dominant, fully penetrant disease caused by the expansion of a repeating trinucleotide sequence (CAG) in the translated portion of a gene called IT15, which is located on chromosome 4p. The gene is expressed widely throughout the body, in general, and the brain, in particular. Thus, its distribution does not account for the regionally selective neurodegeneration found in this disease. The IT15 transcript encodes a 348 kDA protein, known as *huntingtin*, which shows no significant homology with any previously characterized protein (Huntington Disease Collaborative Research Group, 1993). The normal cellular function of huntingtin is unknown; however, it is believed that the disease is not a simple result of loss of normal protein function. Instead, it appears that the mutation results in a 'gain of function', perhaps by virtue of the charged polyglutamine residues encoded by the CAG repeats. This could result in abnormal protein-protein binding or inactivation of specific enzymes.

The major pathological impact of HD is on the striatum (caudate-putamen). The earliest and most striking change is massive atrophy of the caudate nucleus, usually associated with atrophy in the putamen and globus pallidus. In addition to the macroscopic selective vulnerability of striatum, there is a differential, selective susceptibility of striatal neurons to degeneration. Medium-sized aspiny interneurons, containing somatostatin, neuropeptide Y, and the enzyme NADPH diaphorase (identified as nitric oxide synthase; Dawson *et al.*, 1991) are relatively spared, as are large aspiny cholinergic interneurons (Ferrante *et al.*, 1985; Ferrante *et al.*, 1987). In contrast, medium-sized spiny GABAergic projection neurons are selectively vulnerable (Graveland *et al.*, 1985). As mentioned previously, one subset of GABAergic neurons projects to MGP and SNr, while another subset projects to LGP. Both populations of projection neurons are vulnerable to degeneration in HD, but there is evidence for preferential loss of neurons projecting to LGP in the early stages of HD (Reiner *et al.*, 1988) as well as in presymptomatic gene carriers (Albin *et al.*, 1990b, 1992). In later stages of the disease, all striatal projections degenerate (Albin *et al.*, 1990a). Pathological changes, in the form of neuronal loss, can also be observed in the cerebral cortex, particularly in layers III, V, and VI of frontal cortex (Sotrel *et al.*, 1991).

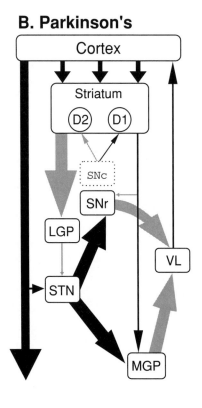

A. Normal   **B. Parkinson's**

FIGURE 32–4

Changes in basal ganglia circuitry after nigrostriatal dopamine depletion. Gray arrows denote inhibitory pathways; black arrows represent excitatory pathways. The relative 'strength' of a pathway is indicated by arrow thickness. **A.** Normal functional anatomy. **B.** After nigrostriatal denervation, striatal GABAergic neurons projecting directly to MGP and SNr become underactive, thus causing a disinhibition of these GABAergic nuclei. In addition, striatal GABAergic neurons projecting to LGP become overactive. Therefore, the firing rate of the LGP GABAergic projection to STN decreases, leading to overactivity of STN which, via its glutamatergic projections, overstimulates MGP and SNr. Thus, in the setting of nigrostriatal dopamine depletion, the activity of the GABAergic output nuclei is increased by two simultaneous, but distinct mechanisms: reduced GABAergic inhibition from the striatum and increased excitatory input from the STN. As a result of the overactivity of the GABAergic projections from MGP and SNr, neurons of the ventrolateral thalamus (VL) that project to cortex become underactive. This reduction in the outflow from the motor thalamus to the motor cortex is believed to underlie many of the clinical manifestations of PD.

Pathogenesis

Excitotoxicity was first suggested to play a fundamental role in HD pathogenesis when it was demonstrated that intrastriatal injection of the glutamate analog, kainate, reproduced many of the neurochemical and histological features of HD (Coyle and Schwarcz, 1976; McGeer and McGeer, 1976). Subsequently, it was shown that intrastriatal injection of *quinolinic acid* (QA), an endogenous tryptophan metabolite and agonist of the NMDA type of glutamate receptor, reproduced a pattern of selective neuronal death more closely reminiscent of that found in postmortem HD brains (Schwarcz et al., 1982; Beal et al., 1986, 1991a). Neuronal death caused by QA can be either apoptotic or necrotic, and apoptotic cells have been found in the striatum of HD patients (Portera-Cailliau et al., 1995). Furthermore, intrastriatal injection of QA induces preferential expression of the IT15 gene in degenerating neurons (Carlock et al., 1995) and of its protein product, *huntingtin*, in surviving neurons (Tatter et al., 1995).

Nevertheless, the specificity of NMDA receptor-mediated toxicity in HD pathogenesis is debated. In the setting of excitotoxicity mediated by the NMDA receptor, a selective depletion of NMDA receptors might be expected. On one hand, selective loss of NMDA receptors in the putamen of postmortem HD brains (Young et al., 1988) or presymptomatic HD gene carriers (Albin et al., 1990b) has been reported. In addition, a decreased density of NMDA receptor-associated glycine binding sites has been found in caudate and frontal cortex (Reynolds et al., 1994). On the other hand, Dure and colleagues (1991) found a similar degree of receptor loss for all subtypes of glutamate receptors in HD brains and, more recently, selective loss of kainate and AMPA, but not NMDA, binding sites has been reported in layer VI of HD frontal cortex (Wagster et al., 1994).

Although intrastriatal injection of QA produces a very useful model of HD, there is a substantial lack of evidence supporting a direct role of this NMDA receptor agonist in HD. Thus, if a direct and exclusive role of excitatory amino acids in HD pathogenesis seems unlikely, it appears more likely that, as already discussed for PD, pre-existing conditions may lower the threshold of neuronal vulnerability to the potentially neurotoxic effects of endogenous substances, such as glutamate.

Bioenergetic Defects and Indirect Excitotoxicity in HD

Defective energy metabolism may play a pivotal role in HD pathogenesis. Glucose and oxygen metabolism are decreased in the caudate and in the cerebral cortex of HD patients (Kuhl et al., 1982; Young et al., 1986; Martin et al., 1992). There is also abnormal mitochondrial function in the caudate nucleus and in platelets (Brennan et al., 1985; Parker et al., 1990; Mann et al., 1990). Intrastriatal injection of mitochondrial toxins, such as aminooxyacetic acid, malonate, and nitropropionic acid, produce selective excitotoxic lesions which replicate many of the histologic

and neurochemical features of HD (Beal et al., 1991b, 1993; Brouillet et al., 1993; Greene et al., 1993, 1995). It has also been reported that inhibition of complex I produces a similar excitotoxic lesion (Storey et al., 1992). Importantly, the vulnerability of the striatum to mitochondrial poisons is age-dependent (Brouillet et al., 1993), and mirrors the age-dependence of HD. Thus, it is possible that the genetic abnormality of HD may be associated in some fashion with impairment of mitochondrial energy metabolism. The fact that NMDA antagonists can prevent these lesions (Greene et al., 1993, 1995) suggests that, as for PD, excitotoxicity may simply be a final common pathway to neuronal death in cells rendered pathologically vulnerable by the primary disease process.

Functional Modification of Basal Ganglia Circuitry in HD

The modifications in the functional anatomy of the basal ganglia which produce HD motor symptoms are not fully understood. Excitotoxic lesion of the striatum does not produce a hyperkinetic movement disorder in rodents; in primates with a striatal lesion, chorea manifests only when dopaminergic agonists are also administered (Ellison et al., 1987; Kanazawa et al., 1986). In monkeys, however, blocking the activity of STN or its output to MGP results in chorea (Crossman, 1987; Robertson et al., 1989). Similarly, infusion of a GABA receptor antagonist into LGP (simulating decreased activity of the indirect pathway) also produces chorea (Crossman et al., 1988). Consistent with this model of basal ganglia function, it has been shown that decreased STN activity is associated with a decrease in the tonic firing of MGP neurons (Hamada and DeLong, 1988). This may result in disinhibition of the thalamus and overflow of thalamocortical feedback (DeLong, 1990).

Thus, chorea in HD may result from selective loss of striatal GABAergic output to LGP (Figure 32–5), which occurs in the early stages of HD, when chorea is most prominent (Reiner et al., 1988). Later in the course of the disease, when chorea diminishes and parkinsonian features appear, there is more widespread loss of striatal output with additional involvement of the direct pathway, which connects the striatum to the basal ganglia output nuclei, SNr and MGP.

Treatment

Current treatment of HD is inadequate. Although chorea can be controlled with dopamine receptor antagonists or agents to deplete dopamine, this generally results in little functional benefit and may cause significant side effects. There is no effective treatment for the dementia of HD. Thus, therapy is presently targeted at the depression and behavioral problems associated with HD. Aggressive treatment of these symptoms can have an enormous beneficial effect. Based on the present knowledge about HD pathogenesis, clinical trials are underway with agents that

A. Normal

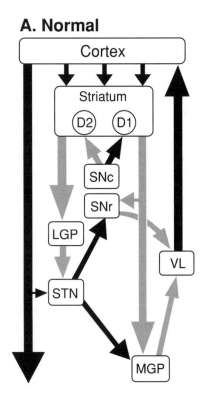

B. Huntington's

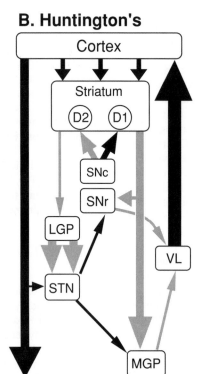

FIGURE   32–5
A. Simplified schematic diagram of normal basal ganglia circuitry. Gray arrows denote inhibitory pathways; black arrows represent excitatory pathways. The relative 'strength' of a pathway is indicated by arrow thickness. **B.** In early HD there is a selective loss of the projections from striatum to LGP. This results in increased activity of inhibitory LGP neurons that project to STN. The resultant decrease in STN output is analogous to that in hemiballism and reduces the firing rates of the output nuclei of the basal ganglia, the SNr and MGP. In turn, the VL is disinhibited and thalamocortical feedback is aberrantly enhanced. This sequence of events may be responsible, in part, for development of chorea.

block excitotoxicity, bolster mitochondrial function, or quench free radicals.

An Overall View

Anatomical and biochemical factors cause the basal ganglia nuclei to be selectively exposed to age-related oxidative stress. This is likely to be exacerbated by the impairment of energy metabolism which occurs with aging. One result is enhancement of neuronal susceptibility to the potentially neurotoxic effects of endogenous substances, such as glutamate. Because the basal ganglia are primarily involved in the control of voluntary movement, degenerative processes associated with aging, which disrupt the functional organization of the basal ganglia, lead to movement disorders.

Selected Readings

Beal, M. F. 1995. Aging, energy, and oxidative stress in neurodegenerative diseases. Ann. Neurol. 38:357–366.

Gerfen, C. R. 1992. The neostriatal mosaic: multiple levels of compartmental organization. Trends Neurosci. 15:133–139.

Ghez, C., and Gordon, J. 1995. Voluntary Movement. In E. R. Kandel, J. H. Schwartz, and T. M. Jessel (eds.) Essentials of Neural Science and Behavior, Norwalk: Appleton & Lange. pp. 529–550.

Graybiel, A. M. 1990. Neurotransmitters and neuromodulators in the basal ganglia. Trends Neurosci. 13:244–254.

Greenamyre, J. T., and Shoulson, I. 1994. Huntington's Disease. In D. B. Calne (ed.) Neurodegenerative Diseases, Philadelphia, W. Saunders Company. pp. 685–704.

Janetzky B., Hauck, S., Youdim, M. B. H., et al. 1994. Unaltered

aconitase activity, but decreased complex I activity in substantia nigra pars compacta of patients with Parkinson's disease. Neurosci. Lett. 169:126–128.

Krige, D., Carroll, M. T., Cooper, J. M., Marsden, C. D., and Schapira, A. H. V. 1992. Platelet mitochondrial function in Parkinson's disease. Ann. Neurol. 32:782–788.

Kure, S., Tominaga, T., Yoshimoto, T., Tada, K., and Narisawa, K. 1991. Glutamate triggers internucleosomal DNA cleavage in neuronal cells. Biochem. Biophys. Res. Comm. 179:39–45.

McBain, C. J., and Mayer, L. 1994. N-methyl-D-aspartic acid receptor structure and function. Physiol. Rev. 74:723–760.

Mizuno, Y., Suzuki, K., and Ohta, S. 1990. Postmortem changes in mitochondrial respiratory enzymes in brain and a preliminary observation in Parkinson's disease. J. Neurol. Sci. 96:49–57.

Orrenius, S., and Nicotera, P. 1994. The calcium ion and cell death. J. Neural Transm. 43:S1–S11.

Parker, W. D., Boyson, S. J., Luder, A. S., and Parks, J. K. 1990. Evidence for a defect in NADH: Ubiquinone oxidoreductase (complex I) in Huntington's disease. Neurology 40:1231–1234.

Schapira, A. H. V., Cooper, J. M., Dexter, D., Clark, J. B., Jenner, P., and Marsden C. D. 1990. Mitochondrial complex I deficiency in Parkinson's disease. J. Neurochem. 54:823–827.

References

Albin, R. L., and Greenamyre, J. T. 1992. Alternative excitotoxic hypotheses. Neurology 42:733–738.

Albin, R. L., Makowiec, R. L., Hollingsworth, Z., et al. 1992. Excitatory amino acid binding sites in the basal ganglia of the rat: a quantitative autoradiographic study. Neuroscience 46:35–48.

Albin, R. L., Reiner, A., Anderson, K. D., *et al*. 1990a. Striatal and nigral neuron subpopulations in rigid Huntington's disease: Implications for the functional anatomy of chorea and rigidity-akinesia. Ann. Neurol. 27:357–365.

Albin, R. L., Young, A. B., Penney, J. B., *et al*. 1990b. Abnormalities of striatal projection neurons and N-methyl-D-aspartate receptors in presymptomatic Huntington's disease. N. Engl. J. Med. 322:1293–1298.

Albin, R. L., Young, A. B., and Penney, J. B. 1989. The functional anatomy of basal ganglia disorders. Trends Neurosci. 12:366–375.

Aldes, L. D. 1988. Thalamic connectivity of rat somatic motor cortex. Brain Res. Bull. 20:333–348.

Allen, K. L., Almeida, A., Bates, T. E., and Clark, J. B. 1995. Changes of respiratory chain activity in mitochondrial and synaptosomal fractions isolated from the gerbil brain after graded ischaemia. J. Neurochem. 64:2222–2229.

Anderson, J. J., Kuo, S., and Chase, T. N. 1994. Endogenous excitatory amino acids tonically stimulate striatal acetylcholine release through NMDA but not AMPA receptors. Neurosci. Lett. 176:264–268.

Beal M. F., Hyman B. T., and Koroshetz W. 1993. Do defects in mitochondrial energy metabolism underlie the pathology of neurodegenerative diseases? Trends Neurosci. 16:125–131.

Beal, M. F. 1992. Does impairment of energy metabolism result in excitotoxic neuronal death in neurodegenerative illnesses? Ann. Neurol. 31:119–130.

Beal, M. F., Brouillet, E., Jenkins, B. G., *et al*. 1993. Neurochemical and histologic characterization of striatal excitotoxic lesion produced by the mitochondrial toxin 3-nitropropionic acid. J. Neurosci.13:4181–4192.

Beal, M. F., Ferrante, R. J., Swartz, K. J., and Kowall, N. W. 1991a. Chronic quinolinic acid lesions in rats closely resemble Huntington's disease. J. Neurosci. 11:1649–1659.

Beal, M. F., Kowall, M. N., Ellison, D. W., *et al*. 1986. Replication of the neurochemical characteristics of Huntington's disease by quinolinic acid. Nature 321:168–171.

Beal, M. F., Swartz, K. J., Hyman, B. T., *et al*. 1991b. Aminoxyacetic acid results in excitotoxin lesions by a novel indirect mechanism. J. Neurochem. 57:1068–1073.

Bennett, D. A., Beckett L. A., Murray, A. M., *et al*. 1996. Prevalence of parkinsonian signs and associated mortality in a community population of older people. N. Engl. J. Med. 334:71–76.

Ben-Shachar, D., Eshel, G., Finberg, J. P. M., and Youdim, M. B. H. 1991. The iron chelator desferrioxamine (Desferal) retards 6-hydroxydopamine-induced degeneration of nigrostriatal dopamine neurons. J. Neurochem. 56:1441–1444.

Bergman, H., Wichmann, T., and DeLong, M. R. 1990. Reversal of experimental parkinsonism by lesions of the subthalamic nucleus. Science 249:1436–1438.

Blandini, F. and Greenamyre, J. T. 1995. Assay of [3H]dihydrorotenone binding to complex I in intact human platelets. Anal. Biochem. 230:16–19.

Blandini, F., and Greenamyre, J. T. 1995. Effect of subthalamic nucleus lesion on mitochondrial enzyme activity in rat basal ganglia. Brain Res. 669:59–66.

Blandini, F., Garcia-Osuna, M., and Greenamyre, J. T. 1997. Subthalamic ablation reverses changes in basal ganglia oxidative metabolism and motor response to apomorphine induced by nigrostriatal lesion in rats. Eur. J. Neurosci. (in press).

Blandini, F., Porter, R. H. P., and Greenamyre, J. T. 1995. Autoradiographic study of mitochondrial complex I and glutamate receptors in the basal ganglia of rats after unilateral subthalamic lesion. Neurosci. Lett. 186:99–102.

Brennan, W., Bird, E. D., and Aprille, J. R. 1985. Regional mitochondrial respiratory activity in Huntington's disease brain. J. Neurochem. 44:1948–1950.

Brouillet, E., Jenkins, B. G., Hyman, B. T., *et al*. 1993. Age-dependent vulnerability of the striatum to the mitochondrial toxin 3-nitropropionic acid. J. Neurochem. 60:356–359.

Brotchie, J. M., and Crossman, A. R. 1991. D-[3H]aspartate and [14C]GABA uptake in the basal ganglia of rats following lesions in the subthalamic region suggest a role for excitatory amino acid but not GABA-mediated transmission in subthalamic nucleus efferents. Exp. Neurol. 113:171–181.

Calabresi, P., Mercuri, N. B., Sancessario, G., and Bernardi, G. 1993. Electrophysiology of dopamine-denervated striatal neurons. Implications for Parkinson's disease. Brain 116:433–452.

Carlock, L., Walker, P. D., Shan, Y., and Gutridge, K. 1995. Transcription of the Huntington disease gene during the quinolinic acid excitotoxic cascade. Neuroreport 6:1121–1124.

Chiba, K., Trevor, A. J., and Castagnoli, N. Jr. 1984. Metabolism of the neurotoxic tertiary amine, MPTP, by brain monoamine oxidase. Biochem. Biophys. Res. Comm. 120:574–578.

Cleeter, M. W., Cooper, J. M., and Schapira, A. H. 1992. Irreversible inhibition of mitochondrial complex I by 1-methyl-4-phenylpyridinium: evidence for free radical involvement. J. Neurochem. 58:786–789.

Conneally, P. M. 1984. Huntington's disease: genetics and epidemiology. Am. J. Hum. Genet. 36:506–526.

Coyle, J. T., and Puttfarcken, P. 1993. Oxidative stress, glutamate, and neurodegenerative disorders. Science 262:689–695.

Coyle, J. T., and Schwarcz, R. 1976. Lesion of striatal neurons with kainic acid provides a model for Huntington's chorea. Nature 263:244–246.

Crossman, A. R. 1987. Primate models of dyskinesia: The experimental approach to the study of basal ganglia-related involuntary movement disorders. Neuroscience 21:1–40.

Crossman, A. R., Mitchell, I. J., Sambrook, M. A., and Jackson, A. 1988. Chorea and myoclonus in the monkey induced by gamma-aminobutyric acid antagonism in the lentiform complex: the site of drug action and a hypothesis for the neural mechanisms of chorea. Brain 111:1211–1233.

Dawson, T. M., Bredt, D. S., Fotuhi, M., Hwang, P. M., and Snyder, S. H. 1991. Nitric oxide synthase and neuronal NADPH diaphorase are identical in brain and peripheral tissues. Proc. Natl. Acad. Sci. USA 88:7797–7801.

DeLong, M. R. 1990. Primate models of movement disorders of basal ganglia origin. Trends Neurosci. 13:281–285.

Dure, L. S., Young, A. B., and Penney, J. B. 1991. Excitatory amino acid binding sites in the caudate nucleus and frontal cortex of Huntington's disease. Ann. Neurol. 30:785–793.

Ehringer, H., and Hornykiewicz, O. 1960. Verteilung von Noradrenalin und Dopamin (3-hydroxytyramin) im Gehirn des Menschen und ihr Verhalten bei Erkrankungen des extrapyramidalen Systems. Klin. Wochenschr., 1236–1239.

Ellison, D. W., Beal, M. F., Mazurek, M. F., *et al*. 1987. Amino acid neurotransmitter abnormalities in Huntington's disease and the quinolinic acid animal model of Huntington's disease. Brain 110:1657–1673.

Erecinska, M., and Dagani, F. 1990. Relationships between the neuronal sodium/potassium pump and energy metabolism. Effects of K^+, Na^+, and adenosine triphosphate in isolated brain synaptosomes. J. Gen. Physiol. 95:591–616.

Ferrante, R. J., Beal, M. F., Kowall, N. W., Richardson, E. P. Jr., and Martin, J. B. 1987. Sparing of acetylcholinesterase-containing striatal neurons in Huntington's disease. Brain Res. 411:162–166.

Ferrante, R. J., Kowall, N. W., Beal, M. F., *et al.* 1985. Selective sparing of a class of striatal neurons in Huntington's disease. Science 230:561–563.

Glynn, I. A. and Karlish, S. J. D. 1975. The sodium pump. Annu. Rev. Physiol. 37:13–55.

Graveland, G. A., Williams, R. S., and DiFiglia, M. 1985. Evidence of degenerative and regenerative changes in neostriatal spiny neurons in Huntington's disease. Science 227:770–773.

Greenamyre, J. T. 1993. Glutamate-dopamine interactions in the basal ganglia: relationship to Parkinson's disease. J. Neural Transm. 91:255–269.

Greenamyre, J. T., Eller, R. V., Zhang, Z., *et al.* 1994. Antiparkinsonian effects of remacemide hydrochloride, a glutamate antagonist, in rodent and primate models of Parkinson's disease. Ann. Neurol. 35:655–661.

Greenamyre, J. T., and Porter, R. H. P. 1994. Anatomy and physiology of glutamate in the CNS. Neurology 44(suppl.8):S7–S13.

Greene, J. G., and Greenamyre, J. T. 1995. Characterization of the excitotoxic potential of the reversible succinate dehydrogenase inhibitor malonate J. Neurochem. 64:430–436.

Greene, J. G., Porter, R. H. P., Eller, R. V., and Greenamyre, J. T. 1993. Inhibition of succinate dehydrogenase by malonic acid produces an 'excitotoxic' lesion in rat striatum. J. Neurochem. 61:1151–1154.

Hamada, I., and DeLong, M. R. 1993. Effects of subthalamic nucleus lesions on pallidal discharge in the primate, Biomed. Res. 14(suppl.1):43–45.

Hollman, M., Hartley, M., and Heinemann, S. 1991. Ca^{2+} permeability of KA-AMPA-gated glutamate receptor channels depends on subunit association. Science 252:851–853.

Huntington's Disease Collaborative Research Group. 1993. A novel gene containing a trinucleotide repeat that is expanded and unstable on Huntington's disease chromosomes. Cell 72:971–983.

Huntington, G. 1872. On chorea. Med. Surg. Rep. 26:320–321.

Jellinger, K. 1989. Pathology of Parkinson's disease. In D. B. Calne (ed.) Handbook of experimental pharmacology. Vol. 88, pp. 47–112. Berlin Heidelberg: Springer-Verlag.

Jellinger, K. A., Kienzl, E., Rumpelmaier, G., *et al.* 1993. Iron and ferritin in substantia nigra in Parkinson's disease. In H. Narabayashi, T. Nagatsu, N. Yanagisawa, and Y. Mizuno (eds.) Advances in Neurology, pp. 267–272. New York: Raven Press.

Jenner, P. 1994. Oxidative damage in neurodegenerative disease. Lancet 344:796–798.

Kaatz, K. W., and Albin, R. L. 1995. Intrastriatal and intrasubthalamic stimulation of metabotropic glutamate receptors: a behavioral and fos immunoistochemical study. Neuroscience 66:55–65.

Kanazawa, I., Tanaka, Y., and Cho, F. 1986. 'Choreic' movement induced by unilateral kainate lesions of the striatum and L-DOPA administration in monkey. Neurosci. Lett. 71:241–246.

Keinanen, K., Wisden, W., Sommer, B., *et al.* 1990. A family of AMPA selective glutamate receptors. Science 249:556–560.

Kieburtz, K., McDermott, M., Feigin, A., *et al.* 1994. A controlled clinical trial of the glutamate antagonist, remacemide hydrochloride, in Huntington's disease. Soc. Neurosci. Abstr., Vol. 20.

Klockgether, T., Turski, L., Zhang, Z. M., *et al.* 1991. The AMPA receptor antagonist NBQX has antiparkinsonian effects in monoamine-depleted rats and MPTP-treated monkeys. Ann. Neurol. 30:717–723.

Klockgether, T. and Turski, L. 1993. Toward an understanding of the role of glutamate in experimental parkinsonism: agonist-sensitive sites in the basal ganglia. Ann. Neurol. 34:585–593.

Kuhl, D. E., Phelps, M. E., Markham, C. H., *et al.* 1984. Cerebral metabolism and atrophy in Huntington's disease determined by 18FDG and computed tomography scan. Ann. Neurol. 42:82–84.

Landwehrmeyer, G. B., Standaert, D. G., Testa, C. M., Penney, J. B. and Young, A. B. 1995. NMDA receptor subunit mRNA expression by projection neurons and interneurons in rat striatum. J. Neurosci. 15:5297–5307.

Langston, J. W., Ballard, P. A., Tetrud, J. W., and Irwin, I. 1983. Chronic parkinsonism in humans due to a product of meperidine-analog synthesis. Science 219:979–980.

Limousin, P, Pollak, P., Benazzouz, A., *et al.* 1995. Effect on parkinsonian signs and symptoms of bilateral subthalamic nucleus stimulation. Lancet 345:91–95.

Marey-Semper, I., Gelman, M., and Lévi-Strauss, M. 1995. A selective toxicity toward cultured mesencephalic dopaminergic neurons is induced by the synergistic effects of energetic metabolism impairment and NMDA receptor activation. J. Neurosci. 15:5912–5918.

Markey, S. P., Johannessen, J. N., Chiueh, C.C., *et al.* 1984. Intraneuronal generation of a pyridinium metabolite may cause drug-induced parkinsonism. Nature 311:464–467.

Martin, W. R. W., Clark, C., Ammann, W., *et al.* 1992. Cortical glucose metabolism in Huntington's disease. Neurology 42:223–229.

McGeer, E. G., and McGeer, P. L. 1976. Duplication of biochemical changes of Huntington's chorea by intrastriatal injections of glutamic and kainic acids. Nature 263:517–519.

Mecocci, P., MacGarvey, U., Kaufman, A. E., *et al.* 1993. Oxidative damage to mitochondrial DNA shows marked age-dependent increases in human brain. Ann. Neurol. 34:609–616.

Meldrum, B., and Garthwaite, J. 1990. Excitatory amino acid neurotoxicity and neurodegenerative disease. Trends Pharmacol. Sci. 11:379–387.

Miller, W. C., and DeLong, M. R. 1987. Altered tonic activity of neurons in the globus pallidus and subthalamic nucleus in the primate MPTP model of parkinsonism. In M. B. Carpenter, and A. Jayrman (eds.) The Basal Ganglia II, pp. 415–427. New York: Plenum Press.

Mitchell, I. J., Clarke, C. E., Boyce, S., *et al.* 1989. Neural mechanisms underlying parkinsonian symptoms based upon regional uptake of 2-deoxyglucose in monkeys exposed to 1-methyl-1,2,3,6-tetrahydropyridine. Neuroscience 32:231–226.

Mithöfer, K., Sandy, M. S., Smith, M. T. and DiMonte, D. 1992. Mitochondrial poisons cause depletion of reduced glutathione in isolated hepatocytes. Arch. Biochem. Biophys. 295:132–136.

Nicklas, W. J., Vyas, I., and Heikkila, R. E. 1985. Inhibition of NADH-linked oxidation in brain mitochondria by 1-methyl-4-phenylpyride, a metabolite of the neurotoxin, 1-methyl-4-phenyl-1,2,3,6-tetrahydropiridine. Life Sci. 36:2503–2508.

Novelli, A., Reilly, J. A., Lysko, P. G., and Henneberry, R. C. 1988. Glutamate becomes neurotoxic via the NMDA receptor when intracellular energy levels are reduced. Brain Res. 451:205–212.

Olney, J. W., Ho, O. L., and Rhee, V. 1971. Cytotoxic effects of acidic amino acids on the infant mouse central nervous system. Exp. Brain Res. 14:61–76.

Parent, A., and Hazrati, L. N. 1995. Functional anatomy of the basal ganglia. II. The place of subthalamic nucleus and external pallidum in basal ganglia circuitry. Brain Res. Rev. 20:128–154.

Parker, W. D., Boyson, S. J., and Parks, J. K. 1989. Abnormalities of the electron transport chain in idiopathic Parkinson's disease. Ann. Neurol. 26:719–723.

Peng, T.-I., Sheu, S.-S., and Greenamyre, J. T. 1995. Visualization of NMDA-induced mitochondrial calcium uptake in striatal neurons using confocal microscopy. Soc. Neurosci. Abstr. 21:1343.

Perry, T. L., and Young, V. W. 1986. Idiopathic Parkinson's disease, progressive supranuclear palsy and glutathione metabolism in the substantia nigra of patients. Neurosci. Lett. 67:269–274.

Porter, R. H., Greene, J. G., Higgins D. S., and Greenamyre, J. T. 1994. Polysynaptic regulation of glutamate receptors and mitochondrial enzyme activities in the basal ganglia of rats with unilateral dopamine depletion. J. Neurosci. 14:7192–7199.

Portera-Cailliau, C., Hedreen, J. C., Price, D. L., and Koliatsos, V. E. 1995. Evidence for apoptotic cell death in Huntington disease and excitotoxic animal models. J. Neurosci. 15:3775–3787.

Ramsay, R. R., and Singer, T. P. 1986. Energy-dependent uptake of N-methyl-4-phenylpyridinium, the neurotoxic metabolite of 1-methyl-4-phenyl-1,2,3,6-tetrahydropiridine (MPTP). J. Biol. Chem. 261:7585–7587.

Reiner, A., Albin, R., Anderson, K. D., et al. 1988. Differential loss of striatal projection neurons in Huntington's disease. Proc. Natl. Acad. Sci. USA 85:5733–5737.

Reynolds, G. P., Pearson, S. J., and Hutson, P. H. 1994. Deficit of [3H]L-689,560 binding to the glycine site of the glutamate/NMDA receptor in the brain in Huntington's disease. J. Neurol. Sci. 125:46–49.

Reynolds, I. J., and Hastings, T. G. 1995. Glutamate induces the production of reactive oxygen species in cultured forebrain neurons following NMDA receptor activation. J. Neurosci. 15:3318–3327.

Robertson, R. G., Farmery, S. M., Sambrook, M. A., and Crossman, A. R. 1989. Dyskinesia in the primate following injection of an excitatory amino acid antagonist into the medial segment of the globus pallidus. Brain Res. 476:317–322.

Robledo, P., and Feger, J. 1990. Excitatory influence of rat subthalamic nucleus to substantia nigra pars reticulata and the pallidal complex: electrophysiological data. Brain Res. 518:47–54.

Sanchez-Ramos, J. R., Overvik, E., and Ames, B. N. 1994. A marker of oxyradical-mediated DNA damage (8-hydroxy-2'deoxyguanosine) is increased in nigro-striatum of Parkinson's disease brain. Neurodegeneration 3:197–204.

Schwarcz, R., Whetsell, W. O., and Mangano, R. M. 1982. Quinolinic acid: An endogenous metabolite that produces axon-sparing lesions in rat brain. Science 219:316–318.

Shoulson, I. 1982. Care of patients and families with Huntington's disease. In C. D. Marsden, and S. Fahn (eds.) Movement Disorders. London: Butterworths. pp. 277–290.

Sian, J., Dexter, D. T., Lees, A. J., et al. 1994. Alterations in glutathione levels in Parkinson's disease and other neurodegenerative disorders affecting basal ganglia. Ann. Neurol. 36:348–355.

Sofic, E., Lange, K. W., Jellinger, K., and Riederer, P. 1992. Reduced and oxidized glutathione in the substantia nigra of patients with Parkinson's disease. Neurosci. Lett. 142:128–130.

Soltis, R. P., Anderson, L. A., Walters, J. R., and Kelland, M. D. 1994. A role for non-NMDA excitatory amino acid receptors in regulating the basal activity of rat globus pallidus neurons and their activation by the subthalamic nucleus. Brain Res. 666:21–30.

Sotrel, A., Paskevich, P. A., Kiely, D. K., et al. 1991. Morphometric analysis of the prefrontal cortex in Huntington's disease. Neurology 41:1117–1123.

Storey, E., Hyman, B. T., Jenkins, B., et al. 1992. 1-Methyl-4-phenylpyridinium produces excitotoxic lesions in rat striatum as a result of impairment of oxidative metabolism. J. Neurochem. 58:1975–1978.

Tallaksen-Greene, S. J., and Albin, R. L. 1994. Localization of AMPA-selective excitatory amino acid receptor subunits in identified populations of striatal neurons. Neuroscience 61:509–519.

Tallaksen-Greene, S. J., Wiley, R. G., and Albin, R. L. 1992. Localization of striatal excitatory amino acid binding site subtypes to striatonigral projection neurons. Brain Res. 594:165–170.

Tatter, S. B., Galpern, W. R., Hooheveen, A. T., and Isacson, O. 1995. Effect of striatal excitotoxicity on huntingtin-like immunoreactivity. Neuroreport 6:1125–1129.

Tohgi, H., Abe, T., Saheki, M., Hamato, F., Sasaki, K, and Takahashi, S. 1995. Reduced and oxidized forms of glutathione and alpha-tocopherol in the cerebrospinal fluid of parkinsonian patients: comparison between before and after L-dopa treatment. Neurosci. Lett. 184:21–24.

Turski, L., Bressler, K., Rettig, K. J., Löschmann, P. A., and Wachtel, H. 1991. Protection of substantia nigra from MPP+ neurotoxicity by N-methyl-D-aspartate antagonists. Nature 349:414–418.

Tzagournissakis, M., Dermon, C. R., and Savaki, H. E. 1994. Functional metabolic mapping of the rat brain during unilateral electrical stimulation of the subthalamic nucleus. J. Cereb. Blood Flow Metab. 14:132–144.

Uitti, R. J., Rajput, A. H., Ahlskog, J. E., et al. 1993. Amantadine treatment is an independent predictor of improved survival in parkinsonism. Can. J. Neurol. Sci. 20(S4):235.

Wagster, M. W., Hedreen, J. C., Peyser, C. E., Folstein, S. E., and Ross, C. A. 1994. Selective loss of [3H]kainic acid and [3H]AMPA binding in layer VI of frontal cortex in Huntington's disease. Exp. Neurol. 127:70–75.

Yamamoto, B. K., and Cooperman, M. A. 1994. Differential effects of chronic antipsychotic drug treatment on extracellular glutamate and dopamine concentrations. J. Neurosci. 14:4159–4166.

Youdim, M. B. H., Ben-Shachar, D., Eshel, G., Finberg, J. P., and Riederer, P. 1993. The neurotoxicity of iron and nitric oxide. Relevance to the etiology of Parkinson's disease. In H. Narabayashi, T. Nagatsu, N. Yanagisawa, and Y. Mizuno (eds.) Advances in Neurology. New York: Raven Press. pp. 259–266.

Young, A. B., Greenamyre, J. T., Hollingsworth, Z., et al. 1988. NMDA receptor losses in putamen from patients with Huntington's disease. Science 241:981–983.

Young, A. B., Penney, J. B., Starosta-Rubinstein, S., et al. 1986. PET scan investigations of Huntington's disease: Cerebral metabolic correlates of neurological features and functional decline. Ann. Neurol. 20:296–303.

Index